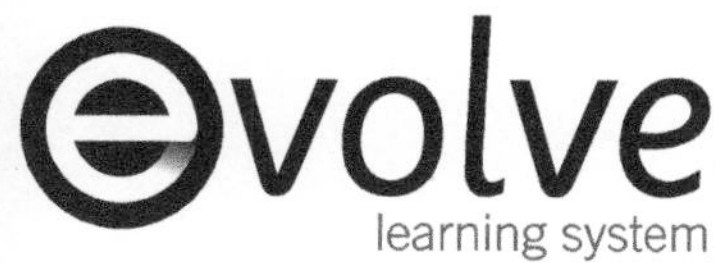

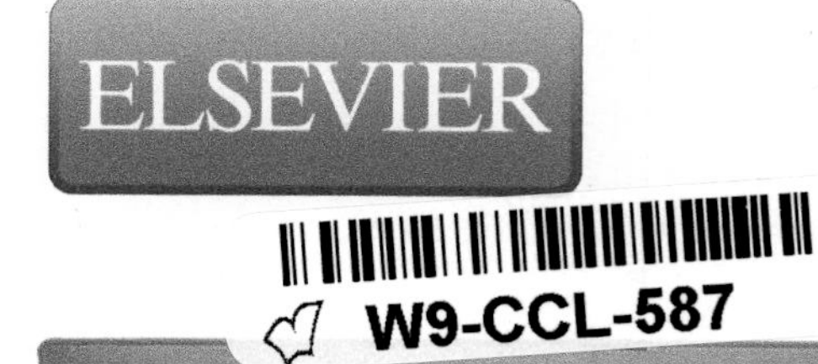

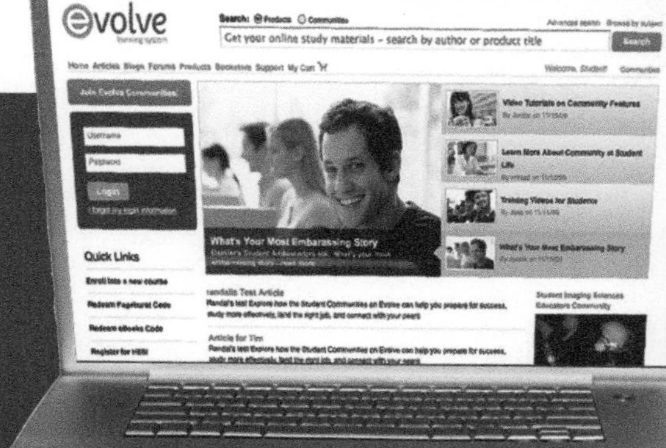

YOU'VE JUST PURCHASED MORE THAN A TEXTBOOK

ACTIVATE THE COMPLETE LEARNING EXPERIENCE THAT COMES WITH YOUR BOOK BY REGISTERING AT

http://evolve.elsevier.com/Cook/essentials/

Once you register, you will have access to your FREE STUDY TOOLS:

- Learning Activities
- Video clips
- Weblinks
- Glossary
- Additional Resources

REGISTER TODAY!

ESSENTIALS OF ASSISTIVE TECHNOLOGIES

ESSENTIALS OF ASSISTIVE TECHNOLOGIES

Albert M. Cook, PhD, PE

Professor, Department of Speech Pathology and Audiology
Faculty of Rehabilitation Medicine
University of Alberta
Edmonton, Alberta

Jan Miller Polgar, PhD, OT Reg. (Ont.)

Associate Professor, School of Occupational Therapy
Chair, Graduate Program in Health and Rehabilitation Sciences
Faculty of Health Sciences
The University of Western Ontario
London, Ontario

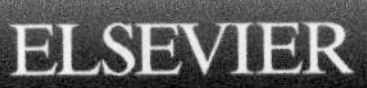

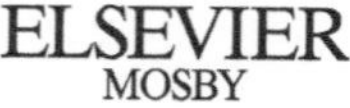

3251 Riverport Lane
St. Louis, Missouri 63043

COOK: ESSENTIALS OF ASSISTIVE TECHNOLOGIES ISBN: 978-0-323-07536-7

International Standard Book Number 978-0-323-07536-7

Library of Congress Cataloging-in-Publication Data
Cook, Albert M., 1943-
Essentials of assistive technologies/Albert M. Cook, Jan Miller Polgar. – 1st ed.
p. ; cm,
Includes bibliographical references and index.
ISBN 978-0-323-07536-7 (pbk. : alk. paper)
I. Polgar, Jan Miller. II. Title.
[DNLM: 1. Self-help Devices. 2. Disabled Persons–rehabilitation. 3. Rehabilitation–methods. WB 320]
617' .033–dc23

2011048561

Vice President: Linda Duncan
Executive Content Strategist: Kathy Falk
Content Manager: Jolynn Gower
Publishing Services Manager: Pat Joiner-Myers
Design Direction: Paula Catalano

Printed in the United States of America

9 8 7 6 5 4 3

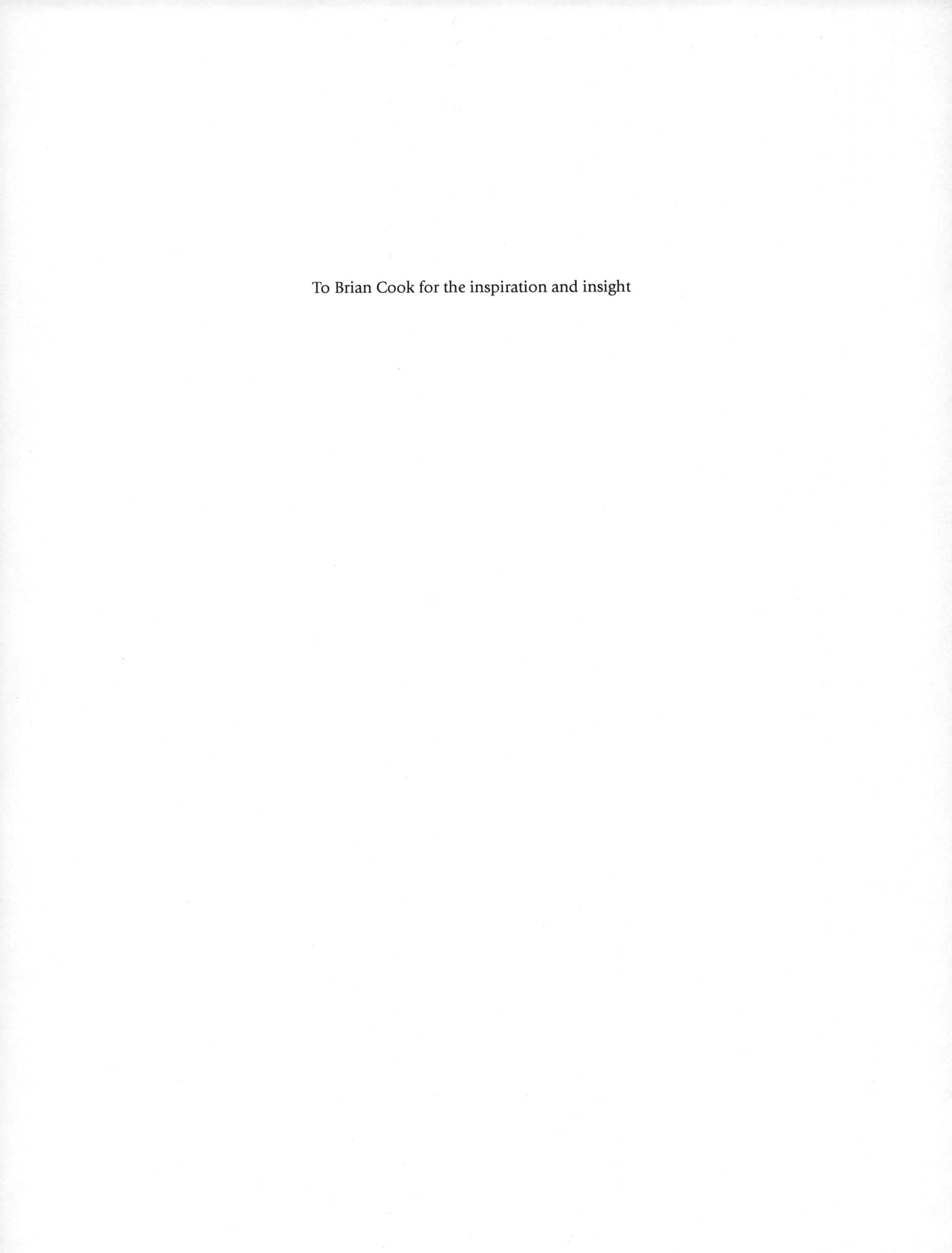

To Brian Cook for the inspiration and insight

Preface

You work in a skilled nursing facility and the rehabilitation staff has recommended some assistive technology for one of your residents. The equipment has arrived and you have been told to make it work and train the resident in its use. What do you do? Well, you can start here. This book has been written for the occupational therapist assistant as well as other rehabilitation assistants such as the physical therapist assistant and speech language pathology assistant (OTA, PTA, SLPA) who work at the front line of assistive technology (AT) application. It is focused on applications of ATs in the home, group home, school, work site, and community. We have included lots of case studies and tips for making AT more useful as well as basic descriptions of the most commonly used assistive devices. As an aid to understanding, we've also included many study questions in each chapter. For those who want more theory or background, we have also included a bit about underlying research, but we separated that from the rest of the text to make it easy to either use or ignore, depending on your preference. Reference lists with each chapter also guide the reader to more information as needed. If your goal is more along the lines of principles and theory than application, we suggest that you consult our text entitled *Cook and Hussey's Assistive Technologies: Principles and Practice*, written with Sue Hussey.

Each chapter begins with a set of learning objectives and key terms—all of which are defined in the Glossary on the Evolve website. Chapter 1 covers basic concepts related to general characteristics of AT, the AT industry, professional practice and ethics, and some information about standards for devices and outcomes of AT use by individuals with disabilities. In Chapter 2 we introduce the HAAT model and illustrate its use in implementing AT systems for individuals. Chapter 3 is about AT service delivery, particularly the implementation of treatment plans that involve AT. We also describe some approaches to evaluating the effectiveness of AT services and systems. A brief discussion of typical funding sources completes Chapter 3. Technologies that aid seating for positioning and comfort are described in Chapter 4, with an emphasis on evaluation of effectiveness and maximizing function. Chapters 5, 6, and 7 will help you make electronic ATs effective for individuals with upper extremity motor disabilities. Chapter 5 concentrates on the ways an individual can control an assistive device, beginning with a discussion of anatomic sites that are typically used for control. This is followed by an explanation of the primary ways that electronic devices can be controlled using one or more switches, a keyboard, or a pointing device. The many different options for these control technologies and how to evaluate their effectiveness is described in Chapter 6. In Chapter 7, alternatives to the use of the mouse or keyboard for computer access are explained. The next chapters address sensory aids, the underlying reasons for their use, and the technologies that aid those with mild to severe limitations in vision (Chapter 8) or hearing (Chapter 9). In both of these chapters we emphasize the needs and approaches associated with aging. Increasingly, ATs have been developed to assist individuals who experience cognitive limitations. These may be mild (e.g., learning disabilities) or severe (e.g., dementia). Chapter 10 is devoted to understanding how ATs can be applied to address cognitive needs across the life span, from a child born with an intellectual disability to a senior who has just sustained a stroke. Communication limitations also affect individuals across the life span. In Chapter 11 we describe the application of ATs designed to augment communication. Mobility limitations are also prevalent across the lifespan, resulting from conditions that are present at birth or those that result from trauma, disease, and, increasingly, lifestyles that result in obesity. We organized the discussion of mobility into two broad areas: personal assistance (e.g., wheelchairs) and transportation (e.g., vehicle safety and driving adaptations). Chapter 12 deals with ATs for personal mobility and includes a discussion of the different types and parts of a wheelchair and considerations for wheelchair setup and training, which are often the responsibility of the rehabilitation assistant. Chapter 13 describes adaptation considerations related to transportation, including devices that are used to restrain infants and young children while travelling in a vehicle, vehicle modifications that aid getting into and out of the vehicle, and safe restraint for individuals with physical disabilities who travel while seated in their wheelchair. A brief discussion of devices to aid driving is included in this chapter. Upper extremity limitations affect activities of daily living as well as control of the environment. Chapter 14 describes both low-tech devices such as adapted cutlery and high-tech devices such as electronic aids to daily living that assist individuals in manipulating objects in their environment.

As a frontline worker, you, along with the client's family, are in the best position to judge whether an assistive device is actually working for the client. You are the one who will interact with the individual on a daily basis and you will know when the way someone completes a daily activity needs to be changed. Your input as part of the rehabilitation team is important. Throughout this book, we have tried to highlight what we believe to be the important aspects of day-to-day interaction with a client who uses an assistive device. We've identified different observations to make, suggested training strategies, and offered tips for regular maintenance of the equipment. We have tried to make this book as practical as possible, for your benefit and that of your client. You play an important role on the rehabilitation team. We hope you will find this book a useful contribution to your role.

Albert M. Cook
Jan Miller Polgar

Acknowledgments

This book is a continuation of a collaborative writing adventure with Jan Polgar. I say *adventure,* because collaboration is always challenging and often produces unexpected outcomes. When that collaboration occurs by phone and email rather than face to face, it can be even more challenging. Jan has made that collaboration special for me and has made it possible for this book to see the light of day. Jan is thoughtful, critical, and highly productive—all attributes that contribute to quality outcomes. An added bonus—that got us through those impossible deadlines—is her sense of humor and her amazing positive attitude. While at times Jan may have questioned the wisdom of her decision to join with me in developing this new project, I have had no regrets. Working with Jan has been a delight from start to finish. She has made many major improvements to the parts that I wrote and has shown her typical insight and care in the parts that she led. Thank you, Jan, for all the effort and for the quality product that resulted. This book is intended to provide assistance to, among others, occupational therapy assistants.

Neither Jan nor I have direct experience in that field. As luck would have it, my daughter Barbara Cook is an OTA. Her thoughtful reading of each word in this book and her constructive criticism not only kept Jan and me honest about our audience, but also increased the quality of the finished product. Thank you, Barbara.

I cannot adequately express the gratitude I have for the continuing support, love, and understanding of my wife Nancy and the support of my daughters Barbara and Jennifer. Finally, my son Brian continues to inspire me to understand the ways in which technology can ameliorate the problems faced by individuals who have disabilities.

Albert M. Cook

This book is the second writing project that I have undertaken with Al Cook. Once again, Al was an amazing coauthor. I appreciate his accommodating my work schedule so that we could have our "virtual coffee breaks" very early in the morning. Our discussions of assistive technology ideas and practice continue to enrich my knowledge of this area. Al continues to be a thoughtful mentor and a wonderful friend. Thanks Al, for all that you do!

Many other people have supported me through this process. My thanks go to Barbara Cook, who read each of the chapters that we wrote and encouraged us to say more about many topics. She was always very kind with her comments, even when suggesting that what I had written really didn't make sense! Also, thank you Laura Titus, doctoral student in Health and Rehabilitation Sciences at the University of Western Ontario and experienced seating clinician. She was very generous in sharing her experience and enhancing the seating and mobility chapters. Jessica Huber, also a doctoral student in the Health and Rehabilitation Sciences graduate program, wrote many of the exam questions that are found on the companion website. Andrea Hickling, future occupational therapist, was an extremely valuable addition to the team at the end of the project. She completed many of the mundane tasks at the end of the writing project, with great care and intelligence, and always with a smile. I want to thank my parents Charles and Evelyn Miller for their continued love and care. Most important, I want to thank my husband Roger, my daughter Andrea, and my son Alex, who make my life worthwhile.

Jan Miller Polgar

There are many individuals who helped us with the preparation of this edition of our textbook, and we would like to acknowledge their valuable contributions. Much of the material in this book is based on Cook and Hussey's Assistive Technology, 3rd edition. Sue Hussey was a major contributor to that text, and her original material and ideas helped in the preparation of this book. Chris Beliveau of the Glenrose Rehabilitation Hospital I CAN Centre in Edmonton provided pictures of devices in use. Rob Hussey provided some of the original artwork used in this book, and Gaëtan LaBelle provided the original artwork portraying the HAAT model in Chapter 2. We are grateful for their creativity. Thank you to Kathy Falk, Executive Content Strategist at Elsevier, for having confidence in us and this project. Jolynn Gower, Content Manager, Mary Tindle, and the production associates at Elsevier provided highly professional support and assistance in the production of this text. Thanks to all of the Elsevier staff for making this project successful.

Albert M. Cook
Jan Miller Polgar

Contents

CHAPTER 1

Introduction and Overview

CHAPTER OUTLINE

LEARNING OBJECTIVES

Upon completing this chapter, you will be able to do the following:

1. Define assistive technology
2. Delineate the characteristics of assistive technologies
3. Describe the components of the assistive technology industry
4. Explain the roles of the consumer
5. Identify several distinguishing features of service delivery programs
6. Identify the roles of those who are associated with the provision of assistive technologies
7. Understand the transdisciplinary approach to assistive technology service delivery
8. Discuss the major professional issues in assistive technology practice

KEY TERMS

Activity
Alpha Testing
Applied Research
Assistive Technology (AT)
Assistive Technology Practitioner (ATP)
Assistive Technology Service
Basic Research
Beta Testing
Consumer of Assistive Technologies
Devices
Direct Consumer Services
Participation
Prototype
Quality Assurance
Telerehabilitation
Transdisciplinary Team Approach
Universal Design

Much of the information available about assistive technologies is intended for those individuals who are assessing and recommending these technologies.[3] There is much less written for the person who is responsible for implementing these recommendations and making assistive technologies work to meet the needs of people who have disabilities. This book has been written to support those front line rehabilitation therapy workers who need basic information about assistive technologies with an emphasis on implementing effective systems in clinical and community settings. We begin in this chapter by providing an overview of assistive technologies and the industry that supports their development and distribution. We also discuss standards of practice in assistive technology and a code of ethics for practitioners.

ASSISTIVE TECHNOLOGIES: A WORKING DEFINITION

The *International Classification of Functioning, Disability and Health* (ICF) is a system developed by the World Health Organization (WHO) that is designed to describe and classify health and health-related states. These two domains are described by body factors (body structures and functions) and individual and societal elements (activities and participation).[19] The ICF is a revision of the previous classification system, the *International Classification of Impairments, Disabilities and Handicaps* (ICIDH).[18] Two primary shifts in philosophy discriminate between the ICIDH and the ICF classification systems: the recognition of the importance of the environment as a mediating factor in the performance of daily function, and the use of more positive language.

Body structures and function refer to the structural and physiological functions of the body. For example, the classification relating to vision lists the anatomical structures of the eye and the sensory and motor as well as perceptual elements of vision. Activity and participation are considered to be a single classification. There is much debate on whether it is possible to differentiate between an **activity** and **participation**. Something that may be considered participation at one stage in life becomes an activity at a later stage. The ICF defines activities as the "execution of tasks" and participation as "involvement in life situations."[19] Examples of the different components of activity and participation include learning and applying knowledge, communication, mobility, self-care, and community, social, and civic life.

The ICF recognizes two contextual factors that modify health and health-related states: the environment and personal factors.[19] The latter are not classified but merely identified and include age, gender, race, lifestyle habits, and social and cultural backgrounds, among other factors. The inclusion of these factors in the ICF recognizes their ability to differentially influence the outcome of the same impairment in two individuals.

The ICF does classify environmental elements. Assistive technologies are located in this classification, most prominently in the products and technology chapter. They are specifically mentioned related to activities of daily living, mobility, communication, religion, and spirituality as well as in specific contexts such as education, employment, culture, recreation, and sport.[19] Many of the remaining environmental chapters have reference to assistive technology, although it is not mentioned explicitly. These chapters include access to public and private buildings; the natural and built outdoor environments; people and animals that provide physical and emotional support (personal care attendants and health care professionals are identified here, service animals are not); attitudes of individuals and others; and services, systems, and policies, including legislation.[19] Scherer and Glueckauf (2005)[13] reviewed the ICF and discussed the implications to assistive technology provision. They concluded that the revised classification system puts the onus on the assistive technology provider to demonstrate positive outcomes for assistive technology recommendations and use.

Definition of Assistive Technology Devices and Services

Dictionaries provide the following definition of "technology":

(1) The science or study of the practical or industrial arts, (2) applied science, (3) a method, process, etc., for handling a specific technical problem.[6,8] Surprisingly, none of these definitions says anything about a "device"; instead the emphasis is on the application of knowledge. This is an important concept, and we shall use the term **assistive technology (AT)** to refer to a broad range of **devices,** services, strategies, and practices that are conceived and applied to ameliorate the problems faced by individuals who have disabilities.

Within this concept there are many ways to define assistive technologies. One widely used definition is that provided in the United States in Public Law (PL) 100-407, the Technical Assistance to the States Act. The definition of an assistive technology device is as follows:

> Any item, piece of equipment or product system whether acquired commercially off the shelf, modified, or customized that is used to increase, maintain or improve functional capabilities of individuals with disabilities.

This definition has several important components and, because we plan to use it as a working definition throughout this book, we need to examine these in some detail. First, the definition includes commercial, modified, and customized devices. By including all types of devices, we encompass an extremely wide range of applications. Second, this definition emphasizes *functional* capabilities of *individuals* with disabilities. Functional outcomes are the only real measure of the success of assistive technology devices, and throughout this text we stress the importance of providing technologies that result in increased functional capability. Finally, the emphasis on individual persons with disabilities underscores the importance of treating each application of technology as a unique circumstance. No two applications are exactly the same in terms of the needs and skills of the person being served, the activities to be accomplished, and the context in which the application takes place.

Public Law 100-407 also defines an **assistive technology service** as any service that directly assists an individual with a disability in the selection, acquisition, or use of an assistive technology device.

The law also includes several specific examples that further clarify this definition. These include (1) evaluating needs and skills for assistive technology; (2) acquiring assistive technologies; (3) selecting, designing, repairing, and fabricating assistive technology systems; (4) coordinating services with other therapies; and (5) training both individuals with disabilities and those working with them to use the technologies effectively. This definition demonstrates the broad spectrum of services inherent in the delivery of assistive technologies.

BOX 1-1 Characteristics of Assistive Technologies

Assistive versus rehabilitative or educational technologies
Low to high technology
Hard technologies and soft technologies
Appliances versus tools
Minimal to maximal technology
General versus specific technologies
Commercial to custom technology

Data from Odor P: Hard and soft technology for education and communication for disabled people, *Proc Int Comp Conf,* Perth, Australia, 1984; Rizer B, Ourand P, Rein J: *How adapted microcomputer technology contributes to successful educational and vocational outcomes.* Presented at Closing the Gap Conference, October 1990, Minneapolis; Smith RO: Technological approaches to performance enhancement. In Christiansen C, Baum C, editors: *Occupational therapy: overcoming human performance deficits,* Thoroughfare, N.J., 1991, Slack; and Vanderheiden GC: Service delivery mechanisms in rehabilitation technology, *Am J Occup Ther* 41:703–710, 1987.

Characterization of Assistive Technologies

In this section we present a characterization of assistive technologies from several points of view. Each of these is a logical outgrowth of the definitions presented earlier, and each is useful in the process of applying assistive technologies. Box 1-1 shows several classifications used to distinguish different types of assistive technologies.

Assistive versus Rehabilitative or Educational Technologies

Technology can serve two major purposes: helping and teaching.[15] Technology that helps an individual to carry out a functional activity is termed *assistive technology.* Our emphasis in this text is on assistive technologies that serve a variety of functional needs. Technology can also be used as part of an educational or rehabilitative process. In this case the technology is usually used as one modality in an overall education or rehabilitation plan. Technology in this sense is used as a tool for remediation or rehabilitation rather than being a part of the person's daily life and functional activities, and we refer to it as *rehabilitative* or *educational* technology, depending on the setting. Often rehabilitative or educational technology (e.g., cognitive retraining software) is employed to develop skills for the use of assistive technologies. We discuss some of these applications in later chapters.

Low to High Technology

The next of these distinctions is between low-technology devices and high-technology devices. Although this distinction is imprecise, we often describe inexpensive devices that are simple to make and easy to obtain as "low" technology and devices that are expensive, more difficult to make, and harder to obtain as "high" technology. According to this distinction, examples of low-technology devices are simple pencil and paper communication boards, modified eating utensils, and simple splints. Wheelchairs, electronic communication devices, and computers are examples of high-technology devices.

Hard and Soft Technologies

Odor (1984)[11] has distinguished between *hard technologies* and *soft technologies.* Hard technologies are readily available components that can be purchased and assembled into assistive technology systems. This includes everything from simple mouth sticks to computers and software. The PL 100-407 definition of an assistive technology device applies primarily to hard technologies as we have defined them. The main distinguishing feature of hard technologies is that they are tangible. On the other hand, soft technologies are the human areas of decision making, strategies, training, concept formation, and service delivery as described earlier in this chapter. Soft technologies are generally captured in one of three forms: (1) people, (2) written, and (3) computer software.[1] Assistive technology services as defined in PL 100-407 are basically soft technologies. These aspects of technology, without which the hard technology cannot be successful, are much harder to obtain because they are highly dependent on human knowledge rather than tangible objects. This knowledge is obtained slowly through formal training, experience, and textbooks such as this one. The development of effective strategies of use also has a major effect on assistive technology system success. Initially the formulation of these strategies may rely heavily on the knowledge, experience, and ingenuity of the assistive technology practitioner. With growing experience, the assistive technology user originates strategies that facilitate successful device use. The roles of both hard and soft technologies as integral portions of assistive technology systems are discussed in later chapters.

Appliances versus Tools

An appliance is a device that "provides benefits to the individual independent of the individual's skill level."[16] Tools, on the other hand, require the development of skill for their use. Household appliances such as refrigerators do not require any skill to operate, whereas tools such as a hammer or saw do require skill. The determining factor in distinguishing a tool from an appliance is that the quality of the result obtained using a tool depends on the skill of the user. For example, eyeglasses or a seating system are appliances since the quality of the functional outcome does not depend on the skill of the user. Success in maneuvering a powered wheelchair or generating a meaningful utterance with an augmentative communication system does depend on the skill of the user, and these are classified as tools. Examples of assistive technology tools and appliances are shown in Table 1-1.

As Vanderheiden (1987)[16] points out, the successful use of assistive technology tools requires training, strategies, and special skills. These are soft technologies. Tools require carefully planned and implemented training programs that lead to skill development. Some appliances

TABLE 1-1 Examples of Assistive Technology Tools and Appliances

Topic (Chapter)	Appliances	Tools
Control interfaces (6)	Keyguards	Joystick
Computer access (7)	Enlarging lens	Enlarged keyboard
Augmentative communication (11)	---	Alphabet board
Manipulation (14)	Environmental control*	Electric feeder
Mobility (12)	Wheelchair armrest	Manual wheelchair push rims
Sensory (8)	Eyeglasses	Long cane

* See text; classification depends on EADL (electronic aid for daily living) and its functions.

may also require training of care providers and the user of the technology. For example, when a new seating system (an assistive technology appliance) is provided (Chapter 4), the care staff must be trained in how to position the person in the seating system and how to position the system in the wheelchair.

People routinely use observation, such as watching someone using a hammer, as a means of learning how to use a tool. Because tools used by persons with disabilities are often different from those used by the general population, the assistive technology user often cannot observe someone using the same device, and she must rely more heavily on personal experience and training to learn to use it effectively.[16] The importance of strategies and skills for assistive device use means that the trainer, most often a rehabilitation assistant such as an occupational therapy assistant (OTA), physical therapy assistant (PTA), and speech language pathology assistant (SLPA), has a large role in the ultimate success of the assistive technology system.

Minimal to Maximal Technology

Assistive technologies are specified and designed to meet a continuum of needs. At one extreme are devices that provide some assistance or augment the individual's ability to perform a task. For example, an individual with cerebral palsy may be able to speak, but on occasion his speech may be difficult to understand. In those instances the individual may clarify his speech using a letter board to spell out words not understood. Or a person with respiratory problems may be able to ambulate inside her house but, because of low endurance, may require a powered wheelchair to be able to do her grocery shopping independently. In fact, many grocery stores now provide powered carts for individuals who need this type of augmented mobility. At the other extreme are assistive technologies that replace significant amounts of ability to generate functional outcomes. For example, some individuals have no verbal communication ability and may require a device to be able to communicate. Likewise, some individuals are totally dependent on a manual or powered wheelchair for their personal mobility. Minimal technologies generally *augment* rather than replace function. Maximal technologies may replace function.

General versus Specific Technologies

We differentiate between assistive technologies that are used in many different applications (general technology) and those that are intended for a specific application. *General-purpose* assistive technologies include (1) seating and positioning systems, (2) control interfaces, and (3) computers. These are classified as general purpose because they are used across a wide range of applications. Body position affects the way an individual uses the assistive technology. Frequently, external support systems, which are an assistive technology, are necessary to achieve a body position that facilitates functional activities. Control interfaces are things such as the joystick on a powered wheelchair or the keyboard on a computer that allow the user to interact with the assistive technology.

Specific-purpose assistive technologies facilitate performance in one application area. Examples include devices for communication, manual and powered wheelchairs, feeding devices, hearing aids, and mobility aids for persons with visual impairments. Because these devices are intended for a specific use, it is possible to design them to maximize their capabilities to meet a particular need.

Commercial to Custom Technology

For many applications, mainstream technologies (computers, mobile phones, tablet computers) with an assistive technology software application are being used to meet the needs of individuals with disabilities. When mainstream devices cannot meet the needs directly, they may be able to be modified to fit the assistive technology application. In many cases, however, the mainstream technology, modified or not, cannot meet the needs and a specially designed assistive technology is required. Many assistive technologies are mass produced and available commercially. We use the term *commercially available* to refer to devices that are mass produced. Commercially produced devices (mainstream and assistive technologies) can generally meet the majority of needs that people with disabilities face. In some cases, however, it is necessary to design and build a completely custom device because no commercially available approach will work. Figure 1-1 illustrates the progression from commercially available devices to those that are completely customized for an individual.

Universal Design

Universal design is the design of products and environments to be usable by all people, to the greatest extent possible, without the need for adaptation or specialized design.[10] The product design includes use of universal design features that make a product more useful to persons who have disabilities. Typical features that are addressed include: larger knobs; a variety of display

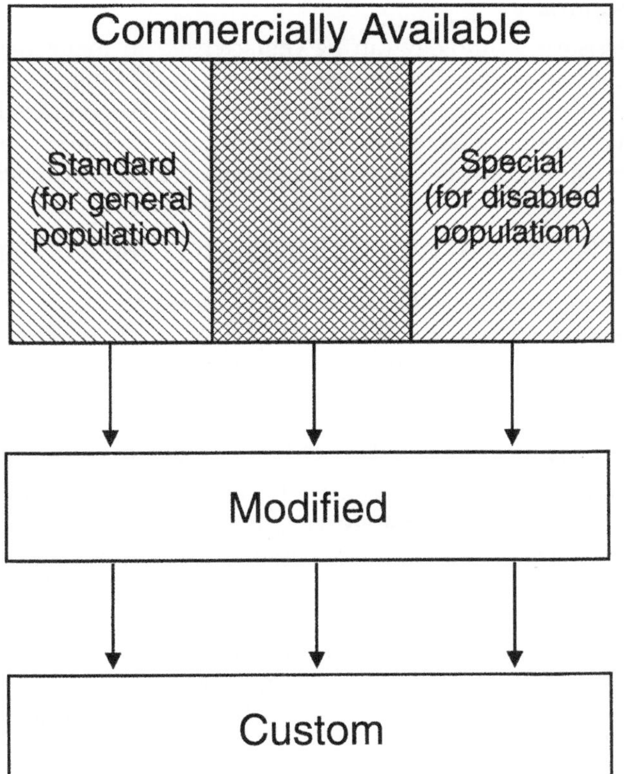

Figure 1-1 This diagram shows the progression from commercially available devices for the general population and commercially available devices for special populations to modified devices and custom devices.

options—visual, tactile, and auditory; and alternatives to reading text such as icons and pictures. This is much less expensive than modifying a product after production to meet the needs of a person with a disability. In some countries, universal design is known as "design for all." A set of universal design principles is shown in Box 1-2.*

BOX 1-2 Principles of Universal Design*

ONE: EQUITABLE USE
The design is useful and marketable to people with diverse abilities.

TWO: FLEXIBILITY IN USE
The design accommodates a wide range of individual preferences and abilities.

THREE: SIMPLE AND INTUITIVE USE
Use of the design is easy to understand, regardless of the user's experience, knowledge, language skills, or current concentration level.

FOUR: PERCEPTIBLE INFORMATION
The design communicates necessary information effectively to the user, regardless of ambient conditions or the user's sensory abilities.

FIVE: TOLERANCE FOR ERROR
The design minimizes hazards and the adverse consequences of accidental or unintended actions.

SIX: LOW PHYSICAL EFFORT
The design can be used efficiently and comfortably and with a minimum of fatigue.

SEVEN: SIZE AND SPACE FOR APPROACH AND USE
Appropriate size and space is provided for approach, reach, manipulation, and use regardless of user's body size, posture, or mobility.

From North Carolina State University, The Center for Universal Design, 1997.
*For complete guidelines, see www.design.ncsu.edu/cud/.

Commercial Assistive Technologies

When an individual's needs for assistive technology cannot be met with a commercial device, we attempt to use mass-produced, commercially available devices that are designed for people with disabilities. Examples include wheelchairs, augmentative communication systems, and many aids to daily living. In some cases a combination of standard and special-purpose technologies is used; this is represented by the crosshatched area of Figure 1-1. For example, a standard general-purpose computer or smart phone may be used with special-purpose software to create an augmentative communication device (see Chapter 11).

Modified Devices

When there are no off-the-shelf commercially available devices that can meet an individual's needs, it is necessary to make modifications so the device fits the need. This modification can vary from simple to very complex. For example, if an individual has difficulty using the keys on a computer keyboard, we can purchase software that facilitates its use. In this case the most expensive and complex part of the system (the computer) is a standard commercial product, and the software is the simplest and least expensive portion of the system. However, the software may have a cost that is much higher than expected relative to its simplicity because it is a special product and all the costs of development must be recovered from the small production run. A commercially available assistive device may be modified as well. For example, a commercially available augmentative communication device may require modification so that it can be mounted on a user's wheelchair.

Custom Devices

When no commercial device or modification is able to meet the need, it is necessary to design and build a device specifically for the task at hand. This approach results in a custom device. One example of such a device is the jigs used for cognitive aids such as the one shown in Chapter 10, Figure 10-8. Because the production

*See also: www.design.ncsu.edu/cud

demands are unique, the jigs must be custom made. Custom devices can be expensive because they are often made for just one person. An important difference between modified or custom devices and commercial devices is the level of technical support that is available. There are sometime volunteers (e.g., retired engineers or electronics technicians) who can make a custom device. A word of caution, however, is that once the device is made the person often disappears, leaving the front line person to repair and maintain the device. Custom devices can also be of lesser quality than commercial devices. The initial lower cost (e.g., of switches) rarely pays off in the long run because custom devices must be replaced far more frequently. A commercially produced device generally has written documentation and operator's manuals available. Modified or custom devices often have little or no written documentation. The manufacturer or supplier of commercial equipment provides technical support and repair. Because modified or custom devices are one of a kind, technical support may be hard to obtain, especially if the original designer and builder is no longer available (e.g., if the user moves to a new area).

Summary

Assistive technology can be characterized in many ways. It is useful to realize, however, that yesterday's high tech is tomorrow's low tech, custom devices become commercial if more than a few people need them, and appliances often enable the use of tools. No categorization is perfect or static.

THE ASSISTIVE TECHNOLOGY INDUSTRY

Figure 1-2 depicts the components of the assistive technology industry and how they are interrelated. Each component in this figure plays an important role in making assistive technologies available to people who have disabilities.

The Consumer and Direct Consumer Services

All the components in Figure 1-2 are focused on the consumer who uses the assistive technology devices and services. The key component linking the consumer to the other components is the delivery system that actually provides the technology to the consumer. Thus, the consumer and direct consumer services are at the center of the figure. However, it is important to note that it is desirable for the consumer to be involved in all aspects of the industry.

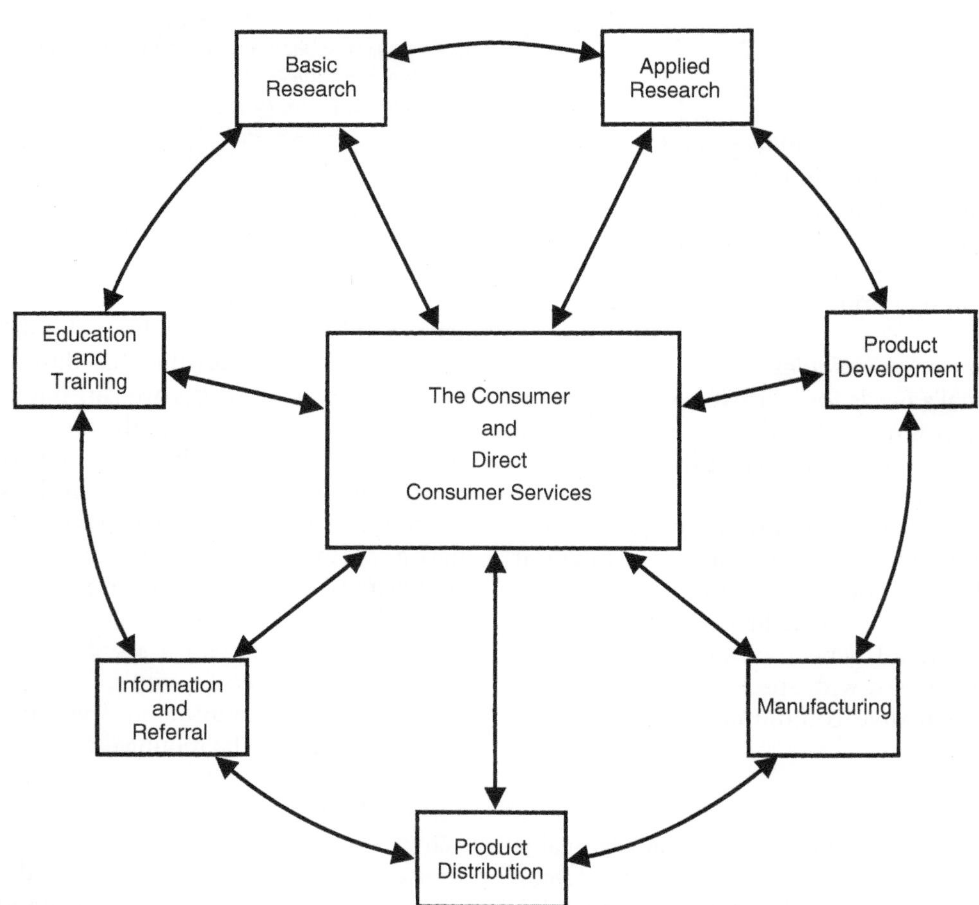

Figure 1-2 The assistive technology industry. The components center around the delivery of devices and services to consumers through direct services. The other industry components are arranged to illustrate their relationships to each other. (Modified from Smith RO: Models of service delivery in rehabilitation technology. In Perlman LG, Enders A: *Rehabilitation service delivery: a practical guide,* Washington, DC, 1987, RESNA.)

Direct consumer services is the component in which a consumer's need for assistive technology is identified, an evaluation is completed, recommendations are made, and the system is implemented. Implementation includes setting up an assistive technology system, training the consumer and support personnel in its use, and following the consumer's progress with the system to make sure that it meets his or her needs.

The Consumer

The **consumer of assistive technologies** is the recipient, or end user, of assistive technology, and all of the industry components should be responsive to the consumer's needs. The true test of effectiveness of assistive technologies is the consumer use of the device in the "real world" outside of the clinic. This use will produce information from the consumer and direct service providers that can impact the other components of Figure 1-2 so that improvements in products and services can be made. The other components also affect the consumer and the direct consumer service providers through research, new product development, and dissemination of information.

The consumer is not, however, solely the recipient of the technology. The consumer must be considered an active participant in the other industry components in order for them to be effective. White et al. (2004)[20] describe the process of *participatory action research* in assistive technology wherein the consumer is involved in all aspects of assistive technology research, development, and implementation.

Because they use assistive devices regularly, consumers are the experts in the use of assistive technologies. They develop skills that exceed those of support personnel, and they can be effective as mentors to others by demonstrating how to effectively use a particular device. The Empowering End Users Through Assistive Technology (EUSTAT) project in Europe has developed guidelines for trainers, a set of critical factors for assistive technology training, and descriptive information on programs that provide assistive technology training for consumers (http://www.siva.it/research/eustat/download_eng.html). One of the documents developed by EUSTAT is written for consumers of AT services and gives practical guidance regarding how to access these services. As you read about each component of the assistive technology industry, think about ways in which consumers can be involved.

Characteristics of Direct Consumer Service Programs

There are a variety of models and different types of settings for assistive technology systems and services. Different types of direct consumer service programs have attributes that distinguish them from each other. There are several distinguishing features of service delivery programs.[14] The primary distinguishing factor, shown in Box 1-3, is the type of administrative setting in which the service delivery

BOX 1-3 Direct Consumer Service Delivery Settings

REHABILITATION SETTING

- Assistive technology services are part of a comprehensive rehabilitation program; may be a part of one of the therapy departments or its own department.
- The primary purpose is to support the other services of the rehabilitation setting; therefore there is usually multidisciplinary team involvement.
- Typical populations served are persons with spinal cord injuries, head injuries, cerebral vascular accidents, and amputations.
- Services are usually billed to third-party health insurance payers.

UNIVERSITY BASED

- Programs in this setting have largely evolved from a research component and may provide direct consumer services, as well as education and training.
- Staff usually consists of personnel capable of performing clinical, research, and educational duties. The types of professionals involved in the team depend on the functional areas addressed by the setting.
- Those settings conducting research provide a national service. The direct consumer service component is usually regionally oriented.
- Funding is largely grant and contract related (particularly for the research component), although portions of the direct consumer services may be billed to third-party payers.

STATE AGENCY PROGRAM BASED

- State agency-based programs are usually a part of vocational rehabilitation departments or special education departments.
- Those programs based in vocational rehabilitation departments are statewide programs developed for the purpose of providing assistive technology services to individuals who need it for attaining or sustaining employment.
- The purpose of programs within special education departments is to facilitate the education of school-aged children. In some instances, school districts have their own multidisciplinary team. In other cases there may be a team that covers the entire state.
- Administration of these programs varies and may be statewide or on a local level.
- Funding is usually mandated at the state or federal level and is designated for these agencies.

PRIVATE PRACTICE

- A small number of assistive technology providers have gone into private practice. They may provide consultation to state agencies or rehabilitation centers.
- The population and functional service area varies and depends upon the professional backgrounds of those involved in the business.

(Continued)

BOX 1-3 Direct Consumer Service Delivery Settings—cont'd

PRIVATE PRACTICE—cont'd

- Operated as a for-profit, small-business venture with fees for service charged. Usually based in one local area.

DURABLE MEDICAL EQUIPMENT SUPPLIER

- Usually these suppliers are for-profit agencies that address a range of equipment needs. Typically they provide walking aids, bathing and toileting aids, wheelchairs, and seating systems. Some suppliers may provide communication and environmental control equipment.
- DME suppliers are reimbursed by third-party payers.
- DME suppliers are known for their technical resources and ability to provide repair and maintenance services.
- There are some DME suppliers that operate on a nationwide basis; others are local operations.

VETERANS' ADMINISTRATION (VA)

- Assistive technology services are provided at many of the Veterans' Administration (VA) hospitals. There is usually a multidisciplinary team approach.
- Research in the field of assistive technology is a large component of the services provided by the VA, and significant contributions have been made in this area.
- The population served is restricted to veterans with service-related disabilities. Veterans with spinal cord injuries have been a major group served by the VA.

LOCAL AFFILIATE OF A NATIONAL NONPROFIT DISABILITY ORGANIZATION

- National organizations such as the United Cerebral Palsy Association (UCPA), Easter Seal Society, Muscular Dystrophy Association (MDA), Association for Retarded Citizens (ARC), and American Foundation for the Blind provide assistive technology services through their local affiliates.
- The purpose of these organizations is often to serve individuals with a particular disability; therefore the populations served and the functional areas are geared primarily toward that disability group.
- Programs of the local chapters are usually administered at the local level, and assistive technology services vary among affiliates. Some local chapters may have a complete assistive technology team to provide services, whereas other chapters may only loan equipment.
- Funding for these agencies is through grants, contracts, donations, and fundraising events.

VOLUNTEER PROGRAMS

- Volunteer organizations in the United States that provide assistive technology services include groups such as the Telephone Pioneers of America, the Volunteers for Medical Engineering, and Rehabilitation Volunteer Network.
- Most of these groups have developed out of private industry and have as their purpose the provision of a philanthropic service.
- These groups usually provide services on a local or regional basis.
- The functional areas served depends on the expertise of the volunteers involved.

Data from Hobson DA, Shaw CG: Program development and implementation. In *Rehabilitation technology service delivery: a practical guide*, Washington, DC, 1987, RESNA Press; and Smith RO: Models of service delivery in rehabilitation technology. In *Rehabilitation technology service delivery: a practical guide*, Washington, DC, 1987, RESNA Press.

program exists. The *purpose and mission* of one service delivery program may be to provide one-time evaluations, whereas other programs may provide comprehensive assistive technology services. The *functional areas* or types of services also vary. Some of the functional areas are augmentative communication, seating and mobility, orthotics and prosthetics, sensory aids, computer access, robotics, and driving.

The *type of population* served by an assistive technology program varies as well. Some programs focus on a particular condition such as spinal cord injury or developmental disability. Other programs serve a particular group such as children or seniors. Service delivery programs also vary by the *geographical area* served. Some programs are community based in that they are set up strictly to serve individuals in rural or urban communities. Other programs provide specialized evaluation services to a large geographical region. Some assistive technology services are delivered through **telerehabilitation** programs. *Telerehabilitation* refers to the use of telecommunications technologies to capture and transmit visual and audio information, biomedical data (e.g., electroencephalograms [EEGs], x-ray films, and ultrasound data), and consumer information.[7] In assistive technology service delivery, telerehabilitation (telerehab) is used for preassessment screening, postassessment training in device use, and the provision of follow-up services. Transmission of telerehab data may be via computer interfaces over the Internet, via telephone lines, or via satellite. For home use there are small units that resemble fax machines.[7] These portable units allow follow-up in a consumer's home.

Funding of assistive technology service delivery programs varies. Some, such as programs based within a rehabilitation hospital, are funded under the general overhead of a larger organization. Other programs are supported by grant funding, whereas others rely on a fee for service charged to third-party payers.

Basic Research

The major goal of **basic research** is the generation of new knowledge. The distinguishing feature of basic research is that the outcomes are not known beforehand, although hypotheses are proposed. Basic investigations help us to better understand how the presence of a disability affects functional performance and how this may be taken into account when designing an assistive device. Throughout this text we describe basic research studies that underlie the successful development and application of assistive technologies.

Applied Research

Applied research in assistive technology typically refers to studies that are clinical or those that focus on device use. Applied research studies can be grouped as follows: (1) testing of assistive devices under various operating conditions; (2) development of new assistive devices based on clinical need, basic research findings, or both; (3) research on the use of assistive technologies by persons with disabilities; and (4) research studies designed to develop new assessment or training approaches or materials.

An example of the testing of devices is the use of performance standards to test wheelchairs or other devices.[4] In some cases, such as wheelchairs, there are accepted standards against which devices are tested (see Chapter 12). There are many applied research studies that focus on the use of assistive technologies. Often these studies involve assistive technologies that rely on user strategies for success. Some of these studies are described in later chapters of this book. For example, McCarthy and Light (2005)[9] evaluated partners' attitudes toward individuals who rely on augmentative communication systems (Chapter 11). Applied research studies have also been carried out to improve the process of assessment, recommendation, and implementation for assistive technologies.

Product Development

Applied research may yield a **prototype** device—a single unit that has been designed and built based on an identified need. The prototype is usually only tested for proper functional capability in an engineering lab. In order to make this prototype into a commercially available product, additional development must be done to make sure it can be used in a clinical environment and that it can be duplicated in production. The next step is production prototype testing, often called **alpha testing**—a process normally conducted in-house by manufacturers. Following successful alpha testing a small production run (as few as 5 or as many as 100) is conducted to verify that the device can be produced. This step both ensures that the device can be produced in quantity and allows for clinical evaluation in what is often referred to as **beta testing** involving clinicians, consumers, and care providers. Beta testing accomplishes several things: (1) identification of as many potential product failures as possible, (2) evaluation of product documentation (e.g., user's manual) to ensure that it is clear and useful, and (3) evaluation of the product with a variety of disabled consumers to identify the target population as accurately as possible.

Manufacturing

Manufacturing is quite different from producing a few beta-test prototype devices that function correctly. It requires repeatable "mass production" of the device. However, on an industrial scale, the production runs in the assistive technology industry are small, and this is the major reason that costs appear high relative to mainstream consumer products with equal or greater functional capability. The production runs necessary for true production automation are approximately 100,000 and higher. This rarely occurs in the production of assistive technology devices. Because of the high cost related to functional capability, the use of assistive technology applications for mainstream technologies (e.g., desktop computers, mobile phones, and tablet or pad computers) is popular.

As the rest of this book illustrates, the assistive technology market is diverse. The variety of needs that can be served by assistive devices is extremely large and the range of disabilities and the effects of those disabilities is extensive. There may be a relatively small number of people with a particular need in any one disability category. This leads to small volumes of production and increased costs per device. It also has the effect of making a device seem more expensive, because it is less complex but costs the same as a consumer device that is more flexible. One approach to the problem of diverse needs is to include many options within one device. These options, often called features or characteristics, make the device much more versatile—but only a few features might be needed by any one individual. This situation places an additional burden on those who work directly with the consumer as each device must be set up for a given individual. The manufacturer provides the options, but the clinician or caregiver must decide which to use and then program the device to function properly for that individual. This situation is most typical of electronic assistive technologies such as computer access (Chapter 7), sensory aids (Chapters 8 and 9), cognitive aids (Chapter 10), alternative and augmentative communication (Chapter 11), powered mobility (Chapter 12), and electronic aids to daily living (Chapter 14). Some non-electronic assistive technologies such as manual wheelchairs (Chapter 12) and seating and positioning systems (Chapter 4) require custom adjustments for many individual consumers.

Distribution of Hard Technologies

Assistive technologies must be marketed and distributed to a highly specialized audience of providers (therapists, rehabilitation assistants such as OTAs and PTAs, SLPAs, and vocational rehabilitation counselors), caregivers, and consumers and their families. Marketing is expensive, but it is also important because it is the primary way in which the intended audience learns about the available assistive technologies. There are several different ways that assistive technologies are distributed. The major distribution options are (1) distribution through a dealer or supplier, (2) direct sales by company representatives, and (3) online catalogs. The choice of one or more of these is highly dependent on the type of product. For wheelchairs, seating and positioning systems, aids to daily living, and home care products, most distribution is through assistive technology or home health care suppliers, often on the recommendation of a rehabilitation professional. For augmentative communication devices the larger companies have direct sales representatives—often speech-language pathologists—who market the devices. Sensory aids are generally available online, but are supported with information from large organizations serving individuals who have visual or auditory limitations. For many low-tech devices, computer software, and some other products, online purchasing is the favored method of distribution. This method of distribution is most effective for products for which there is no fitting or need for a prepurchase trial by the consumer. Some rehabilitation facilities may have an approved list of vendors that they will purchase from. Government agencies also often have contracts with particular vendors based on the lowest bid. These arrangements can interfere with the matching of the appropriate device to the needs of an individual consumer.

Information and Referral

The ability to readily obtain current information on assistive technology services and products is essential for both service providers and consumers. The Internet has a large amount of information available in many areas, including assistive technologies. This is the good news; the bad news is that much of this information is not validated by an independent source, so both the quality and accuracy of the information accessed must be carefully evaluated. The best way to evaluate it is to check several sources and see if you get the same information. Also, the certification programs for both individuals and vendors listed later in this chapter can help ensure quality control. The Appendix found at the end of this book contains a list of Web sites that is intended to provide some initial information; however, it is not meant to be all-inclusive.

ABLEDATA* is the largest and most well known general source of information on commercial products, noncommercial prototypes, one-of-a-kind customized products, and do-it-yourself designs for individuals with disabilities. It has more than 32,000 listings of devices (21,000 currently available products). ABLEDATA listings include sensory and motor aids, low- and high-tech devices, and applications ranging from home care to usage classified by intended function or any special features it possesses. ABLEDATA topics and categories are shown in Table 1-2.

Written publications such as conference proceedings, periodicals, directories, and catalogs are another way to

*http://www.abledata.com/abledata.cfm

TABLE 1-2 ABLEDATA Topics and Categories

Topics	Major Categories
Aids for Daily Living: Products to aid in activities of daily living.	Bathing, Carrying, Child Care, Clothing, Dispenser Aids, Dressing, Drinking, Feeding, Grooming/Hygiene, Handle Padding, Health Care, Holding, Reaching, Smoking, Toileting, and Transfer.
Blind and Low Vision: Products for people with visual disabilities.	Computers, Educational Aids, Health Care, Information Storage, Kitchen Aids, Labeling, Magnification, Office Equipment, Orientation and Mobility, Reading, Recreation, Sensors, Telephones, Time, Tools, Travel, Typing, and Writing (Braille).
Communication: Products to help people with disabilities related to speech, writing, and other methods of communication.	Alternative and Augmentative Communication, Headwands, Mouthsticks, Signal Systems, Telephones, Typing, and Writing.
Computers: Products to allow people with disabilities to use desktop and laptop computers and other kinds of information technology.	Software, Hardware, and Computer Accessories.
Controls: Products that provide people with disabilities the ability to start, stop, or adjust electric or electronic devices.	Environmental Controls and Control Switches.
Deaf and Hard of Hearing: Products for people with hearing disabilities.	Amplification, Driving, and Hearing Aids, Recreational Electronics, Signal Switches, Speech Training, Telephones, and Time.
Deaf and Blind: Products for people who are both deaf and blind.	[no categories listed]
Education: Products to provide people with disabilities access to educational materials and instruction in school and in other learning environments.	Classroom, Instructional Materials.

TABLE 1-2 ABLEDATA Topics and Categories—cont'd

Topics	Major Categories
Environmental Adaptations: Products that make the built environment more accessible.	Indoors, Outdoors, Vertical Lift, Houses, Specialties, Lighting, and Signs.
Home Management: Products to assist in cooking, cleaning, and other household activities as well as adapted furniture and appliances.	Food Preparation, Housekeeping, and Furniture.
Orthotics: Braces and other products to support or supplement joints or limbs.	Head and Neck, Lower Extremity, Torso, and Upper Extremity.
Prosthetics: Products for amputees.	Lower Extremity and Upper Extremity.
Recreation: Products to assist people with disabilities in their leisure and athletic activities.	Crafts, Electronics, Gardening, Music, Photography, Sewing, Sports, and Toys.
Safety and Security: Products to protect health and home.	Alarm and Security Systems, Childproof Devices, Electric Cords, Lights, and Locks.
Seating: Products that assist people to sit comfortably and safely.	Seating Systems, Cushions, and Therapeutic Seats.
Therapeutic Aids: Products that assist in treatment for health problems and therapy and training for certain disabilities.	Ambulation Training, Biofeedback, Evaluation, Exercise, Fine and Gross Motor Skills, Perceptual Motor, Positioning, Pressure/Massage Modality Equipment, Respiratory Aids, Rolls, Sensory Integration, Stimulators, Therapy Furnishings, Thermal/Water Modality Equipment, and Traction.
Transportation: Products to enable people with disabilities to drive or ride in cars, vans, trucks, and buses.	Mass Transit Vehicles and Facilities, Vehicles, and Vehicle Accessories.
Walking: Products to aid people with disabilities who are able to walk or stand with assistance.	Canes, Crutches, Standing, and Walkers.
Wheeled Mobility: Products and accessories that enable people with mobility disabilities to move freely indoors and outdoors.	Wheelchairs (Manual, Sport, and Powered), Wheelchair Alternatives (Scooters), Wheelchair Accessories, Carts, Transporters, and Stretchers.
Workplace: Products to aid people with disabilities at work.	Agricultural Equipment, Office Equipment, Tools, Vocational Assessment, Vocational Training, and Work Stations.

find information on assistive technology services and products. Most manufacturers have websites that contain the latest product information, updates, and applications. Unless a prescription is required, in many cases it is possible to purchase the product directly through the company Web sites. Many of the centers that provide services in assistive technology maintain Web sites as well.

Electronic and social media are becoming increasingly popular means of sharing information about assistive technology. Electronic listservs are formed by individuals with common interests. Each user accesses the information from their own e-mail system, and all messages are available to all members of the list. There are many listservs that address various areas of assistive technology applications. Some are maintained by professional associations (e.g., RESNA,* American Occupational Therapy Association [AOTA], American Speech-Language Hearing Association [ASHA], American Physical Therapy Association [APTA]), whereas others are established and maintained by rehabilitation centers or universities. There are also user- or consumer-oriented listservs, which address either specific issues (e.g., one particular disability) or general issues. These listservs are often useful places to gain information regarding specific assistive technology questions.

Social media provides more flexible options for sharing information. This media allows members to share information in a variety of ways, including text, video, and links to other published materials or media. Members are able to provide commentary on the information that is provided and upload related information easily. This format is very useful for organizations to provide up-to-date information to those individuals who follow their site. Social media differs from a listserv in that it does not tend to be monitored, as most listservs are, with the result that inappropriate comments may be posted to the site. Online conferencing is another media that is emerging that will provide educational and information-sharing opportunities for people who are

*Rehabilitation Engineering and Assistive Technology Society of North America, www.resna.org

geographically dispersed. This software enables individuals to participate online as a collective group, view common materials, and contribute to a discussion. Participants have a way of signaling the session monitor that they wish to make a comment and then are able to comment either via text or voice.

Four of the most useful U.S.-based conferences (all annual) are the California State University at Northridge (CSUN) International Technology and Persons with Disabilities Conference (held in March in Southern California; http://cfp.csuncod.org/overview.php); Closing the Gap (held in October in Minneapolis; www.closingthegap.com); Assistive Technology Industry Association (October, Chicago; January, Orlando, FL; www.atia.org); and RESNA (June, various locations; www.resna.org). International conferences include the Australian Rehabilitation & Assistive Technology Association (even years; http://www.arata.org.au/conf.php); the Association for the Advancement of Assistive Technology in Europe (odd years; http://www.aaate.net/); the International Seating Symposium (held yearly, alternating between Vancouver and a U.S. location; www.iss.pitt.edu for the U.S. event and www.interprofessional.ubc.ca for the Canadian event); and the Japanese Conference on the Advancement of Assistive and Rehabilitation Technology (odd years) sponsored by the Rehabilitation Engineering Society of Japan (http://www.resja.gr.jp/eng/). There are also specialty conferences in specific areas of assistive technology such as the International Association for Augmentative and Alternative Communication (even years; http://www.isaac-online.org/) and the International Seating Conference (annual; http://www.iss.pitt.edu/).

Education

Most front-line workers (e.g., OTAs, PTAs, and SLPAs) who are responsible for implementation of assistive technology systems learn about these technologies on the job. These care providers come from a variety of backgrounds. For those currently in practice, *in-service* educational activities in assistive technologies are sometimes available. Typically this type of educational activity is very focused and of short duration. Some workshops that are offered by industry focus on a specific product or product line. Others are offered by rehabilitation centers or universities and may include one or more areas of application (e.g., seating and positioning, augmentative communication, and computer access). Some workshops will have an emphasis on assistive technology applications for a particular population (e.g., AT for the aging). Often workshops are offered in conjunction with major conferences of professional associations. There are also assistive technology courses and educational programs offered at a distance (including online and teleconference formats). Many professional organizations require continuing education as part of the recertification process. Often AT-related courses and seminars can count toward that requirement.

Preservice educational programs practiced in specific disciplines such as occupational therapy assistant, physical therapy assistant, speech assistant, and other similar disciplines may include some assistive technology material in a formal course. The scope of assistive technology instruction in preservice educational programs varies widely. There may be required or elective courses or subjects in assistive technology, or assistive technology material may be included within another course. The most common programs are those that include some assistive technology material in other courses; the least common are programs that specialize solely in assistive technology. With the increasing role of technology in the lives of individuals with disabilities, it is crucial that newly trained professionals entering their respective fields have some level of formal training in assistive technology applications.

PROFESSIONAL PRACTICE IN ASSISTIVE TECHNOLOGY

This section describes the person who provides assistive technology and the issues surrounding his or her professional practice. Three broad issues are discussed in this section: (1) ethics of practice, (2) quality assurance, and (3) liability. Each of these has implications both for the individual practitioner and for the organizations involved in the assistive technology industry. We begin with a description of the person providing assistive technology services and devices.

Who's on First?—Providers of Assistive Technology Services

Beukelman et al. (2008) have identified a personnel framework for the provision of alternative and augmentative communication (AAC) services.[2] We have generalized this framework to apply to the broad range of assistive technology (AT) services in Box 1-4. Each of the roles shown in Box 1-4 can be played by several different types of people. Some roles require specialized training in AT, others do not. Some roles require clinical skills, some can be provided by family or friends. Some of the roles in Box 1-4 are well developed, while others had not been formally identified before Beukelman and colleagues provided the AAC personnel framework.

One of the previously unidentified roles, but one that is crucial, is the *AT finder*. Finders have several critical roles.[2] One of their most important roles is to identify people who have significant unmet motor, sensory, or cognitive needs. Finders also have enough awareness of AT to recognize when it could be helpful in addressing a need. Finders can also prepare family, friends, and other care providers for the possibility of an AT intervention. Finally, finders may help with obtaining funding for AT devices and services. The finder role may be played by a variety of individuals, including program directors in skilled nursing facilities, physicians, nurses, or family

BOX 1-4 A Personnel Framework for Assistive Technology Services

AT FINDER
Identify persons with unmet needs in areas related to AT
Be aware of current, appropriate AT options for individuals with complex motor, sensory or cognitive needs
Prepare potential decision makers
Organize decision-making process to seek AT assessment
Refer to appropriate AT intervention provider(s)
Certify AT prescription(s) (when appropriate)

GENERAL PRACTICE CLINICIAN
Implement multi-modality interventions
Integrate low-tech AAC materials in restorative/ developmental and compensatory interventions
Implement appropriate low-tech AT options
Implement routine high-tech AT options
Monitor impact of individual AT interventions
Prepare and support AT facilitators
Instruct those who support those with AT needs

AT INTERVENTION SPECIALIST
Implement multi-modality interventions
Integrate low-tech AT materials in restorative/ developmental and compensatory interventions
Implement appropriate low-tech AT options
Implement complex or unique high-tech AT options
Monitor impact of individual AT interventions
Obtain funding for intervention technology
Prepare and support AT facilitators
Support general practice clinicians
Provide continuing education to AT finders
Collaborate to support technology transfer
Collaborate to support AT research
Support AT professional organizations and activities
Provide expert testimony for legal and policy proceedings

AT FACILITATOR
Support implementation of multi-modality interventions
Instruct those who support those with AT needs (e.g., care providers, family, and communication partners)
Support unfamiliar listeners
Maintain AT technology
Prepare low-technology materials
Serve as a liaison with other AT personnel and commercial companies

AT EXPERT
Promote, sustain, and enhance AT services at program or agency level
Preprofessional preparation of AT finders
Continuing education of AT finders
Preprofessional preparation of general practice clinicians
Continuing education of general practice clinicians
Preprofessional preparation of AT intervention specialists
Continuing education of AT intervention specialists
Preprofessional preparation of AT experts
Continuing education of AT experts
Development of AT policies
Execution of AT research
Collaborate to support technology transfer
Prepare AT educational materials
Participate in the leadership and management of AAC professional organizations
Support AT professional organizations and activities
Provide expert testimony for legal and policy proceedings

Adapted from Beukelman DR, Ball LJ, Fager S: An AAC personnel framework: adults with acquired complex communication needs, *Augmentative and Alternative Communication*, 24:255–267, 2008.

members. The AT knowledge and skill of the finder is limited to awareness that AT exists and information about how to refer someone for services.

The second category includes *general practice clinicians* such as OTs or PTs or SLPs, rehabilitation assistants (OTAs, PTAs, and SLPAs), physicians, nurses, vocational rehabilitation counselors, teachers, and educational assistants. These individuals provide a range of clinical services but they do not specialize in AT services.[2] Their needs relative to AT are to have skills and knowledge to address low-tech AT applications and to understand the operation of high-tech AT as it applies to their patients or clients.

The *AT interventionists* are those care providers who are responsible for making AT systems functional for consumers on a daily basis. This group of practitioners requires the same AT knowledge and skills as the AT finders and general practice clinicians plus a level of AT intervention expertise to provide training and other specialized AT intervention services (e.g., adjustment of wheelchair seating systems, programming of AAC devices with new vocabulary, and set-up of computer access systems). These individuals are also responsible for follow-up evaluation to ensure that intervention goals are met.

The *AT facilitators* are those who assist an individual AT user by setting up an AT system (including customizing an electronic system), providing training to both the user and those who support him (family, friends, or care providers) in the operation and successful application of the AT. The actual identity of the AT facilitator depends on the needs of the individual, the available personnel, the setting and the capabilities of the user.[2] The rehabilitation assistant (OTA, PTA or SLPA) is often placed in the role of AT facilitator. In a long-term care setting, the AT facilitator could be a rehabilitation assistant (OTA, PTA, or SLPA); nursing assistant; or other therapy assistant. The AT facilitator also must maintain a relationship with the suppliers of AT devices and with the AT interventionist and AT expert who are responsible for the assessment and recommendation of the AT system. As the front-line person, the AT facilitator is often in a position to note problems with the AT system or its use. She can often address those directly or contact the AT supplier, AT expert, or AT interventionist for assistance. The AT facilitator will also develop an ongoing relationship with the consumer and his family. This relationship will be helpful in determining the degree to which the AT system is actually meeting the consumer's needs.

The *AT expert* is generally a person who has developed a broad understanding of AT devices, the assessment process, how to recommend the appropriate technologies, and how to develop intervention programs including training and follow-up. In some jurisdictions (e.g., the United States) the individuals in this category will be certified as an **assistive technology practitioner (ATP).** The ATP typically has a professional background in one of several areas, including engineering, occupational therapy, physical therapy, recreation therapy, special education, speech pathology, and vocational rehabilitation counseling. ATPs should be well grounded in their disciplines and should have knowledge and skills in assistive technology and familiarity with the scope of the assistive technology industry. ATPs are generally specialized in one or more components of assistive technology application such as AAC, seating and positioning, mobility, computer access, and electronic aids to daily living. ATPs are involved in the needs assessment, evaluation, implementation, training, and follow-up of assistive technology services in various functional areas. AT experts also include university professors, researchers, policy makers, AT program directors, and developers of AT.[2]

Because of the number of factors and the complexity involved in the delivery of assistive technology systems to the consumer, a team approach is desirable. This team may consist of as few as two professionals working together. Each individual team member brings knowledge and skills from his or her area of expertise that can be applied to the assistive technology service delivery process. Although it is tempting to view each functional service area (e.g., augmentative communication, seating, or mobility) as being in the domain of one or two specific disciplines, service delivery is most effective when a **transdisciplinary team approach** is used.

Ethics and Standards of Practice

Ethics is defined as "the study of standards of conduct and moral judgment ... and the system or code of morals of a particular ... profession."[8] When applied to a field of professional endeavor such as assistive technology delivery or a discipline such as OTA, PTA, or SLPA, the ethical conduct of practitioners is embodied both in a code (or canons) of ethics and in standards of practice. Each of the AT providers discussed in the previous section must comply with the code of ethics for his or her discipline. The code of ethics for a discipline is typically developed by the professional association serving it. As we have discussed, AT personnel have responsibilities in assistive technology service delivery that are not specified by their individual discipline's code of ethics. For this reason, it is important to have a code of ethics that addresses the specific issues related to the application of assistive technologies. Standards of practice differ from codes of ethics in that they describe more specifically what is and is not considered to be good practice in a given discipline.

A Code of Ethics for Assistive Technologies: The RESNA Code of Ethics

RESNA is an interdisciplinary professional association whose activities focus on assistive technologies. Its members come from many disciplines and a variety of settings, and their activities involve the full scope of assistive technology applications. RESNA has adopted the code of ethics shown in Figure 1-3. This code is similar to those of other disciplines involved in rehabilitation and is based on several of them. However, it provides the only AT-specific ethics guidelines. This code of ethics is presented as a reminder of the obligations that AT personnel have to their consumers and those who work with and care for them, the general public, and the profession as a whole.

Standards of Practice

Because each assistive technology practitioner belongs to his or her own discipline, it is important that the standards of practice pertaining to that specialty be met. These standards are often the basis for professional certification programs. RESNA has developed the standards of practice shown in Box 1-5 for personnel working in delivery of AT services and devices.

Quality Assurance

Quality assurance is a broad area of fundamental importance to the safe and effective application of assistive technologies. It involves two basic considerations: (1) the quality of the services rendered, and (2) the quality of the devices supplied.[5] Quality assurance is closely tied to reimbursement, and as the number of devices and practitioners increases, third-party payers are requiring some indication that the services and devices are necessary, safe, and effective. A comprehensive quality assurance program addresses these issues. The quality of services can be measured and evaluated by certification (of individual practitioners) and accreditation (of facilities and programs). The efficacy of devices is measured by adherence to device performance standards and good manufacturing practices (GMPs). Ultimately the quality of assistive technology services and devices is determined by measurement of outcomes resulting from both the provision of the services and devices, the adherence to standards of practice and relevant legislation such as that governing privacy and consent, and the utilization of the technologies to facilitate functional improvement and improved quality of life for the individual consumer.

RESNA Code Of Ethics

RESNA is an interdisciplinary association for the advancement of rehabilitation and assistive technology. It adheres to and promotes the highest standards of ethical conduct. Its members:

- *Hold paramount the welfare of persons served professionally.*
- *Practice only in their area(s) of competence and maintain high standards.*
- *Maintain the confidentiality of privileged information.*
- *Engage in no conduct that constitutes a conflict of interest or that adversely reflects on the profession.*
- *Seek deserved and reasonable remuneration for services.*
- *Inform and educate the public on rehabilitation/assistive technology and its application.*
- *Issue public statements in an objective and truthful manner.*
- *Comply with the laws and policies that guide the profession.*

Figure 1-3 RESNA code of ethics. (Modified from RESNA Ethics Committee: RESNA code of ethics, Arlington, Va., 1991, RESNA.)

BOX 1-5 RESNA Standards of Practice for Assistive Technology Practitioners and Suppliers

These Standards of Practice set forth fundamental concepts and rules considered essential to promote the highest ethical standards among individuals who evaluate, assess the need for, recommend, or provide assistive technology. In the discharge of their professional obligations assistive technology practitioners and suppliers shall observe the following principles and rules:

1. Individuals shall keep paramount the welfare of those served professionally.
2. Individuals shall engage in only those services that are within the scope of their competence, considering the level of education, experience and training, and shall recognize the limitations imposed by the extent of their personal skills and knowledge in any professional area.
3. In making determinations as to what areas of practice are within their competency, assistive technology practitioners and suppliers shall observe all applicable licensure laws, consider the qualifications for certification or other credentials offered by recognized authorities in the primary professions which comprise the field of assistive technology, and abide by all relevant standards of practice and ethical principles, including RESNA's Code of Ethics.
4. Individuals shall truthfully, fully and accurately represent their credentials, competency, education, training and experience in both the field of assistive technology and the primary profession in which they are members. To the extent practical, individuals shall disclose their primary profession in all forms of communication, including advertising that refers to their credential in assistive technology.
5. Individuals shall, at a minimum, inform consumers or their advocates of any employment affiliations, financial or professional interests that may be perceived to bias recommendations, and in some cases, decline to provide services or supplies where the conflict of interest is such that it may fairly be concluded that such affiliation or interest is likely to impair professional judgments.
6. Individuals shall use every resource reasonably available to ensure that the identified needs of consumers are met, including referral to other practitioners or sources which may provide the needed service or supply within the scope of their competence.
7. Individuals shall cooperate with members of other professions, where appropriate, in delivering services to consumers, and shall actively participate in the team process when the consumer's needs require such an approach.
8. Individuals shall offer an appropriate range of assistive technology services that include assessment, evaluation, recommendations, training, adjustments at delivery, and follow-up and modifications after delivery.
9. Individuals shall verify consumer's needs by using direct assessment or evaluation procedures with the consumer.
10. Individuals shall assure that the consumer fully participates, and is fully informed about all reasonable options available, regardless of finances, in the development of recommendations for intervention strategies.

(Continued)

BOX 1-5 RESNA Standards of Practice for Assistive Technology Practitioners and Suppliers—cont'd

11. Individuals shall consider future and emerging needs when developing intervention strategies and fully inform the consumer of those needs.
12. Individuals shall avoid providing and implementing technology [that exposes] the consumer to unreasonable risk, and shall advise the consumer as fully as possible of all known risks. Where adjustments, instruction for use, or necessary modifications are likely to be required to avoid or minimize such risks, individuals shall make sure that such information or service is provided.
13. Individuals shall fully inform consumers or their advocates about all relevant aspects, including the financial implications, of all final recommendations for the provision of technology, and shall not guaranty the results of any service or technology. Individuals may, however, make reasonable statements about prognosis.
14. Individuals shall maintain adequate records of the technology evaluation, assessment, recommendations, services, or products provided and preserve confidentiality of those records, unless required by law, or unless the protection of the welfare of the person or the community requires otherwise.
15. Individuals shall endeavor, through ongoing professional development, including continuing education, to remain current on all aspects of assistive technology relevant to their practice including accessibility, funding, legal or public issues, recommended practices and emerging technologies.
16. Individuals shall endeavor to institute procedures, on an on-going basis, to evaluate, promote and enhance the quality of service delivered to all consumers.
17. Individuals shall be truthful and accurate in all public statements concerning assistive technology, assistive technology practitioners and suppliers, services, and products dispensed.
18. Individuals shall not invidiously discriminate in the provision of services or supplies on the basis of disability, race, national origin, religion, creed, gender, age, or sexual orientation.
19. Individuals shall not charge for services not rendered, nor misrepresent in any fashion services delivered or products dispensed for reimbursement or any other purpose.
20. Individuals shall not engage in fraud, dishonesty or misrepresentation of any kind, or any form of conduct that adversely reflects on the field of assistive technology, or the individual's fitness to serve consumers professionally.
21. Individuals whose professional services are adversely affected by substance abuse or other health-related conditions shall seek professional advice, and where appropriate, withdraw from the affected area of practice.

From RESNA, 1700 North Moore Street, Suite 1540, Arlington, VA 22209-1903; phone: (703) 524-6686 (www.resna.org).

Overview

Patterson (1989)[12] presented the following overview of quality assurance from the perspective of The Joint Commission (TJC). The consumer, practitioner, and purchaser (of services or devices) each has a unique view of what constitutes quality. The consumer views it from his or her own point of view and, in the case of assistive technologies, judges the quality on how daily performance is improved in the specific areas of application. The practitioner generates measures of performance and then attempts to judge the quality of the services and devices against these measures. The practitioner evaluates both the technologies and the consumer, since motivation, amount of effort spent on training, and so forth can impact the success of any device or service. The purchaser of services or devices asks the most basic of questions: Are the services and devices cost effective? This question also implies the existence of a measurable outcome, and often purchasers require the practitioner to develop such measures before funding is approved.

Patterson cites several reasons why quality assurance programs are necessary. The most important is to ensure that practice is effective and appropriate to the consumer's needs. A good quality assurance program improves practices and outcomes, as well as consumer satisfaction. In addition, quality assurance programs are necessary to ensure accountability to the public and conformance with codes of ethics.

Quality assurance programs are implemented through both internal and external factors. Organizations that provide assistive technology services and equipment must have a philosophical commitment to quality assurance that is reflected in their mission statements, and there must be internal monitoring and evaluation. External monitoring is also important to ensure objectivity in meeting quality assurance goals. External monitoring can be accomplished through standards required by organizations that accredit the facility (such as JCAHCO); certification of individual practitioners; standards developed by third-party reimbursement organizations; and local, state (provincial), or federal legal requirements.

Standards for Service Providers

Professional certification is a voluntary process in which a professional organization measures and reports the degree of competence of an individual practitioner.[17] In order to establish a certification program, there must be an agreed-upon body of knowledge unique to the practitioners in the area to be certified. Once the body of knowledge is adequately described, a set of professional competencies must be established and a method for evaluating an individual's knowledge in these competency areas (usually a written examination) must be developed and implemented. As Warren points out, the examination process must be developed in such a way as to reflect how a person performs on the job, and it must reflect knowledge actually required for satisfactory job performance.[17] Within the assistive technology field, the challenge of establishing a valid and useful certification program is complicated by the great diversity of disciplines involved. RESNA developed a voluntary certification program in assistive technologies that addresses the special requirements of this field and that builds on other disciplines' certification and licensure requirements, such as those required for specific disciplines. The *assistive technology practitioner certificate* is intended for providers of AT services and devices. The assistive technology certification focuses on the skills and knowledge for AT personnel described Table 1-2. The certification process is further described on the RESNA Web site (www.resna.org).

The National Association of Medical Equipment Suppliers (NAMES), an association of suppliers of rehabilitation and home health care equipment, maintains the NAMES National Registry of Rehabilitation Technology Suppliers (NRRTS; www.nrrts.org), which has a goal of providing a mechanism for consumers, clinicians, and third-party payers to identify qualified suppliers of high-quality rehabilitation technology and related services to people with physical disabilities. Registry is restricted to rehabilitation technology suppliers who provide equipment for wheeled mobility, seating and positioning, ambulation assistance, and activities of daily living. NRRTS awards the Certified Rehabilitation Technology Supplier Certificate to an NRRTS member in good standing who has successfully completed the RESNA ATP examination.

Standards for Devices

There are several types of standards that can be developed for assistive devices. The manufacture and production of assistive technologies and other medically related equipment is regulated by federal legislation in the United States, Canada, and many other countries. These regulations include the specification of good manufacturing practices and classify devices based on the risk of their use. The Food and Drug Administration (FDA) classifies medical devices in these categories: Class I devices (e.g., wheelchair accessories) are minimal risk. Class II devices require performance standards to be met (e.g., powered wheelchairs, standup wheelchairs, and special grade wheelchairs, as well as motorized three-wheel vehicles). Class III devices require premarket approval (e.g., a stair-climbing wheelchair) (21 C.F.R. 890.3890). The Canadian system for medical devices is almost identical to this, with the same risk-based classification system, but ranging from I through IV. Most assistive technologies are judged to be minimal risk (Class I or Class II), and this reduces the restrictions on their development and testing, as well as on their approval for sale by prescription.

Devices can also be rated by development of both compatibility and performance standards. *Compatibility standards* are developed to ensure that devices from different manufacturers can be used together. In assistive technologies, compatibility standards exist for control interfaces, computer emulation interfaces, powered wheelchair controllers, and other devices. For example, control interfaces have connectors on the end of their cables that allow them to be plugged into electronic assistive technologies. In order for a control interface from one manufacturer to be used with a device from another manufacturer, they must both adhere to a compatibility standard that specifies the type of connector, which pins have which functions, and so on. These standards are voluntary, but it is in the best interest of a manufacturer to adhere to them to maximize the use of its products.

Performance standards are also voluntary. These standards specify how a device should perform and provide a set of tests to be used for comparing similar products from different manufacturers. The International Organization for Standardization (ISO) establishes standards that embody reasonable expectations of performance and address issues of safety and efficacy. These standards are developed by expert committees for specific types of products, including a variety of assistive technologies.

Whether standards are informal or formal, or address compatibility or performance, they have an impact on the success of assistive technology utilization only to the degree that they are voluntarily adopted by industry. The motivation for this adoption is both economic (e.g., increased sales) and altruistic (e.g., concern for safety and functional improvement). Assistive technology practitioners need to work with industry to ensure that standards are meaningful. They also need to insist that the products they recommend have met applicable standards. These activities help to ensure that meaningful product standards are developed and used.

Outcomes of Assistive Technology Delivery

Assistive technologies create unique challenges in quality assurance. For many therapies, a service is provided in a clinical rehabilitation setting and the success of the outcome is based on measures such as functional improvement, reduced hospitalization, or the ability to work at average productivity. It is not possible to apply these measures directly to assistive technology services and devices because the goals of the service are different. In assistive technology service delivery, the selection of a device is based on what a person is able to do now, not what she or he will be able to do upon completing a program of therapy. Outcome evaluation in this area is highly individualized and it is based on the goals that were determined in collaboration with the client during the initial assessment process.

A device that is expected to meet the needs of the person is then recommended, and the individual consumer decides whether or not to use it. The device is used not in a well-controlled clinical environment, but in the larger context of employment, school, and community. To evaluate the effectiveness of this entire process, we must focus not on the service or device individually, but on the entire assistive technology system, which includes the user, the technology, the activities being carried out, and the context (environment) in which the system is being used. The determination of the "success" of the service delivery process is based on measurement of outcomes related to the success the consumer achieves using the assistive technology system. *Outcome measures* are objective criteria, usually developed during the assessment and recommendation process, that can be used to judge the effectiveness of both devices and services during the training and follow-up phases of the service delivery process. In Chapter 2 we develop a framework for assistive technologies that provides the basis for outcome measures. In Chapter 3 we identify some of the standardized measures that have been developed specific to the outcome of assistive technology use. We also discuss a structure that the rehabilitation assistant can use when interacting with the client that provides useful information when determining the outcomes of the provision of AT.

SUMMARY

The definitions, history, legislation, and industry and professional issues presented in this chapter provide the foundation for our discussion of assistive technologies and their application. In the remainder of this text, we present a set of principles, some of which are general and some of which apply to a specific need. In addition, the practices that underlie successful application of assistive technologies are described in detail. Many specific assistive devices are also characterized in succeeding chapters.

STUDY QUESTIONS

1. Distinguish between the WHO ICF and the 1980 ICIDH from the point of view of assistive technologies.
2. What is meant by a "low-tech" and a "high-tech" assistive device? Give an example of each.
3. Distinguish between hard and soft technologies.
4. Give three examples of assistive technology appliances and three examples of assistive technology tools.
5. What is the difference between minimal and maximal technology? Give an example of each.
6. Refer to Figure 1-1. Why are standard commercially available products less expensive than special commercially available products? Why are the latter less expensive than modified or custom-designed devices? Give examples of all four classes.
7. Why do we distinguish assistive technologies from rehabilitative and educational technologies? Can one device play a role in both areas?
8. Distinguish between specific purpose and general purpose technologies.
9. Why should the consumer be considered a "co-developer"?
10. Define the characteristics of direct consumer service settings in assistive technology.
11. List the types of assistive technology providers. What is the role of each?
12. Describe how you would carry out an ABLEDATA search if (1) you know the manufacturer, (2) you know the name of the device, and (3) you only know the general name of a device.
13. Describe the benefits of a transdisciplinary team.
14. Why is it necessary to have codes of ethics?
15. How does a code of ethics differ from standards of practice?
16. What are the major elements of a quality assurance program?
17. Describe how certification and accreditation differ. What is the purpose of each?

REFERENCES

1. Bailey RW: *Human performance engineering*, ed 3, Upper Saddle River, N.J., 1996, Prentice Hall.
2. Beukelman DR, Ball LJ, Fager S: An AAC personnel framework: adults with acquired complex communication needs, *Augmentat Altern Commun* 24(3):255–267, 2008.
3. Cook AM, Polgar JM: *Cook and Hussey's assistive technologies: principles and practice*, ed 3, St Louis, 2008, Mosby.
4. Cooper RA: Wheelchair Standards: it's all about quality assurance and evidence-based practice, *J Spinal Cord Med* 93–94, 2006.
5. Enders A, Hall M: *Assistive technology sourcebook*, Washington, DC, 1990, RESNA Press.
6. Guralnik DB, editor: *Coles concise English dictionary*, Toronto, 1979, Coles Publishing.
7. Kim H: The long view: selling providers on telerehab, *Team Rehabil Rep* 10(4):15–19, 1999.
8. McKechnie JL: *Webster's new twentieth century dictionary of the English language*, New York, 1983, Simon and Schuster.
9. McCarthy J, Light J: Attitudes toward individuals who use augmentative and alternative communication: research review, *Augment Altern Commun* 21(1):41–55, 2005.
10. North Carolina State University, The Center for Universal Design: *Principles of universal design*, Raleigh, N.C., 2001.
11. Odor P: Hard and soft technology for education and communication for disabled people. In *Proc Int Comp Conf*, Australia, 1984, Perth.
12. Patterson C: *Overview of accreditation and certification*. Presented at the RESNA Annual Conference Quality Assurance Forum, Washington, DC, June 1989.
13. Scherer M, Glueckauf R: Assessing the benefits of assistive technology for activities and participation, *Rehab Psych* 50(2):132–141, 2005.

14. Smith RO: Models of service delivery in rehabilitation technology. In *Rehabilitation technology service delivery: a practical guide*, Washington, DC, 1987, RESNA.
15. Smith RO: Technological approaches to performance enhancement. In Christiansen C, Baum C, editors: *Occupational therapy: overcoming human performance deficits*, Thoroughfare, N.J., 1991, Slack.
16. Vanderheiden GC: Service delivery mechanisms in rehabilitation technology, *Am J Occup Ther* 41:703–710, 1987.
17. Warren CG: Quality assurance: credentialing providers of assistive technology services, *RESNA News* 3(1):8, 1991.
18. World Health Organization: *International classification of impairments, disabilities and handicaps*, Geneva, 1980, WHO.
19. World Health Organization: *International classification of functioning disability and health-ICF*, Geneva, 2001, WHO.
20. White GW, Suchowierska M, Campbell M: Developing and systematically implementing participatory action research, *Arch Phys Med Rehabil* 85(4 Suppl 2):S3–S12, 2004.

CHAPTER 2

Framework for Assistive Technologies

CHAPTER OUTLINE

LEARNING OBJECTIVES

Upon completing this chapter you will be able to do the following:

1. Describe the components of an assistive technology system
2. Describe and discuss the Human Activity Assistive Technology (HAAT) model
3. List the major performance areas in which assistive technology systems are applied
4. Discuss the contexts in which assistive technologies are used
5. Delineate the major considerations in designing an assistive technology system
6. Describe the application of the HAAT model in the process of designing an assistive technology system

KEY TERMS

Activity
Assistive Technology System
Contexts
Extrinsic Enablers
Function Allocation
Human Activity Assistive Technology (HAAT) Model
Life Roles
Occupation
Occupational Competence
Performance Areas
Tasks

In Chapter 1 we defined an assistive technology *device* as "an item, piece of equipment, or product system . . . that is used to increase, maintain, or improve functional capabilities of individuals with disabilities" (Public Law 100-407). In this chapter we build on this base by defining an **assistive technology system** as consisting of an assistive technology device, a human operator who has a disability, and an environment in which the functional activity is to be carried out. In this chapter we formalize this concept of a system and lay the groundwork for applying it to specific applications in later chapters.

HUMAN PERFORMANCE AND ASSISTIVE TECHNOLOGIES

At the most fundamental level, assistive technology systems represent someone (a person with a disability) doing something (an activity) somewhere (within a context). The major goal of the provision of assistive technology is to enable an individual with disabilities to meet specific needs, consistent with his or her skills and the unique functions within the contexts of that person's daily life. This assistive technology system selection process emphasizes use of available function (human component) to accomplish what is desired (activity) in a given context (place, environment, and other people). We are not concerned as much with remediation of a disability as we are with enabling functional results and helping the individual to achieve what he or she wants to accomplish. Enabling functional results requires that we maximize the skills of the person with a disability, which places human performance at the center of our system. The primary outputs of the assistive technology system are communication, mobility, manipulation, and cognition. In this chapter we discuss means of achieving these outputs in a general sense. More specific applications that may facilitate performance in these areas will be discussed in subsequent chapters.

This book is directed toward rehabilitation assistants (e.g., OTAs, PTAs, and speech assistants) that interact with persons with disabilities on a frequent, often daily, basis. Consequently, rehabilitation assistants are in an excellent position to report on the daily activities and function of a person with a disability. They can provide information on daily and long-term performance, such as how a person's function changes over the course of the day, perhaps as fatigue affects functional performance, or the effect of a social context or activity on function—for example, for a person with dementia singing with other residents may encourage more function than watching a movie.

Let's start with a case study of an individual who uses an assistive device for communication. It provides a brief illustration of a situation of an individual with a disability who uses assistive technology to communicate. It hints at factors that influence whether or not a device will be useful in a given context and how individuals within the environment can affect the use of a device. It raises several issues involving the person using the device, the device itself, and the context in which it is used. It also points to the need for an effective evaluation that will enable selection of the most appropriate device and suggests that the interaction between the person, the device, and the contexts will influence the performance of a desired activity.

CASE STUDY – MARION (Part 1)

Marion is a teenaged girl who has spastic cerebral palsy that affects all four limbs. Because of these motor impairments, she is unable to speak or write. She is also unable to control her facial expressions. When her motor behavior is observed, it appears that her arm movements are random. During conversation, her facial expressions do not appear to mirror her feelings, and it is difficult to interpret what she is feeling from either her arm movements or her facial expressions. Marion uses a language board (an assistive device) that allows her to communicate by pointing to letters and spelling out words. It is clear from our interaction with her that she is capable of using this device to carry out an intelligent conversation. Output using the communication board is slow. Marion is also able to use a voice output communication aid (VOCA) that generates speech electronically, thus increasing her rate of communication.

Marion communicates with others in many different contexts including with friends and peers at school and in social situations, with family at home and teachers at school, and with other less familiar individuals in a variety of contexts. When she communicates with friends in a social situation, the communication board may be the most effective device. Here, both the communication partners and the context are familiar so it is not necessary to spell out individual words. Friends can anticipate what Marion wants to say, thus increasing the rate of her communication. In less familiar situations, or with unfamiliar adults, the VOCA may be the most effective communication aid because the communication partners cannot be depended on to anticipate what Marion intends to say.

Foundation for a Human Activity Assistive Technology Model

Before we describe a model that guides the selection and evaluation of assistive technology, two generic models will be presented that provide a foundation for one specific to assistive technology. These models are the World Health Organization's (WHO) International Classification of Functioning, Disability and Health (ICF) (2001)[37] and the Canadian Model of Occupational Performance and Engagement (CMOP-E).[33] Both of these models include elements of the person, an activity, and the environment to understand a specific construct (health domains and health-related domains in the first instance and occupational performance in the second).

The ICF was described in more detail in Chapter 1. The ICF was derived from the World Health Organization's International Classification of Disability and Handicap (1980),[36] with the addition of environmental factors and use of more inclusive language being two main distinctions between the two versions. It "provides a description of situations with regard to human functioning and its restrictions and serves as a framework to organize this information."[37] Two components comprise factors of health and health-related states: body structures and functions, and activities and participation. The framework includes two contextual factors: environmental and personal factors.

The term "body functions" refers to the functions of various systems in the body such as vision, sensation, and movement. Body structures include the anatomical structures that support the body functions (e.g., nerves, organs, and bones). Activity refers to the performance of a task or action by a person, while participation involves performance of the activity within an individual's life roles or situation.[37] The environmental context includes elements related to the physical, social, attitudinal, and institutional components. Finally, the personal factors include aspects such as age, sex, and lived experiences that have the potential to affect activity and participation.[37]

Another model that is useful for understanding the relationship between the person and their activity and environment is the Canadian Model of Occupational Performance (CMOP),[10] which was revised as the Canadian Model of Occupational Performance and Engagement (CMOP-E) in 2007.[33] It conceptualizes the relationship between these three elements and their combined influence on occupational performance (the choice, organization, and satisfactory completion of daily activities) and engagement in occupations, which is defined as the choice, organization, and satisfactory completion of daily activities.[10] Components of the person factor include physical, affective (emotional), and cognitive elements. **Occupation** is composed of self-care, productivity, and leisure; while the environment consists of physical, social, cultural, and institutional elements. The dynamic interaction of these elements influences an individual's performance in chosen or required occupations.[10]

Both of these models are similar in that they include elements of the person, his or her activities, and environment. The ICF mentions assistive technology as an aspect of the environment, specifying products and technology for personal use in daily living for purposes such as personal indoor and outdoor mobility and transportation, communication, education, employment, and culture, recreation, and sport.[37] It is not specifically mentioned in the CMOP. These models are useful in understanding assistive technology because they identify factors that affect participation in daily activities across the lifespan. However, they are limited as the role and considerations of assistive technology are not specified. A model is now presented that explicitly includes assistive technology as a component of the completion of daily activities. This model is intended to be used as a framework for the selection, implementation, and evaluation of assistive technology systems.

A Human Activity Assistive Technology Model

The **human activity assistive technology (HAAT) model** is proposed as a framework for understanding the place of assistive technology in the lives of persons with disabilities, guiding both clinical applications and research investigations. The model has four components—the human, the activity, the assistive technology, and the context in which these three integrated factors exist. The human component includes physical, cognitive, and emotional elements; activity includes self-care, productivity, and leisure; assistive technology includes intrinsic and extrinsic enablers; and the context includes physical, social, cultural, and institutional contexts. Each of the components shown in Figure 2-1 plays a unique part in the total system. Consideration of each of these elements and their interaction is necessary for the design, selection, implementation, and evaluation of appropriate assistive technology and for research into various aspects of assistive technology development and use. The characterization of the model—with the elements of human, activity, and assistive technology forming a collective that is nested within a physical, social, cultural, and environmental context—is intended to show the dynamic interaction between the initial three factors and the pervasive influence on them, both individually and collectively, of the various contexts. The interaction among the components of the HAAT model can be illustrated through application to our case study of Marion.

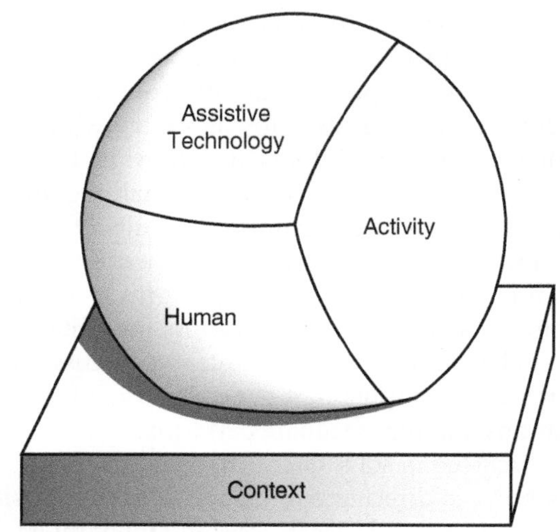

Figure 2-1 HAAT model.

CASE STUDY – MARION (Part 2)

One activity in which Marion needs and wants to engage is communication. She communicates in a variety of different settings, including school, home, in social situations with friends, with others with whom she is familiar, and with strangers. Without the use of a communication aid, Marion's speech is not readily understood by many of her communication partners. She is limited in her ability to engage in conversation, relay her needs, and express her opinions and ideas.

The communication board (the assistive technology) enables her communication by providing a means of conveying her ideas other than by spoken or written language. The communication board is particularly useful in certain contexts in which she communicates with partners with whom she is familiar and who are familiar with her use of the board. In these situations, communication can be a very quick and satisfactory process. However, the communication board is less useful with unfamiliar partners who are not familiar with its use or who may not have the patience to wait as Marion accesses the symbols on the board. Shortcuts that Marion has devised on the board will not be useful with unfamiliar partners. A voice output communication aid provides more effective communication in this latter situation, because the output is clear and audible and Marion can pre-program phrases and text for quick retrieval. However, there are settings in which the VOCA would not be appropriate, such as a very noisy environment or one in which its use would disturb others, such as a movie theatre.

This brief example illustrates how the user's abilities are enhanced or augmented by the assistive technology in order to complete a desired activity. It also demonstrates that an assistive technology solution that works in one context is not as effective in another. The illustration shows that aspects of the person, the desired activity, the assistive technology, and the environment in which the technology will be used must be considered to ensure a satisfactory means to engage in daily living. What works for one person in a particular setting for a particular activity may not be successful for another person in different circumstances. Indeed, a solution that works in one context may not transfer to another context for the same person.

THE ACTIVITY

The **activity** is the fundamental element of the HAAT model shown in Figures 2-1 and 2-2 and it defines the overall goal of the assistive technology system. The activity is the process of doing something, and it represents the functional result of human performance. Activities are carried out as part of our daily living, are necessary to human existence, can be learned, and are governed by the society and culture in which we live.[10]

The profession of occupational therapy is based on the use of occupation, or activity, in the daily lives of individuals. Both the American Occupational Therapy Association (2002) and the Canadian Association of Occupational Therapists (2002) define these terms in the same way:

> [A]ctivities . . . of everyday life, named, organized, and given value and meaning by individuals and a culture. Occupation is everything people do to occupy themselves, including looking after themselves . . . enjoying life . . . and contributing to the social, and economic fabric of their communities. . . .[2,10]

Activities are categorized in three basic **performance areas:** activities of daily living, work and productive activities, and play and leisure.[10] Activities of daily living include dressing, hygiene, grooming, bathing, eating, personal device care, communication, health maintenance, socialization, taking medications, sexual expression, responding to an emergency, and mobility. Included in work/productive activities are home management activities, educational activities, vocational activities, and care of others. The play and leisure area includes activities related to self-expression, enjoyment, or relaxation. While these lists suggest that certain activities form specific categories, in reality the meaning an individual gives to an occupation determines in which performance area it is placed.[10,25] For example, gardening may be a productive activity for one person and a leisure activity for another. Further, the meaning of an activity may vary depending on the role the individual assumes at the time the activity is performed. Christiansen and Baum (1997)[12] define roles as "positions in society having expected responsibilities and privileges" (p 54).

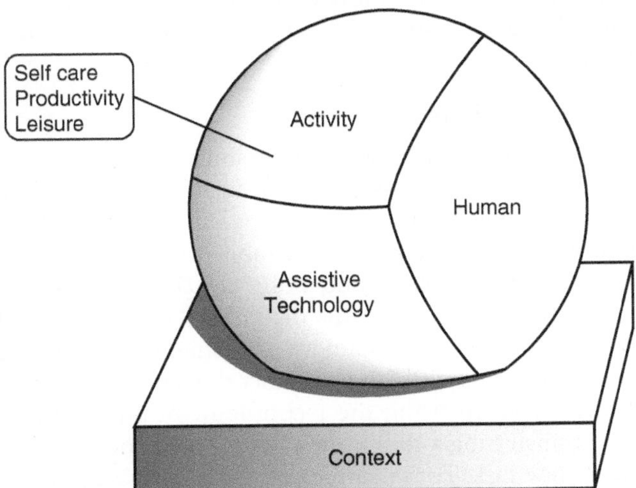

Figure 2-2 HAAT model with elements of activity component identified.

A person can have multiple roles simultaneously, and roles change throughout the person's life span. Examples of roles we hold during our lifetime include student, parent, son or daughter, sibling, employee, friend, and homemaker. Performance of an activity may differ depending on the nature of the role in which it is performed. For example, a parent reading to her child reads in a different way than when the reading is completed as part of the role of worker or student. Activities can be broken down into smaller **tasks**. The skills and abilities intrinsic to the human allow the individual to complete a series of tasks to produce the functional outcome of the activity. These skills may require any combination of physical or cognitive abilities or emotional aids for their successful completion. When an individual lacks the capacity to complete a task, the manner in which that task is completed, including the use of assistive technologies, must be changed. Understanding the activity is part of the assistive technology selection process because it requires identifying the tasks, skills, and abilities required for successful completion; the meaning the individual gives to the activity; and the different roles in which the individual uses the activity. Returning to the case study of Marion, communication is identified as the activity in which she needs to participate. She has the cognitive skills to complete the activity but not the physical ones. Further, the contexts in which she must communicate, including with different communication partners, affects her performance of this activity. Careful analysis of the activity of communication for Marion is required to identify the communication device that is most useful to her.

THE HUMAN

The model in Figure 2-1 represents someone doing something someplace. Who is doing it? The individual with a disability is "operating" the system. Figure 2-3 highlights the human component of the HAAT model. Two theoretical approaches are useful when considering

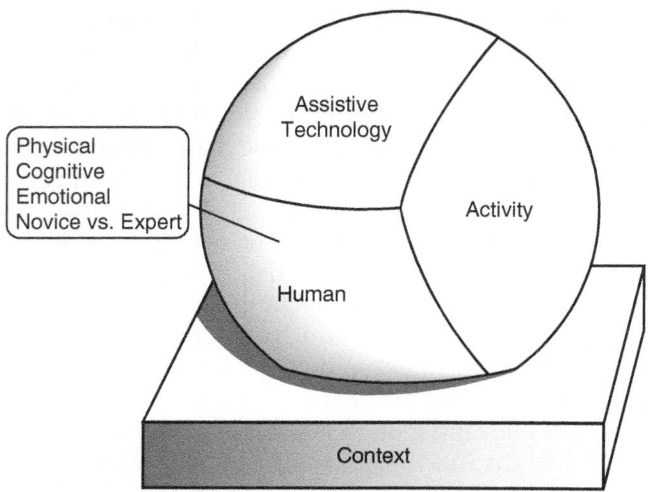

Figure 2-3 HAAT model with elements of the human component identified.

the human operator and his or her ability to use assistive technology: (1) the conceptualization of the person from the Canadian Model of Occupational Performance (CMOP)[10] and (2) occupational competence.[24] The CMOP conceptualizes human abilities as comprised of three elements: physical, cognitive, and affective.[10] Physical abilities include strength, coordination, range of motion, balance, and other physical properties. Cognitive components include attention, judgment, problem solving, concentration, and alertness, while affect includes emotional elements. It is important to understand a person's abilities in each of these areas as they relate to the use of the desired technology. An appropriate match is needed between the person's abilities and the requirements of the technology to ensure effective use.[31] Where a mismatch occurs, devices will be misused or abandoned, as they do not meet the user's needs.

In the HAAT model, the motor outputs of communication, mobility, and manipulation are required in order to accomplish the goals defined by activities. These three areas require that the human operator possess motor output skills as well as sensory function to perform these activities. These are akin to the physical domain of CMOP. For example, visual or auditory input is typically required for communication. If these skills are impaired, assistive technology systems can provide assistance by requiring different skills. For example, when a hearing aid compensates for reduced hearing thresholds or a Braille output system avoids the need for visual reading, the assistive technology provides replacement or augmentation of a sensory system. Finally, central processing is required for the successful completion of activities. Components of central processing include perception, motor control, and cognition, similar to the CMOP cognitive domain. If the human's capabilities are limited, then assistive technology systems can often provide assistance in this area as well. For example, procedures for device operation may be simplified for an individual who experiences difficulty in sequencing tasks, or recall aids may be incorporated to assist someone who has memory deficits. Psychological function (referred to as "affect" in CMOP) influences performance of activities, for example, through motivation, self-efficacy, and perception of the value of the activity. These human performance components of the HAAT model are examined in detail in Chapter 3.

Occupational competence gives a dynamic context to the understanding of human abilities and how a person changes and adapts their engagement in activity in response to environmental demands and changes in their own abilities. While CMOP is useful to conceptualize human behavior at a given point in time, occupational competence helps understand behavior across the life span. Five constructs are important to the notion of occupational competence.[24] Capacity refers to the potential skill, ability, or knowledge that an individual can apply to a given activity. Capacity changes with development and aging, as well as with trauma or illness. Effectance is the extent to which the individual reaches or uses their capacity in a given task. When a person is motivated to perform well in an activity, effectance approaches capacity. Affordances are those environmental elements that can facilitate performance of a task, providing the individual perceives them as a facilitator. Self-efficacy is a well-known concept described by Bandura (1977)[5] that refers to an individual's belief that they can be successful in a particular situation. Finally, competence is the self-perception of satisfactory performance as compared to some defined standard.

Collectively, these constructs contribute to occupational competence, i.e., the ability to meet the demands that are required for successful engagement in various **life roles**.[24] Thus, expectations by and of the individual, relative to performance of an activity, change as the person grows and acquires new skills, or conversely, as they age or experience illness or trauma and lose skills. This notion of occupational competence illustrates the dynamic elements of physical and cognitive capacities and how they are influenced by the individual's attitudinal and motivational characteristics to meet the demands of various life roles.

Skills and Abilities

We can distinguish between a person's skill and his or her ability. An *ability* is a basic trait of a person, what a person brings to a new task, whereas a *skill* is a level of proficiency, which is comparable to "effectance" as described by Matheson and Bohr (1997).[24] In assistive technology applications, this distinction is important. It is usually possible to obtain an assessment of a person's abilities, but it is difficult to predict the level of skill that she will develop using the technology. Ability can also mean transferring a skill from a related area and applying it to a new task. For example, a person with a disability might develop skill in the use of a joystick as a computer interface and then transfer this motor skill to the use of a power wheelchair. In this type of situation, the acquired skill in the first task becomes an ability that can be used in the second task.

Although it is possible for most humans to *perform* more than one task at a time, it is generally necessary to concentrate on one task in order to *learn* it. For example, a beginning user of an augmentative communication system may need to concentrate initially on the development of motor skills necessary to make selections using a keyboard. Eventually, he will have mastered this motor task sufficiently so that he can perform it reliably while also concentrating on the language content of his message.

In Chapter 1 we defined soft technologies as "the human areas of decision making, strategies, training, and concept formation." In particular, strategies are part of the human skills required for the success of an assistive technology system. As Enders (1999)[15] has pointed out, people who have disabilities use strategies to complete tasks. These can often either replace assistive technologies completely or compensate for deficiencies in the technology. For example, Marion uses strategies to enhance her augmentative communication system functionality. She may wave instead of typing "hi," or at times she may use pre-stored words to increase her speed and spell at other times to increase the participation of her communication partner. As in other aspects of the assistive technology system, the strategies used are highly dependent on all the other aspects of the assistive technology (AT) system. The context determines which strategies are important and useful; the characteristics of the technology affect which strategies are important to success; and the activity dictates the choice of strategies. Enders has proposed that strategies make up one side of a three-pronged approach to assistive technology applications that she calls "a human accomplishment support system." This framework is consistent with the HAAT model. The other two aspects of the framework are personal assistants and assistive technology devices.

Novice versus Expert User

In the selection or evaluation of assistive technology, another consideration related to the person is whether they are a novice or expert user of the specific technology. The term *novice* describes a user of an assistive technology system who has little or no experience with that particular system or the task for which it is used. As the user practices and gains more experience, she may become an *expert* user, i.e., she demonstrates a high degree of skill in the use of the system. What differentiates an expert from a novice? The novice is more likely to use the system in prescribed ways, relying on soft technologies to use it effectively. She is less likely to generalize use of the system from one task to another and must use more conscious effort to control it. An expert takes more risks with the equipment in terms of stretching the way it is used and trying new activities with the system. For example, a skilled manual wheelchair user will take his chair up or down an escalator rather than use an elevator. A skilled communication aid operator will develop strategies to increase their rate of communication.

Understanding the differences between a novice and expert user has important implications for teaching people how to use a system and the development of strategies (soft technologies). An expert user exerts less conscious effort in the operation of the system—because she doesn't need to do so. Analysis of the strategies of an expert user and translation of these into teaching programs can be an effective means of assisting a novice to become an expert user of a system.

THE CONTEXTS

Over the past several decades the models used to describe disability and the disablement process have changed dramatically.[29] In the 1950s the focus was on the disabled person's "problem" of an inability to participate in work, play, education, and daily activities of living; this problem was "in the person"; that is, it was strictly the result of the impairment. More recently, there has been an increasing awareness that the difficulties experienced by individuals with disabilities result as much from environmental factors as from the impairment itself. Initially the focus was on the physical or built environment, with much effort to make curb cuts, install elevators, and so on. As individuals with disabilities began to participate more fully in society, it became evident that the social and attitudinal barriers were just as great as the physical ones. A "minority group model" of disability emerged in which the attention was shifted away from the impairment to the social, political, and environmental disadvantages forced on people who have disabilities.[9] Bickenbach et al. (1999) conceptualized disability in a different way.[6] In their view, disability was a universal experience if a person lives long enough. Contrary to the minority group model, which advocated for special status for individuals with disabilities, the universalism concept advocated for broader social justice and policies that were more inclusive of persons with disabilities, actions that would benefit a broader segment of society. With these new perspectives, problems of societal participation were no longer attributed to the impairment of the person with a disability. Rather, lack of participation in society was viewed as resulting from limitations in the social and physical environments. The emphasis on participation in ICF is indicative of the move away from a "problem in the person" concept to a "problem in the environment" model. In the HAAT model we have captured these external influences in the *context*.

As shown in Figure 2-4, the context includes four major considerations. These are (1) the physical context, including natural and built surroundings and physical parameters, (2) the social context (with peers and with strangers), (3) the cultural context, and (4) the institutional context including formal legal, legislative, and socio-cultural institutions such as religious institutions.

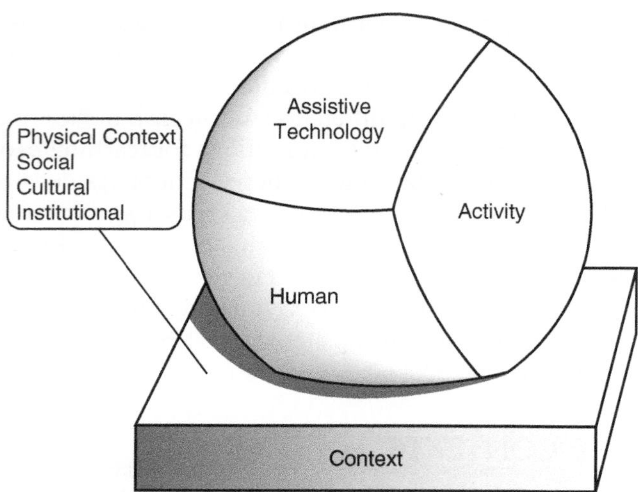

Figure 2-4 HAAT model with elements of the context identified.

The **contexts** in which the human carries out the activity can be determining factors in whether the person successfully uses an assistive technology system. The supports and barriers in these environments are important considerations in the selection and evaluation of these systems.

One further distinction is important in the consideration of context, which is the level of the environment. Three levels of environments have been described in the literature: microenvironment, meso environment, and macro environment.[17,22] The microenvironment refers to the closest, most intimate environments in which a person functions, such as their home, school, or work setting. Here the person and their abilities are known, roles are defined and rules and expectations are understood. The meso environment describes those settings in which a person functions less frequently and includes various community facilities such as community centers, shopping malls, and churches. The macro environment refers to the broader social and cultural contexts that impose a legislative and moral behavioral framework on the person.[22] Each of these environments influences the use of assistive technology systems. It is important to understand how each aids or hinders the use of assistive technology.

Physical Context

Perhaps the easiest environmental component to understand is the physical context. This context involves the physical attributes of the environment that enable, hinder, or affect performance of daily activities, either with or without assistive technology. It is important to identify the physical attributes of the environments in which the individual intends to use an assistive device to determine whether or not the device is compatible with those environments. In some cases, a device will work in one environment but not in another. Voice recognition software is an example of a device that does not readily transfer from one environment to another. In the relative quiet of an individual's home, voice recognition software may be an excellent alternative to direct input of computer keystrokes. However, it may not work in an office environment where noise interferes with the software and its use may interfere with the work of colleagues in close proximity to the individual.

A distinction that is important to understanding the physical environment is between the natural and built surroundings. The natural surroundings include non–man-made elements such as parks. Conversely, built surroundings include those structures or elements that are man-made, such as buildings and sidewalks. It is critical to know whether the individual intends to use an assistive device in both built and natural surroundings because it will affect the technology selection and performance. A wheelchair with tires that facilitate travel over uneven and loose surfaces should be recommended for a person who intends to use a chair both indoors and outdoors on unpaved areas. One with smooth tires will not be useful for outdoor travel.

Assessment of the physical environment for selection or evaluation of assistive technology begins with the activities the person wants or needs to do and in which environments those activities will be performed. Within buildings, a person needs to enter and exit the building, access various locations, possibly move between levels, and perform a variety of daily activities. Further, a person needs to move from one environment to another (e.g., home to place of employment). Some of the physical aspects of the environment that should be considered include the width of hallways or doorways; distances between locations the person must navigate; surfaces (e.g., carpets, transitions, and floor surfaces); the height and weight of devices and objects (e.g., doors) that the person must manipulate; and sensory cues (visual or auditory) required to successfully complete daily activities. Physical safety is an important consideration when assessing the environment.

Three commonly measured parameters of the physical environment—heat (related to temperature), sound, and light—most directly affect the performance of assistive technologies. Many materials are sensitive to temperature and are affected by excessive heat or cold. For example, the properties of foams and gels used in seat cushions can change under conditions of very high or very low temperatures. Liquid crystal displays are affected by temperature as well as by ambient (existing) light.

Ambient light in classrooms or work environments can affect the use of assistive technologies. Some displays emit light and are better in conditions of reduced ambient light, whereas others reflect light and are better used in bright light. For example, lighting that is appropriate for normal classroom work may be too bright for the use of some displays, such as computer screens, because of glare.

Ambient sound (including noise) can have a major effect on the intelligibility of voice synthesizers or voice recognition systems. Sounds generated by devices such as printers, power wheelchairs, voice output communication aids, and auditory feedback from computer programs can be disruptive in a classroom. Church and Glennen (1992)[13] discuss ways of controlling sound and lighting to avoid interference in the classroom while still facilitating the functional gains provided by the assistive technology.

Social Context

For assistive technology use, the social aspects of the context can be the most important. The social context refers to those individuals who interact with the individual that uses assistive technology, either directly or indirectly. Their acceptance or rejection of the assistive technology or their understanding of the purpose and need for the assistive technology is a critical component of whether or not the individual will be successful with their technology use. As Fougeyrollas (1997)[16] points out, social influence on individuals is related to what is considered normal or expected. Individuals who have disabilities may be stigmatized because of their disability. A frequent comment by persons with disabilities is that it is often the social environment (i.e., the attitude of others) that creates more of a handicap than the physical barriers in the environment. The use of assistive technologies can contribute to this stigmatization and lead to further isolation. For these reasons, it is important to understand the social aspects of the environments in which the individual will use the technology. If others in the environment do not support the use of the technology, the individual faces greater challenges to successful use of the device.

Relationships with others in the environment affect the use of technology. Those close to the individual, such as family, friends, teachers, or co-workers, have a better understanding of the person's capacities so use of technology is often easier. With unfamiliar people, technology use may be more complex as expectations differ as well as the level of understanding of how the technology works. For these reasons, it is important to determine who provides assistance to individuals using assistive technology in various environments, but most importantly in key environments such as the home, school, and workplace. Technology use, and consequently function, is easier when assistance is received from consistent individuals such as family or personal care attendants, as these individuals understand both the AT user's needs and the function of the AT. When assistance is provided by several attendants, the result may be inefficient and incorrect use of the AT, because each successive attendant must learn the AT user's preferred method of completing activities and how the AT is integrated into daily activities. In such situations, the AT user or caregiver should be able to provide instruction to the attendants.

Let's return to Marion and examine how her use of communication devices differs with various communication partners.

CASE STUDY – MARION (Part 3)

Marion may use her communication systems with her friends (familiar peers) or with her teacher (familiar nonpeer) or with a salesperson at the shopping mall (stranger). In each case her choice of vocabulary, her use of slang, and the ease with which she communicates is different. In Marion's case, she may have some stored slang words or phrases that are typically used by her friends. She may also have some more formal stored phrases that she can use in class or in a store. Additionally, because Marion and her familiar communication partner know each other well, her friend anticipates what she is spelling, which increases Marion's rate of communication as well as her effectiveness. A stranger who is unfamiliar with Marion's system would not anticipate, and the overall rate of communication would be slower. The social context directly affects total system performance. The effectiveness of her communication system is measured by the degree to which it accommodates these varied needs. Effective assistive technology systems are flexible and accommodating.

Communication systems are not the only type of assistive technology affected by social context. Brooks (1998)[9] asked 595 disabled scientists and engineers to evaluate the assistive devices they used. She found that users applied devices in a variety of social settings, but use varied depending on the specific setting. For example, intimate, essential devices, such as those for personal hygiene, are not as frequently used as are those devices that assist in employment. Brooks interpreted this result as a reflection of the complex ties between the human (especially self-esteem), the technology, the activity, and the social setting. It is not possible, nor is it desirable, for us to separate the contexts (social and physical) from the other components of the assistive technology system.

A final point to consider relative to the social context is that the degree to which various types of assistive technologies contribute to stigma differs. Stigma is defined as mark of shame; an attribute that discredits the person who possesses it.[18] Certain devices such as hearing aids and power wheelchairs seem to convey greater disability than others such as spectacles or manual wheelchairs. Consequently, persons with disabilities may choose not to use a particular assistive technology in a social environment because of the stigma it conveys. If others in an environment perceive an individual as generally incapacitated because of the presence of a specific disability, an individual may reject the use of an assistive device that brings additional attention to that disability. Consider an office worker, Ted, who has the capacity to use a manual wheelchair but could choose to use a power chair because of the physical energy savings it affords. The behavior of certain colleagues in the office suggests that they perceive Ted to be less competent in performing his job tasks than he actually is. Ted's reaction may be to minimize the appearance of his disability by choosing to use a manual wheelchair, although this might result in negative consequences such as excessive energy expenditure and fatigue in the short-term, and shoulder injury in the long-term.

Cultural Context

The effectiveness of assistive technology systems is closely related to and influenced by the *cultural context.* Krefting and Krefting (1991)[21] define culture based on three concepts: (1) "culture is a system of learned patterns of behavior"; (2) it is "shared by members of the group rather than being the property of an individual"; and (3) it includes effective mechanisms for interacting with others and with the environment (p 102). The first of these two are closely related to our definition of activity or occupation. The third concept, interaction with the external world both socially and physically, illustrates the relationship of culture to the social and physical aspects of assistive technology context. Thus these three elements of culture clearly couple it with the HAAT model and emphasize the importance of cultural considerations in the design and implementation of assistive technology systems.

Krefting and Krefting[21] point out that we all view the world through a "cultural screen" (p 105) that is the product of our experiences, family relationships, heritage, and many other factors. This cultural screen differs for each of us, and it biases the way we interact with others and the ways in which we perceive various activities, tasks, and life roles. For example, in some cultures leisure is recognized as a desirable and socially acceptable pursuit. However, in other cultures pursuit of leisure time is thought to indicate laziness and lack of productivity. If the ATP, rehabilitation assistant, and the consumer have differing cultural screens, they may have difficulty establishing and achieving mutual goals. For example, if the rehabilitation assistant views leisure as a desirable and satisfying occupation, she may encourage use of assistive technology systems that enable leisure activities, which could include modified computer or video games or an adapted wheelchair for tennis or other sports. However, if the consumer is from a culture in which leisure is viewed as being nonproductive, he may reject these assistive technology systems as frivolous.

There are many cultural factors that must be considered when applying assistive technology systems. Box 2-1 lists factors that affect how assistive technology systems are perceived and used by consumers from different cultures.[21] These factors must be kept in mind by the rehabilitation assistant when interacting with the client. For example, consider three of these cultural factors: importance of appearance, independence and its importance, and family roles. The importance of appearance is seen in the attention that wheelchair manufacturers give to how the chair looks. Wheelchairs are made now in a variety of colors, the designs are streamlined, and options exist that allow customization of the chair (e.g., caster wheels that light up as the person moves). These features allow the person using the wheelchair to express their personality and avoid the "institutional chrome" appearance of some chairs.

BOX 2-1 Cultural Factors That Affect Assistive Technology Delivery

Use of time
Balance of work and play
Sense of personal space
Values regarding finance
Roles assumed in the family
Knowledge of disabilities and sources of information
Beliefs about causality
View of the inner workings of the body
Sources of social support
Acceptable amount of assistance from others
Degree of importance attributed to physical appearance
Degree of importance attributed to independence
Sense of control over things that happen
Typical or preferred coping strategies
Style of expressing emotions

Modified from Krefting LH, Krefting DV: Cultural influences on performance. In Christiansen C, Baum C, editors: *Occupational therapy,* Thoroughfare, N.J., 1991, Slack, p 107.

An example that illustrates cultural aspects of independence and family roles involves Frank, who has amyotrophic lateral sclerosis (ALS).[26] Before his disability, Frank was dominant as head of his family. He was fiercely independent and he valued his role as provider. As he lost the ability to speak because of his ALS, he used a small typewriter-like device to interact with his family. It allowed him to retain his head-of-household role. He used his communication device to make investment decisions, plan legal affairs, and make shopping lists. His family provided the legwork to carry out his directions. As his ALS progressed, his motor control deteriorated until he could only raise his eyebrows. A new communication device, which used this limited movement, was obtained for him, but he was not interested in using it. After repeated unsuccessful attempts to provide support for the use of this new device, those working with Frank began to realize that his role in the family had changed. Because of his dependence on aids and the difficulty in communicating with the new device, he lost all interest in his family role. His wife became the family leader, and she began to make decisions that had always been reserved for him. These changes in the family, a difficult concept for Frank because of his cultural perception of family roles, led to his withdrawal and the failure of the assistive technologies to meet his needs.

Institutional Context

The institutional context refers to larger organizations within a society that are responsible for policies, decision-making processes, and procedures. CMOP-E includes economic, legal, and political components such as government-funded services, legislation, and political regulations and policies.[10] The World Health Organization's ICF section that categorizes similar aspects is labeled "Services, systems and policies."[37] Services are "benefits, structured programs and operations in various sectors of society" that meet the needs of individuals.[37] Systems refer to the administrative and organizational layer, at all levels of government or other authorities, that plan, implement, and monitor services. Policies are "rules, regulations, conventions and standards" that regulate systems, and again, exist at all levels of government or other organizations.[37]

The institutional context has major implications for the acquisition and use of assistive technology. Funding is probably the most influential element in this context. Funding policies and regulations establish who is eligible to receive assistance for the purchase of devices, which devices are supported in funding schemes, and who (i.e., which professional group) serves as the funding gatekeepers. Government programs also provide regulation and support for environmental modifications that enable the inclusion of persons with disabilities.

Legislation in many countries establishes laws, policies, and regulations that enable persons with disabilities to engage in activities in various contexts with both their local community and more broadly. These laws specifically comment on environmental access issues; modifications required in employment, educational, and other community settings; and the responsibility of the employer or educational system in providing accommodations for eligible individuals, including the provision of assistive technology. Examples of such legislation include the Americans with Disabilities Act,[3] Ontarians with Disabilities Act,[27] Accessibility for Ontarians with Disabilities Act,[1] and the Individuals with Disabilities Education Act (IDEA).[19]

A final implication of the institutional environment on assistive technology is legislation and standards that govern product design, function, and safety standards. In order for a product to be marketed and, in particular, for it to be included as a device for which funding assistance is provided, the developers or manufacturers must ensure that testing and other measures have been undertaken to ensure that the product meets certain technical standards. Standards for individual types of assistive technologies are discussed in later chapters.

EXTRINSIC ENABLERS: THE ASSISTIVE TECHNOLOGIES

The final component shown in Figure 2-1 is assistive technology. We presented a detailed characterization of this component in Chapter 1 (see Box 1-1). We also describe assistive technologies as **extrinsic enablers** because they provide the basis by which human performance is improved in the presence of disability. The components shown in Figure 2-5, *B*, represent the flow of information and forces among the assistive technologies and the other components of the HAAT model. Interaction with the human is via the *human/technology interface* component of the assistive technology. This component represents the boundary between the human and the assistive technology. This is a two way interaction; that is, information and forces may be directed from the human to the technology, or vice versa. In order for the technology to contribute to functional performance, it must

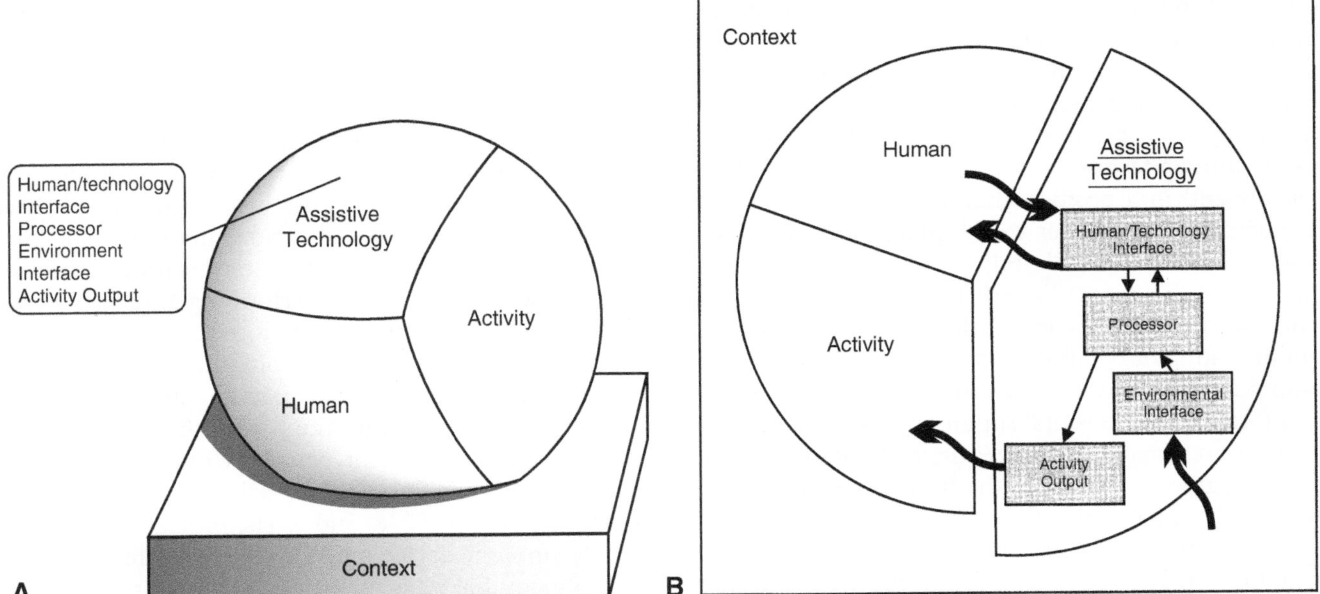

Figure 2-5 **A**, HAAT model with assistive technology elements identified. **B**, The assistive technology component of the HAAT model includes both the specific purpose and general purpose technologies.

provide an output, which is accomplished by the *activity output* component. The human/technology interface and activity output are linked by the *processor*, which translates information and forces received from the human into signals that are used to control the activity output. Finally, some assistive technologies (e.g., sensory aids) must also be capable of detecting external environmental data. The *environmental interface* accomplishes this function. Once the external data are detected, the *processor* interprets and formats them so they can be provided to the user through the human/technology interface. Not all assistive technologies have all the components of Figure 2-5. However, all of them have at least one of the components, and most have two or three.

Different sets of the components shown in Figure 2-5 are required to meet the needs of different consumers. These components function together to facilitate the completion of tasks that underlie specific activities. Because the use of assistive technologies has the effect of adapting the skills required for the task to match those of the human, these technologies enable the human operator. The specific characteristics of the assistive technology components are determined by the person's needs and skills together with the goals determined by the activities to be performed. This process is described in Chapter 3 as part of the needs assessment procedure.

Human-Technology Interface

All the interactions between the human user of the technology and the device occur through the human-technology interface. As we have said, these interactions can occur in either direction (e.g., from human to technology or from technology to human), and they include both forces and information. Sometimes separate components are used to provide input to and output from the device. For example, a computer keyboard is used for typing, and the monitor provides feedback to the typist. Sometimes bidirectional interaction occurs in one component. For example, the computer keyboard provides tactile, auditory, and visual feedback to the typist.

Positioning devices, or *postural support systems,* are one type of human-technology interface. Any person must be stable and in a position that allows interaction with her environment in order to complete functional tasks. Some individuals with disabilities have insufficient postural control to support the efficient and effective movements needed for this interaction. Provision of some form of seating or positioning system can influence their postural control. As we discuss in Chapter 4, the human exerts forces on the postural support system, and the postural support system exerts forces on the human. This two-way interaction also involves the human sensory system. For example, if paralysis causes absence of sensation, the human may not detect the forces exerted by the human-technology interface (e.g., a seat cushion). If the pressures exerted on the human user by the human-technology interface are too high, or unrelieved for too long, they can lead to tissue damage. Likewise, if the human user reduces the forces that her body exerts on the device's human-technology interface (e.g., through performance of weight shifts), the total pressure at the human-technology interface is reduced and this decreases the possibility of tissue damage.

Another commonly employed human-technology interface is called the *control interface.* The control interface is the boundary between the user and an electronic or mechanical assistive technology device that allows the individual to operate, or control, the device. For electronic assistive technology systems, control interfaces include joysticks for power wheelchairs, keyboards for computers and communication devices, and single switches used to control household devices such as lights or radios. In addition to the motor output to the control interface exerted by the human user, sensory feedback is provided to the user during operation. This bidirectional interaction is essential to effective performance (see Chapter 7). The ways in which persons with disabilities are assessed for control interfaces, how the control interfaces are selected, how they are used, and how training can be accomplished are also described in Chapters 3 and 7.

Displays that provide information to the human user are another type of *human-technology interface.* Displays are used in a wide range of technologies, including power wheelchairs, computers, augmentative communication devices, environmental control systems, and sensory aids. Examples include the lighted display of remaining battery power on a power wheelchair and the lights used in a scanning display for augmentative communication. The major types of displays are visual, auditory (including synthesized speech), and tactile (e.g., Braille). Visual and tactile output modes are discussed further in Chapters 7 and 8. Speech output is discussed in Chapter 11.

Processor

Many assistive technology devices require control and processing of data in order to accomplish the desired functional task. The processor, often a computer, performs these actions. Many assistive devices (e.g., power wheelchairs, environmental control units) contain computers as integral components. These greatly increase flexibility and adaptability in performing functional tasks. They also allow systems to be tailored to individual needs much more readily. Personal computers, tablet computers, and smart phones also play an important role in increasing access to education, work, financial management, and recreation for persons with disabilities. The role of computers in assistive technology systems is discussed in Chapters 7, 8, and 9. The processor in an assistive technology device may also be a simple mechanical component that links the control interface to the activity output. A common manipulation device is a mechanical reacher, which extends the user's reach. The user controls the reacher through a hand grasp, which is coupled with a mechanical linkage that closes a gripper to grasp and carry the object. In this case the mechanical linkage is the processor.

Activity Outputs

The *activity outputs* include communicating; moving from place to place; manipulating objects for self-care, work, school, or recreation; and performing cognitive activities. Each of these activities can be either replaced by a functional equivalent (e.g., a computer word processor for someone who cannot use a pencil and paper) or augmented (e.g., a holder that allows someone with limited grip to manipulate the pencil). The activity output for communicating is transmission of information, usually provided via voice synthesis, visual display, or printed copy. Devices for manipulation are either special purpose (e.g., a modified spoon, brush, or shoe horn) or general purpose (e.g., environmental control units or robotic systems). Wheelchairs, modified driving aids for vehicles, and similar devices provide mobility outputs. Memory aids, computer sensors within the home, and computer software such as word recognition provide cognitive outputs. Assistive technology systems may provide one or more activity outputs that facilitate performance.

Environmental Interface

The final component of the assistive technology, the environmental interface, provides the link between the device and the external world, represented by the context. This interface supports sensory performance: seeing, hearing, and feeling. A camera capable of imaging the information to be input to the human is used to augment or replace vision. Two broad classes of performance are typically aided: reading and orientation, and mobility for persons with visual impairments. Relevant assistive technologies for persons with visual impairment are discussed in Chapter 8. Systems for aiding hearing often use a microphone as an environmental interface. Systems that are used by persons with hearing impairment are discussed in Chapter 9. Finally, systems designed to assist with tactile input (feeling) use transducers to detect external pressures or forces. The environmental interface is linked to the human/technology interface by a processor, often a computer.

Soft Technologies as Extrinsic Enablers

The extrinsic enablers that we have described for general and specific purposes are hard technologies. Soft technologies can serve as extrinsic enablers in addition to their role as strategies that we include as part of the human component of the HAAT model. For example, performance aids, written instructions, and training are all extrinsic enablers. Performance aids are often conceptual (e.g., a method of remembering vocabulary in a communication system by using pictures that can have multiple meanings). Marion, our augmentative communication system user, benefits from the use of soft technologies. With the electronic communication system, Marion must use codes to represent words or phrases. If she has many codes or difficulty remembering the codes, a list of the codes can be displayed on the device, and is referred to as a *performance* aid.

Training is often required in order to make a system useful. Not only the user but also the caregivers and family must be included in this training process. When adequate training in the use of an assistive device is provided to both the user and caregivers, that device is more likely to be used properly, with less likelihood of abandonment.[11] Written instructions and other documentation can make the difference between success and failure in the use of an assistive device. Training programs and written materials should be developed with feedback from the user, family, and caregiver. Some form of evaluation is important to determine the effectiveness of these programs. The rehabilitation assistant is frequently the person responsible for implementing a training program, and therefore plays a key role in its development and monitoring.

Assistive Technology Devices for Specific Applications

Specific application devices for mobility, communication, or manipulation have a *human/technology interface,* a *processor,* and an *activity output.* For example, for a manual wheelchair system, the human/technology interface includes positioning components and the push rims used for turning the wheels. The processor consists of the mechanical linkages between the push rims and wheels, and the activity output is mobility. For augmentative communication, the human/technology interface has two parts: a control interface and a user display. The processor is typically a computer with a software program that relates the control interface to stored vocabulary and controls the outputs. The output is synthetic speech, print, or visual display. An environmental control unit for television, lights, telephone dialing, and control of other appliances typically has a keypad or single switch and display as the human/technology interface. The processor is an electronic circuit, possibly a computer. The output is a signal or signals used to control the appliance and replace direct physical manipulation of its controls (e.g., television channel change or volume control).

Sensory aids have an *environmental interface,* a *processor,* and a *human/technology interface.* For example, a hearing aid uses a microphone as an environmental sensor, an amplifier as a processor, and a speaker (often called a receiver) as a human/technology interface. A reading machine for persons with severe visual impairments uses a camera as an environmental sensor, a computer as a processor, and a speech synthesizer as the human/technology interface.

APPLICATION OF THE HAAT MODEL: DESIGNING ASSISTIVE TECHNOLOGY SYSTEMS FOR SUCCESSFUL OUTCOMES

To meet the needs of an individual, an *assistive technology system* must be designed, although this idea does not refer to the research and design process that results in the development of a new product. Rather it means the ultimate recommendation of assistive technology and how it will be used by a certain person within relevant contexts. An assistive technology system is designed through the process of assessing a consumer's needs, goals, and skills, using these to determine the necessary characteristics that an assistive technology system must have, conceiving of and planning the system for that individual, delivering the device and training in its use, and following up to evaluate success. In this section we define the assistive technology system and then describe a process for designing such systems.

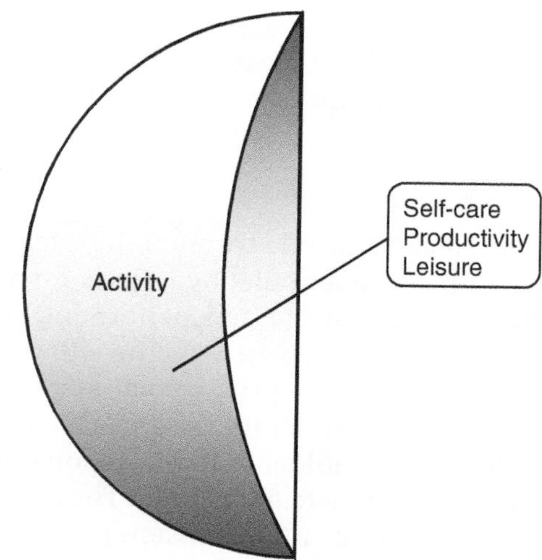

Figure 2-6 The first step in designing the assistive technology system is to define the key activities.

Assistive Technology System

In the previous sections each of the four components of the assistive technology human performance model was discussed. We defined the assistive technology system as the four components shown in Figure 2-1. Needs arise from all aspects of a person's life, and the assistive technology system goals are defined by the chosen activities (see Figure 2-2). The tasks required by the activity, together with the contexts of use (see Figure 2-4) and the human operator's skills, determine the characteristics of the assistive technologies. The tasks must be matched to the human operator's abilities and skills to be completed successfully. This match is facilitated through the assistive technologies, which replace or augment the human operator's function that would be precluded by his disability. The choice of the assistive technology characteristics (see Figure 2-5) and the matching of them to the skills and needs of the consumer complete the design process and the specification of the assistive technology system.

Define Key Activities

The first step in the process of designing the assistive technology system is the identification of an activity or activities that are meaningful to the consumer (Figure 2-6). These are activities that he either needs or wants to do. The categories of self-care, productivity, and leisure, described earlier, are useful to help organize the evaluation and ensure that relevant activities are identified. The Canadian Occupational Performance Measure[23] is a useful tool to assist with this identification. It involves the client and the ATP in a process that identifies important activities in self-care, productivity, and leisure areas and is useful to initiate a discussion of how and where these activities occur. The rehabilitation assistant is one person who is able to provide feedback on a client's daily activities and factors that affect their performance of these activities.

There are a number of questions that help define the activity. Who will perform the activity? Is it important for the client to perform the activity independently or will he accept assistance from others or technology? When he does accept assistance from others, it is important to determine whether this assistance can be provided by family, friends, or a personal care attendant. If the activity is a sensitive one, such as toileting, the consumer may be very particular about the person from whom he will accept this assistance.

It is important to determine the meaning of the activity to the consumer and what adaptations he will accept to that activity. Klinger and Spaulding (1998)[20] identified several different ways in which an activity can be adapted, including changing how it is completed, who does it, when and how frequently it is completed, stopping the activity, and substituting one activity for another. The consumer's acceptance of adaptation of an activity will depend on the meaning that engagement in that activity has for him. For example, a consumer who performed an activity, such as a competitive sport, at a highly skilled level may not find satisfaction with involvement in the same activity if his performance no longer meets previous standards. The meaning given to the activity will be a predictor of whether or not the consumer will accept technology as an alternate means to its completion.[32]

An additional factor that helps to define the activity relates to time. How frequently does the consumer engage in that activity and will she accept a change in that activity? One that is completed regularly and frequently is of higher priority than something that is only done infrequently. It is also useful to ask how long it takes the person to complete the task and whether she is willing to invest that amount of time in it.

A thorough occupational or activity analysis is important for identification of the task demands. These demands are considered to be physical, cognitive, or affective skills, knowledge, or behaviors that are required for successful completion of the activity. Although they are attributes of the human, they are independent of the attributes of any specific individual. Rather, the analysis describes the skills, behaviors, etc., required to successfully complete the activity and its sub-tasks. Several schemes for conducting an occupational or activity analysis are found in the literature.[7,35]

Consider the Perspective of the User

Once the activities have been defined, with input from the user, the focus of the system design process shifts to the human (Figure 2-7). The activity and the human are linked and it is artificial to separate the activity from the person. In this section the focus is on the attributes, perceptions, and preferences of the specific individual who will use the assistive technology. A thorough assessment should be completed of the user's physical and cognitive abilities and her affective state. Elements of the physical, cognitive, and affective domains and assessment specific to each of the types of assistive technologies are discussed in subsequent chapters.

Individual choice is important to determine at this stage. The consumer participates in the choice of activities in which to engage and the choice of how to adapt a specific activity. The assistive technology practitioner contributes expertise that assists the consumer in the choice of assistive technologies but must recognize the consumer's right to exercise that choice. The rehabilitation assistant provides input into the current engagement and performance of activities in such situations as a skilled nursing facility (SNF) or educational setting. How much input to provide depends on many things, such as whether the consumer is a novice or expert assistive technology user and the capacity of the consumer and her caregivers to understand the implications of the use of the assistive technology.

Choice is also seen in how a consumer completes an activity. Denison (2003)[14] theorized that assistive technology users choose between performing a task themselves, using technology, or seeking assistance from others. For any given activity, the person may choose a combination of these three components. Let's return to the case of Marion presented at the beginning of this chapter. In some situations, she chooses to use a voice output communication aid for oral communication. When she uses this device, she performs some of the task herself (physically accessing the device), she may rely on another person to set up the device for her, and she relies on the device for oral output. In this situation, she primarily chooses to use her own abilities and the device to complete the task of communication.

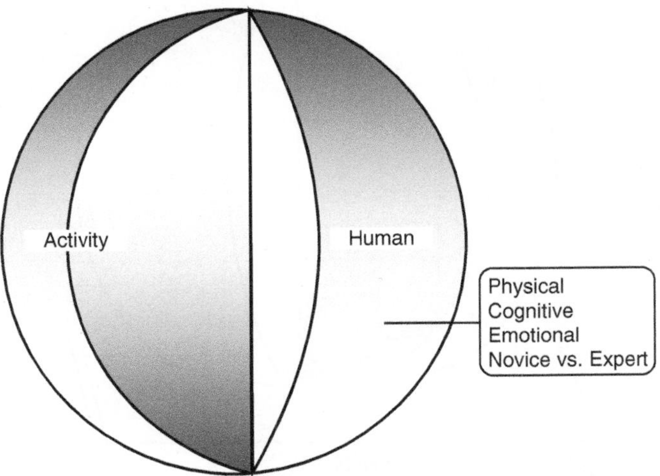

Figure 2-7 Once the activities are defined, the skills and perspective of the human user should be investigated.

What are some of the factors that influence a person's choice to complete an activity themselves, receive assistance from another, use technology, or use, as in the previous example, some combination of the three? These factors are unique to the individual user and are outside of the person's actual physical and cognitive abilities. The individual may choose to complete an activity, or part of it, themselves when they perceive themselves to have the ability to do so (i.e., their self efficacy[5]). Conversely, when the person does not believe she has the ability to perform a task, she is more likely to avoid doing it altogether or rely on someone else even when she actually has the ability.

People make choices in their activities partially based on the amount of energy they are willing to expend on the activity. For example, a person with a spinal cord injury that resulted in quadriplegia, who works outside the home, may choose to have a personal care attendant assist with bathing and dressing in the morning, when these activities would require a significant time and energy investment to be completed independently. So, even when a person is physically capable of completing a task on her own, it might not be worth the energy consumption if it leaves her tired and unable to engage in activities that she values highly. To some extent, people make choices based on short- and long-term benefits and risks. The person with a spinal cord injury might be physically capable of propelling a manual wheelchair independently. However, evidence is confirming that long-term manual wheelchair use results in repetitive injuries to the shoulder[8,30] that affect not only wheelchair propulsion but other important activities such as transfers. Thus, even though she is physically capable of propelling a manual wheelchair, she might choose to use a power chair to conserve the integrity of her joints and reduce her energy consumption, both for the short-term gain of engaging in meaningful activities and the long-term benefits of retaining her physical abilities.

Features of the device itself will determine whether or how the individual chooses to use it to complete an activity. A device that is reliable, i.e., performs the task for which it is intended in a consistent manner, and that is simple and intuitive to use is more likely to be used than one that is not.[28] If use of a device conveys a stigma, then it is less likely that the person will choose to use it. Aesthetics, portability, maintenance, and affordability are other device features that have been shown to influence whether a person will choose to use a device or not.

Elements of the social environment also affect a person's choice of how to complete an activity. Assistance is more likely to be received from another person when that person is knowledgeable in, and effective with, the assistance he provides. In the example of Marion, her decision to use a communication board versus a VOCA was made, in part, on the basis of her specific communication partner. The communication board requires more assistance from another person (as he must interpret the symbols or understand her abbreviations), so it was only used with more familiar partners. The VOCA, which requires less effort on the part of the communication partner, was used with less familiar partners.

Others in the environment can influence the choices an individual makes regarding task completion. For some individuals the notion of "use it or lose it" results in them expending more of their own effort on a task. Another common example is the use of a power versus a manual wheelchair. A person who chooses power over manual mobility may be seen as lazy by others, including family or therapists, even when the power chair enables more independence in other functional areas. Others may only focus on a single activity, in this case wheelchair propulsion, rather than seeing the larger picture, which may be, for example, the energy expenditure of a university student propelling herself across campus. In this case, the person may be so tired from propelling the chair that she has difficulty concentrating on the academic tasks.

Finally, the choice may be dependent on what the environment will support. If another person is not available to provide assistance to someone with a disability in a certain environment, then another means of completing a task must be found. For example, a student with a visual impairment may not be able to take notes in class. In some situations a note taker is provided. When the educational institution cannot provide a note taker, then other means, such as use of a recording device, can be implemented to accomplish the activity of note taking. Further, different environments support the use of technology in different ways. A power wheelchair may be an excellent mobility choice when moving about the community but may be less effective for mobility within the confines of a home. Voice recognition software may be a very effective means of entering information at home or in a private office where ambient noise and the proximity of others are limited.

Together, the personal attitudes of the user, the effectiveness of the technology in supporting the activity, and the ability of the environment to support the activity all influence the choice that the individual makes when determining how she will complete an activity. The assistive technology provider's role is to ask the questions and serve as a resource for the individual to assist them with this decision-making process.

Consider the Environment

When designing the assistive technology system, there are a number of important questions to answer when considering the environment. Figure 2-8 shows the influence of the context on the human user's performance of desired activities. We discussed the effect that the environment has on the user's choice of how to complete the activity. Some additional questions include: Where will the assistive technology be used? Does the consumer expect to use it in a single environment (e.g., the home or workplace) or does he need to use it in, and thus transport it to, different locations, in which case portability and flexibility are important? If the technology is to be used across many different environments, the effect of the environment on its use must be considered. For example, the extremes of temperature that are experienced will affect the performance of the materials used to construct seating systems. In northern climates, extreme cold has the potential to alter the material properties, therefore influencing the ability of the device to distribute pressure. Similarly extremes of temperature will have a detrimental influence on any device with electronic components. Available light and sounds within the environment will also influence device performance.

The effect of the environment on the performance of the activity is another consideration. What are the differences in how an activity is or can be performed across all pertinent environments? Environments that incorporate universal design principles (see Chapter 1) facilitate performance of activities by individuals with a variety of abilities. Institutional policies and procedures can be

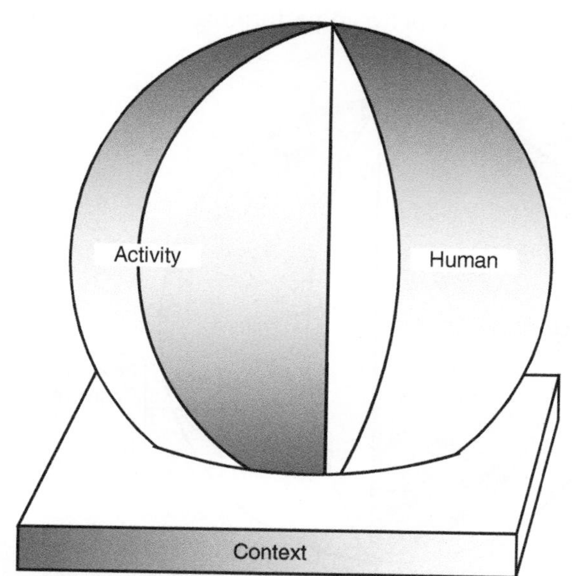

Figure 2-8 Consider the influence of the context on the human user's performance of desired activities.

barriers or enablers to performance of an activity and may even determine whether an individual has access to necessary technology.

When a device must be used in a variety of environments, the complexity of its setup is an important consideration. A device that is very complex to set up may not be used across various environments because the setup is too time consuming and the potential for error is great. Even when device setup is simple, such as replacing a seat cushion into a wheelchair, there is a potential for misuse if the individual replacing it is not familiar with its use. Most rehabilitation assistants have seen wheelchair cushions placed backwards in the wheelchair, obviously compromising their performance.

Funding is another reason why it is important to determine where the device will be used. Under some funding schemes, a person is only eligible to receive a device if it is used in a specific environment, such as the home. In such a situation, the initial assessment for the device will determine that the device and the environment in which it is to be used are compatible. Issues such as physical access and social support for use of the device are important considerations here.

Up to this point, we have discussed definition of the activities in which the person wants to participate, an assessment of the abilities of the user along with his personal choice in how to complete an activity, and the influence of the environment on the use of assistive technology. Now, we will discuss selection of the assistive technology.

Selecting the Assistive Technology

Two issues will be discussed relative to selecting the assistive technology. The first is a hierarchy of assistive technology described by Trefler and Hobson (1997)[34] (Box 2-2). The second is the notion of function allocation[4] that comes from human factors engineering.

The device abandonment literature suggests that assistive technology that is simple to use is less likely to be abandoned than that which is more complex. Trefler and Hobson[34] describe a hierarchy that moves from simple, relatively easy-to-obtain devices to those that are more complex and more difficult to obtain. Their premise is that the device recommended should be as simple as possible yet still meet the client's needs. As you can see from Box 2-2, these devices range from those that are commercially available for general consumption to those that are custom made for a single individual. While it is tempting sometimes to recommend or purchase a device that promises to perform a wide variety of functions, unless the user needs or wants all the functions, a simpler device is usually the better option. Think about all the various functions that are available on current smart phones. Most people don't use all these functions, even though they add to the cost. The same holds true for assistive device selection.

BOX 2-2 A Hierarchy for Assistive Technology Selection

Adapt the activity or task.
Select a device that is commercially available for persons without disabilities.
Select commercially available rehabilitation products.
Combine commercially available rehabilitation products in innovative ways.
Modify existing commercially available rehabilitation products.
Design and create a new device for a specific individual.

Modified from Trefler E, Hobson D: Assistive Technology. In Christiansen C, Baum C, editors: *Occupational therapy: enabling function and well-being*, Thoroughfare, N.J., 1997, SLACK, p 490.

Allocation of Functions

In any human/device system we can allocate some functions to the human, some to the device, and some to the Personal Assistant Services (PAS). Bailey (1996)[4] defines several approaches to **function allocation** that are used in general human factors design. Several of these are applicable to the design of assistive technology systems and are useful for both the user and others when determining how and what type of assistive technology will be beneficial to the individual. The simplest approach is *comparison allocation.* Here each task to be carried out is assigned completely to the human or the device. The user's skills define the tasks that can be assigned to her, and the characteristics of the technology determine which capabilities are assigned to it. For example, a standard telephone is designed with the assumption that the user can hold the handset, press the buttons to dial, hear the other person, and speak into the telephone. These are all functions assigned to the user. However, if the user cannot perform any of these tasks, the assistive technology must provide an alternative set of capabilities. For example, assume that a particular consumer is able to carry out all the functions except holding the handset and dialing. A speaker phone, which avoids the need to hold the handset, combined with a mouth stick for dialing could be used. These constitute the assistive technology component of this system. We often use comparison allocation when matching characteristics of technology to a consumer's skills.

A second allocation approach is *leftover allocation,* in which as many functions as possible are assigned to the human and the device carries out the remainder. In assistive technology system design, this approach is often followed to give the consumer as much natural control over his activities as possible, but to provide assistance when needed. For example, some manual wheelchairs are equipped with power assist wheels that amplify the user's propulsion strokes. Thus a person who has limited strength and endurance can propel the wheelchair manually but the power assist wheels augment their abilities.

A third approach is *economic allocation,* in which the basic consideration is whether it is cheaper to select, train, and pay a personal assistant to do the activity or to design an assistive technology system for this purpose. Often the economic analysis initially favors the personal assistant because the purchase cost of the technology is relatively high. However, if the technology cost is amortized over its useful life, the technological approach may be significantly less expensive, since the personal assistant cost (salary) rises over time.

The final approach that we use when designing an assistive technology system is *flexible allocation.* In this approach the consumer can vary his or her degree of participation in the activity based on skills and needs. Whenever possible, we use this approach in assistive technology systems, and we couple the use of the AT system with PAS. The human and technology components are not fixed in scope; they change based on the specific activities and tasks to be carried out. Initially the novice operator may rely more heavily on intuitive skills to perform the desired tasks. As knowledge of the device operation increases and strategies are developed, the tasks carried out by the human operator change and system operation becomes more efficient. The role of PAS may also change over time. As an example of allocation of functions, consider the case of Pat.

CASE STUDY – PAT

Pat sustained a high-level spinal cord injury that resulted in quadriplegia. He has good control of his head, but he has no functional use of his arms or legs. He uses an electronic pointing device attached to a headband to substitute for using his fingers to type on the computer keyboard. This device must be placed on his head, and a personal assistant must set up the computer. Because of his underlying disabilities, Pat will always need to rely on PAS to place the device on his head. Pat will also rely on PAS as a backup if his electronic pointing system becomes inoperative. The particular device that Pat is using is equipped with a word prediction feature, which presents a choice of words based on the keys he enters. Pat's assistant may also help with some system functions as Pat is learning to use the system. As Pat gains more skill in using the system, this assistance will not be necessary. Initially Pat will use just the letter-by-letter input mode, since he is familiar with that method from previous use of a keyboard. However, as he begins to learn what words are likely to be predicted when he types certain sequences of keys, he'll start using the word completion feature to speed up his selections. The advanced features of his system—in this case, word prediction—are not used until the basic features have become familiar. As Pat learns to use the advanced features, he will need to make fewer entries because the device has taken over a larger portion of the total system functions. As Pat becomes more and more skilled, he will be able to allocate more functions to the system and reserve his own energy for thinking and decision making.

Flexible allocation also allows for the system to change to account for decreasing human function, as in the case of degenerative disease. For example, an individual with muscular dystrophy generally regresses from walking to using a manual wheelchair and then to a powered wheelchair as his disease progresses. This loss of function often requires two new systems, a manual and a powered wheelchair. However, there are add-on power units that can be attached to a manual wheelchair. The use of an add-on unit makes the basic manual wheelchair more flexible and allows the transfer of functions from the human (upper body strength to propel a manual wheelchair) to the device (an electric motor to power the wheelchair). Similar considerations apply to individuals whose abilities, and resulting performance, fluctuate throughout the day or from day to day because of changing neuromuscular capabilities (e.g., muscle tone, strength, or attention) or fatigue. Often this fluctuation in abilities is great, and the system must compensate for these changes. If the system is able to reallocate functions flexibly, the consumer will be able to accomplish tasks with greater device assistance when she is tired, and she will be able to exert more control and independence when she is well rested.

Some extrinsic enablers are more flexible than others, and they allow continual alteration in the allocation between the human and technology. For example, computer-based devices can be altered by software to perform many functions with the same control interface. On the other hand, some extrinsic enablers, including some seating and postural support systems, are less flexible, and they must be redesigned or adjusted if the human component changes significantly (e.g., when a child goes through a growth phase).

APPLICATION OF THE HAAT MODEL: A CASE STUDY

The following case study demonstrates the application of the HAAT model from the perspective of the rehabilitation assistant. While much more detail could be provided in this analysis, the key elements have been portrayed to facilitate understanding of how the HAAT model can guide device selection and use. Each component of the HAAT model is considered separately, and then the total system is described.

The case considers the role of the rehabilitation therapy assistant who is asked to participate in a multidisciplinary team that will evaluate Andy, a 38-year-old man who lives in an apartment. He receives in-home personal support. Andy has difficulty producing speech and the team has been asked to make a recommendation for an augmentative communication device (see Chapter 11).

Define the Key Activities (The Activity)

Andy receives assistance for activities of daily living in his home from the in-home support service personnel. He uses a computer to access the Internet, watch movies, and read. Computer use and watching TV are his primary activities at home. During the day, he attends an adult day program, which offers physical therapy, occupational therapy, speech therapy, social work and nursing services, and social activities. Andy's favorite activities are the book club, relaxation group, computer time to go online, and chances to go out to the center's garden with the occupational therapy garden group. The day program is the setting in which the evaluation will occur and where the rehabilitation assistant works.

Andy attends a community-based coffee house regularly. He also enjoys attending rock concerts, game nights at friends' homes, and going to the library to get books for the book club. What types of communication are important during these activities? In his home, Andy likely provides direction to his in-home support service worker when he receives assistance during activities of daily living. He presumably engages in conversation with the worker and with peers and staff at the day hospital. In the community, Andy needs to communicate with unfamiliar partners when he interacts with staff at the coffee house or the library. These activities suggest that a communication system needs to be portable and allow him to converse both with people who are familiar with this technology and those who are not.

Consider the Perspective of the User (The Human)

Andy experienced hypoxia at birth, which resulted in cerebral palsy. As a young adult, he was involved in a motor vehicle accident that further affected his physical abilities. He has athetoid movements in both his upper and lower extremities. His movements are neither smooth nor accurate. Fine motor movement is very imprecise. His right hand is more accurate than his left. He finds it difficult to keep his head upright and close to midline, but can do so with lots of verbal cuing. When Andy becomes frustrated in his daily activities, he will flail his arms and sometimes pound the table.

His speech is severely dysarthric, which makes it difficult for even regular communication partners to understand. He has great difficulty communicating with unfamiliar and occasional communication partners. Without a communication device, Andy's speech is highly unintelligible. The staff members agree that it is very hard to understand Andy. They report that they all communicate with Andy using yes/no questions to decrease Andy's frustration and to allow them time with other clients. Staff members find that Andy prefers to type out a response on the computer when he is given the option and is near the computer.

Cognitive abilities are strengths, as shown by his great sense of humor and his participation in postsecondary education. He dropped out of college because of communication difficulties rather than an inability to complete the academic work. He has experienced depression in his adult years.

Andy is an experienced computer user. Once he is set up with his computer, he uses it to receive and send e-mail or participate in social media, surf the internet, and play games. His primary mode of mobility is a power wheelchair, which he uses at home, at the day hospital, and in the community, when possible. He has well-developed power wheelchair skills. On the occasions when he must use a manual chair, he demonstrates few skills, becoming fatigued easily when propelling the chair. Typically, someone else propels the manual chair. He has never used any form of augmentative communication.

What are the key personal aspects for Andy that will influence the choice of a communication system? He is an experienced computer user who can access a keyboard with a keyguard. His cognitive abilities are strengths. He has athetoid movements in his upper extremities that make it difficult for him to use controlled, accurate movements when accessing a communication device. His right hand is more functional than his left. He shows his frustration in ways that have the potential to damage equipment. These elements suggest that Andy has the cognitive abilities to use an augmentative communication device that is sufficiently flexible to allow him to engage in conversations of varying complexity and purposes. Attention needs to be paid to how he will access the device due to his lack of fine motor control.

Consider the Environment (The Context)

Three primary environments are identified from the consideration of the key activities: his apartment, the day hospital, and community venues, including the coffee house and library.

Physical Context

Andy lives in an apartment that is fully accessible. He lives alone, with twice daily visits from an in-home personal support worker to provide assistance for activities of daily living (ADLs). The day program is similarly accessible. Andy has transportation to and from the day program by a company that provides accessible transportation. Community facilities vary in terms of their accessibility. Andy or some other person commonly calls ahead to a facility when a trip is planned to determine the level of physical accessibility.

Social Context

People forming the social context of his home and the day program are familiar both with Andy and with the technology. These individuals can be viewed as natural supports, individuals who can assist with setup and use.

They are also likely to be comfortable talking with someone who uses an augmentative communication device. In the community, social barriers may be evident as Andy comes into contact with individuals who have little to no experience with augmentative communication systems.

Other aspects of the social context include the policies and procedures of the day program, the transportation company, and other organizations. The transportation company does not always bring Andy's power wheelchair to the day program. On these occasions, Andy only has use of his manual wheelchair. Similarly, when the program takes trips to the community, the power wheelchair cannot be transported, so Andy again uses his manual chair. The ability of the staff to receive necessary training in the use of a communication device, which might be unique at the institution, will influence both Andy's ability to use the device and the staff's ability to communicate with him. If the staff members have familiarity and skill in the use of the device, they can assist him if he experiences difficulty. Their level of skill and familiarity are examples of soft technology, which was discussed in Chapter 1.

Policies of the day program related to the care and transportation of the device also are considered with the social context. Currently, the day program keeps similar devices on site rather than sending them home with the client, which limits the client's use and access to function with the device in other contexts.

Institutional Context

The primary institutional context element concerns funding, in particular funding that comes from some form of government. The funding regulations typically stipulate eligibility requirements that include the abilities of the person who will use the device; where the device will be used (e.g., whether it needs to be used in more than one location, or whether it must be used in the home); who actually owns or keeps the device (for example, in the provision of devices for educational uses, the device remains with the child, so that if she moves from one school to another, the device will move with her); and requirements for documentation and justification in order to obtain the device.

•••••••

How do these aspects of the context affect device selection and use?

Physical Context

Noise elements will be different across the environments. The home is likely to be quiet, enabling the use of an electronic augmentative communication device. Other environments, particularly the coffee house, will be much noisier, affecting use of the system. The noise may make it difficult for Andy to signal to another person that he wants to initiate a conversation or for the communication partner to hear the output from the device. In the library, the output from the device might be distracting to other patrons, although probably no more so than the voices of other patrons as they interact with library staff.

Social Context

The institution's policies concerning staff continuing education will affect Andy's ability to learn and develop skills in the use of the technology. If the staff members do not have support to learn how to use the device, they will not be able to assist Andy. The transportation company's lack of consistency of transporting the power chair places significant limitations on Andy's communication function. If the device is mounted on the power chair, then whenever he is without the chair, he is also without the device. In these situations, staff members need to devise alternate strategies to foster communication. Finally, if the day program persists with the policy of keeping the communication device on site, then Andy is denied access to communicative functions when away from the facility.

Institutional Context

The team will need to consider the funding eligibility requirements when making the recommendation of a specific system. The rehabilitation assistant may assist with the development of a letter or assembly of documentation to justify the request for funding. Her observation of Andy's function and his daily activities, particularly at the day program, will provide important justification for the device recommendation.

Selecting the Assistive Technology (the AT)

What are some of the key elements from the integration of Andy's activities, personal attributes, and environments that affect the assistive technology selection? First, let's consider the AT that he currently uses. He uses a desktop computer with a keyguard to prevent accidental activation of unwanted keystrokes. He uses a mouse with a large trackball. The computer is set up so that all necessary control elements are within his reach so he can use it independently. He is also an experienced user of a power wheelchair with a right-side joystick controller. He has a manual wheelchair that he uses when transportation is not available for the power wheelchair. He also owns an adapted van that supports personnel drive.

Andy wants to use the device at home, at the day program, and in the community, where he will engage with both familiar and unfamiliar communication partners. His communication will include providing direction to personal care attendants, interaction with staff at community venues, and talking with peers and staff in all environments. Andy requires a device that will allow him to easily access switches and one that will provide flexibility to accommodate all of his various communication needs. The device should be easily controlled with one hand, and positioned so that he can easily reach it with his right hand. The device should be portable and mount to his power wheelchair, while still enabling access to his adapted van. Consideration of how the device will be mounted to the power wheelchair should include whether it has an influence on Andy's transfers into and out of the chair, mobility in the chair (e.g., weight shifts), and mobility in other environments. Consideration should also be given to how the device will be stowed when not in use and whether Andy can do so independently. The device also needs to provide sufficient flexibility for use in environments with varying noise levels.

What information can the rehabilitation assistant provide? Andy's ability to control devices or perform activities may change during the day. The rehabilitation assistant can provide feedback on his function at different times of the day. She can also report on his ability to locate a target, and to reach and program similar devices, such as a computer. She will likely be familiar with the computer-based activities in which Andy engages and the assistance that he needs in order to perform them. She can also provide insight to situations that cause him frustration and comment on the different communication activities in which Andy engages, primarily in the day program setting where she is located. The rehabilitation assistant might also interact with the in-home personal support worker, who can provide valuable information about home activities as well as observing Andy as he enters and exits his van.

Once Andy has received his communication device, the rehabilitation assistant can provide valuable information about his ability to use the device.

SUMMARY

In the previous sections we discussed each of the four components of the assistive technology human performance model. We defined the assistive technology system to be the four components shown in Figure 2-1. Needs arise from all aspects of a person's life, and the assistive technology system goals are defined by the chosen activities (see Figure 2-2). The tasks required by the activity, together with the contexts of use (see Figure 2-4) and the human operator's skills, determine the characteristics of the assistive technologies. Tasks must be matched to the human operator's abilities and skills to successfully complete desired activities. Facilitation of this match is accomplished through the assistive technologies, which enable the consumer to complete tasks that would be precluded by his disability. The choice of the assistive technology characteristics and the matching of them to the skills and needs of the consumer, with consideration of the context, complete the design process and the specification of the assistive technology system. Figure 2-5 illustrates this integrated assistive technology system.

The following chapters will expand on aspects of human performance and evaluation of the assistive technology system, and then describe specific types of assistive technology in greater detail.

STUDY QUESTIONS

1. Describe the three elements common to the ICF, CMOP, and HAAT models. How does the HAAT model differ from the other two? What is the purpose of the HAAT model?
2. What are the three basic performance areas defined in the HAAT model? Give an example of each.
3. Describe the relationship between tasks and activities. How is this knowledge applied to assistive technology selection?
4. Describe the five components of occupational competence and discuss how they affect the use of assistive technology.
5. What is meant by the terms *novice* and *expert*, and how do they affect assistive technology application?
6. Distinguish between *ability* and *skill*.
7. Describe the role that strategies play in the use of assistive technology systems. How can strategies compensate for the absence or inadequacy of an assistive technology?
8. Describe the four major parts of the context and how each can affect overall assistive technology system performance.
9. What are the three physical parameters of the physical context of the HAAT model? How do they affect the performance of assistive technology?
10. How do cultural considerations affect the application of assistive technology systems?
11. Explain the shift in thinking regarding societal participation by persons who have disabilities; that is, where is the "problem" with this participation thought to lie? What implications does this have for assistive technology applications?
12. What is meant by the term "institutional environment" in relation to considerations of the context of assistive technology application?
13. What are the four components of the assistive technology portion of the HAAT model?
14. Why do we refer to assistive technologies as *extrinsic* enablers?
15. Describe three factors that affect users' decisions of whether or not to use assistive technology to assist with daily activities.
16. Describe the process of evaluating the effectiveness of an assistive technology system.
17. Define the term "stigma." How does it affect assistive technology selection and use?
18. What is the influence of the environment on assistive technology selection and use?
19. What is meant by the term *function allocation*, and how is it applied to assistive technology systems?
20. What are the major approaches to function allocation? What are the strengths and weaknesses of each approach when used in assistive technology system design?

REFERENCES

1. Accessibility for Ontarians with Disabilities Act (AODA): S.O. 2005, Chapter 11.
2. American Occupational Therapy Association : Occupational therapy practice framework: domain and process, *Am J Occup Ther* 56:609–639, 2002.
3. Americans with Disabilities Act of 1990, 42 U.S.C. §§ 12101 et seq.
4. Bailey RW: *Human performance engineering*, ed 3, Upper Saddle River, N.J., 1996, Prentice Hall.
5. Bandura A: *Social learning theory*, Englewood Cliffs, N.J., 1977, Prentice-Hall.
6. Bickenbach J, Chatterji S, Badley EM, et al: Models of disablement, universalism and the international classification of impairments, disabilities and handicaps, *Soc Sci Med* 48:1173, 1999.
7. Blesedell Crepeau E: Analyzing occupation and activity: a way of thinking about occupational performance. In Blesedell Crepeau E, Cohn ES, Boyt Schell BA, editors: *Willard and Spackman's Occupational Therapy*, ed 10, Philadelphia, 2003, Lippincott, Williams & Wilkins, pp 189–198.
8. Boninger M, et al: Pushrim biomechanics and injury prevention in spinal cord injury: recommendations based on CULP-SCI Investigations, *J Rehabil Res Dev* 42:9–20, 2005.
9. Brooks NA: Models for understanding rehabilitation and assistive technology. In Gray DB, Quatrano LA, Lieberman ML, editors: *Designing and using assistive technology: the human perspective*, Baltimore, 1998, Paul H. Brookes, pp 3–11.
10. Canadian Association of Occupational Therapists: *Enabling occupation: an occupational therapy perspective*, ed 2, Ottawa, ON, 2002, CAOT Publications/ACE.
11. Chen T, Mann WC, Tomita M, et al: Caregiver involvement in the use of assistive devices by frail older persons, *Occup Ther J Res* 20:179, 2000.
12. Christiansen C, Baum C: Person-environment occupational performance: a conceptual model for practice. In Christiansen C, Baum C, editors: *Occupational therapy: enabling function and well being*, ed 2, Thoroughfare, N.J., 1997, Slack.
13. Church G, Glennen S: *The handbook of assistive technology*, San Diego, Calif, 1992, Singular Publishing Group.
14. Denison I: Technology: how much is enough? In *Proceedings of the Canadian Seating and Mobility Conference*, Toronto, ON, 2003.
15. Enders A: *Technology for the next millennium: building a framework for collaboration*. Presented at the 1999 conference of the Association for the Advancement of Assistive Technology in Europe (AAATE), Dusseldorf, Germany, November 1999.
16. Fougeyrollas P: The influence of the social environment on the social participation of people with disabilities. In Christiansen C, Baum C, editors: *Occupational therapy: enabling function and well being*, ed 2, Thoroughfare, N.J., 1997, Slack, pp 378–391.
17. Fougeyrollas P, Gray DB: Classification systems, environmental factors and social change. In Gray DB, Quatrano LA, Lieberman ML, editors: *Designing and using assistive technology: the human perspective*, Baltimore, 1998, Paul H. Brookes, pp 13–28.
18. Goffman E: *Stigma: notes on the management of spoiled identity*, New York, 1963, Simon & Schuster.
19. Individuals with Disabilities Education Act Amendments of 1997, U.S.C.A. § 600, et seq.
20. Klinger L, Spaulding S: Chronic pain in the elderly: is silence really golden? *Phys Occ Ther in Geriat* 15:1–17, 1998.
21. Krefting LH, Krefting DV: Cultural influences on performance. In Christiansen C, Baum C, editors: *Occupational therapy*, Thoroughfare, NJ, 1991, Slack.
22. Law M: 1991 Muriel Driver Lecture. The environment: a focus for occupational therapy, *Can J Occup Ther* 58:171–180, 1992.
23. Law M, et al: *Canadian Occupational Performance Measure*, ed 3, Toronto, ON, 1998, CAOT/ACE Publications.
24. Matheson LN, Bohr PC: Occupational competence across the life span. In Christiansen C, Baum C, editors: *Occupational therapy: enabling function and well-being*, ed 2, Thorofare, NJ, 1997, SLACK, pp 428–457.
25. Miller Polgar J, Landry J: Occupations as a means for individual and group participation in life. In Christiansen C, Townsend E, editors: *Introduction to occupation*, Upper Saddle River, N.J., 2003, Prentice Hall, pp 197–220.
26. Murphy JW, Cook AM: Limitations of augmentative communication systems in progressive neurological diseases. In *Proc 8th Ann Conf Rehabil Technol*, Washington, DC, June 1985, RESNA, pp 120–122.
27. Ontarians with Disabilities Act, Bill 118, Chapter 11 of Statutes of Ontario, Legislative Assembly of Ontario, 2005.
28. Pape TL, Kim J, Weiner B: The shaping of individual meanings assigned to assistive technology: A review of personal factors, *Disabil Rehabil* 24:5, 2002.
29. Pope A, Brandt E, editors: *Enabling America, Assessing the role of rehabilitation science and engineering*, Washington, DC, 1997, National Academy Press.
30. Sawatsky BJ, et al: Prevalence of shoulder pain in adult- versus childhood-onset wheelchair users: a pilot study, *J Rehabil Res Dev* 42:1–8, 2005.
31. Scherer M: The impact of assistive technology on the lives of persons with disabilities. In Gray DB, Quatrano LA, Lieberman ML, editors: *Designing and using assistive technology: the human perspective*, Baltimore, 1998, Paul H. Brookes, pp 99–115.
32. Spencer J: Tools or baggage? Alternative meanings of assistive technology. In Gray DB, Quatrano LA, Lieberman ML, editors: *Designing and using assistive technology: the human perspective*, Baltimore, 1998, Paul H. Brookes, pp 89–98.
33. Townsend E, Polatajko H: *Enabling occupation II: advancing occupational therapy vision for health, well-being & justice through occupation*, Ottawa, ON, 2007, CAOT Publications ACE.
34. Trefler E, Hobson D: Assistive technology. In Christiansen C, Baum C, editors: *Occupational therapy: enabling function and well-being*, Thoroughfare, N.J., 1997, SLACK, pp 482–506.
35. Watson DE: *Task analysis: an occupational performance approach*, Bethesda, Md., 1997, American Occupational Therapy Association.
36. World Health Organization: *International classification of impairments, disabilities, and handicaps: a manual for classification relating to the consequences of diseases*, Albany, NY, 1980, World Health Organization Publication Center.
37. World Health Organization: *International classification of functioning disability and health-ICF*, Geneva, 2001, World Health Organization Publication Center.

CHAPTER 3

Delivering Assistive Technology Services to the Consumer

CHAPTER OUTLINE

LEARNING OBJECTIVES

Upon completing this chapter, you will be able to do the following:

1. Describe principles related to assessment and intervention in assistive technology service delivery
2. Describe the methods used to gather and analyze information during assistive technology assessment and intervention
3. Identify and describe each of the steps in assistive technology service delivery
4. Understand the need for training and describe strategies for the development of an effective training program
5. Describe the purpose of formal evaluation of assistive technology service outcomes
6. Describe the rehabilitation assistant's role in the informal evaluation of assistive technology service outcomes
7. Describe different types of funding sources for assistive technology and considerations to make when determining eligibility for funding

KEY TERMS

Activity Output
Aesthetics
Assessment
Auditory Function
Clinical Reasoning
Cognitive Skills
Criteria for Service
Criterion-Referenced Measurement
Cultural Context
Device Characteristics
Environmental Interface
Evaluation Phase
Feedback
Follow-along

Follow-up
Formal Evaluation
Funding
Implementation Phase
Informal Evaluation
Institutional Context
Language Skills
Needs Identification
Norm-Referenced Measurements
Outcome Measures
Operational Competence
Performance Aid
Physical Construction
Physical Context
Physical Properties
Physical Skills
Qualitative Measurement
Quantitative Measurement
Referral and Intake
Sensory Functions
Social Context
Somatosensory or Tactile Function
Strategic Competence
Technology Abandonment
Visual Perception
Visual Skills

Service delivery is the provision of hard and soft assistive technologies to the consumer. In Chapter 1 we delineated the components of the assistive technology industry, which has at its core the consumer and service delivery programs. This chapter describes the process by which the consumer obtains assistive technology devices and services. Chapter 2 described a model that is used as the basis for assistive technology assessment and intervention (the Human Activity Assistive Technology [HAAT] model) and it discussed the principles of assistive technology system design. This chapter builds on the HAAT model by delineating systematic methods of assessment and intervention that help the team utilize components of the model and integrate them into an effective assistive technology system for each individual consumer. This chapter provides information on the full range of service delivery aspects, highlighting those elements in which the rehabilitation assistant has a primary role. To effectively provide these services to the consumer, the rehabilitation assistant should be knowledgeable in the following areas:

1. The principles related to assessment and intervention and methods of gathering and interpreting information.
2. The service delivery practices used to determine the consumer's needs, evaluate his skills, recommend a system, and implement the system.
3. The measurement of outcomes of the assistive technology system that indicate whether the identified goals have been achieved.
4. The identification and attainment of funding for services and equipment.

PRINCIPLES OF ASSISTIVE TECHNOLOGY ASSESSMENT AND INTERVENTION

The assistive technology intervention begins with an **assessment** of the consumer. Through this assessment, information about the consumer is gathered and analyzed so that appropriate assistive technologies (hard and soft) can be recommended and a plan for intervention developed. Information is gathered regarding the skills and abilities of the individual, the activities she would like to perform, and the contexts, including social, physical, and institutional elements, in which she will be performing these activities. The assessment also yields information regarding the consumer's ability to use assistive technologies. Based on the assessment results, a plan for intervention is developed. This plan includes recommendation and implementation of the system, follow-up, and follow-along. Basic principles that underlie assessment and intervention in assistive technology service delivery are listed in Box 3-1.

Assistive Technology Assessment and Intervention Should Consider All Components of the HAAT Model: Human, Activity, Assistive Technology, and Context

Often AT assessment focuses on the assistive technology only, which can lead to later rejection or abandonment of the technology. One way to reduce the probability of abandonment or misuse is to consider systematically all four parts of the HAAT model. Needs and goals are often defined by a careful consideration of the activities to be performed by the individual. However, it is rare that the activity will be performed in only one

BOX 3-1 Principles of Assessment and Intervention in Assistive Technology

- Assistive technology assessment and intervention should consider all components of the HAAT model: the human, the activity, the assistive technology, and the context.
- The purpose of assistive technology intervention is not to rehabilitate an individual or remediate impairment, but to provide assistive technologies that *enable* an individual to perform functional activities.
- Assistive technology assessment is ongoing and deliberate.
- Assistive technology assessment and intervention require collaboration.
- Assistive technology assessment and intervention require an understanding of how to gather and interpret data.

context, so it is important to identify the influence of the physical, socio-cultural, and institutional elements in the contexts in which the activities will be performed (see Chapter 2). Thus the careful evaluation of the activities to be performed and the contextual factors under which that performance will occur are keys to success. Once the goals have been identified, an assessment of the skills and abilities of the human operator (the consumer) must be identified. Only after consideration of these three components (activity, context, and human) can a clear picture emerge of the assistive technology requirements and characteristics. The assessment process must also include an assessment of the degree to which these characteristics match the consumer's needs. Chances of success in implementation of an assistive technology system are enhanced by attention to all four parts of the HAAT model during the service delivery process.

Assistive Technology Intervention Is Enabling

The *primary* purpose of assistive technology intervention is not remediation or rehabilitation of an impairment, but provision of hard and soft technologies that *enable* an individual with a disability to be functional in the activities of daily living. This principle places the focus on functional outcomes. Through the application of the HAAT model we can develop goals for the assistive technology intervention, and these goals ultimately are used to measure the functional outcomes of the intervention. Approaching intervention from this perspective requires that the team determines the individual's strengths and capitalizes on them instead of focusing on deficits or impairments. For example, consider the functional activity of computer input. If we were to use a rehabilitation approach, the goal would be to improve hand and finger control sufficiently to allow for input, with the intervention focusing on exercises and activities for the fingers and hands. From an assistive technology perspective, however, the objective becomes enabling the person to perform the functional activity of computer input using available motor abilities. The impairment in the hands and fingers that causes the disability is not necessarily addressed. The disability of being unable to use a computer keyboard is what is addressed in the assistive technology approach. Through the use of assistive technology, alternatives to the typical way of using the fingers for input, such as using a mouthstick, head pointer, or a speech recognition system, are considered.

This focus on function does not mean that an individual's potential for improvement is ignored. The *parallel interventions model*[1,44] demonstrates how technology can be used to promote the dual objectives of enabling function and improving an individual's skill level. In one track, assistive technologies are provided that are based on the consumer's current skills and needs in order to maximize his function. Simultaneously, a second track provides intervention that focuses on improving his skill level so as to minimize his reliance on technology. Some individuals who have a severe physical disability may have never had the opportunity to develop their motor skills, and training to develop these skills can take months or years.[8] A common example is an individual whose evaluation shows that she is able to use her head to activate a single switch to make simple choices on a computer. With training and a period of experience in using this switch, her head control may improve to the point where she can use a light beam positioned on her head to make direct choices with a dedicated communication device. The latter means of control provides access that is faster and much less demanding cognitively.

Assistive Technology Assessment Is Ongoing and Deliberate

Although assessment is typically considered a discrete event in the direct service delivery process, it is actually an ongoing process. Assistive technology assessment entails a series of activities linked together and undertaken over time. The activities that occur and the decisions that are made during the intervention are deliberate rather than haphazard. Information is gathered and decisions are made from the moment of the initial intake referral through follow-along.

Progression toward the goals of the intervention plan is ongoing, with revisions to the plan as necessary. For example, during training, observation may reveal that the consumer can access the control interface more effectively if it is positioned at an angle instead of flat. This observation will result in adjustment to the position of the computer interface. The ideas of client-centered practice highlight the importance of involving the client at all stages of assessment, from the initial framing of the activities in which the client wishes to engage to the recommendation of an AT system.[6] The client refers to the individual and others in their environment such as family and caregivers.[6] Assessment is ongoing not only while the consumer is actively involved in the service delivery process, but also potentially throughout the consumer's life. Because many individuals have lifelong disabilities, they will be in need of assistive technology throughout their lives. It is important not only to recommend assistive technology that enables the individual today but also to predict the technology that will be necessary to enable the individual in the future. The components of the HAAT model change over each individual's lifetime. Changes may occur in the individual's skills and abilities, life roles, and goals; in the capabilities of technology; and in the context in which the assistive technologies are used. Using the HAAT model as a framework, the team can predict some of these changes and plan for the consumer's future technology needs.

Assistive Technology Assessment and Intervention Require Collaboration and a Consumer-Centered Approach

Given the nature of assistive technology and its impact on the consumer's activities of daily living, it is essential that the assessment and intervention be a collaborative process. McNaughton (1993)[31] defines a collaborator as "one who works with another toward a common goal" (p 8). Furthermore, she states that collaboration requires that (1) all participants be equal partners; (2) a problem-solving attitude be shared by all participants; (3) there be mutual respect for each other's knowledge and the contributions each person can make, as opposed to the titles he or she holds; and (4) each participant has available the information necessary to carry out his or her role.[31] These ideas are supported in the ideas of client-centered practice.[6]

There are several people who are key collaborators in the assessment and ongoing evaluation process. Central to this group is the consumer who will be the primary user of the technology and his caregivers/family who will be assisting with care and use of the technology on a regular basis. Other collaborators include teachers, vocational counselors, employers, therapists, and representatives from the funding source. The assistive technology assessment and intervention is more successful when these significant others are identified and involved at the beginning of the process.

There is a delicate balance between the "opinion" and "expertise" of the team (based on technical knowledge and experience with a variety of individuals) and the "opinion" and "expertise" of the consumer and family relating to their specific needs and goals. The consumer and family come to the assessment process with expertise in their daily lives, including the activities in which they need and want to engage, as well as expertise in the modifications and strategies they employ in the performance of these activities. The role of the team is to educate the consumer on the choices available to her so that she can make decisions related to the assistive technology in an informed manner. The challenge for the ATP is to do so without unduly influencing her choice. As identified above, AT is one component of the process of enabling activities. It may not be the consumer's preferred method of performing activities. Beukelman and Mirenda (2005)[4] discuss the importance of building consensus among the user, family members, and other team members. Negative consequences—such as a lack of vital information needed for the intervention; lack of "ownership" of the intervention, resulting in poor follow-through with the recommendations; and distrust of the service provider—may result if the process of consensus building is not begun during the initial assessment. Initiating this process early on helps to avoid problems in the future with regard to the acceptance and utilization of a device.

Assistive Technology Assessment and Intervention Require an Understanding of How to Gather and Interpret Data

The assessment process (either initial or ongoing) involves determination of what needs to be assessed and the most effective method of completing the assessment. It occurs in both formal and informal manners, using a variety of methods. Commonly, formal assessments involve use of standardized instruments, following the protocol established by the instrument developers.[32] Informal assessment tends to occur on an ongoing basis, often involving observation or interview as the client is engaged in daily activities. Assessment includes gathering information on the client's physical, sensory, language, and cognitive skills and emotional state; his performance in functional activities; the details of the settings in which these activities occur, including physical accessibility issues; social support; and institutional elements such as funding and policies around AT use and maintenance in those settings.

The rehabilitation assistant may be involved in the data-gathering process using a standardized assessment providing that she has established competence in the administration of the assessment and that the use of the assessment is not restricted to specific professionals.[45] For example, some cognitive tests are limited to use and score interpretation by only registered psychologists. More commonly, she will be involved in informal data gathering, particularly during the implementation phase of the AT service delivery process. The data gathered by the rehabilitation assistant provides useful information to guide the device selection process; thus she needs to be able to present her findings effectively in both written and verbal formats.[45] She also needs to understand issues of measurement to appreciate the implications of the conclusions that are drawn from the data she has gathered.[32] A framework to guide this data collection will be presented and discussed later in this chapter. A more thorough discussion of assessment formats, different types of measurements, and data gathering and interpretation follows in the section on initial evaluation of the AT service delivery process.

OVERVIEW OF SERVICE DELIVERY IN ASSISTIVE TECHNOLOGY

Figure 3-1 illustrates the basic process by which delivery of services to the consumer occurs. The first step is **referral and intake**. Referral can be initiated by many different people, depending on the service delivery context. The consumer or a family member, a physician or another health care professional, or a teacher or other professional may make a referral for an AT assessment. The service provider gathers basic information and determines whether there is a match between the type of services he provides and the identified needs of the consumer.

Once the criteria for intake have been met, the **evaluation phase** begins. The first step involves an interview with the consumer and relevant others to identify their concerns about the consumer's engagement in daily activities, which results in a *needs identification*. Following a thorough identification of the consumer's needs, the consumer's sensory, physical, language, and cognitive skills are evaluated. Technologies that match the needs and skills of the consumer are identified and, ideally, a trial

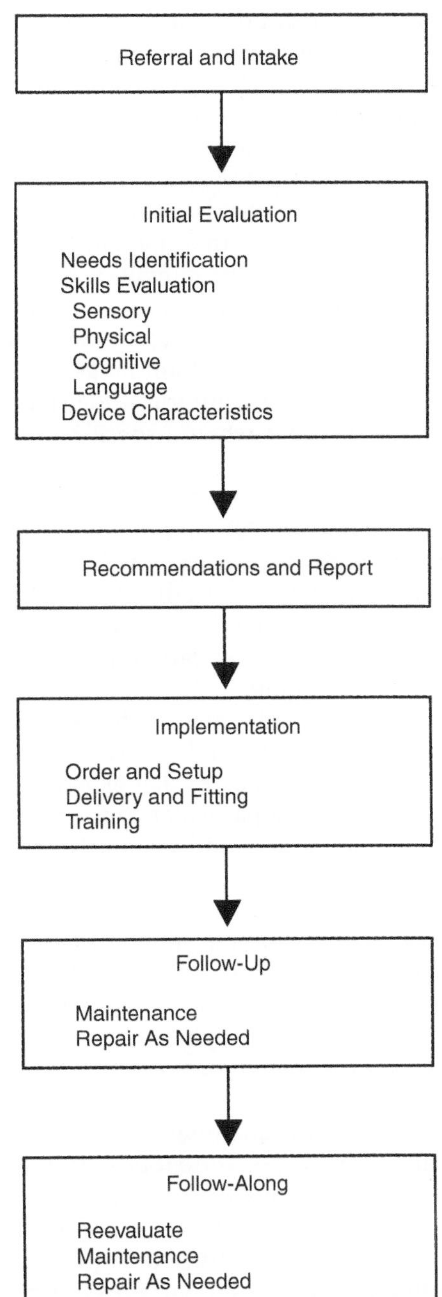

Figure 3-1 Steps in the service delivery process.

evaluation of these technologies takes place. The evaluation results are summarized and *recommendations* for technologies are made based on consensus among those involved. These findings are summarized in a written *report,* which is used frequently to justify funding for the purchase of the assistive technology system.

When funding is secured, the consumer proceeds with the intervention in the **implementation phase**. At this phase, the equipment that has been recommended is ordered, modified, and fabricated as necessary; set up; and delivered to the consumer. Initial training on the basic operation of the device and ongoing training of strategies for using the device also take place during this phase. The rehabilitation assistant plays a primary role at this phase. Her feedback provides important information in monitoring the successful outcome of the technology use.

Once the device has been delivered and training has been completed, we need to know whether the system as a whole is functioning effectively. This step normally occurs during the follow-up phase, in which we determine whether the consumer is satisfied with the system and whether the goals that have been identified are being met. The follow-up phase actually closes the loop by putting in place a mechanism by which regular contact is made with the consumer to see whether further assistive technology services are indicated. When further AT services are required, the consumer returns to the referral and intake phase, and the process is repeated. Building this final phase into the service delivery process ensures that the consumer's needs are considered throughout her lifespan. Now let's take a more in-depth look at each of these steps.

Referral and Intake

The purpose of the **referral and intake** phase is to (1) gather preliminary information on the consumer, (2) determine whether there is a match between the needs of the consumer and the services that can be provided by the ATP, and (3) tentatively identify services to be provided.[19]

The consumer, or the person making the referral on the consumer's behalf, recognizes a need for assistive technology services or devices, which triggers the referral to the ATP. These identified needs are called **criteria for service**, and they define the objectives for the intervention. A third-party funding agency, such as a state vocational rehabilitation agency, may be involved at this stage. They will have a set of policies and procedures that governs who is eligible to seek assistive technology intervention and what devices and services they cover. Depending on the policies of the service provider, referrals are accepted from a variety of sources. These sources include the consumer, a family member or care provider, a rehabilitation or educational professional, or a physician. At this time, information regarding the consumer's background and perceived assistive technology needs is gathered for the initial database. This information includes personal data (e.g., age, place of residence), medical diagnosis and health information, and educational or vocational background. Information related to the individual's medical diagnosis and health information that may guide the assessment includes whether or not the condition is expected to remain stable, improve, or decline. The appropriateness of the referral is viewed from the perspective of both the ATP and the referral or funding source. When exchanging information about the consumer's needs and the services provided by the ATP, each party can determine whether there is a match. For example, the needs of a consumer with complex seating and mobility needs may not match the services provided by the ATP if the ATP does not have the necessary expertise in this area. For the consumer's benefit, this mismatch should be acknowledged and the consumer referred to another source that can more appropriately address her needs. The assistive technology provider should have a policy within the organization's mission statement that establishes what services are provided and who is eligible to receive those services. For example, some assistive technology service providers specialize in certain disabilities (e.g., visual impairment), and others focus on specific technologies (e.g., seating technologies). Professional codes of ethics and standards of practice (see Chapter 1) require that ATPs practice within their specialization and not try to provide services outside of this realm.

The other outcome is that there is a match between the needs of the consumer and the services provided by the ATP. In this case, plans are made to move forward with the initial evaluation, starting with a thorough identification of the consumer's needs. In some jurisdictions funding must be secured prior to the initiation of the evaluation. From the information provided, the ATP also determines the level of service that would be most beneficial to the consumer. There are a number of scenarios. First is the individual who has never used or been evaluated for assistive technologies, which could be an individual who is newly disabled or someone with a long-standing disability. An individual with a long-standing disability who may not have previously received assistive technology services may now be able to access assistive devices because of recent advances in technologies. In this situation an in-depth assessment is warranted. Referrals may also be received from consumers who have used assistive technology for some time and would like to evaluate current commercially available technologies. If this person's functional status has remained stable, it may not be necessary to conduct a complete evaluation. In some cases the assistive technology is not working or has been abandoned by the consumer and he is seeking a referral to see if modifications to the system can aid in making it more functional. Sometimes the consumer may only require further training or reevaluation of how she is using her current system to see whether training in new strategies would be beneficial. Similarly, there may be a new care provider who needs training or technical assistance.

Initial Evaluation

Through a systematic evaluation, the ATP gathers information and facilitates decisions related to eventual device use. Because of the cost of the assistive technology to the consumer (or third-party funding source), it is essential that the team be able to assist the consumer in making informed decisions in the selection of a device. Current knowledge of the available technology and use of a systematic process facilitate the decision-making process. This section focuses on the type of information gathered and the procedures used during the evaluation. We start with some background information on measurement.

Quantitative and Qualitative Measurement

Throughout the assistive technology intervention, the team can gather information by either **quantitative measurement** or **qualitative measurement.** The philosophies of qualitative measures and quantitative measures are quite different. Quantitative measures assign a number to an attribute, trait, or characteristic.[34] The assumption of quantitative measures is that the construct of interest can be measured in some meaningful way. For example, a test can be constructed that measures the joint range of motion (the construct) available to an individual to control a computer access device. Joint range is expressed as degrees of motion and a common understanding exists regarding what is meant when a specific joint range of motion is described. Here the construct can be assigned a number that is meaningful to individuals both using and interpreting the test. Alternatively, a test can be constructed that intends to measure boredom. For example, it is possible to develop a four-point scale and have individuals rate their boredom on it. But what does a score of "4" mean on such a scale? We can assign a number but it doesn't carry any meaning.

Qualitative assessments assume that each individual has a different experience and that it is important to provide the opportunity to capture that experience. There is no attempt to measure a particular construct. Rather, the purpose is to describe and understand the user's experience with the technology. Qualitative assessments may include observation, either directly or via videotape, or interviews with the client and others. Qualitative assessments often capture those experiences which cannot be directly quantified or for which quantification holds little meaning. They provide the client with the opportunity to identify issues, experiences, or goals that may not have been previously identified on a quantitative measure.

Both qualitative and quantitative assessment formats are important in the AT assessment process and for evaluation of the outcomes of AT use. Quantitative measures allow comparison of experiences of a large number of individuals, and a well-constructed instrument is essential in building evidence to support the efficacy of AT use. Qualitative methods provide a rich description of AT user experiences that may not be readily apparent from the use of quantitative instruments alone. Together these methods can provide strong support for AT use, both on an individual and collective basis.

Norm-Referenced and Criterion-Referenced Measurements

Two commonly used standards are employed for measuring performance (for both the human and the total system): norm referenced and criterion referenced. In **norm-referenced measurements** the performance of the individual or system is ranked according to a sample of scores others have achieved on the task. Norm-referenced measures usually produce a percentile rank, a standardized score, or a grade equivalent that indicates where the individual stands relative to others in the representative sample.[49] It is important to review how the norms were developed when selecting a norm-referenced test for use. Norms need to be relevant to the population with which the instrument is being used. They need to be recent and representative.[48] In other words, the characteristics of the sample used to develop the norms must be similar to those of the client group with which the assessment is being used. The items that form the instrument need to be relevant to the client group. For example, assessing visual-perceptual skills using blocks is not relevant for most adults. Similarly, the use of outdated questions or materials will not give an accurate picture of the client's abilities. For example, testing keyboarding skills on a typewriter will give some information on keyboarding skills but does not cover the full range of skills required to use a computer.[32] An alternative way to assess human or system performance is to rate the performance according to a specified criterion or level of mastery, which is referred to as **criterion-referenced measurement,** and the person's own skill level in using the system is used as the standard. Criterion-referenced measurement requires that different degrees of competence in the functional ability to be measured can be expressed. One standardized method of achieving this description is through Goal Attainment Scaling (GAS).[21] This method involves a consensus-driven process where a target behavior is identified and five levels of competence are clearly articulated. These are coded on a 5-point scale from −2 to +2. The zero point on the scale represents basic or minimum competence. The points below zero represent inadequate performance and those above zero are better than expected performance. Goals are specific, measureable, and time specific. Benefits to using GAS are that it is flexible, identifies performance over time, and is individualized to the client. However, it is time consuming and, because it is individualized, may not easily capture a range of functional activities. An example of GAS goals is shown in Box 3-2.

When we use the criterion-referenced approach to measurement, we accomplish two desirable goals. First, we base our assessment of progress on the person's unique set of skills and do not attempt to relate this performance to a normalized standard. The second goal we accomplish by using the person's own performance as a standard is that we have a way of measuring progress.

BOX 3-2 An Example of Goal Attainment Scaling Goals

Target Behaviour: Client will be able to self-initiate a wheelie with their manual wheelchair and hold the position momentarily.

+2: Client is able to self-initiate a wheelie with their manual wheelchair and propel the chair forward for a short duration. [Client achieves target behavior and demonstrates a high level of competence.]

+1: Client is able to self-initiate a wheelie with their manual wheelchair and hold the position for one minute. [Client achieves the target behaviour and demonstrates a moderate level of competence.]

0: Client is able to self-initiate a wheelie with their manual wheelchair and hold the position momentarily. [Client achieves target behavior.]

−1: Client is able to hold a balanced wheelie position for one minute if another person assists her to assume the wheelie position [Client does not achieve the target behavior but is successful with a somewhat less difficult skill.]

−2: Client is unable to hold a balanced wheelie position when another person assists her to assume the wheelie position. [Client is unable to self-initiate the wheelie position. This level is often the client's starting skill level.]

Needs Identification

Through the **needs identification** process we determine the individual's needs and goals, which provide the basis for the assistive technology intervention. Identifying the needs of the consumer is the most critical component of the service delivery process and must be completed at the onset of evaluation. The information collected during needs identification is the cornerstone for measuring the effectiveness of the final outcome. Therefore it is important to take this step seriously and ensure that there is a consensus among those involved both as to the nature and scope of the problem to be addressed by the assistive technology intervention and the goals identified to target these problem areas.

Information gathered during needs identification is also used by the ATP to justify purchase of services and equipment. Third-party payers who fund services and equipment want to know what the problem or need is and how the equipment is going to address the need. Finally, the needs identification process results in the development of a plan for completing the remainder of the evaluation, which includes composition of the evaluation team, determination of needed evaluation tools and devices, and identification of further information required (either through evaluation of the consumer or by request from outside sources).

The purpose of the initial interview is to establish the needs and goals of assistive technology intervention. In this interview the consumer and/or caregivers frame the performance issue that brings them to the assistive technology service. The ATP guides this interview to determine the activities of self-care, work, and leisure in which the client wishes to engage and identify those aspects of performance for which assistive technology has potential benefit. Information is secured about the consumer's medical information, daily activities, settings in which these activities occur, and current or past experience with assistive technology. Information is also gathered about current or potential sources of funding. Depending on the service delivery model, a more in-depth assessment will be conducted during the same session as this initial interview. In other models, this initial interview serves to determine the appropriateness of the referral and then funding is required to proceed with further stages of the intervention process. The components of an in-depth assessment will be described in the following sections.

The information for the needs assessment can be derived from an interview or through a written questionnaire completed by the consumer or his representative. Instruments such as the Matching Person and Technology Assessment[42] can also be used by the ATP to identify the areas of the individual's needs and his predisposition to use assistive technology. If the information is gathered through a written questionnaire before actually meeting the consumer, it should be reviewed at the time of the first meeting with the consumer. The purpose of reviewing this material at the first meeting is to ensure that all the necessary information has been provided and to analyze the information to develop the goals. In addition, the provider needs to ascertain that the consumer understands the questions that were asked. The total team should also be present at this meeting, and everyone's input regarding the needs and goals of the consumer can be discussed and a consensus reached.

Once the client has clarified their activity needs, a more detailed evaluation of specific components follows. This evaluation includes assessment of basic skills, including sensory, physical, cognitive, affective (emotional), and communication skills; performance in functional activities; and relevant aspects of the context in which the client engages in activities. Some of the evaluation data are gathered from reports of other professionals, such as assessment of visual function by an optometrist or ophthalmologist. Other data are gathered by a collaborative effort of the team, including the rehabilitation assistant. The integration of all of the evaluation information is important for the rehabilitation assistant to understand because it influences her involvement in the implementation and follow-up stages.

Skills Evaluation: Sensory

The rehabilitation assistant needs to understand the **sensory functions** that are available to the client when using assistive technologies. If the primary disability is sensory, an alternative sensory pathway may need to be used and we need to know what the consumer's sensory capabilities are. For example, in the case of a consumer who is blind and who needs to read, the ATP must evaluate tactile and auditory skills that can substitute for vision during reading.

In other cases a consumer may have a sensory disability secondary to either a physical or cognitive limitation. For example, if a consumer is hard of hearing, the ATP needs to know how this will affect interaction with technology, including everything from hearing warning beeps when a computer error is made to understanding voice synthesis on a communication device. The chapters that describe assistive technology for specific activity outputs discuss the implications of sensory limitations to the use of the technology and how modifications can be made to accommodate for these limitations.

Evaluation of Functional Vision

The most critical **visual skills** needed for assistive technology use are sufficient acuity to see the symbols used in the system of choice, or to identify small objects in the environment; adequate visual field to allow receipt of information from a display (e.g., the keyboard or the monitor) or the environment; and sufficient visual tracking ability (e.g., for reading or tracking a moving cursor). Known visual problems should have been identified during the initial interview. A visual evaluation by a vision care professional will provide information about the following visual functions.

A *visual field deficit* can be experienced in two ways: loss of peripheral vision or loss of central vision (Figure 3-2). Peripheral vision loss results in a narrowing of the visual field, commonly an age-related deficit.[38,41] This type of loss makes it increasingly difficult to see objects to the side, potentially causing difficulties when maneuvering a wheelchair through a crowded environment. A central field loss has more significant functional implications because the individual loses the ability to see something they are looking at directly. Age-related macular degeneration and diabetic retinopathy are two common central field deficit disorders.

Visual acuity refers to the clarity with which a person can see objects in the environment.[38] The loss of this visual function is probably the best understood as it occurs so frequently in the population. There are three types: myopia (near-sightedness); far-sightedness; and presbyopia (the inability to focus on a near object), which is an age-related visual change. All of these functions result from an inability to focus the image on the retina. In most cases, functional vision is restored with the use of corrective lenses (glasses or contact lenses) or laser surgery. Chapter 8 discusses assistive technology to assist individuals with low vision or blindness, for whom these common interventions are inadequate.

Visual tracking refers to the ability to track a moving object with the eyes; for example, tracking the movement of a cursor on a computer screen.[15,38] Evaluation of visual tracking includes the coordination of both eyes, tracking ability in vertical and horizontal planes, smoothness of the movements, delay in the initiation of visual tracking, and the ability to track without moving the head. *Visual scanning* refers to the ability to scan the environment to gather visual information. In this situation, the object doesn't move; instead, the eyes are moving.[15] Visual scanning is most commonly used when reading text. Clients who have had a stroke may have a visual scanning impairment if they also have a neglect of one side of the body. In this situation, the eyes do not move past midline, so visual information on the affected side of the body is not detected.

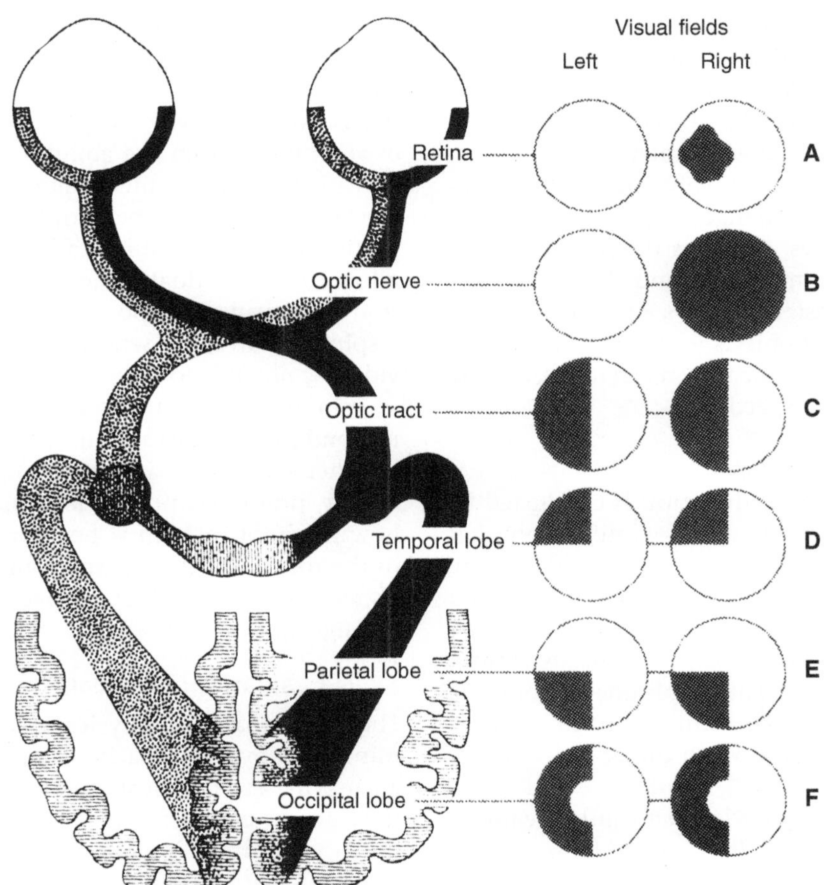

Figure 3-2 Types of visual field deficits. **A,** Retinal lesion: blind spot in the affected eye. **B,** Optic nerve lesion: partial or complete blindness in that eye. **C,** Optic tract or lateral geniculate lesion: blindness in the opposite half of both visual fields. **D,** Temporal lobe lesion: blindness in the upper quadrants of both visual fields on the side opposite the lesion. **E,** Parietal lobe lesion: contralateral blindness in the corresponding lower quadrants of both eyes. **F,** Occipital lobe lesion: contralateral blindness in the corresponding half of each visual field, but with macular sparing. (From Umphred DA, Burton GU, Lazaro RT, Roller ML, eds: *Neurological Rehabilitation*, ed 5, St. Louis, 2007, Mosby, page 977. Courtesy Smith Kline & French Laboratories, Philadelphia.)

Visual contrast is required to differentiate a figure from its background, and is commonly used during reading and in retrieval of information from a display.[41] With age and other visual impairments, contrast needs to be enhanced in order for the user to detect the information. *Visual accommodation* is the ability of the eyes to re-focus when shifting attention between different locations[38]; for example, shifting attention from the board to a notebook when taking notes during class or shifting attention from the road to displays on the vehicle instrument panel while driving. This function requires coordination of the small muscles of the eye.

Evaluation of Visual Perception

Visual perception is the process of giving meaning to visual information. Visual perceptual skills that need to be considered during the AT assessment include depth perception, spatial relationships, form recognition or constancy, and figure-ground discrimination. Visual perception is an important consideration when considering the client's ability to interpret information presented in a visual display or to safely navigate a mobility device in their environment. Formal testing of the consumer's visual perception may have been completed before the assistive technology assessment, and the results of this evaluation can be reviewed during the initial interview. The rehabilitation assistant may have completed parts of the visual perception assessment. It is necessary to observe the consumer during functional tasks and note any apparent perceptual problems. If there is still some concern regarding the exact nature of the problems, a formal evaluation such as the Motor-Free Visual Perception Test can be used.[7]

Figure-ground perception refers to the ability to discriminate between an object in the foreground and the background on which it rests. For example, recognizing that a white sock is different from the white sheet on which it rests is an indicator of intact figure-ground perception. Vision is certainly a key element of this skill, but other aspects such as recognition of the object and form constancy affect the ability to differentiate an object from the background. Figure-ground perception is also an element of hearing, and refers to the ability to discriminate a sound from background or ambient noise.

Spatial relations involve understanding basic concepts such as up/down and right/left as well as understanding the relationship of objects to each other (e.g., on top of, or in front of, another object). This perceptual function is key to safe movement in the environment.

Form constancy or recognition involves the understanding that an object does not change, despite being viewed from different perspectives, either as the object itself is moved or as the person moves around the object. For example, intact form constancy allows a person to recognize the size and shape of objects in the environment as well as to recognize that an object hasn't changed, despite viewing it from various perspectives.

Evaluation of Auditory Function

Formal evaluation of **auditory function** is conducted by an audiologist. Any significant auditory impairment that has been previously diagnosed should be identified in the initial referral or during the needs assessment. In cases of suspected hearing loss, referral should be made to an audiologist. She will determine *auditory thresholds*, including *frequency* and *amplitude*. The amplitude of sound is measured in decibels (dB). This minimum threshold is equivalent to the ticking of a watch under quiet conditions at a distance of 20 feet.

The typical range of frequencies that can be heard by the human ear is 20 to 20,000 hertz (Hz).[2] However, the ear does not respond equally to all frequencies in this range. A combination of frequency and amplitude determine the auditory threshold. Pure tone audiometry presents pure (one frequency) tones to each individual to determine the threshold of hearing for that person. The intensity of the tone is raised in 5-dB increments until the stimulus is heard. It is then lowered in 5-dB decrements until it is no longer heard. The auditory threshold is the intensity at which the person indicates that she hears the tone 50% of the time.[3]

Evaluation of Tactile Function

Somatosensory or tactile function enables the individual to perceive information through touch, either via actively touching something or passively receiving touch.[14] There are three particular circumstances in which attention needs to be paid to the evaluation of tactile sensation. These occur when conducting seating and positioning assessments, when evaluating tactile input for the use of control interfaces, and when considering the use of tactile alternatives to vision or hearing. The rehabilitation assistant may be involved in the assessment of tactile function.

Tactile functions that are included in a somatosensory protocol include: one-two point discrimination, perception of light touch versus deep pressure, perception of temperature, joint position sense (or proprioception), and localization of tactile stimulation. *One-two point discrimination* involves the ability to detect a single tactile stimulus from two points that are applied simultaneously. Areas such as the fingertip are able to detect, due to requirements for manipulation, two points that are quite close together; while other areas, such as the back, only detect two points when they are quite distinct.[14] *Perception of touch* varies from the ability to detect a stimulus that is feather weight to the ability to detect deep pressure, the lack of which can be harmful. This tactile function is particularly important in seating. *Temperature* perception allows the individual to detect hot and cold. This function is particularly important to assess for someone with a spinal cord injury. Serious harm can result if the individual is not able to detect hot temperatures.

Pain perception refers to the ability to detect and respond to a noxious stimulus.[14] Commonly the stimulus is either sharp (e.g., a pinprick) or dull (deep pressure). Finally, proprioception or joint position sense refers to how the joint or limb is positioned in space. Receptors in the muscles, tendons, and joints provide information about where the limb is in space and how it is moving through space.

Skills Evaluation: Physical

The overall goal of the **physical skills** evaluation is to determine the physical capacity of an individual to perform an activity, and the most functional position or positions in which to conduct that activity related to gross motor function, and manipulation and device access related to fine motor function. At a very basic level, physical skills include range of motion, muscle strength, muscle tone, and the presence of obligatory movements. Many protocols exist for evaluation of range of motion.[18,22,25] Both passive and active range of motion are assessed. Range of motion is important when considering positioning needs for function and the amount of movement available to access a device or perform a task. Related to range of motion is muscle strength. Again, many protocols are available for testing muscle strength.[18,23] Muscle strength is graded in a range from unable to move independently, moves with gravity eliminated, able to move against gravity, and moves against different degrees of resistance. The presence of a neurological disorder such as cerebral palsy, stroke, or traumatic brain injury will affect both range of motion and muscle strength. Typical protocols for testing these components are not generally useful for these populations because the position of the individual affects their muscle tone and, subsequently, range of motion and muscle strength. For example, a child with cerebral palsy may seem to have limited flexion range of motion in their lower extremities when lying in supine. However, when turned on her side, the ability to flex the legs is much easier. In supine, the influence of the tonic labyrinthine reflex increases extensor tone. This influence is not present in side lying, making flexion much easier.

Muscle tone and the presence of obligatory movements, or reflexes, are important considerations for individuals with neurological disorders. As described above, the position of the individual affects the movements that are available. Muscle tone is assessed in various functional positions, particularly prone, supine, sitting, and standing. Obligatory movements are assessed to determine how they might affect function. Key reflexes or obligatory movements include the asymmetrical and symmetrical tonic neck reflexes, tonic labyrinthine, extensor thrust, bite, and grasp reflexes. The ability to right the head when moved out of a vertical alignment, either lateral or in the anterior-posterior plane, is another component. Postural control is a related component that refers to the ability to maintain the trunk in a vertical alignment. When completing an assessment to determine function in various positions, it is important to handle the client and to challenge his balance and postural control to determine both the degree of support he will need to work in a given position and the movement available in that position.

Sitting and standing balance are additional considerations. The ability to maintain balance in these positions is determined through observation of the ability to maintain the position independently and the response to challenges to balance in these positions. Sitting balance is described as hands-free, where the individual can maintain her balance and function without using her hands to support herself; hands-dependent, where she needs to support herself with one or both hands to maintain sitting; and propped or dependent sitting, where she cannot sit without external support. Sitting balance is an important component of a seating and mobility assessment (Chapters 4 and 12).

Gross and fine motor assessments generally test higher-level motor skills. Gross motor skills include: balancing on one foot; performing symmetrical and asymmetrical movements of the upper and lower extremities; coordinating one side of the body; lifting and carrying objects; rapidly alternating movements; and running, skipping, and hopping. The Bruininks-Oseretsky Test of Motor Proficiency[5] and the Movement ABC[20] are two examples of comprehensive motor evaluations appropriate for children. The Gross Motor Function Test[40] is designed specifically for children with neurological impairments. Once again, if a neurological condition is present, it is important to remember that function is dependent on the client's position. The Assessment of Motor and Process Skills is a standardized test of motor control in adults.[17]

Fine motor assessment includes: rapidly alternating finger movements, performance of isolated finger movements, manipulation of objects of different sizes, and performance of specific fine motor tasks. Examples of fine motor evaluations include the Erhardt Developmental Prehension Assessment,[16] the Crawford Small Parts Dexterity Test,[10] the Jebsen-Taylor Hand Function Test,[21] and the Minnesota Rate of Manipulation Test.[26]

Motor planning is a higher-order motor function that involves executive planning of complex motor skills. Motor planning is key to the successful use of all assistive technology. Assessment of motor planning involves asking the client to demonstrate how they would use a common device, for example, a pen or a hammer, with and without the actual implement present. A client may also be asked to describe how to use a particular implement or device. The ability to detect and repair errors made during the execution of a motor act is another aspect of motor planning.[46]

Skills Evaluation: Cognitive

Assessment of **cognitive skills** is important when determining whether the client will be able to learn how to use the technology as well as whether they have the capacity to use it effectively in the long term. The main cognitive dimensions to be assessed include orientation, attention, memory, and executive functions. *Orientation* refers to orientation to self, place, and time. In other words, the client is asked who she is, where she is (home, hospital, or specific location in a facility such as the geriatric day hospital), and a temporal question (e.g., day and month). This function is very basic and usually is intact in most people except those experiencing severe dementia.

There are many aspects to *attention*. The simplest component is the ability to attend to a stimulus when it is presented (e.g., looking at a picture when it is presented on a display). Selective attention refers to the ability to focus on a desired stimulus and filter out any extraneous input. For example, selective attention is involved when we pay attention to a communication partner while in a crowded room. Sustained attention refers to the ability to focus on a task for a length of time, which varies depending on the age of the individual (young children have a short attention span) and the presence of an impairment that affects the ability to attend (e.g., developmental delay or traumatic brain injury). Divided or shifting attention refers to the ability to alternate focus on different stimuli. For example, a driver exhibits divided attention while driving his vehicle and conducting a conversation with a passenger at the same time.[46]

Memory involves working memory, which is recall of information immediately after it is received.[46] Long-term memory refers to recall of information that was learned or experienced in the recent or distant past. Memory involves three processes: (1) encoding or input of information, (2) storage of information and (3) retrieval of information.[46] Memory impairment can occur due to interruption of any of these processes.

Finally, *executive functions* refer to higher-order cognitive abilities. They refer to abilities such as judgment, insight (or self-awareness), problem solving, planning and organizational skills, and self-monitoring. Clients who exhibit impairment of executive function may have difficulty planning a task (e.g., figuring out the proper sequence of steps to make a bed); may not recognize functional limitations (a common example involves drivers who are no longer safe because of a cognitive impairment, but who do not recognize that they are no longer safe drivers); and may exhibit impulsive behaviors such as attempting to cross a busy intersection when it is not safe to do so.[46]

Skills Evaluation: Language

The evaluation of **language skills** required for the use of assistive technology devices focuses on both expressive and receptive abilities. In addition, the abilities to sequence items, use symbol systems, combine language elements into complex thoughts, and use codes are important in operating various types of assistive technologies. Whereas the most extensive language evaluation is carried out for augmentative communication system recommendations (see Chapter 11), language skills and use are also important in employing other assistive devices such as cognitive aids (see Chapter 10), mobility systems (see Chapter 12), or systems for manipulation (see Chapter 14). Also, language and hearing are closely coupled, and assistive technologies intended for persons with hearing impairments must address language as well as auditory skills (see Chapter 9).

Specific areas that are evaluated include categorization, sequencing, matching, social communicative skills (e.g., degree of interaction), receptive language skills (e.g., recognition of words or symbols, understanding of simple commands), motor speech skills, and pragmatic language skills. Advanced language capabilities (e.g., syntax and semantics) are also evaluated when possible. The evaluation of these skills for augmentative communication device use is discussed in Chapter 11.

Past Experience with Assistive Technology

The consumer's prior history with technology should also be discussed as part of the assessment process. Useful information can be gathered from the consumer's previous success or failure with using assistive technology. Has he had experience in using technology before and, if so, what technology was used and was the experience successful? If not, why? If a student attempts to turn pages of different books with the use of a mouthstick, which turns out to be unsuccessful, it is important to identify and discuss why the mouthstick did not work out for him. It is important to identify and discuss reasons why the mouthstick did not work out for the individual. Perhaps the mouthstick was cumbersome and uncomfortable to use for any extended period, or perhaps he could physically perform the task with the mouthstick but didn't like the aesthetics of it.

Evaluation of the Context

Evaluation of the context includes consideration of physical, social, cultural, and institutional elements (See Figure 2-4). Where possible, an assessment in the client's home is critical in order to determine how the assistive technology will be used and integrated into the home setting. If an actual home visit is not possible, then a discussion needs to occur during the assessment. While an assessment of the home is critical for mobility devices that might not physically fit into the home, it is equally important to have knowledge of how other devices such as communication aids, computers, and EADL devices will be set up and accessed in the home.

The **physical context** includes consideration of the physical aspects in the settings and transportation between settings. The ATP and team need to identify the settings in which the device will be used. Typically, there will be a primary setting where the device is used most of the time (e.g., home, work, and school) and other settings where it is used less often (e.g., a community setting). Within the primary setting, it is important to determine access into and out of the building, access through the building (including through doorways), travel within a room, the need to go up or down stairs, and access to key features in the home such as the toilet, shower, etc. Attention is given to safety issues in the home such as clutter that might result in a fall.

Physical elements in the setting that affect the use of technology include light, temperature, and noise. Light affects the use of devices that have a display. The brightness of light in a room, from either artificial or natural sources, may make it easier to see a display. However, too much light might cause a glare on a screen. Temperature in a setting is often not extreme enough to affect the performance of a device, although where the device is stored (e.g., garage or shed) might expose the device to temperature extremes. Ambient noise in the setting might affect the ability to use some devices. For example, the reliability of a voice recognition system may be diminished if other conversations or noise are present. Similarly, the user may not be able to hear auditory output if there is too much noise in the background.

Transportation is considered here because it is an important consideration for portable devices and in particular for mobility devices. How a device is to be transported needs to be determined to ensure integration of the device with the transportation method. For example, some configurations of a powered wheelchair will not fit into an adapted van (e.g., wheelchairs for clients who are obese may be too wide to fit into the opening of a side-loading van). Who will be transporting the device is also important if they need to load and unload the device from the vehicle.

The **social context** refers to who is in the setting and the type of interaction they will have with the user. Individuals in the setting may have regular and close contact with the user, such as family members, caregivers, staff in a supported nursing facility or group home, teachers, classmates, and co-workers. Other individuals have less frequent interaction (e.g., an employer, facility administrator, or school principle). However, their actions and attitudes can have a significant effect on the access and use of assistive technology. The social context is particularly import for sensory aids and augmentative communication and cognitive-assistive technologies.

In the social setting, it is important to consider who is available to assist the user, as needed, and the skills and abilities of these particular individuals. For example, an older adult who has had a stroke and relies on others to assist with mobility or cognitive activities may have a caregiver who is also an older adult, typically a spouse. The caregiver is also likely to have some form of age-related functional change that poses a challenge to providing assistance. An older spouse may not be physically capable of assisting with the use of a mobility device or may not have the knowledge to assist with the use of a device that supports cognitive skills.

Beukelman and Mirenda (2005)[4] discuss the need to identify actual or potential "opportunity barriers" and "access barriers" for the consumer. Although their model specifically targets consumers with augmentative communication needs, it also holds true for other area of assistive technology. *Opportunity barriers* are imposed by individuals or situations that are not under the consumer's control. Generally, the provision of assistive technology does not result in the elimination of these barriers. Beukelman and Mirenda[4] identify five types of opportunity barriers: policy barriers, practice barriers, attitude barriers, knowledge barriers, and skill barriers. Policies and practice barriers are described under the institutional context later in this chapter. In the social context, attitude, knowledge, and skill barriers apply to those individuals with whom the consumer interacts and on whom the effective use of the device depends. If the consumer's job supervisor has a negative attitude regarding the use of automatic speech recognition because it is distracting to other workers, it is an attitude barrier that prevents the consumer's participation in that job. Alternatively, the supervisor may have insufficient knowledge or skill regarding a device characteristic such as automatic speech recognition to ensure that it is effectively installed and made available to the consumer.

Access barriers are barriers related to the abilities, attitudes, and resource limitations of the consumer or her support system.[4] Known constraints related to user and family preferences and the attitudes of communication partners are other access barriers that should be identified. A potential barrier to accessing technology—one commonly seen during augmentative communication assessments—is resistance on the part of parents to pursuing an augmentative communication device because they are worried that the use of such a device will inhibit the child's development of natural speech, a concern that is not supported by current research. As we discuss later in this chapter, the ability to find funding for assistive technology systems and services may also pose a barrier.

Cultural context refers to the client's cultural background and its implications for acceptance and use of technology. In particular, the assessment should consider the cultural perspective of disability and how this influences the family's view of the individual. For example, the family may believe that a person with a disability should not be expected to be independent and so might reject technology in favor of providing assistance from another person for daily activities. A culture that values independence highly may similarly reject technology, viewing its use as a sign of weakness or laziness.

Cultural views of acceptance of outside help will also influence whether support will be sought for an assistive technology evaluation. The role of the user of the assistive technology in the home may also affect whether it is accepted or used. The ATP and team need to be sensitive to how the provision and use of assistive technology affects the perception of the user relative to their position in the family.

The components of the **institutional context** are similar to policy barriers defined by Beukelman and Mirenda (2005)[4] as the legislative, regulative, or agency policies that govern situations in which consumers find themselves. For example, there are regulations in some school districts that restrict the use of school-purchased assistive technology to use only in the school, preventing it from being taken home. Practice barriers refer to routine activities that are not dictated by policy but that constrain the use of assistive technologies. If the school's policy doesn't *require* that the device stay in the school, but the local teacher or principal has the practice of keeping the devices in the school, the result is the same as if it were a policy. Legislative barriers refer to laws that govern access to assistive technology (e.g., who is eligible to receive the technology, what technology is provided, who pays for the technology, where it can be used, and another aspects of the use of the technology) as well laws that govern access to services and physical structures.

Matching Device Characteristics to the User's Needs and Skills

The assessment process we have described to this point provides the basis by which the ATP and the rest of the assistive technology service delivery team carefully define the goals to be accomplished and determine the skills the consumer has available for assistive technology system use. It is necessary to systematically transform these goals and skills into characteristics of assistive technology devices. We use the term **device characteristics** to refer to general properties of the technology. A *feature* is a particular implementation of a characteristic. Characteristics of automobiles include, for example, engine, color, size, performance (acceleration, gas mileage), and doors. Features for these same characteristics might include a four-cylinder engine, blue color, compact size, 35 miles per gallon, and two doors. As consumers, we have certain needs, and we match those needs to general characteristics to select specific features of interest to us. We also have skills that apply to our selection. For example, we may not be able to use a standard manual transmission and therefore choose only automatic transmission cars for consideration. Life roles also play a part in our selection decision. For instance, parents with small children may choose a minivan rather than a compact car.

In assistive technology service delivery, we can use a similar matching process to choose features that match the consumer's needs and skills. In some areas of assistive technology applications (e.g., augmentative communication)

BOX 3-3 Assistive Device Characteristics

HUMAN/TECHNOLOGY INTERFACE
Physical properties
User feedback
Number of inputs
Selection methods
Selection set

PROCESSOR
Commands
Control parameters
Data or information processing

ACTIVITY OUTPUT
Magnitude
Precision
Flexibility

ENVIRONMENTAL SENSOR
Range
Threshold

PHYSICAL CONSTRUCTION
Mountability
Portability
Packaging

this process is referred to as *feature matching*. This systematic approach is superior to using trial and error with all the possible devices that *may* work and then trying to pick one. To use this approach, however, we must first define a set of characteristics to be considered. A generic set of assistive technology device characteristics is listed in Box 3-3. The categories in this box parallel those used in Figure 2-5 to describe the components of the assistive technology portion of the HAAT model. In the following chapters we consider more specific characteristics for certain areas of assistive technologies: seating systems, control interfaces, computer adaptations, augmentative communication systems, mobility devices, manipulation devices, and sensory aids.

The Human/Technology Interface

The human/technology interface is the portion of the device with which the consumer directly interacts. Examples of an interface include a keyboard, joystick, control unit for an EADL, access switch, and seating system. The most general human/technology characteristics, applying to all devices, are the **physical properties**. These include the size and weight of the interface, its texture, hardness, size and brightness of the display, loudness of any auditory feedback, and the force required to use the interface. The human/technology interface provides **feedback** to the user. Feedback can be visual, auditory, or tactile. In some cases, the feedback is a direct consequence of the interface. For example, the comfort of a seat cushion is a type of feedback that is only determined over time as the client uses the seat. In other cases user feedback is intentionally built into the device to provide specific information to the user, such as a flashing light indicator on a television control or a tactile display on a reading device for a person with total visual impairment. Feedback is described in terms of the characteristics of magnitude, type, and origin. For example, the *magnitude* of a visual display is the brightness of the light. The *types* of human/technology interface feedback are other characteristics and include visual, auditory, and tactile varieties. The *origin* refers to the source of the feedback, such as that provided by a seat cushion or the voice output provided from the screen reader.

The next three characteristics listed in Box 3-3 apply to human/technology interfaces used with electronic assistive devices (including power mobility). The *number of inputs* required to operate any device is a characteristic. The most appropriate control interface for any given consumer is largely determined by the physical and interface assessments that are described here and in Chapter 6.

Depending on the size of the input domain related to the consumer's needs and skills, a *selection method* can be chosen. In Chapter 7 we describe two basic selection methods: direct and indirect. In direct selection, all the choices are presented to the user at one time and the user has the physical ability to choose any one element directly. With indirect selection, there are intermediate steps required for the user to make a selection. Direct selection requires greater physical skill than indirect selection; however, indirect selection requires greater cognitive, visual, perceptual, and possibly auditory abilities. Selections are made from a *selection set* consisting of the choices available to the consumer. Features of this set include size, number of choices, format (e.g., print, tactile), and type of symbol (real objects, pictures, computer icons, line drawings, traditional orthography, or symbols used to represent an idea). The type of symbol system that is most appropriate to a given individual is determined during the language assessment.

The Processor

Recall that the processor is the element of the assistive technology device that relates the human/technology interface to the other components. Sometimes this is simply a mechanical linkage (e.g., in a reacher), and in such cases there are not many choices in characteristics. However, processors for electronic devices have several characteristics. The first of these is the basic set of *commands* that are necessary to operate the device. For example, in a powered wheelchair system the basic commands are forward, backward, left, and right. In a communication device, some basic commands include printing a document and speaking. In an EADL the commands may include lights on and off, TV channel selection, and telephone dialing. These are essential for operation. The greater the number of commands, the more flexible the system is to the user. However, the more commands included, the more confusing the system can become. The consumer, family, care providers, and ATP need to evaluate the effect of a specific command set size during the assessment.

A second characteristic of the processor is the *control parameters*. In contrast to commands, control parameters allow adjustments to be made to the system; they are nice to have but not always essential. Control parameters include such things as variable speeds for forward and reverse, or indoor and outdoor speed levels in a powered wheelchair. In an augmentative communication device, control parameters adjust the voice synthesizer pitch, voice type, and rate to affect the way the speech output sounds. A control parameter also provides the ability to switch between different applications for multiple activity outputs. For example, it is possible to operate an EADL, communication device, and computer-access system from a powered-wheelchair controller. Individual control parameters need to be presented to the consumer for the systems being considered, and both the consumer and the ATP need to evaluate their effectiveness.

The final general processor characteristic is *data or information processing*. In this case the device is internally processing information rather than dealing with commands or control signals. One example, used in augmentative communication systems and screen readers for the blind, is the generation of spoken output from text using software programs. Another example of information processing is word prediction, in which the software program guesses at the desired word based on the entries the consumer makes. This type of application can also adapt to the user by learning her most frequently used words.

Information processing is also used in sensory systems to convert the input from the environmental sensor to a form that can be presented to the user. For example, a hearing aid uses a microphone to detect voices, amplifies them (data processing), and presents the amplified signal to the ear (see Chapter 9). Different hearing aids have different data processing, and this characteristic can be evaluated by the consumer.

Activity Output

The **activity output** is what the system accomplishes for the consumer (e.g., communication, mobility, or manipulation). The first characteristic that describes the activity output is its *magnitude*. This includes the volume for a speech synthesis system, the force or torque generated by a powered wheelchair, and the brightness of a video screen display. *Precision* is a measure of how accurately the system performs the functions and how exactly it accomplishes its task. For example, a reacher may be able to pick up a cup but not a button. If the consumer needs to pick up the button, then this particular reacher has insufficient precision to accomplish the task. If an output can be used in different contexts or can be used to accomplish different goals for the consumer, we would say that it is *flexible*. Flexibility can be an important factor when the consumer has many tasks that he wishes to perform.

The Environmental Interface

The **environmental interface** is that portion of the assistive technology system that is used to take in information from the external world for use in a sensory substitution system. For example, when the person has a visual limitation, we use a camera, and when a person has an auditory impairment, we use a microphone. Characteristics that apply to this element include the *range* of the input signal (i.e., how big or small the signal can be and still be detected). The smallest signal that can be discerned from background noise is the *threshold*. As an example of how these characteristics can be applied, consider the two problems of reading and mobility for persons with severe visual impairments. For reading, the device needs very little range because only one letter or line of text needs to be viewed at a time. However, for mobility the environmental sensor needs to take in a variety of sizes (e.g., from a dish to a tree). For reading, the threshold is low (a letter in fine print), but for mobility the threshold can be much higher.

Physical Construction

The final category of characteristics is **physical construction**. This category refers to the properties of the device that allow it to be mounted or positioned so that the client has reliable access to it, the portability of the device, its size and weight, and its aesthetics (appearance and color). No matter how well a system works in an assessment session, it will not be effective in everyday use unless the person has access to it at all times. This is determined primarily by the *mountability* of the system. The device might be mounted to a piece of furniture, such as a desk, or to another assistive device, as in the case of mounting a communication system on a powered wheelchair. In the latter case, consideration must be given to the compatibility of the two devices. The ability to remove the device when finished with its use is another mountability consideration. *Portability* is a measure of the degree to which the device can be moved from place to place. This characteristic includes a consideration of its size, weight, and power source. For electronic devices, portability often requires that the device be battery operated and that it be small and lightweight enough to be carried or attached to a wheelchair. If the person is ambulatory, her ability to carry the device needs to be assessed. Battery size, weight, and charge duration influence portability. A device with a large, heavy battery is less likely to be moved from one setting to another. Similarly, a device is likely to be left at home if the duration of charge is short, resulting in concern that the device will become inoperable. Portability for mobility devices involves consideration of how they will be transported and who is responsible for lifting them in and out of a vehicle. A final consideration involves the **aesthetics** of the device, including aspects like colour, size, and style that make the device look more like a mainstream device rather than looks institutional. This characteristic is often overlooked in the design of the system, yet it carries a significant meaning to the user.[33] The look of the device may convey an unintended meaning of vulnerability, frailty, or stigma. A device that is aesthetically appealing is more likely to be used than one that is not.

Evaluating the Match between Characteristics and the Consumer's Skills and Needs

At this point in the evaluation process, information has been gathered about the activities, the human (the client), the context, and the elements of the technology. These are the components that drive the decision rather than a specific device. The team can now identify different technologies and determine the match between the consumer's skills and needs and the characteristics of the device. There are two primary ways in which the team can evaluate specific technologies for use by the consumer: (1) trial using the actual device and (2) simulation of device characteristics.

Ideally the consumer will have the opportunity to try the devices being considered and evaluate their usefulness before a recommendation is made. However, because of the expense, lack of availability of trial equipment, and institutional or funding policies, this option is not always available. It is beneficial for the team to have available a set of devices that represents a broad range of characteristics. The service delivery program typically has a range of devices that can be used for assessment purposes or a manufacturer's representative may provide equipment to trial. Other manufacturers and service delivery programs might lease devices for this purpose. If these devices are available, it is helpful to demonstrate the various features to the consumer and have the consumer try them. There may be two or three devices being considered, and, if possible, each device should be tried and evaluated by the consumer. The trial period should be sufficiently long to give the consumer the opportunity to use the device in a variety of situations and for different purposes. For example, a communication device should be trialed with different communication partners and in different settings. Similarly, a wheelchair should be used in different settings to determine access. A number of device use aspects should be considered during the trial including: (1) how easy the device is to use and learn to use, (2) the ability of the consumer and family to transport the device as necessary, (3) relevant positioning aspects, (4) comfort when using the device, and (5) a preliminary determination of whether the device is assisting the consumer to meet his goals.

In lieu of having the actual device available, the ATP can simulate device characteristics. Simulation requires that the team members be knowledgeable about the characteristics and features available for specific assistive technologies. For computer-based products, the assistive technology adaptations are often software based, and demonstration disks can be obtained from manufacturers or downloaded from a manufacturer's Web site. These demonstration programs illustrate the essential features of the software, but they are not fully functional and their use is time-limited. To position a control interface for simulation during assessment, universal mounting systems can be used that can be adjusted and placed in various positions. This step is important to ensure that the control interface is in a functional position for the consumer and remains stable during the assessment.

Decision Making

The team is now at the point where the assessment is complete and the client has had some opportunity to trial the equipment (or at a minimum has had some hands-on experience with it). A recommendation for a specific technology is made at this stage. The most important principle in this process is the relationship between the tasks that the client will use the assistive technology device to accomplish, the skills and abilities of the client, and the characteristics that must be contained in the device for those tasks to be accomplished. Each goal may be accomplished only if a set of essential characteristics is included in the assistive technology system. For example, the goal may be mobility, and the characteristics of the type of cushion, wheelchair type, and wheelchair color all contribute to the accomplishment of this goal.

It is important to recognize that the features that are most limiting must be considered first, followed by those that are less restrictive. For example, in an augmentative communication system, the type of symbol system is often the most limiting characteristic. If a consumer requires pictures as a symbol, many devices are eliminated immediately. In contrast, spoken output as a characteristic is not as limiting, since most devices use similar speech output. For each type of assistive technology, it is important for the team to identify a set of general characteristics (or features) that fit within the categories of Box 3-3. The major advantage of the assessment methods described here is that they are based on a consideration of the goals and skills first, and a consideration of assistive technology system characteristics second. Thus the system is matched to the consumer (within the limits of current technology), rather than the consumer being forced to adapt to the system. Without a structured approach like the one presented here, however, it is very difficult to meet consumer's goals.

The decision making process is also guided by the **clinical reasoning** of the professionals involved. Four types of clinical reasoning have been identified in the literature: procedural, interactive, conditional, and narrative.[13,29,30] Procedural reasoning considers the influence of the condition that resulted in the need for assistive technology. For example, using procedural reasoning, the professional understands the influence of cerebral palsy on the ability to sit, move, speak, and manipulate objects. Interactive reasoning engages the actual client. This type of reasoning builds on the procedural reasoning by understanding the individual client with cerebral palsy and his specific situation and needs. Conditional reasoning engages the collective clinical experience of the professional (or the team). This type of reasoning draws on past experience to guide the decision making in the moment. For example, if a particular type of communication device has been beneficial for clients with a similar level of function and needs in the past, then conditional reasoning leads the clinician to consider this type of device in the present situation.

Finally, narrative reasoning is the ongoing relationship of the consumer and the team and their joint understanding of the goals of the client. Collectively, these forms of clinical reasoning support the decision-making process.

Recommendations and Report

The recommendations summarize the information gathered during the evaluation and suggest a design for the assistive technology system. At the conclusion of the assessment, everyone involved should sit down to review it and come to a consensus regarding the final recommendation. A written report is prepared that details the assessment and recommendations for an assistive technology system. The written report synthesizes the assessment process and starts out by defining the needs and goals that have been addressed. A summary of the consumer's skills applicable to device use is provided, with a description of the generic characteristics to be incorporated into a device. This is followed by specific recommendations for equipment, including descriptions, part numbers (if applicable), manufacturer's name, any modifications that need to be made, and cost. Recommendations for soft technologies are also included in the written report. These may include recommendations for developing skills that are necessary before purchase of a device, training once the device has been purchased, and strategies for incorporating the technology into the individual's context. Finally, a plan for implementation of the recommendations is provided. This includes logistics such as seeking funding from the appropriate sources and designating who will take responsibility for implementing the recommendations.

Often the written report is aimed at various individuals, thus presenting a unique challenge for the professionals writing it. The report, first of all, needs to be geared toward the consumer, who may not be familiar with medical or technical jargon. Rehabilitation or educational professionals who will be working with the consumer may also be receiving the report and its recommendations. These professionals typically need information on what the consumer's skills have been in using the technology and what skill areas they may need to address to facilitate the use of the device. Some of these professionals may be very knowledgeable in assistive technology, but for others this may be their first experience with it. The contact person for the funding source will also be reading the report, and his or her interest is typically in the "bottom line," or what it is going to cost. This person wants evidence that the system recommended is going to meet the consumer's needs at the lowest possible cost. In the section on funding in this chapter, we describe how to write a report to a third-party payer in order to justify the purchase of an assistive technology system.

IMPLEMENTATION

Once the recommendations have been made and funding is obtained, the implementation phase begins. This aspect of the delivery process consists of ordering specified equipment, obtaining commercially available equipment or fabricating custom equipment, making needed modifications, assembling or setting up equipment, thoroughly checking it as a system, fitting the device to the consumer, and training the consumer and care givers in its use.

Ordering and Setup

Many recommended interventions have components from several manufacturers, and these must be integrated into a total system. Some of these may be standard commercially available components and others may be commercial assistive technologies. These devices are ordered from the manufacturer or equipment supplier and may take a significant amount of time to be received after ordering. The recommendation may have also included a custom device or devices that require an adaptation. Examples of custom modifications include mounting a switch to a wheelchair or table, making a cable for connecting two devices together (e.g., a communication device and an EADL), programming a device for unique vocabulary, setting up a wheelchair to provide the appropriate degree of stability and mobility, and adapting a battery-powered toy so it can be controlled with one switch. The design and fabrication of these system components can occur during the waiting time for the delivery of the commercially available technologies. Once all the individual devices and adaptations are available, it is necessary to assemble them into a total package. For example, a wheelchair obtained from one source and a seating system from another will need to be interfaced to each other. The complexity of this assembly process varies widely, and some systems require much more effort than others.

Delivery and Fitting

Once the equipment is obtained, modified, or adapted as necessary and integrated into a system, the system is ready to be delivered to the consumer. This may occur in a clinic setting, in a school or at a job site, or in the consumer's living setting. The choice of locations depends on the nature of the equipment, the ease of transport of the consumer, and the complexity of the system (i.e., what support services of technicians and tools are required). We refer to all system deliveries as a "fitting" because we are interfacing the human (consumer) with the rest of the system. In some cases, such as custom seating systems, the process resembles a fitting for an orthotic or prosthetic device. In other cases the fitting focuses on installation of the system, mounting the control interface and the device to a wheelchair, and interconnection of the various components. The fitting phase may also include some amount of assessment as adjustments are made to optimize the consumer's ability to utilize the system. An example of this is the use of head switches to control a powered wheelchair. The head switches must be attached to the wheelchair and wired into the controller unit. This is done before the fitting; and during the fitting, the location of the head switches (e.g., how close they are to the consumer's head) is adjusted to maximize performance.

As much as possible, the fitting should be accomplished by a clinician and a technician who can make adjustments. When a significant amount of time has elapsed between ordering and receiving the equipment, changes may have occurred in the client's function or body size. The fitting session must, therefore, assess whether the recommendations made at the time the device was ordered still work. If not, adjustments are made at the fitting session.

The complexity of many assistive technology systems may require more than one session to obtain all the proper adjustments, mountings, and fittings. Often it is the rehabilitation assistant (OTA, PTA, SLPA) who first identifies the need for adjustments and initiates the process with the vendor or other personnel. The ATP must be prepared to continue making adjustments and adaptations in the system until the consumer's goals and needs are met. This phase of the delivery process often involves some reassessment, but its success is directly related to the quality of the initial assessment and recommendations, and difficulties experienced at this time can often be traced to incomplete or inaccurate assessments.

Facilitating Assistive Technology System Performance

A major concern of everyone involved in the delivery of assistive technology services is whether the recommended device is going to meet the stated goals. It *cannot* be assumed that intervention ends with the delivery of the device. Most users of technology, even those with previous technology experience, require assistance in facilitating their performance with the device. The ATP is responsible for developing the plan for facilitating the client's performance. It is commonly the rehabilitation assistant who implements that plan. The degree of independence the rehabilitation assistant has in the implementation process depends on the practice of the clinical setting, the experience of the assistant, and any professional regulatory issues. This section discusses three general strategies that the rehabilitation assistant can use to facilitate development of skills in the use of the assistive technology: training, performance aids, and written instructions.[2] Training engages the client as well as her family and caregivers. Performance aids are those soft technologies that aid in the use of a device, including things such as stored phone numbers in a telephone controller. Written instructions can be provided in multiple formats, and we will present some considerations in the development of these instructions.

Training

Training in the use of an assistive technology has been identified as one of the most crucial factors that predicts continued use and acceptance of the device. It is also the component of the service delivery process in which the rehabilitation assistant commonly has the greatest role. Yet, training is often the element that is either missing or inadequate due to funding issues that drive practice. Clients who receive a device while they are in a clinical setting are more likely to receive training than those who receive the device once they've returned to the community. What we discuss here is considered to be an ideal situation.

Training typically occurs in a face-to-face situation, either individually or in a group. A client who is new to the use of the device is most likely to receive individual training. Clients with some experience with device use are more likely to benefit from group sessions because they are already familiar with the basic functions of the device. Wheelchair "camps" that teach specific wheelchair skills or drama programs that involve children who use communication devices are two examples of group training methods.

We will describe six strategies that can be implemented in training: (1) familiarize the client with the basic functions of the device, (2) start simple and build to complex, (3) build in success, (4) start with an activity that is of primary importance to the client, (5) involve the client (and caregivers) in establishing goals and plans at all stages, and (6) build in informal evaluation throughout the process (Box 3-4). These strategies were derived from a review of suggested training strategies for assistive technology.[24,28]

Familiarizing the client with the features of the device and how they work is an important first step. As suggested in Chapter 1, we often learn skills by observing others. Assistive technology use is not a common activity, so a client receiving a device for the first time does not have prior knowledge of its use from observing others. For example, scanning as a selection method is not a common means of controlling commercial devices. A client first using scanning needs to learn about the scanning pattern, control of the speed, and how to make a selection. Similarly, a client first receiving a manual wheelchair needs to know how to apply the brakes, propel

BOX 3-4 Tip Box: Training Strategies for the Implementation of Assistive Technology

1. Familiarize the client with the basic functions of the device.
   a. Identify the different controls for the device.
   b. Show the client what the device does.
2. Start simple and build to complex
   a. Don't assume that the client has prior knowledge with this type of device; start with a task that involves minimal control steps.
   b. Add complexity and the need for problem solving as the client gains skills with the device.
   c. The rehabilitation assistant is responsible for safety in the clinical environment.
3. Build in success—know the client's skill level and work at or just above that level. Provide a level of challenge that maintains motivation but doesn't result in frustration.
4. Start with an activity that is of primary importance to the client.
5. Involve the client and caregivers in establishing goals and plans at all stages.
6. Build in informal evaluation throughout the process.

the wheels to go in a straight line or make a turn, or how to remove the foot and armrests in order to complete a transfer. Knowing how the device works is a first step toward successful use. This aspect of the training has been called **operational competence**.[35]

The rehabilitation assistant's clinical reasoning guides the determination of a simple activity that can be used to initiate training and ensure success.[13] For example, use of a single switch that turns a toy or TV on when pressed once, and off when pressed a second time, teaches the client the basic function of the switch. Providing an environment that is free of obstacles so that a client can freely propel a wheelchair allows him to safely move the chair without the need for accuracy. Interactive and conditional reasoning are employed by the rehabilitation assistant to assist with the identification of activities in the implementation of a training program that pose the right degree of challenge to the client and enable his success in the use of the device. Training that facilitates the client's use of the AT in increasingly complex situations and that incorporates his problem solving in unfamiliar situations is termed **strategic competence**.[35]

As with all of the other steps in the service delivery process, training involves understanding the goals of the client and including them in the planning and decision making of the process. Working with the client on her goals ensures that training is a collaborative process and engages the client. For example, a client who has a spinal cord injury that has resulted in limited physical function will be more engaged in learning to use an electronic aid to daily living if it allows her to control a music device if listening to music is important to her. Similarly, a client who enjoys being outside and walking with her spouse will engage in wheelchair skills training if the training involves activities that enable her to resume this activity with her spouse.

Informal evaluation of the client's performance needs to occur throughout the process. Initial work in uncovering clinical reasoning in rehabilitation revealed tacit (or subconscious) reasoning that occurred during intervention as the clinician was constantly adjusting the activity in response to the client's performance or feedback. These adjustments might include knowing when to provide assistance versus stepping back when the client is successfully using the device, making necessary positioning adjustments or adjustments to device controls, or modifying or changing the activity to accommodate the needs of the clients. Often these adjustments happen without conscious thought during the session. It is during the record keeping or charting that occurs following the session that these adjustments, the rationale for them, and their outcome often come to the forefront. It is important to reflect on the session and record the information in order to document progress and guide the next steps.

Performance Aids

A document or device containing information that an individual uses to assist in the completion of an activity is called a **performance aid**. By decreasing the amount of information to be remembered, the performance aid reduces the amount of cognitive processing required to complete an activity. With a performance aid, the user does not have to rely as much on long-term memory, which results in reduced errors, increased speed for certain tasks, and a reduction in the amount of training required. Performance aids do not necessarily have to be written; picture symbols can also be effective for individuals who cannot read. Bailey (1996)[2] describes five quality standards for performance aids: (1) accessibility, (2) accuracy, (3) clarity, (4) completeness and conciseness, and (5) legibility.

Performance aids are commonly used with individuals who have memory deficits as a result of damage to the brain. One type of performance aid is simple step-by-step instructions that assist the user in carrying out a sequence of tasks. For example, Tim is a young man who has sustained a head injury. He uses a computer to complete school assignments but has problems remembering the sequence of steps to get into his computer's word-processing program. The steps to complete this task have been simply written and are posted next to his computer. Because Tim also has visual acuity problems, the instructions are printed in large, bold letters. For Tim, this simple performance aid has meant the difference between success and failure in using his computer.

Another type of performance aid assists in remembering several items of information. An example of this type of aid is a printed list of codes with their meanings, which an individual may have stored in her augmentative communication system. Often such a list is attached to the side of the device so the user can easily view it as needed. Sometimes codes and their meanings are built into software programs and presented on the screen each time the user selects a letter.

Instructions

Instructions should be considered an integral part of the system and should be available to the user at the time of the system delivery. These are available in many different formats, including print and digital media. Instructions are helpful when step-by-step directions with detailed information are required or when graphic information needs to be presented. The rehabilitation assistant must not assume that the instructions provided by the manufacturer are going to be adequate. Instructions provided by the manufacturer of the system may include too little or too much information; they may assume a basic knowledge level or they may be difficult to follow by the user. It is recommended that instructions from the manufacturer be reviewed and supplemented as needed. When the manufacturer's documentation is overwhelming, the rehabilitation assistant can review the documentation and condense it into a quick reference sheet that provides simplified and frequently used information.

The rehabilitation assistant should consider a few factors when developing performance aids or supplementing the manufacturer's instructions. Consideration should be given as to the most useful format for the client. As the case of Tim illustrated, a large-print written system might be most appropriate. Some clients may not be comfortable reading instructions from a computer or tablet screen, necessitating the translation of instructions in electronic format to print format. Other clients may need oral rather than visual instructions. In some cases, multiple sets of instructions are necessary to meet the needs of the client, the family, and other caregivers.

The accessibility and usability of instructions should be considered. Information that is presented via print material should be analyzed for reading level and clarity of instructions. Font size and color contrast are important for clients and caregivers who have vision limitations. In this instance, simpler is better—black letters on white background, or reverse, are the easiest to read. Consideration should be given to alternate delivery modes when the user has a visual impairment that limits their ability to read. Usability of the instructions should be checked with the client and other users to determine whether they understand the instructions that have been written.

FOLLOW-UP AND FOLLOW-ALONG

Once the system has been implemented, it is tempting to think that the intervention has been completed. This perception, however, is totally false; the delivery of the system marks the beginning of the time of use, and it therefore signals the beginning of the evaluation of system effectiveness. We use the term **follow-up** to refer to activities that occur during the period immediately following delivery of an assistive technology system and that address the effectiveness of the device, training, and user strategies. The term **follow-along** is used to describe those activities that take place over a longer period. This phase addresses factors such as changes in needs or goals, availability of new devices, and other concerns.

We include a formal follow-up phase in our delivery process for several reasons: (1) assistive devices can seldom be used right out of the box without ever needing to be adjusted; (2) electronic devices are not 100% reliable, and a significant portion of them require repair during the first year of use; (3) training programs seldom proceed flawlessly, and questions arise during the initial period of use; and (4) perceived device failures are often the result of operator error caused by a lack of device understanding. A carefully developed follow-up program will identify these problems easily and address them quickly.

Repair and maintenance are often conducted during the follow-up phase. *Repair* refers to action taken to correct a problem in a system. *Maintenance*, on the other hand, is a systematic set of procedures that is aimed at keeping the device in working order. Examples of maintenance functions are proper battery charging, cleaning, tightening mounting hardware, and lubrication of moving mechanical parts. A regular schedule will ensure that necessary maintenance takes place. Assistive technology system failures result in a major disruption of the consumer's life. For example, a consumer depends on his powered wheelchair for mobility. If it fails, he may have a manual wheelchair as a backup, but his independence is significantly reduced. Repair of assistive technologies is most often carried out either through manufacturer's representatives or directly through the manufacturer. In the latter case the device must be returned to the factory for repair, and the consumer may be without it for several days or even longer. Prompt attention to repair needs of consumers is an important part of follow-up.

As part of a formal follow-up program, contacts with the consumer (via telephone, email, on the job site, in the home, or in the clinic) are desirable on a regular basis, such as at 1, 3, 6, and 12 months after delivery. These contacts occur whether there is a perceived problem or not, and they are in addition to other activities such as training or repair. This regularly scheduled contact is important because there may be unnoticed problems, or more often there are underutilized features that are discovered during the follow-up sessions. As we have defined it, follow-along has a much longer time frame than follow-up. Whereas follow-up typically covers the first year of operation of an assistive technology system, follow-along is carried out over the individual's lifetime. Consumers may return for service after a period of years for several reasons. They may have found that the device is not working as they would like and is not meeting their functional goals. Another reason is to obtain information about advances in technology since they obtained their device. In other cases the consumer may have changed in significant ways. This change is often seen in children who have grown significantly and need a revision in their seating system. Change can also be the result of a degenerative condition such as amyotrophic lateral sclerosis, and in these cases the device may need to be altered to accommodate decreased physical function. In other cases the change in consumer condition is a result of the development of new skills that make it possible to consider new device features. For example, a consumer who has suffered a traumatic brain injury (TBI) may initially receive a communication device that is based on very simple replay of sentences. As she recovers, her ability to spell effectively may improve and a device with this capability should be considered.

There are other reasons for follow-along. One of the most important of these is a change in the life roles and context of the consumer. For example, Martin, who has severe cerebral palsy and has used an augmentative and alternative communication (AAC) device for several years, decides to move into an apartment on his own. The success of this transition could depend heavily on the availability of assistive technologies. An EADL would allow him to control lights and appliances; answer and dial the telephone; and control the television, DVD player, and other entertainment devices. This reevaluation is dictated not by changes in his condition, but by changes in his life roles and the context in which he will be using his technology.

The Effects of Errors in Assistive Technology Systems

Identification of errors and determination of their source is another component of the process of evaluating the match between the device characteristics and those of the consumer. There are two types of errors that are of concern in assistive technology systems. *Random errors* are infrequent and are generally chance occurrences. An example of a random error is the inability to understand a voice synthesizer because of high amounts of ambient noise. If the noise is not present, there is no error, and even if there is noise it may not lead to an error in interpretation. It is only the random co-occurrence of the need to use the voice synthesizer, the presence of noise, and a listener who doesn't understand the output that creates the error. Random errors may reoccur, but they are not consistently present in the system. We can do very little to avoid this type of error in the assistive technology system design process.

Of greater concern are *periodic*, or regular, *errors*, which occur under predictable conditions. These errors may also be infrequent, but they are foreseeable. As an example, many letter-to-speech software programs make mistakes in pronunciation when used with voice synthesizers. The mispronunciation always occurs whenever the particular word is entered. This type of error can be dealt with in the design process. For our example of mispronunciation, exception tables are typically used so that the utterance sounds correct even though the letter-to-speech rule makes an error. There are several effects of errors on assistive technology system performance, including loss of information, injury, and embarrassment. All three of these can occur in the same system, and they may be due to the human, the activity, the context, the assistive technology, or the interaction of some or all of these components. For example, a power wheelchair will not function if the user does not regularly charge the batteries. The user must somehow cause the action that results in the batteries maintaining a charge and the power wheelchair system must provide accurate information about the degree to which the batteries are charged. Error-free function here relies on the successful integration of the human with the technology.

Loss of information is a common effect associated with augmentative communication systems (see Chapter 11) and sensory aids (see Chapters 8 and 9). Loss of information refers to an interruption in the output of the system, whether the interruption is visual or auditory, as in a voice output communication aid, or physical, as in the power to propel an electrically powered wheelchair. It can occur because the human operator makes an error in motor, sensory, or cognitive performance, or as a result of a device error. Although the net effect on system performance of either of these errors (human or device) may be the same, it is important to distinguish between them to correct the problem.

When the human operator makes the errors, the distinction needs to be made as to whether the cause is lack of capacity (e.g., inability to control excessive tremor resulting in erroneous selections, or visual limitations in reading a display) or lack of skill (inadequate experience or practice in using the device). If the problem is the capacity of the user, then modifications must be made in the system (e.g., using a keyguard to prevent erroneous entries or an enlarged display screen to improve visibility). If the problem is one of skill, training may help reduce the number of errors.

Physical injury is a more serious effect of a system error. This type of error can occur in a mobility system (see Chapter 12) if, for example, a braking system fails or a motor fails to turn off. Consideration of this type of error leads us to the concept of "failsafe" design. This approach attempts to anticipate the types of errors and to ensure that if they do occur the probability of injury is minimized. For example, if a powered wheelchair controller fails, it should fail in the "off" state. If it fails in the full "on" state, the user may be injured because the chair cannot be controlled. Similar to loss of information, the capacity or the skill of the user can cause physical injury. Another example is the failure of a mobility aid for a person who is blind. If the device fails to identify an obstacle or a hazard such as a drop off, the individual could suffer a serious injury.

A final general effect of assistive technology system errors is embarrassment. This effect is somewhat unique to assistive technologies, and it is a direct result of the role that assistive technology systems play in the daily life of the user who has a disability. Because the tasks being performed cannot be accomplished without the system, its use is continual throughout the day. Over a long period, system errors leading to embarrassment are inevitable. The embarrassment may be relatively minor, such as a manipulation system dropping a spoonful of food. In other contexts, it may be much more significant. For example, an augmentative communication device may fail and produce the wrong utterance. If the context is a presentation in an important meeting and the mistaken utterance is an obscenity, the consequences are potentially very negative. To place the importance of this type of error in perspective, recall that the device is often perceived by both the user and other people as being a part of the user. Thus the user is held responsible for an inappropriate utterance just as if she had used her own voice to produce it.

The errors and their resulting effects may arise from any of the components of the assistive technology system or their interaction. The human error may be related to capacity or skill. The device may malfunction, in which case the error is related to the design. The context may cause an error. For example, the pressure relief properties of a wheelchair cushion may be impaired if the cushion is exposed to extremely cold environments for a prolonged time and the cushion materials freeze. An example of an error that is caused by the interaction of the components of the HAAT model relates to devices that have many functions and require complex commands for successful activation. In part, the error is caused by the capacity of the user to learn how to operate the device. It is also caused by the design of the device that requires complex actions for successful operation. Some of the concepts related to human factors that were discussed in Chapter 2 are relevant here.

It is clear from this discussion that identification and reduction of errors can occur at several points in the assistive technology process. Initially, incorporating a design and accompanying soft technologies that are congruent with universal design principles can minimize errors. Errors can be identified and possibly corrected through use of a thorough evaluation that leads to a suitable device recommendation, coupled with a trial period. Finally, errors in the assistive technology system are identified and reduced through follow-up with individual users and post-marketing research into the effectiveness of the system.

EVALUATING THE EFFECTIVENESS OF ASSISTIVE TECHNOLOGY SERVICES AND SYSTEMS

Evaluation of the effectiveness of assistive technology services and systems is important for many reasons. First and foremost, it provides the team with an indication of the benefits of the assistive technology service to the individual client and her family. It can provide the client with a measure of their improved function and quality of life. Formal outcome evaluation may be a condition of the funder—both in terms of outcomes for the individual client and for obtaining funding in the future. In the latter case, cumulative documentation of positive outcomes of device use, using formal assessment instruments, provides justification that the device makes a difference and thus supports provision of the device to other clients in the future. In this section we provide information about formal assessments, which are typically completed by the ATP, and a framework for informal assessment, which is often completed on an ongoing basis by the rehabilitation assistant.

One important reason for outcome measurement is to limit device abandonment and misuse. We will consider this situation next, before proceeding to a discussion of evaluation.

Assistive Technology Abandonment

One of the most tangible indicators of lack of consumer satisfaction is when the consumer stops using a device even though the need for which the device was obtained still exists. We call this situation **technology abandonment**, and it is useful to look at some of the factors that lead to it. Phillips and Zhao (1993)[37] surveyed more than 200 users of assistive technologies and identified four factors that were significantly related to the abandonment of assistive technologies: (1) failure of providers to take consumers' opinions into account, (2) easy device procurement, (3) poor device performance, and (4) changes in consumers' needs or priorities.

More recent research examined personal and social factors that predict AT abandonment. Pape, Kim, and Weiner (2002)[36] conducted a review of the literature related to AT abandonment to look at how the personal meaning attributed to assistive devices influences their integration into the user's daily life. They found that psychosocial and cultural variables were primary factors in determining the meaning individuals assigned to AT. In particular their expectations of how the device would function, the social costs of using the device (i.e., cost/benefit of device use), and an outlook that disability did not define themselves as a person were the primary factors that contributed to whether a person integrated AT into her life or not.[36] Reimer-Weiss and Wacker (2000)[39] examined factors that predicted AT use in individuals with disability. They found that the relative advantage of the AT in the user's life and the user's involvement in the device selection process were predictors of device use or discontinuance.

Scherer (1998)[42] has developed a group of measures that help determine the match between the individual and technology. The Matching Person and Technology (MPT) assessment is described shortly. A recent study examined the validity of the assumptions that guided the development of this instrument. The results of the study supported these assumptions, specifically that personal characteristics related to mood, self-esteem, self-determination and motivation, and psychosocial characteristics related to friend and family support (as examples) were significant predictors of device use.[43] Collectively, the earlier studies such as Phillips and Zhao (1993)[37] and the more recent work of Pape et al. (2002),[36] Reimer-Weiss and Wacker (2000),[39] and Scherer et al. (2005)[43] provide evidence that characteristics of the device, the person, and their environment predict whether the client will use a device or abandon it.

Formal Evaluation

Formal evaluation of assistive technology service delivery consists of **outcome measures** that evaluate general function and those that evaluate specific components of assistive technology use. Outcome measurement in assistive technology has gained more attention over the past decade. Instruments are being developed that enable outcome measurement related to use of specific technology such as communication devices and wheelchairs. Examples of these assessments will be described in following chapters that discuss these types of technology. Box 3-5 lists four common evaluations that can be used to evaluate AT service delivery outcomes. Two of these measure general function and are designed to be used at the initial assessment and then again at the end of service delivery in order to determine change in function following the implementation of the device. These two assessments are the Canadian Occupational Performance Measure[27] and the Functional Independence Measure™.[47]

Two further instruments are specific to assistive technology, intended to evaluate psychosocial outcomes. These are the Psychosocial Impact of Assistive Devices

BOX 3-5 Common Assistive Technology Outcome Measures

GENERAL PERFORMANCE MEASURES—NOT SPECIFIC TO ASSISTIVE TECHNOLOGY

Canadian Occupational Performance Measure (COPM)[27]

The COPM measures the client's perception of the importance of self-identified occupational performance goals and their satisfaction with that performance. Goals are identified for self-care, productivity, and leisure. The COPM is designed to be used both pre- and post-intervention.

Functional Independence Measure™[47]

The FIM™ instrument is a widely used rehabilitation outcome measure that measures performance under the categories of self-care, bowel and bladder management, transfers, locomotion, communication, and cognition. An individual who uses AT cannot receive the maximum score, which is awarded only to individuals who perform the activity unaided. It is used pre- and post-intervention.

ASSISTIVE TECHNOLOGY–SPECIFIC PERFORMANCE MEASURES

Psychosocial Impact of Assistive Devices Scale (PIADS)[11]

The PIADS measures three psychosocial constructs related to the use of assistive technology. These constructs include: competence (functional independence, performance, and productivity); adaptability (the enabling and liberating effects of a device); and self-esteem (extent to which a device has affected self-confidence, self-esteem, and emotional well-being).

Quebec User Evaluation of Satisfaction with Assistive Technology (QUEST)[12]

The QUEST involves three parts. The first part provides the context in which satisfaction with the AT is evaluated. The second part asks the user to rate the importance of a number of different variables. The third part organizes the results of part 2 into three global categories: environment, person, and assistive technology. The final part enables the determination of areas of low satisfaction with device use.

Scale[11] and the Quebec User Evaluation of Satisfaction with Assistive Technology.[12] Both of these assessments are used after implementation of the assistive device system.

Gathering data with these instruments, as well as with those that are specific to a certain type of assistive technology, provides the consumer, the team, the organization delivering the service, and third-party funders with information on the effectiveness of the intervention. As indicated earlier in this chapter, the rehabilitation assistant may participate in this aspect of data gathering and contribute to the collective interpretation of the information. The rehabilitation assistant is often in a unique position of providing more detailed information on the client's use of technology through her frequent interactions with the client. In the next section, we describe a framework that can be used to guide the rehabilitation assistant's observations.

Informal Evaluation

Box 3-6 lists two primary areas related to assistive technology use that the rehabilitation assistant should consider in an **informal evaluation** of the assistive technology outcome. Many of these elements will have been evaluated, formally and informally, during the initial assessment process as well as during the implementation aspect of the service delivery process. These elements can be determined through observation and interview with the consumer during their regular interaction. While these elements are described separately, the process of gathering information about each of them is integrated. They are only separated here to achieve greater clarity.

The first element to consider is the actual use of the technology. What activities are completed with the device? The needs assessment and implementation process was based on client-determined goals that in part identified activities that would be completed using the device. During the evaluation, the rehabilitation assistant determines whether the consumer is using the AT for those activities. If not, what are the reasons that the device isn't being used? What affects the consumer's choice of these activities? Perhaps they haven't mastered

BOX 3-6 Informal Evaluation of Assistive Technology Use

USE OF THE ASSISTIVE TECHNOLOGY

- What activities are completed with the device?
- What affects the consumer's choice of these activities?
- When is the device used?
- What affects the consumer's choice of when to use the device?
- Does the assistive technology do what it is supposed to do?
- How long does the consumer use the device?
- Can they use it for the duration of the intended activity?
- Do they become fatigued when using the device? Is there some aspect of the device use that is causing the fatigue?
- What assistance does the consumer need to set up the device?
- Is the consumer independent in completion of the activity once the device is set up?
- Can the device be easily transported from one location to another? Within a setting? Across settings?

HUMAN/ASSISTIVE TECHNOLOGY INTERFACE

- Is the device properly positioned so the consumer can access it easily?
- Can the consumer see necessary components of the device? (E.g., visual display, control switches.)
- Can the consumer hear auditory output of the device?
- Does the consumer have the physical strength, range of motion, and dexterity to use the device?
- Is the consumer comfortable when using the device over the long term?
- Can the consumer detect and repair errors when using the device?
- Is the error a result of consumer capacity or skill?

the use of the device, so they find it is easier to ask for assistance from another person or to complete the activity themselves.

A related consideration is when the device is used. Time of day is a consideration here because the device might only be used when the person feels alert and able to operate it or, alternately, uses it to support function when they are fatigued. Another consideration is the social aspect. Does the consumer use the device only in settings where they are alone or with familiar other people? Do they choose not to use the device in a setting with unfamiliar people? If so, the rehabilitation assistant needs to uncover the meaning to the consumer of the use of the device because feelings of embarrassment or vulnerability may be associated with device use, limiting function in certain settings.[33]

An important consideration, which seems obvious, is whether the device does what it is supposed to do. Is the device reliable? Does the device enable the function as it is intended? This observation should have been made during the trial period and initial implementation phase.

The rehabilitation assistant should document how long the consumer uses the device, what support is required to set up and use the device, and any changes in these elements as the consumer becomes more proficient with the device use. Similarly, any issues with transportation of the device within the setting or across settings should be documented. As mentioned earlier, transportation may be affected by the physical effort needed to move the device from one place to another as well as institutional policies that limit the device from being removed from one setting and used in another (e.g., some schools do not allow students to take technology from the school to their home).

The second major aspect of this informal evaluation is the consideration of the human/technology interface. Here, the rehabilitation assistant considers whether the device is properly positioned so the consumer can access it (e.g., use controls on a communication device or the joystick control of a wheelchair). In addition to evaluating the positioning of the device for control access, the rehabilitation assistant evaluates positioning of the device for comfort. Consider whether the consumer is comfortable using the device (or sitting in a seating system) for the length of time needed to complete necessary activities.

The physical and sensory aspects of the human/technology interface include observation and documentation of whether the consumer can see the controls and the display during use; whether he can hear the output or feedback from the device; and whether he has the necessary strength, range of motion, and dexterity to use the device. While each of these components was evaluated during the initial assessment, the client's abilities may have changed between recommendation and receiving the technology. Further, the client's functional abilities may change over time if they have a progressive condition. A child's growth, either physically or developmentally, may change the skills and/or needs for the use of the assistive technology.

Finally, the rehabilitation assistant should note errors the client makes when using the device. These errors may be due to the client's capacity (e.g., her strength may have declined so she no longer has the physical capacity to exert sufficient force to use the technology). Alternately, the errors may be due to the client's skill level, suggesting the further training is required. The rehabilitation assistant should further note whether the client can detect the errors they make and repair them. For example, if she initiates a turn too soon when propelling her powered wheelchair, does she recognize this error and make adjustments to avoid hitting the wall? Does she learn from this error and initiate the turn at the proper time when making subsequent turns?

It is the rehabilitation assistant's responsibility to synthesize and record these observations. He also needs to articulate these observations as they provide valuable information for the ATP. These observations will also be useful to the rehabilitation assistant to guide his interaction with the client and her use of the assistive technology in the future.

A FINAL WORD ABOUT FUNDING

Assistive technology is expensive. If the consumer and her family had to bear the full cost, it would result in a significant burden. In many jurisdictions, **funding** is available for certain types of assistive technology. This section will familiarize the rehabilitation assistant with the different sources of funding for assistive technology and will include a list of factors that need to be considered regarding third-party funding.

Public Funding

Governments in many jurisdictions provide full or partial funding for some devices. Funding may come from national (federal), state (provincial), or municipal governments. It may target particular groups, such as veterans, children, seniors, first nation groups, or individuals who are on some form of social assistance. Public funding may also be specific to a setting such as an educational or work setting. Funding is often based on medical necessity. Examples of public funding include Medicaid and Medicare in the United States, the Assistive Devices Program in Ontario, Canada, and the Program of Appliances for Disabled People in New South Wales, Australia. Details of funding programs in these three countries are described by Cook and Polgar (2008).[9]

Private Funding

Private health insurance is often an employment benefit, although individuals can also purchase an insurance policy on their own. Although insurance policies may vary considerably, benefits such as durable medical equipment (see definition of assistive devices in Chapter 1) are often included. In some situations, private health insurance can be used to "top up" the funding that is received from a government source.

Other Sources of Funding

Alternative sources of funding that are not included in public funding or private insurance include service clubs, private foundations, and volunteer organizations. Various community service clubs (e.g., Kiwanis, Rotary Club) may be a source of funding for a local individual who has no other means of funding. In addition, there are foundations related to specific disability groups that directly supply equipment and services to individuals with that particular disability.

Determining Eligibility for Funding

It is important to determine eligibility requirements when determining appropriate funding sources. While it is commonly the ATP who determines eligibility for funding, the rehabilitation assistant can provide information that helps determine if the client meets these eligibility requirements. Some of these requirements include the age of the client and their functional status. For example, some programs require that the client be able to propel a wheelchair independently for a certain distance to be eligible for funding support. Eligibility may be limited to specific settings. Some programs will only fund devices used in the school or work settings. Most funding programs list eligible device categories. For example, Medicare in the United States only funds durable medical equipment, as defined in Chapter 1. Some funding organizations define a specific timeframe in which the client is expected to use the device in order to be eligible for funding. For example, a client who has had a total hip replacement and is only expected to need a walker for six weeks is not likely eligible for funding to support the purchase of the walker, because of the temporary nature of its use. Finally, the rehabilitation assistant needs to understand the process for procuring funding and the points in the process when prior approval is required.

SUMMARY

This chapter describes the principles of assessment and intervention and the process of service delivery to the consumer. The steps in the process include referral intake, needs assessment, evaluation, recommendation, implementation, follow-up, and follow-along. A framework for structuring observations of the client when using assistive technology is described.

STUDY QUESTIONS

1. Describe the five principles for assistive technology assessment and intervention.
2. Distinguish between quantitative and qualitative assessment procedures.
3. List the steps involved in assistive technology service delivery and write a brief description of each one.
4. List the four major categories of skill evaluation and provide two examples of each category.
5. List four considerations of the context relevant to the assistive technology assessment?
6. Describe the difference between opportunity barriers and access barriers. Give an example of each.
7. List six training strategies and give an example of each.
8. Describe considerations that are important when determining whether written instructions are useful to the client and caregivers.
9. Discuss the four factors that influence whether an assistive technology will be used or abandoned.
10. Describe the difference between formal and informal evaluation.
11. Describe two main elements of an informal evaluation of assistive technology use and give two examples of each element.
12. Describe three sources of assistive technology funding.
13. Discuss aspects that need to be considered when determining a client's eligibility for funding.

REFERENCES

1. Angelo J, Smith RO: The critical role of occupational therapy in augmentative communication. In American Occupational Therapy Association, editor: *Technology review '89: perspectives on occupational therapy practice*, Rockville, Md, 1989, American Occupational Therapy Association, pp 49–53.
2. Bailey RW: *Human performance engineering*, ed 3, Upper Saddle River, NJ, 1996, Prentice Hall.
3. Ballantyne JC, Graham JM, Baguley DM: *Ballantyne's deafness*, ed 7, Chichester, UK, 2009, Wiley Blackwell.
4. Beukelman DR, Mirenda P: *Augmentative and alternative communication, supporting children and adults with complex communication needs*, Baltimore, 2005, Paul H Brookes.
5. Bruininks RH: *Bruininks-Oseretsky Test of Motor Proficiency*, Circle Pines, MN, 1978, American Guidance Service.
6. Canadian Association of Occupational Therapists: *Enabling occupation: an occupational therapy perspective*, ed 2, Ottawa, ON, 2002, CAOT Publications/ACE.
7. Colarusso RP, Hammill DD: *Motor-free visual perception test manual*, Novato, Calif., 1972, Academic Therapy Publications.
8. Cook AM: Development of motor skills for switch use by person with severe disabilities, *Developmental Disabilities Special Interest Section Newsletter* 14(2), 1991.
9. Cook AM, Polgar JM: *Cook and Hussey's assistive technologies: principles and practice*, St. Louis, 2008, Mosby.
10. Crawford J: *Crawford Small Parts Dexterity Test*, London, 1981, Psychological Corporation.
11. Day H, Jutai JW: Measuring the psychosocial impact of assistive devices: The PIADS, *Can J Rehabil* 9:159–168, 1996.
12. Demers L, Weiss-Lambrou R, Ska B: Development of the Quebec User Evaluation of Satisfaction with Assistive Technology (QUEST), *Assist Technol* 8(1):3–13, 1996.
13. Doyle Lyons K, Crepeau EB: The clinical reasoning of an occupational therapy assistant, *Am J Occup Ther* 55(5): 577–581, 2001.
14. Dunn W: Sensation and sensory processing. In Crepeau EB, Cohn ES, Schell BAB, editors: *Willard and Spackman's Occupational Therapy*, ed 11, Philadelphia, 2009, Lippincott Williams & Wilkins.

15. Eby DW, Molnar LJ, Pellerito JM: Driving cessation and alternative community mobility. In Pellerito JM, editor: *Driver rehabilitation and community mobility: principles and practice*, St. Louis, MO, 2006, Mosby.
16. Erhardt RP: *The Erhardt Developmental Prehension Assessment*, Maplewood, MN, 1994, Erhardt Developmental Products.
17. Fischer AG: *Assessment of Motor and Process Skills*, Fort Collins, CO, 2003, Three Star Press.
18. Flinn NA, Trombly Latham CA, Podolski CR: Assessing abilities and capacities: range of motion, strength, and endurance. In Radomski MV, Trombly Latham CA, editors: *Occupational Therapy for Physical Dysfunction*, ed 6, Philadelphia, 2007, Lippincott, Williams & Wilkins.
19. Gaster LS: *Continuous quality improvement in assistive technology*, Presented at RESNA International Conference, Toronto, June, 1992.
20. Henderson SE, Sugden DA: *Movement ABC*, London, 1992, Psychological Corporation.
21. Jebsen RH, et al: An objective and standardized test of hand function, *Arch Phys Med Rehabil* 50(6):311–319, 1969.
22. Killingsworth AP, Pedretti LW: Joint range of motion. In Pendleton HM, Schultz-Krohn W, editors: *Pedretti's occupational therapy: practice skills for physical dysfunction*, ed 6, St. Louis, 2006, Mosby.
23. Killingsworth AP, Pedretti LW: Evaluation of muscle strength. In Pendleton HM, Schultz-Krohn W, editors: *Pedretti's occupational therapy: practice skills for physical dysfunction*, ed 6, St. Louis, 2006b, Mosby.
24. King GA, et al: Goal attainment scaling: its use in evaluating pediatric therapy programs, *Phys Occup Ther Pediatr* 19(2):31–52, 1999.
25. Kirby RL: *Wheelchair Skills Program v. 3.2*, 2005. Available from: www.wheelchairskillsprogram.ca.
26. Lafayette Instrument: *Minnesota Rate of Manipulation Test, Test Manual, Revised*, Lafayette IN, 1998, Author.
27. Law M, et al: *Canadian Occupational Performance Measure*, ed 3, Toronto, ON, 1998, CAOT/ACE Publications.
28. Light J: Toward a definition of communicative competence for individuals using augmentative and alternative communication systems, *Augment Altern Commun* 5(2):137–144, 1989.
29. Mattingly C: The narrative nature of clinical reasoning. In Mattingly C, Fleming MH, editors: *Clinical reasoning: forms of inquiry in a therapeutic practice*, Philadelphia, 1994, FA Davis.
30. Mattingly C, Fleming MH: *Clinical Reasoning: forms of inquiry in a therapeutic practice*, Philadelphia, 1994, FA Davis.
31. McNaughton S: Connecting with consumers, *Assist Technol* 5(1):7–10, 1993.
32. Miller Polgar J: Critiquing assessments. In Crepeau EB, Cohn ES, Schell BAB, editors: *Willard and Spackman's occupational therapy*, ed 11, Philadelphia, 2009, Lippincott Williams & Wilkins.
33. Miller Polgar J: The Myth of neutral technology. In Oishi MMK, Mitchel IM, Van der Loos HFM, editors: *Design and use of assistive technology: social, technical, ethical, and economic challenges*, New York, 2010, Springer.
34. Nunnally JC, Bernstein IH: *Psychometric Theory*, ed 3, Toronto, ON, 1994, McGraw-Hill.
35. Pallin M: *Techniques for the successful use of augmentative communication systems*, Presented at *Demystifying Technology Workshop*, Sacramento, Calif, 1991, Assistive Device Center.
36. Pape TL, Kim J, Weiner B: The shaping of individual meanings assigned to assistive technology: a review of personal factors, *Disabil Rehabil* 24(1/2/3):5–20, 2002.
37. Phillips B, Zhao H: Predictors of assistive technology abandonment, *Assist Technol* 5(1):36–45, 1993.
38. Quintana LA: Assessing abilities and capacities: Vision, visual perception, and praxis. In Trombly CA, Radomski MV, editors: *Occupational therapy for physical dysfunction*, ed 5, Baltimore, MD, 2002, Lippincott Williams & Wilkins.
39. Reimer-Weiss ML, Wacker RR: Factors associated with assistive technology discontinuance among individuals with disabilities, *J Rehabil* 66(3):44–50, 2000.
40. Russel DJ, et al: *Gross Motor Function Measure*, Cambridge, 2002, Cambridge University Press.
41. Scheiman M: *Understanding and managing vision deficits: a guide for occupational therapists*, ed 2, Thorofare, NJ, 2002, Slack Inc.
42. Scherer M: *Matching person and technology: a series of assessments for evaluating predispositions to and outcomes of technology use in rehabilitation, education, the workplace and other settings*, Webster, NY, 1998, The Institute for Matching Person & Technology.
43. Scherer MJ, Sax C, Vanbiervliet A, et al: Predictors of assistive technology use: the importance of personal and psychosocial factors, *Disabil Rehabil* 27(21):1321–1331, 2005.
44. Smith RO: Technological approaches to performance enhancement. In Christiansen C, Baum C, editors: *Occupational therapy*, Thorofare, NJ, 1991, Slack.
45. Smith V, Early MB: Occupational therapy process: evaluation and intervention in physical dysfunction. In Early MB, editor: *Physical dysfunction practice skills for the occupational therapy assistant*, St. Louis, 2006, Mosby.
46. Toglia JP, Golisz KM, Goverover Y: Evaluation and intervention for cognitive perceptual impairments. In Crepeau EB, Cohn ES, Schell BAB, editors: *Willard and Spackman's occupational therapy*, ed 11, Philadelphia, 2009, Lippincott Williams & Wilkins.
47. Uniform Data System for Medical Rehabilitation (UDS): *Functional Independence Measure, version 5.1*, Buffalo, NY, 1997, Buffalo General Hospital, State University of New York.
48. Wiersma W, Jurs SG: *Educational measurement and testing*, ed 2, Boston, 1990, Allyn and Bacon.
49. Witt JC, Cavell TA: Psychological assessment. In Wodrich DL, Joy JE, editors: *Multidisciplinary assessment of children with learning disabilities and mental retardation*, Baltimore, 1986, Paul H Brookes.

CHAPTER 4

Seating Systems as Enablers of Function

CHAPTER OUTLINE

LEARNING OBJECTIVES

On completing this chapter, you will be able to do the following:

1. Identify the potential outcomes of seating for postural control, tissue integrity, and comfort
2. Describe a comprehensive seating assessment
3. Describe key biomechanical principles related to sitting and seating technologies
4. Describe the principles of seating for postural control
5. Describe the factors that contribute to the development of pressure ulcers
6. Describe the different characteristics of seating materials
7. Discuss the different classifications of materials used to construct seats

KEY TERMS

Center of Gravity
Center of Mass
Center of Pressure
Compression
Dampening
Density
Envelopment
Equilibrium
Fixed Deformity
Flexible Deformity
Force
Frictional Forces
Fulcrum
Gravitational Line
Linear

Line of Application
Mobility
Pelvic Obliquity
Pelvic Rotation
Planar
Pressure
Pressure Ulcer
Recovery
Resilience
Restraint
Rotational
Scoliosis
Shearing
Sliding Resistance
Stability
Stability Zone
Stiffness
Tension
Windswept Hip Deformity

A comfortable position that promotes function is a prerequisite for involvement in any activity. Seating devices assist users to function in activities across all performance areas (self-care, work or school, and play or leisure) in many different environments; for this reason, they are considered to be general-purpose extrinsic enablers. Throughout this chapter, the role of the rehabilitation assistant in the use and maintenance of seating devices and the proper positioning of clients is discussed.

The first part of this chapter describes the needs served by seating systems, evaluation of individuals for seating, and biomechanical principles related to seating. The remainder of the chapter provides in-depth information on each of the three categories of seating needs (seating for postural control, tissue integrity, and comfort), including related principles and the technologies used for intervention. Seating components are typically used with some type of mobility base. For purposes of this text, however, these two systems are separated. Mobility is viewed as a specific-purpose extrinsic enabler (see Chapter 12).

THE ROLE OF THE REHABILITATION ASSISTANT

The rehabilitation assistant (OTA or PTA) is often involved with clients on a more frequent basis than other members of the health care team. This frequency puts him in a strong position to know the client's functional abilities and their use of assistive technology. The rehabilitation assistant is often responsible for setup and adjustment of the individual and her technology on a daily basis. Additional roles of the assistant in the use of technology are to ensure that the technology is used in a safe manner and that it is properly maintained, both on a daily and long-term basis; and also to provide feedback and information on any changes in the client's function that would require an adjustment to existing technology or a change to new assistive technology.

OVERVIEW OF NEEDS SERVED BY SEATING

Three distinct areas of seating intervention have emerged, each serving a particular consumer need. These three categories of seating intervention are (1) seating for postural control, (2) seating for pressure redistribution, and (3) seating for comfort.[18]

Adults and children who have neuromuscular disorders such as cerebral palsy or stroke frequently require seating systems that aid postural control. Abnormal muscle tone, muscle weakness, or uncoordinated movements associated with neuromuscular disorders frequently impair the ability to maintain an upright posture when sitting. Impaired motor control affects the person's ability to participate in activities of daily living, can compromise their general health status, and can result in skeletal deformities.

The primary population served by the category of seating interventions for pressure redistribution is individuals with spinal cord injury. These individuals can have partial or complete paralysis and reduced or absent sensation below the level of their lesion. As a result, they are susceptible to breakdown of the tissue (skin, fat, and muscle) over bony prominences on weight-bearing surfaces. Also benefiting from the technologies in this category are individuals with multiple sclerosis, those with muscular dystrophy, the elderly, and others who have limited mobility or cognitive function, or sensory impairment, and therefore a reduced ability to relieve pressure from weight-bearing surfaces.

The third category of seating addresses the need to improve an individual's level of physical comfort through postural accommodation. Persons in this category include the elderly, individuals with limited endurance for walking (e.g., people with cardiac or pulmonary conditions), and individuals with amputations or arthritis. They may or may not use a wheelchair on a regular basis and typically have normal or near-normal sensation; however, any prolonged sitting causes discomfort from which they are unable to obtain relief. Therefore, they have unique needs and are not completely served by either category previously described. Specialized seating can help to alleviate this chronic discomfort and maximize function. Box 4-1 shows some of the potential outcomes of seating intervention for these populations.

EVALUATION FOR SEATING

The process of assessing individuals for the purpose of recommending seating technologies requires a systematic method that includes consideration of many factors. The

BOX 4-1 Potential Outcomes of Proper Seating and Positioning

Facilitation of optimal postural control to enable engagement in functional activities
Provision of an optimal balance between stability and mobility in the seated position
Maintenance of neutral skeletal alignment
Prevention of skeletal deformities
Maintenance of tissue integrity
Maintenance of a position of comfort
Decreased fatigue
Enhance respiratory and circulatory function
Facilitate caregiver activities

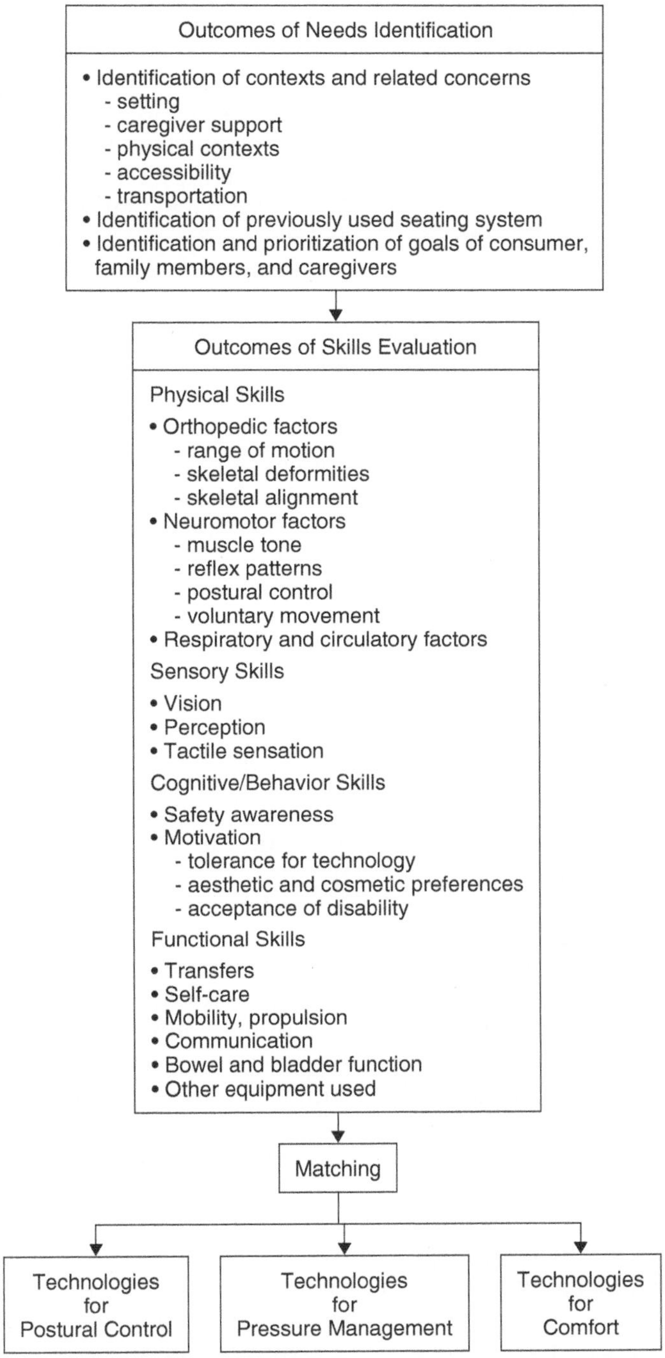

discussion of the design of an assistive technology system in Chapter 2 gave a general framework to guide assessment. The purpose of this section is to describe the factors that are considered when evaluating a client for seating technology. Figure 4-1 depicts a framework showing the process of this evaluation. The rehabilitation assistant's role in this process is to provide information about the client's daily activities, physical and cognitive function, and emotional state, particularly noting any changes that might affect the client's seating needs.

Overview of Assessment Process

The first element of the HAAT model requires the team to understand the activities in which the client wants or needs to participate. Figure 4-1 lists the desired outcomes of the identification of needs. An ATP is usually responsible for completion of the assessment to determine seating needs and the most appropriate technology recommendation. However, others provide important information to support this information. Any assessment with the goal of identifying seating needs and recommended technology starts with discussion of the occupations the user wants and needs to complete while using the seating system. A general measure such as the Canadian Occupational Performance Measure[28] provides a systematic means of discussing key occupations in the areas of self-care, productivity, and leisure. There are some measures that are specific to seating and wheeled mobility, including the Functioning Everyday in a Wheelchair measure[37] and the Wheelchair Outcome Measure,[34,38] that consider function in self-care, productivity, and leisure specifically from the view of an individual who uses seating and mobility devices.

Understanding the client's abilities is a second important element in the process guided by the HAAT model. Functional skills, including transfers to and from different surfaces (e.g., bed to wheelchair, car to wheelchair), self-care skills (e.g., feeding, dressing), wheelchair mobility, written and verbal communication skills, and bowel and bladder care should be evaluated. Equipment the person will use while in the seating system needs to be taken into consideration. For example, respiratory equipment and augmentative communication devices are frequently mounted on the wheelchair and need to be in a position that is functional for the user. The level of assistance an individual requires to use the seating system is an important consideration in the assessment. Consideration must be given to whether an individual can transfer to the system and fasten any straps. The complexity of the system and the ease of access influence the demands placed on an individual providing assistance with a transfer. It is equally important to consider the abilities of the

Figure 4-1 Framework for seating and positioning decision making.

individual providing the assistance and their capacity to provide the support required. Many older adults who use assistive devices live with their spouses who may have conditions that limit their ability to provide assistance. Ideally, the individual's ability to perform functional activities should be evaluated both in the existing system and in the proposed system. Here, a rehabilitation assistant can provide useful information by recording their observations of the client's function in both systems as they go about their daily activities. These observations give context to the client's function in different situations, where the client experiences limitations, and the strategies they currently use to complete functional activities. A rehabilitation assistant who interacts with clients for longer periods of time in situations such as a school setting or long-term care facility is in a unique position to understand how the client functions during the day and what elements affect their function. This information is highly informative in the assessment process.

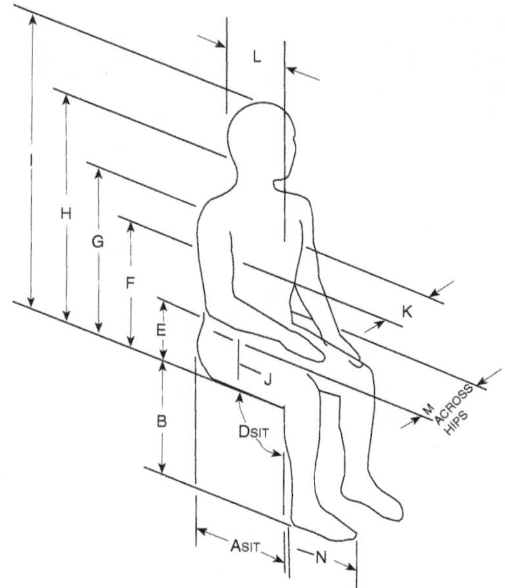

Figure 4-2 Joint angle and body measurements taken during the evaluation. *ASIT* (R and L), behind hips/popliteal fossa; *B* (R and L), popliteal fossa/heel; *DSIT*, knee flexion angle; *E*, sitting surface/pelvic crest; *F*, sitting surface/axilla; *G*, sitting surface/shoulder; *H*, sitting surface/occiput; *I*, sitting surface/crown of head; *J*, sitting surface/hanging elbow; *K*, width across trunk; *L*, depth of trunk; *M*, width across hips; *N*, heel/toe. (From Bergen AF, Presperin J, Tallman T: *Positioning for function: wheelchairs and other assistive technologies*, Valhalla, NY, 1990, Valhalla Rehabilitation Publications.)

Human Factors

Physical Skills or Mat Assessment

The physical evaluation includes assessment of orthopedic factors, postural control, and respiratory and circulatory factors (see Figure 4-1). It is recommended that evaluation of physical skills take place with the person both in a sitting position and supine on a flat surface such as a mat.

Musculoskeletal Factors

Orthopedic evaluation involves measurement of joint range of motion and assessment of skeletal deformities and skeletal alignment to determine optimal angles for sitting. Obtaining information regarding limitations in range of motion and deformities is necessary to determine whether the goal of the seating system will be to prevent deformities, correct deformities, or accommodate deformities.[55]

Starting with the consumer supine on the mat, mobility of the lumbar spine and pelvis are assessed, followed by range of motion measurements of the hips, knees, ankles, upper extremities, and neck. Joint angle and body measurements as shown in Figure 4-2 are made at this time. Alignment of the individual's head, shoulders, and trunk with the pelvis is determined next. Range of motion and skeletal alignment should also be assessed with the individual in a sitting position to determine how the body parts are affected by gravity. Bergen, Presperin, and Tallman (1990)[1] describe in detail a process for measuring joint angles and assessing skeletal alignment.

The skeletal deformities present may be fixed or flexible. In a **fixed deformity,** permanent changes have taken place in the bones, muscles, and other structures that restrict the normal range of motion of the particular joint. When fixed deformities are present, the alignment of the other joints is also affected. For example, a fixed deformity of the pelvis will affect spinal alignment. In such situations, the seating system is designed to accommodate the deformity. Muscle tightness can cause individuals to assume certain postures so that they may appear to have a deformity. When the joint is stretched passively in the opposite direction, however, it is possible to move the joint and reduce the deformity. In this situation, the person is considered to have a **flexible deformity** at that joint. Depending on the situation, the seating system may be designed to correct a flexible deformity. Specific deformities and their effects on sitting posture are described in the section on seating principles for postural control.

Postural Control

A key element to assess is the user's postural control, particularly for children developing motor control, individuals recovering motor function after a neurological injury (such as traumatic brain injury), or someone losing motor control as a consequence of a progressive illness such as ALS. Two important aspects are considered: the individual's ability to control their posture in a sitting position (i.e., how much support is required to maintain a comfortable sitting position with a reasonable amount of effort) and the response to various positional changes. The most effective way to assess these aspects is with the client seated on a mat, with their feet supported either on the floor or on other support such as a bench.

The client's sitting ability is described by the amount of support required to maintain a seated position. *Hands-free sitters* are those who do not need to use their hands to support themselves to maintain sitting, whereas

BOX 4-2 Levels of Postural Control in Sitting

THE HANDS-FREE SITTER

Can sit for prolonged periods without using the hands for support.

Seating system is designed primarily for mobility, to provide a stable base of support, and to be comfortable.

THE HANDS-DEPENDENT SITTER

One or both hands are used to maintain support while sitting.

Seating system is designed to provide pelvic or trunk support to free the person's hands for functional activities.

THE PROPPED SITTER

Lacks any ability to support self in sitting.

Seating system provides total body support.

hands-dependent sitters do need to use their hands. These individuals could not perform a seated activity using the hands without some type of external support. A *dependent sitter* does not have sufficient motor control to support herself in sitting at all. A dependent sitter (or propped sitter) requires more support from a seating system in order to maintain the sitting position.[54] Box 4-2 defines these levels of postural control.

The amount of external control required to assist an individual to maintain a seated position is an important determination. Kangas (2006)[24] recommends that only the minimal amount of external support needed by the client to remain in an upright position be used. This strategy enables the client to use the postural control they have and also gives them freedom of movement that they wouldn't have when held more tightly with straps. Support may vary with the activity. Less support may be needed when the individual is engaged in a sedentary activity, such as watching television. Alternatively, more support is needed when the individual is using his hands for an activity and the focus of attention is on the activity. The individual should not need to divert attention to the maintenance of posture when engaged in an activity.

It is also important to understand the client's response to changes in posture. The assessment considers the client's muscle response and function when the pelvis is placed in various positions (e.g., neutral, anterior-tipped, or posterior-tipped); when the lower extremities are in different positions; or with different degrees of spinal flexion or extension. The client's response to these position changes will influence the configuration of the seating system.

Tissue Integrity

The mat assessment also includes examination of the skin to determine any areas at risk for pressure ulcers or indications that a pressure ulcer might develop. This examination is particularly important for clients who have limited ability to move independently, including those clients with limited sensation. Limited cognitive abilities along with limited motor function impair their awareness of the need to perform weight-relieving movements. Particular attention is paid to the areas over bony prominences, such as the buttocks, spine, elbows, and ankles.

Respiratory and Circulatory Factors

The person's respiratory status and circulation are other factors addressed during the evaluation. With skeletal deformities, pulmonary and cardiac function can be compromised. It is important to know whether certain positions enhance or limit respiration. For example, a client with weak trunk muscles may sit with increased trunk flexion, which makes it difficult to fully expand the lungs on inhalation. A seating system that helps the user maintain an upright trunk position will make breathing easier. Circulation, particularly in the lower limbs, needs to be considered as well. Some individuals may have a condition, such as diabetes, that predisposes them to circulatory problems. Care should be taken for these consumers that the seating system doesn't cause pressure or restrict movement because these may compromise circulation, resulting in a pressure ulcer or edema. It is particularly important to observe the area around the knee to ensure that there is no pressure behind the knee and that the lateral aspects of the knee are not in contact with the wheelchair. Similarly, it is important to ensure that the ankles and feet are not exposed to excess pressure against any of the wheelchair components. Observe the position of the lateral supports on the trunk to ensure that they are not causing undue pressure on the trunk and to ensure that they are not too high, causing pressure in the axilla (armpit).

Sensory and Perceptual Skills

Vision and visual perception contribute to a person's balance and sitting posture, and deficits in these areas are considered during the evaluation. The configuration of the seat can affect the user's line of vision. For example, an individual with poor postural control who is unable to maintain spinal extension with consequent neck flexion may not be able to maintain her head in an upright position if the seat-to-back angle is set at 90 degrees. The user's line of vision will be downward in this seating configuration as her head falls forward.

Proprioception and vestibular function influence body posture. With vision, these functions assist the client to keep the head in an upright and midline position. Further, they provide feedback to the client regarding the position of the trunk, with proprioception providing information about the position of the limbs. These senses assist the client to maintain an optimal biomechanical position for daily activities.

Tactile sensation is another factor to consider. Some individuals may react defensively to the touch of certain textures or positioning components on the body. Other individuals lack tactile sensation, which can contribute to skin breakdown. The assessment should provide the rehabilitation assistant with information about any known decrease in sensation, particularly in the buttock area, or history of redness, skin abrasions, or pressure ulcers.

Cognitive Skills

Cognitive skills such as problem solving and motor planning are not as much of an issue in seating as in mobility. However, there are a few areas that require consideration. Individuals with poor safety judgment may not be aware of the need to keep a positioning belt fastened, and special considerations may be necessary. When the seating system is complex, understanding the client's cognitive abilities will aid the decision whether to teach the client or the caregiver about the proper use of the system. If a person relies on an augmentative communication device or on yes/no responses, these modes of communication should be used during the evaluation process. If it is known that the consumer is not reliable in his or her responses, then the ATP should seek assistance from a caregiver in interpreting the consumer's responses to the seating system.

Psychosocial Factors

The meaning that technology holds for the individual is an important factor to explore with the user, although it is more significant for the mobility component of a seating and mobility system (see Chapter 12). Many clients prefer technology that does not draw attention to a disability. This preference will be a factor in the selection of a seating system. Aesthetics, or the appearance of the device, is an important factor in acceptance or rejection of the technology.[36,41] Behavioral problems, such as an agitated person who throws himself against the back of the chair, can also present a safety problem that needs to be addressed. Working together with the consumer and the caregiver to address these concerns is essential.

Environmental Considerations

Physical Context

The extent to which the seating system will be used outdoors is an important factor to consider because extreme heat or cold will affect the function of many materials, limiting their ability to meet the goals set for use of the system. Extreme heat can soften some materials, limiting their ability to provide support. Other materials will freeze if left in a car for a length of time in cold temperatures. A more complete discussion of the effect of temperature on materials used in seating systems follows. Exposure to light sources may affect some materials used to cover a system component, altering their properties and, again, affecting the function of the system.

Social Context

The consumer may be assisted by many people during the day, including family, other caregivers, and rehabilitation assistants. The social context influences the instructions given to the users of the system and influences considerations with respect to the frame weight, complexity, and maintenance (e.g., cleaning and sanitation issues) of the system. Misuse or inadequate maintenance of the system will reduce its effectiveness in meeting the client's needs. The user and any caregivers need to be familiar with proper use and care of the seating system. Adequate instruction reinforced over time is key to preventing misuse of the system. Often the rehabilitation assistant is responsible for ongoing education of the consumer and their caregivers.

Individuals who routinely lift and carry a seating system must be able to do so with good body mechanics to decrease the risk of injury. OTAs and PTAs spend a lot of time on caregiver training to ensure that proper technique is understood and used. Materials used to construct seating systems have changed in recent years, in part to decrease the weight. However, some custom-made systems (such as foam in place, which will be discussed later) can be quite heavy. Maintenance of the system is another consideration. Air-filled cushions require careful attention to ensure that they are properly inflated and free of punctures. As mentioned previously, the properties of some materials are affected by extremes of temperature, so whoever is responsible for maintenance of the system must take care to avoid damage to it by not leaving it in a location where it would be exposed to temperature extremes (e.g., in a car on a hot summer day or a cold winter night). An individual maintaining a system should also take care not to use harsh or abrasive chemicals when cleaning the device because these can also cause damage. In some situations, the system that is most ideal for the client cannot be recommended because of the inability of the caregiver to use and care for it.

Institutional Context

Funding implications are a key institutional consideration. General considerations with respect to funding were described in Chapter 3. The ATP has the responsibility for providing the necessary documentation to secure funding but may rely on the rehabilitation assistant to provide important information about the client's function to include in the documentation.

Another type of legislation has unique implications for seating products: the use of restraints. The Centers for Medicare and Medicaid Services define a **restraint** as "any manual method or physical or mechanical device, material or equipment attached or adjacent to the resident's body that the individual cannot remove easily which restricts freedom of movement or normal access to one's body."[9] Certain legal jurisdictions have legislation that regulates the use of restraints with individuals residing in institutional settings. The intent of this legislation is to limit inappropriate use of restraints, such as tying an individual into a chair simply to prevent him or her from moving around. This legislation has implications for the use of straps, pelvic belts, and sub–anterior-superior iliac spine (ASIS) bars, trays, and tilt systems (as part of the wheelchair set up) that are used in seating systems for positioning and safety reasons. The legislation typically regulates how restraints are used in institutional settings, requiring most institutions to have a plan and a documented process when restraints are used. Box 4-3 provides information on what to look for in an institution's guidelines and care plan concerning restraint use.[11,44] The rehabilitation assistant should be familiar with the restraint use policies of the institution, how these policies affect their practice, and what is required of them when interacting with a client whose seating system includes elements listed above that are considered to be restraints.

Restraints are frequently used to prevent falls. However, there is little evidence to suggest their use actually does result in any significant reduction in the incidence of falls.[53] The rehabilitation assistant should monitor the client for any adverse outcomes to the use of restraints. These outcomes include increased agitation if the client becomes upset by the restriction of movement, redness, skin abrasion or pressure ulcer formation, or undue limitation of functional activities if the client's movement is overly restrained by seating components.

Matching Device Characteristics to a Consumer's Needs and Skills

The final component of the evaluation process involves the matching of the client and the technology. Box 4-4 lists a number of questions that are important in the determination of whether the recommended technology is appropriate. Because the rehabilitation assistant engages with the client for several hours a day, over several days, she is in an excellent position to provide information that contributes to the evaluation of the technology as it is used by the client. The rehabilitation assistant can observe the client over time to determine if he is able to maintain a functional position that is comfortable and minimizes the risk of pressure ulcer development. She can observe the client if various daily activities and note whether the seating technology enables their performance in these activities. Interaction with the client over the long term can provide information on whether the technology is sufficiently durable and flexible to meet the client's changing needs. Finally, interactions with caregivers provide important information about their ability to cope with caregiving demands, including their ability to use and maintain the seating technology.

BOX 4-3 Considerations for Use of Restraints with Clients in Institutional Setting

RESTRAINT GUIDELINES*

- The least restrictive device should be used.
- Client's response to the restraint should be reassessed frequently as being restrained can increase agitation.
- Client should be reassessed frequently to determine whether continued restraint is required.
- Restraints should be removed periodically.
- Facility's guidelines for documenting use of restraints need to be followed.
- Depending on jurisdiction, a physician's order is required at regular intervals for continued use of restraints.

CARE PLAN

- Reposition the client frequently; monitor the client's position to ensure that they are neither at risk of injury because of their position nor at risk for a pressure ulcer from immobility due to the restraint.
- Perform skin care routine on a regular basis, including observation of the skin for areas of redness that might indicate formation of a pressure ulcer.
- Perform range of motion exercises (active or passive as the client is able) frequently during the day.
- Provide assistance with activities of daily living; if the client remains in a restraint during these activities, ensure that the restraint is not limiting their performance.
- Ensure ongoing assessment by the team to monitor the need for continued use of the restraint.

ALTERNATIVE STRATEGIES

- Observe the client to determine if behavior that prompted the use of the restraint is triggered by something in the environment, for example:
  - Another person in the environment may trigger agitated behavior so limiting the interaction may be calming.
  - If restraints are used to prevent falling out of bed, lower the bed and use mats to reduce the risk of injury in the event of a fall.
  - Provide stimulating activities that engage the client to encourage calmer emotions.
- When possible include the individual in a group so they can be observed and assisted on an ongoing basis.
- Be aware of the effect of your style of communication and interaction on the client's emotions as these may increase agitation.
- Use a positioning alarm on the bed that alert the staff when a client tries to climb out of bed.
- Enhance exercise programs.
- Ensure that staff is familiar with the client, their needs and abilities.
- Ensure that the client is comfortable in bed.

*Data from Collins LG, Haines, C, Perkel RL: Restraining devices for patients in acute and long-term care facilities, *American Family Physician* 79: 254–256, 2009; Registered Nurses Association of Ontario (RNAO): Risk assessment and prevention of pressure ulcers (revised), Toronto, ON, 2005: RNAO.

BOX 4-4 Critical Questions for Evaluating Seating Technologies

Does the seating system as simulated meet the consumer's goals and needs (e.g., postural control, deformity management, pressure relief)?
Does the seating system provide stability and allow for maximal performance in functional activities (e.g., transfers, weight shifts, activities of daily living)?
Is the seating system comfortable for the consumer?
Is the seating system durable enough to meet the consumer's needs for a reasonable period?
Is the seating system sufficiently flexible to meet the consumer's changing needs (e.g., change in functional abilities, disease progression, growth changes in children, or predicted weight loss)?
Are there resources available to ensure appropriate maintenance of the seating system?
Can the consumer or a third-party payer finance the cost of the seating system?

BIOMECHANICAL PRINCIPLES

It is important for the rehabilitation assistant to understand some of the aspects of body position and movement when they position a client in their seating system and interact with that client during the day. Biomechanics is the study of body position and movement. This section presents the major concepts of biomechanics that are fundamental to an understanding of seating and positioning systems for persons with disabilities. There are additional aspects of biomechanics that are pertinent to this area. A lengthier discussion of relevant biomechanical principles can be found in Cook and Polgar (2008).[13]

Kinematics: Study of Motion

When seating systems are designed, the position of the consumer, the position of the seating system components, and the movements of both the consumer and system components should be considered. The term kinematics describes movement. The term displacement is used to define the position of a body in space; a change in displacement results in a new position. For example, in a postural support system, one goal is to bring the trunk to a midline position. This action may require a displacement from the client's preferred resting position to a midline position by application of an external lateral trunk support. The rate of change in displacement is called velocity. It is also important to know how fast the velocity is changing (increasing or decreasing); this change is called acceleration. One of the most common accelerations is that of gravity. The term gravity actually refers to the acceleration of an object toward the center of the earth. Acceleration of an object is directly related to the force generated by the object's movement.

There are two fundamental types of displacement: linear and rotational. When all parts of a body move in the same direction, at the same time, and for the same distance, the movement is **linear.**[30] For example, a person generates translational movement when walking. Displacements caused by external positioning components can also be translational. If the direction, distance, and time of the movement occur simultaneously, but the movement is through an angle instead of in a straight line, the movement is called **rotational.** Rotational movements occur around an axis called the **fulcrum.** The majority of body movements are rotational, such as hip or elbow flexion and shoulder flexion or extension. Some positioning components cause rotational displacements (e.g., reclining the back of a wheelchair causes rotation at the pelvis and hip).

Kinetics: Forces

Force is a major element in both biomechanics and seating for individuals with disabilities. **Force** is anything that acts on a body to change its rate of acceleration or alter its momentum.[30] It is described by both magnitude and direction.[49] Forces always occur in equal and opposite action-reaction pairs between bodies. Forces can be applied to the body internally or externally. Internal forces are generated inside the body, such as muscle contractions that cause movement of the joints. Externally applied forces (such as the shearing of skin against the wheelchair cushion during transfers) come from outside the body and act on it in some way. One example is the forces applied by a support surface and components of a seating system such as lateral supports. The force resulting from the acceleration of gravity is another external and ever-present force that acts on the body and influences its posture and movement.[49] This force on the body acts along a line called the **gravitational line,** and its effect is localized around a point in the body called the **center of gravity.** The center of gravity changes as posture changes from standing to sitting and in different sitting positions. Figure 4-3 shows the change in the position of the center of gravity with different positions.

The four properties of force ultimately determine its result. These properties are magnitude, direction, line of application, and point of application. Magnitude is the amount or size of the force measured in newtons, pounds, or kilograms. Forces are applied in some direction, either pushing or pulling, and are applied along a particular **line of application.** The force acts at a particular point on the body, called the point of application.[30]

Types of Forces

There are three different types of force. Each of these types produces different effects on the body, and it is beneficial to understand these differences when considering the client's use of seating and positioning systems. **Tension** forces act in the same line but away from each other (pulling apart), such as the force applied on the antagonist muscle during contraction of the agonist muscle.

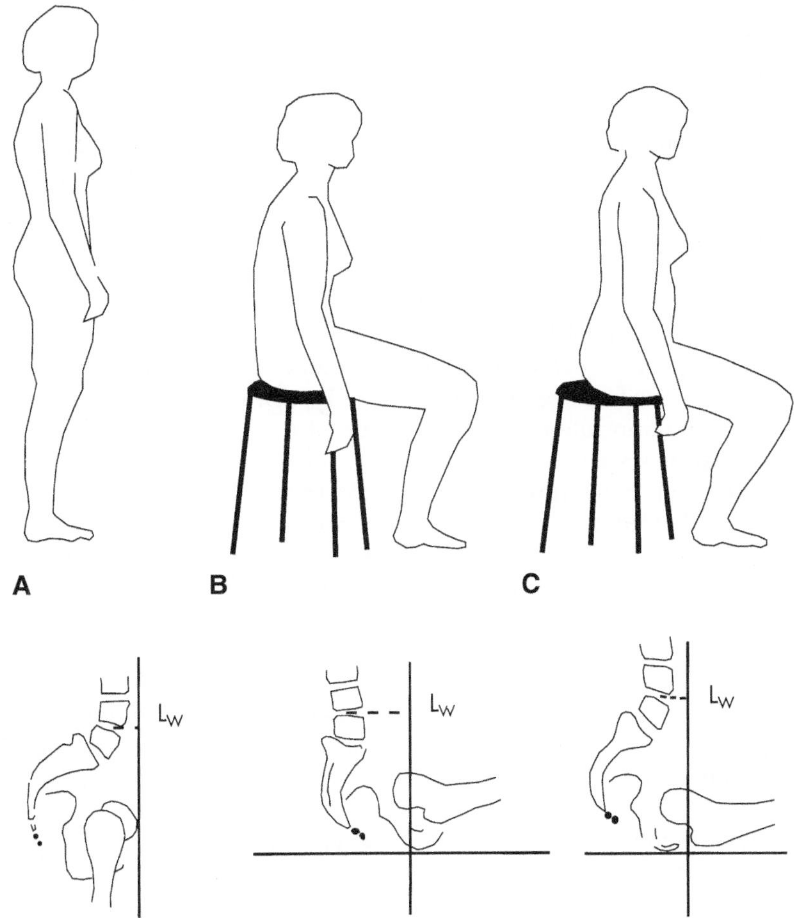

Figure 4-3 **A,** Line of gravity in erect upright standing. **B,** Relaxed unsupported sitting resulting in backward tilt of the pelvis and flattening of the lumbar lordosis. **C,** Erect sitting with reduction in backward pelvic tilt and increased lordosis. L_W, Lever arm. (From Frankel VH, Nordin M: *Basic biomechanics of the skeletal system,* Philadelphia, 1980, Lea & Febiger.)

A tension force can be understood by considering the effect of gravity on the leg of someone sitting in a wheelchair. Gravity will exert a downward force on the lower leg, which is not supported by the seat cushion. When a contracture is present, for example a flexion contracture of the knee, the tension force resulting from the pull of gravity may cause discomfort. Adjustment of the client's position may be required to minimize the effect of gravity on the lower limb.

Compression occurs when forces act toward each other (pushing together), such as the force of the vertebrae on the discs in the spinal column. Compression is the force experienced on skin and other tissues between bony prominences, such as the ischial tuberosities, and the seat cushion.

Shearing occurs when the forces are parallel to each other (sliding across the surfaces). This last force is increasingly recognized as an important cause of pressure ulcers. Shear occurs when the client is transferred from one surface to another or shifts his weight. Older clients with fragile skin may experience skin breakdown easily if they are not transferred with care. Shear forces may also be experienced on the buttocks and lower back when a client is moved into a recline position.

Pressure

Every force is applied over a surface area. **Pressure** is defined as force per unit area, which means that a force applied over a very small area generates more pressure than the same force applied over a larger area. Imagine a 10-pound cat lying on your stomach. The force generated by the cat is applied over the entire surface of its body and the pressure is uniform. Now imagine the same cat standing on your stomach. The force of the cat is the same, but the pressure at each of the cat's paws is much greater (and it hurts more) because the area of application (the paw) is much smaller than when the force is distributed over the whole surface area of the cat. This basic concept of distributing pressure by increasing the area of application is applied extensively in seating and positioning systems.

Newton's Laws of Motion

The English scientist Sir Isaac Newton formulated three laws relating to forces on bodies at rest and in motion. Newton's first law states that a body at rest tends to remain at rest and that a body in motion in a straight line tends to remain in motion, unless external forces act to change either of these states. In other words, a body likes to continue what it is doing, whether moving or resting. This law defines inertia. Newton's second law defines force. Force is equal to mass (in kilograms) multiplied by the acceleration of the object (force = mass × acceleration). This means that the greater the force, the greater the acceleration; or, conversely, the greater the mass for the same force, the smaller the acceleration. Newton's third law states that if one body exerts a force on another, there is an equal and opposite force, called a reaction, exerted on the first body by the second.[30] This law is applied to seating systems with the assumption that every force exerted by the human body while sitting in a wheelchair or seating system is balanced by an opposite force exerted by the sitting surface on the person.[49] The force generated by the body is equal in magnitude and opposite in direction to the force generated by the seating system, a state often referred to as **equilibrium.** When a body is at rest and all internal and external forces are balanced, the body is then in a state of static equilibrium. When forces are balanced around a body during movement, resulting in a constant velocity, it is described as a state of dynamic equilibrium. Both types of equilibrium are important in seating and positioning systems.

Friction

Frictional forces exist between two bodies in contact moving in opposite directions.[49] These forces result in resistance to movement between the two bodies. Two types of friction are defined: static friction and dynamic friction. Static friction is that force that must be overcome to start a body in motion. Static friction is proportional in magnitude to the perpendicular (compression) force holding the two bodies together. Static friction is independent of the area of contact between the two bodies. Once motion is initiated, the resistive force is generally smaller than when at rest, and it takes less force to keep the bodies moving relative to each other than to start movement. Friction during movement is called dynamic friction. Both of these frictional forces are affected by surface conditions such as moisture, heat, texture, and lubricants, and both are important considerations in the recommendation, design, and on-going evaluation of seating surfaces.

Sitting Posture and Center of Pressure

Stability and mobility are two related dimensions of seated postural control. For example, **stability** allows an individual to maintain an upright seated position while mobility allows movement that enables function. **Mobility** allows the individual to lean forward to reach out to shake a friend's hand. Seating interventions for postural control must achieve an optimal balance between stability and mobility.

Two constructs are important to consider when discussing postural control: center of gravity and center of pressure. The location of the center of gravity is fairly well defined in the standing position. Its location is described as passing through the mastoid processes of the jaw, a point just in front of the shoulder, a point just behind the center of the hip joints, a point just in front of the center of the knee joints, and approximately 5 to 6 cm in front of the ankle joints (Figure 4-3). In this posture the pelvis is in a neutral position and there is a natural lordosis of the lumbar spine.[59] The location of the center of gravity in sitting is more difficult to determine, but it is usually considered to be lower, with the buttocks and thighs forming the base of support. The individual must maintain the center of gravity over the base of support to maintain an upright posture in either sitting or standing. Seating interventions for postural control assist the client to keep the center of gravity within the limits of the base of support.

Typically, the center of gravity is defined by its position in the frontal, lateral, and coronal planes. However, in the clinic we are only able to capture the location of the **center of pressure** location in the frontal and lateral planes. This location can be identified and monitored in the clinic by using a pressure mapping system (see Figure 4-16). These systems use various technologies to monitor the pressure between the individual and a support surface (i.e., between the client's buttocks and thighs and the seat cushion). They are most commonly used to show pressure distribution when pressure redistribution cushions are evaluated, so their function will be described in greater detail in that section.

As mentioned previously, the aim of postural control in seating intervention is to provide the client with a functional upright position (i.e., provide enough support to enable her to retain a seated position but also to enable sufficient movement to promote function in sitting). The ideal location of the center of pressure is midway between the ischial tuberosities. Dunk and Callaghan (2005)[14] found that the location of the center of pressure in the frontal plane varied between men and women. They studied various sitting postural parameters of university students engaged in computer activities while sitting on different office chairs. They found that the center of pressure was behind the **center of mass** of the chair (i.e., the point in the object where its mass is concentrated and the object is balanced) for men and ahead of it for women. This finding, although it has not been explored, has interesting implications for seating interventions.

Parkinson, Chaffin, and Reed (2006)[42] describe the **stability zone** or limit, which they define as the balance limits for a person in either sitting or standing. They investigated this idea in a study with persons without a disability. Participants were asked to reach in different directions while sitting unsupported. They were able to reach further in the forward and lateral directions versus reaching backward. The authors' work also suggests that the greater trochanters, age, and hip breadth affect the stability zone. A seat back and laterals or armrests will affect the stability limits in sitting when a seat or wheelchair is used.

The center of pressure is an interesting phenomenon that has been explored recently, primarily in a nonclinical population. The studies described previously suggest that differences exist in parameters related to center of pressure between men and women,[14] body mass, and age.[42] These studies did not include individuals with disabilities, so the implications of the findings to this group are not clear. Further study is needed to explore the relationship between center of pressure and function and the effect of various seating interventions on this relationship.

PRINCIPLES OF SEATING FOR POSTURAL CONTROL

Earlier in this chapter we identified three categories of sitting skills—hands-free sitting, hands-dependent sitting, and propped sitting.[54] These categories are important to consider for seating someone who has a neuromuscular impairment. Someone who can sit without supporting themselves with their hands may only require a seat cushion to allow them to engage in activities while in this position. Someone who is dependent on external support to sit will require more extensive postural support. The aim here is to provide the minimum support that will assist the person to maintain an upright position but not limit their ability to move.

Guidelines for Postural Control

Seating systems designed to assist postural control aim to augment the client's ability to exercise control in this position. The following ideas guide positioning of an individual in a seating system. Box 4-5 lists the main guidelines for positioning for postural control. The most important positioning principle related to postural control is that proximal stabilization, near the center of the body, facilitates movement and control of the head and the extremities (e.g., function). During normal development, the infant achieves stability in the proximal joints (e.g., spine and shoulders) before using the distal limbs (e.g., hands) for manipulation. For example, before a baby can successfully reach out and grab a toy while sitting, he must have mastered the ability to maintain a balanced sitting posture.[4,19,20,47] Otherwise the hands must be used to maintain balance.

When any type of external support is provided, care needs to be taken so that the individual is not excessively restrained. We need to keep in mind that sitting is a dynamic activity. We often associate sitting with relaxation and lack of activity and movement, when in fact many activities are performed while sitting, including writing, driving, talking on the phone, and typing. Even during quiet sitting an individual frequently shifts weight to maintain comfort. It is not uncommon to see individuals with disability "properly" positioned to the point that they are no longer able to use the motor movements they have used in the past to complete functional tasks. The fewest restraints necessary to optimize function should be used.[24] In this section we present a set of general guidelines for positioning a client who uses a seating system.

BOX 4-5 Guidelines for Positioning for Postural Control

1. Proximal stabilization (i.e., a stable pelvis) is important for trunk and head control and use of the upper and lower extremities.
2. Sitting is a dynamic activity. Seating for postural control should enable the client's movement rather than restrict it.
3. The pelvis is a key point of control as its position affects posture in the rest of the body.
4. The lower extremities should be neutral with respect to internal/external rotation, abduction, and adduction.
5. The trunk should be upright and in a midline position (i.e., limited lateral flexion and rotation).
6. The head should also be in a midline position, with neutral neck position (for neck flexion and extension, rotation, and lateral flexion).
7. The shoulders should be down and forward with a neutral position with respect to internal/external rotation and abduction and adduction. Elbows should be supported at about a 90° angle.

Pelvis and Lower Extremities

We have described important ideas such as center of pressure, center of gravity, and proximal stabilization. These ideas are all related to the position of the pelvis, which is a key point of control. Its position affects the posture of the rest of the body. Therefore, alignment and stabilization of the pelvis is normally the first area addressed in positioning an individual. A position with the pelvis in neutral or in a slight anterior tilt is desired.[31] The pelvis should be level and in midline.

Research examining the role of pelvic stability in the facilitation of function supports the assertion of starting with the pelvis when an appropriate seating system in being determined. Two studies investigated the effect of two methods of pelvic stabilization: a regular lap belt, typically using hook and pile fastening, versus a rigid pelvic stabilizer (a sub-ASIS bar in one case and the Embrace™ Pelvic Positioner [Body Tech NW, Mukilteo, WA, www.bodytechnw.com/pelvic_positioners.php] in the second) on function of children with cerebral palsy.[35,45] Both these studies compared daily function, as perceived by the participants and their families, when using the typical lap belt versus the rigid pelvic stabilizer. Results were comparable in both, although better function and greater perceived posture and comfort were found with the rigid pelvic stabilizer compared to the lap belt. The results of these studies are limited by the small sample size, but the similarity of their findings provides evidence for the practice of controlling the pelvis in seating for postural control.

A position with the hips flexed at approximately 90 degrees is recommended for most individuals.[2,54,55] This angle of hip flexion helps to inhibit extensor tone and reduces posterior tilt of the pelvis, thus keeping the individual positioned back in the seat. In some instances it is necessary to increase the amount of hip flexion (thus reducing the angle to less than 90 degrees) to further inhibit extensor tone. Hip flexion is achieved, in part, through the seat-to-back angle of the seating system. It is important to understand here that the seat-to-back angle results in a more acute hip flexion angle; for example, a 95° seat-to-back angle may result in a 90° hip flexion angle, depending on how the client sits in their system.

The most suitable hip angle will have been determined in the mat assessment. The rehabilitation assistant should monitor the effect of pelvis position and hip angle on the client's upper body when positioning them in their wheelchair or other seat. Some individuals with high muscle tone will benefit from a hip angle that is less than 90 degrees to minimize their tendency to extend out of the seat. Others will benefit from a hip angle that is greater than 90 degrees as it will allow them to maintain extension of the spine in order to sit upright.

In some instances 90 degrees of hip flexion is not achievable (because of deformity). Tight hamstrings may prevent achievement of 90 degrees at the knees. Be aware of the effect of musculoskeletal deformities and muscle tone on both function and comfort in the sitting position. Asymmetrical postures that may be present in the pelvis and hips include pelvic obliquity, pelvic rotation, pelvic tilt, and windswept hips. These postural asymmetries are often interrelated. There may be inflexible postures or fixed bony deformities that restrict the mobility of the pelvis and limit the attainment of the recommended pelvic position.

An individual with a **pelvic obliquity** has one side of the pelvis higher than the other when viewed in the frontal plane (Figure 4-4, *A*). The obliquity is named for the side that is lower; for example, with a left pelvic obliquity, the left side is lower than the right. This deformity is often accompanied by **pelvic rotation,** where one side of the pelvis is forward of the other side (Figure 4-4, *B*). **Windswept hip deformity** manifests itself with one hip adducted and the other hip abducted. Often there is a scoliosis of the spine as the body attempts to compensate for the musculoskeletal deformities. The hip on the high side is typically dislocated, and the opposite hip may or may not be dislocated[29] and there may be significant pain with this deformity. When fixed deformities such as these are present, the seating system should be designed to accommodate them rather than to attempt to correct them.[31]

Support to the pelvis can be provided from under, behind, in front, or from the sides. At the very least, a firm seating surface for the individual to sit on will level and stabilize the pelvis. Other technology includes contour of the seat, contour of the back in the lumbar area, lateral support at the level of the pelvis, and sub-ASIS or similar technology at the front of the pelvis. Individuals with moderate to severe neuromuscular involvement typically need more support for stabilization. This support can be provided by contours around the buttocks and up into the lumbar area.

A contoured seat provides additional support in different ways. A preischial block is one option used to control excessive extensor tone (Figure 4-5). With this approach, a cushion is formed with a depression under the buttocks that accommodates the pelvis and limits forward movement. Supports to prevent lateral shifting of the pelvis or external rotation of the hips can be provided either by contouring the seat to provide channels that position the thighs or with some form of lateral support at the pelvic level.

Various types of pelvic positioning belts or bars are used to support the pelvis from the front. The placement of the belt is important to effectively maintain pelvic position. Depending on the person's pelvic mobility, comfort, and positioning needs, the pelvic positioning belt is placed at an angle ranging from 45 to 90 degrees to the seating surface, as shown in Figure 4-6. In most cases, a belt with an angle of pull at 45 degrees sufficiently maintains the pelvis in position. If there is excessive hip extension or a need for anterior pelvic mobility, positioning the belt at a 90-degree angle of pull is more effective.

Pelvic positioning belts can be soft and flexible (e.g., webbing or padded vinyl) or rigid when more support is required. A rigid pelvic positioning device, also called a sub-ASIS bar (Figure 4-7), is typically a close-fitting,

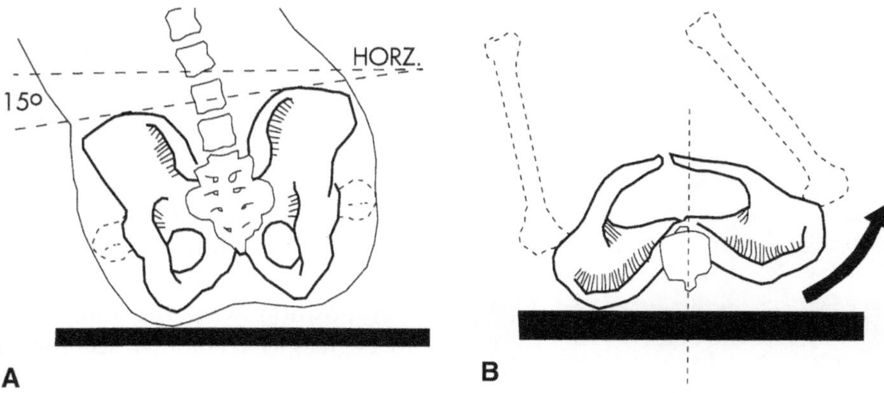

Figure 4-4 **A,** Pelvic obliquity viewed in the frontal plane. **B,** Pelvic rotation. (From Siekman A: The biomechanics of seating: a consumer's guide, *Action Dig* March/April:8–9, 1992.)

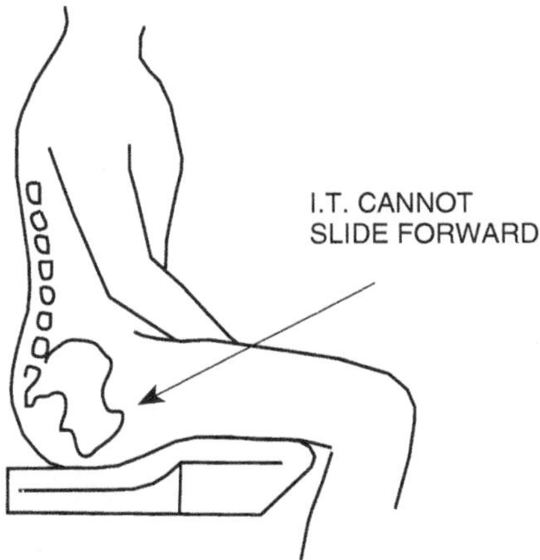

Figure 4-5 Antithrust seat. (From Bergen AF, Presperin J, Tallman T: *Positioning for function: wheelchairs and other assistive technologies,* Valhalla, NY, 1990, Valhalla Rehabilitation Publications.)

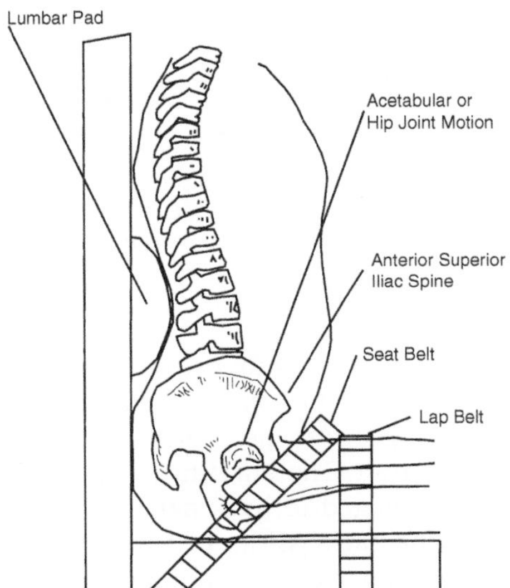

Figure 4-6 Pelvic positioning belts can be applied at 45 degrees (seat belt) or at 90 degrees (lap belt). (From Church G, Glennen S: *The handbook of assistive technology,* San Diego, 1992, Singular Publishing Group.)

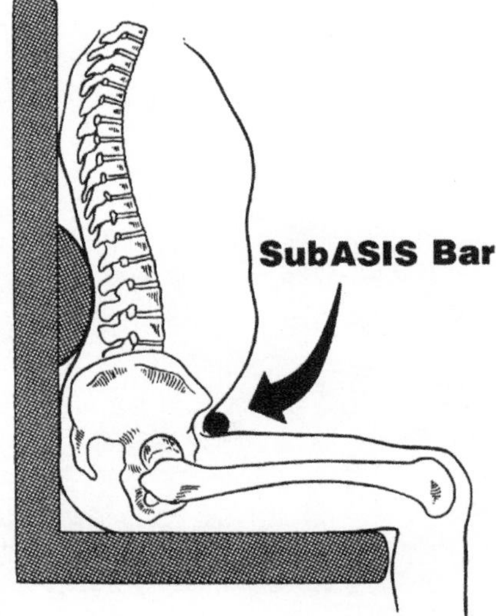

Figure 4-7 Sub-ASIS bar. (From Margolis SA, Jones RM, Brown BE: The subASIS bar: An effective approach to pelvic stabilization in seated positioning, *Proceedings of the RESNA Eighth Annual Conference,* pp 45–47, June 1985.)

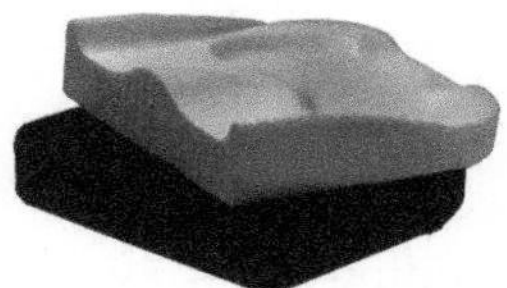

Figure 4-8 Example of sculpted foam cushion to maintain pelvic and femur alignment. (Courtesy of Invacare Corp., www.invacare.ca.)

padded metal bar that is attached to the wheelchair frame or seat insert to position the pelvis below the individual's ASIS. It is designed to be used in conjunction with a complete seat and back system for individuals who require greater control to maintain the neutral position of the pelvis and to prevent pelvic rotation.

Adequately positioning the lower extremities helps to maintain the pelvic and hip positions. It is recommended that the legs be positioned so that the femurs are neutral with respect to abduction and adduction and rotation and with approximately 90 degrees of knee flexion, although there are some exceptions that will be noted below. Some form of sculpting is frequently used in the seat to keep the femurs in a neutral position and to limit adduction and internal rotation (Figure 4-8). A frequently encountered problem in the lower extremities is hamstring tightness, which may or may not result in flexion contractures of the knees. Recall that these muscles are closely related to the position of the pelvis. Attempts to position the individual to stretch these muscles and reduce the flexion contracture can result in posterior pelvic tilt and a sliding forward in the chair into a sacral sitting position. Instead, it is best to accommodate this problem by modifying the seating surface (shortening the seat depth or undercutting the front edge) so that the legs are allowed to flex under the seating surface. This maintains the correct pelvic position.

Support for the feet is important for maintaining hip and knee position, for preventing deformities in the ankles, and for distributing pressure. If the feet are left to hang or are positioned too low, pressure increases under the distal thigh area, which can cut off blood flow. Positioning the feet too high places excess pressure on the ischial tuberosities and the sacrum, which can cause a pressure ulcer. It is recommended that the feet be positioned flat and with 90 degrees of ankle flexion.[31] Support surfaces for the feet can be one or two platforms and come in different sizes, depending on the person's needs. Increasing the thickness of the foot support under the shorter leg serves to accommodate unequal lower leg length. Foot platforms can be angled to accommodate fixed plantar flexion contractures of the ankle. Various strapping systems can be used to maintain the desired

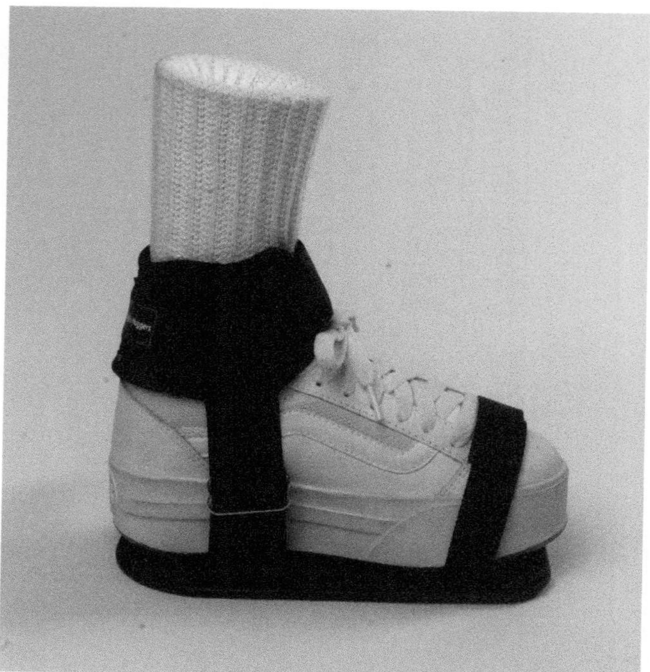

Figure 4-9 Example of an ankle positioning system that attaches to the footplate of a wheelchair. (Courtesy Bodypoint Designs, Inc., www.bodypoint.com.)

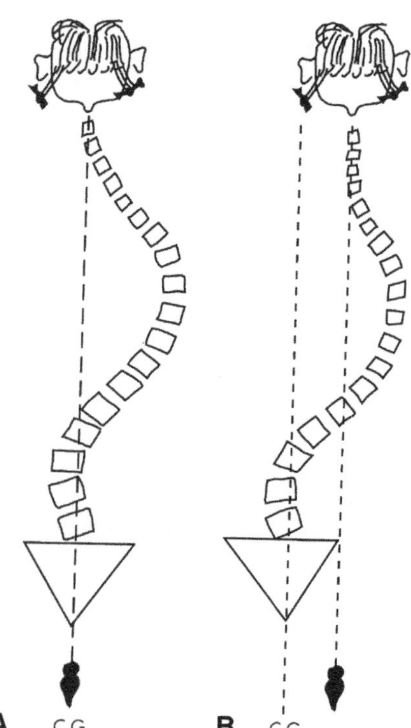

Figure 4-10 **A,** Development of compensatory curve in scoliosis. **B,** Uncompensated scoliotic curve. CG, Center of gravity. (From Cailliet R: *Scoliosis: diagnosis and management,* Philadelphia, 1975, FA Davis Co.)

ankle position, including straps over the top of the foot, behind the heel, and enclosing the ankle (Figure 4-9). These systems are more commonly used with children than with adults. When they are used, it is important to monitor the client to: (1) ensure that the straps are not causing pressure, (2) ensure that they are positioned in the correct location on the client's body, and (3) be aware of any changes in the client's health. For example, an infection might affect muscle tone, thus changing the effectiveness of these devices.

Trunk

Once the desired position in the pelvis and lower extremities has been obtained, the trunk is considered. An upright position with the trunk aligned in midline is desirable. This position may not be attainable if the individual has fixed deformities. Possible spinal deformities are (1) scoliosis, (2) lordosis, (3) kyphosis, or (4) a combination of these. **Scoliosis** of the spine occurs when there is lateral curvature or rotation of the vertebral column. Scoliotic curves are further defined according to the anatomical site in the vertebral column that is involved, that is, cervical, thoracic, or lumbar. Compensatory (or secondary) curves develop as a result of the head's attempting to maintain its upright position (Figure 4-10, *A*).[8] Figure 4-10, *B*, shows an uncompensated curve with the spine unbalanced and the head lateral to the center of gravity. Rotation of the vertebrae is also frequently found in scoliosis and can cause greater respiratory difficulty than lateral curving.[8] A rotary component to the scoliosis causes compression of the chest wall on one side, limiting the ability to fully expand the lung on that side.

The amount of trunk support required depends on how well the client can control their trunk. As in the pelvis, trunk support can be provided from behind, at the side, or in front. The amount of support provided from behind is related to back height and contouring. The height of the backrest can be varied, depending on the amount of upper body support needed. Someone who requires minimal support can use a lower backrest height, whereas a higher backrest is necessary for the individual with a need for greater support. Contouring accommodates the individual's body shape and provides optimal support. If the person has a kyphosis, the back needs to be recessed so that he or she is not pushed forward in the seat. For a lordosis, lumbar support can be added to bring the seat back in contact with the person. In cases where the shoulders are retracted, wedged blocks can be added to the back to position the shoulders forward.

When a person has difficulty maintaining a midline position (side to side) of the trunk, lateral support is provided (Figure 4-11). The positioning of the lateral supports depends on how much control the person has. Lateral supports placed high on the trunk and close to the body provide greater control than those placed lower on the trunk.[31] Because the forces placed on the body by the lateral supports can be great, care should be taken in placement of these components. Laterals should be well padded to prevent tissue damage. If there is scoliosis, the application of force at three positions on the body is one means to attempt to limit the progress of

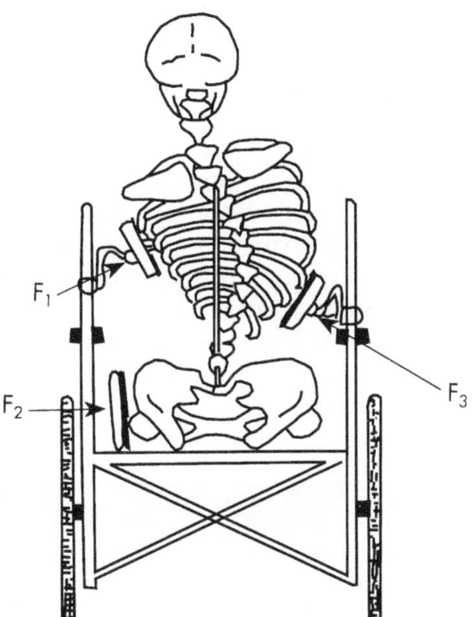

Figure 4-11 Three-point system of control for reducing the effects of scoliosis. (From Nwaobi OM: Biomechanics of seating. In Trefler E, editor: *Seating for children with cerebral palsy: a resource manual,* Memphis, 1984, University of Tennessee.)

the scoliosis, although there is limited evidence to support or refute this use. This three-point system uses the principles of equilibrium of forces to stabilize and align the trunk. As shown in Figure 4-11, one pad is applied under the apex of the curve on the convex side (F_3), with two other pads opposing it to provide resistance (F_1 and F_2). One of these pads is placed up high under the armpit and the other point is on the pelvis.[7,55]

Tilting the seating system back slightly can eliminate some of the effects of gravity for individuals with spinal deformities, low tone, decreased strength in the trunk, or poor head control and can also help the individual maintain a more symmetrical posture. The force of gravity is reduced in the tilt position, making it easier to maintain the trunk in midline and increasing the comfort of the laterals. The positive effects of tilt on trunk position must be evaluated by the limitations this position can place on function. Vision, the ability to eat, use of equipment on a tray, and social engagement are just some activities that can be compromised when the wheelchair seat is tilted.

When control is required to prevent forward trunk flexion, anterior supports can be used. This type of support is necessary for individuals who need to be in an upright position for a functional or therapeutic activity but who do not have the ability to maintain this position independently. The most common approaches used in the seating system are straps, chest panels, and rigid shoulder supports. Tilt-in-space systems for wheelchairs, which also promote an upright trunk position, are described in Chapter 12. One simple approach is to use straps that are attached to the seat back below shoulder level, come up over the shoulders, and attach to the seating system near the hips (Figure 4-12, *A*). The chest restraint must be well maintained because it poses a safety concern if the lower attachment becomes loose and allows the strap to constrict around the neck.[55] Another approach is a solid chest panel in a butterfly, "X," or "I" shape with straps that attach to the seating system as described above (Figure 4-12, *B*). The final approach is to use rigid shoulder components (Figure 4-12, *C*) that come over the clavicle and hold the shoulder girdle back against the seating system. These components should be adjustable and well padded to ensure stabilization without excessive pressure. These last components can be uncomfortable because they provide rigid control of posture. The rehabilitation assistant should monitor the client's tolerance of these devices over several days. Often it is appropriate to combine approaches to control of trunk flexion so the client is more comfortable.

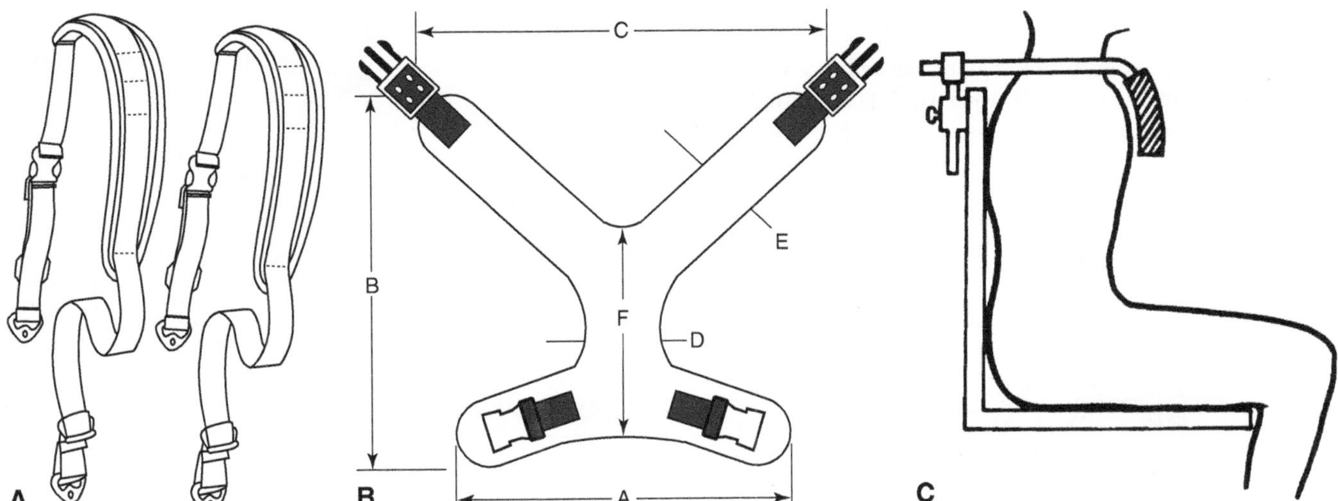

Figure 4-12 A, An example of a chest strap that attaches to the seat back below shoulder level, comes up over the shoulders, and attaches to the seating system near the hips. (Courtesy Bodypoint Designs, Inc., www.bodypoint.com.) **B,** Solid chest panel in an X design. (Courtesy Daher Manufacturing, Inc., www.daherproducts.com.) **C,** Rigid shoulder supports. (From Bergen AF, Presperin J, Tallman T: *Positioning for function: wheelchairs and other assistive technologies,* Valhalla, NY, 1990, Valhalla Rehabilitation Publications.)

Head and Neck

With the pelvis, lower extremities, and trunk positioned, head and neck positions are considered next. The position of the head is important in inhibiting abnormal reflexes and maximizing the visual skills of the individual. In some cases a headrest is necessary only part of the time, when, for example, the individual becomes fatigued or during transportation. The most common problems leading to the need for positioning of the head include hyperextension of the neck, which is commonly seen in individuals with cerebral palsy, weak neck musculature, lateral neck flexion, and neck rotation. In addition, support may be required to right the head to midline when the person has been reclined or the wheelchair is in the tilt position (Chapter 12). As in the positioning of other body segments, posterior, anterior, or lateral components are used for support. Figure 4-13 shows examples of components for each of these types of support. Posterior support can range from a high backrest (for those requiring minimal support) to headrests of different types. With any posterior head support, it is important to avoid triggering extension or pushing the head forward into flexion. Lateral supports can be incorporated into a headrest or be provided as separate components. They can be applied at the temporal area, at the neck, or at the side of the face just in front of the ear. The seating system headrest can be used as a control interface for an augmentative and alternative communication system or for switch use (see Chapter 6 for a more extensive discussion). In this situation it is important to monitor the position of the client's head and the pain or discomfort and fatigue levels while she controls these other devices.

Upper Extremities

Finally, it is time to position the upper extremities. Support of the upper extremities is an essential component of the seating system. A lack of support for the arms can adversely affect head and neck position. Additionally, arms that are left to hang can sustain injury if caught on some object in the environment, in the wheels of the chair, or pinched between the wheelchair and furniture or a wall. The client may acquire a subluxation of the glenohumeral joint of the shoulder if the arm is not well supported. Using an upper extremity support surface, such as a lap tray, helps with positioning of the head and neck, reduces the likelihood of damage to the arms and shoulder joints, and places the hands in a midline position that facilitates bilateral manual activities. The height of the lap tray depends on the needs of the consumer. Commonly the tray is mounted so that it allows the forearms to rest on it with the elbows bent at a 90-degree angle. For individuals with spasticity, a tray mounted higher will help to reduce upper extremity tone.[55] Some individuals do not want a lap tray but still require positioning of the upper extremities. For these situations, individual arm troughs (Figure 4-14) mounted to the armrests of the wheelchair are available that provide channeling and support for the arms.

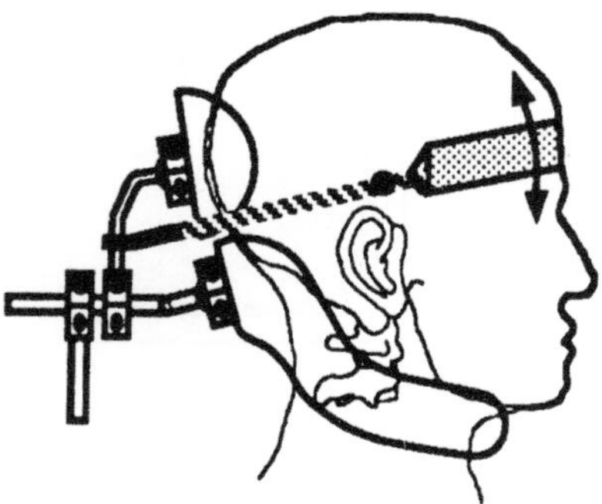

Figure 4-13 Head positioning components include headrest, lateral supports, and headband. One or more of these components are included in head supports. (Courtesy Whitmyer Biomechanix, Inc.)

CASE STUDY – JILLIAN

Jillian is a happy 5-year-old girl with cerebral palsy resulting in severe motor impairment. Jillian is nonverbal and uses a smile or an eye blink to indicate "yes." She is very alert and aware of her environment. She will be attending kindergarten in the fall. She does not have a wheelchair and has never been evaluated for a seating system. Her parents carry her from place to place or use an umbrella stroller for her as needed. She receives therapy with a neurodevelopmental treatment approach three times a week. When they made the initial phone referral, Jillian's parents stated to you that they have put off getting a seating system for Jillian because they did not want her to "look handicapped." With Jillian soon to be attending school, they have decided it is time to get her a wheelchair and seating system. You are the educational assistant in the classroom that Jillian will be attending.

Jillian has mixed tone. Her lower extremities, particularly her ankles, have increased tone. The tone in her upper extremities is increased as well. Her trunk and neck are hypotonic. She exhibits a startle reflex and the symmetrical tonic neck reflex. She does not have any apparent musculoskeletal deformities. She is unable to keep her head up for any length of time unless she is reclined slightly. Jillian can use a switch with her right hand when her head is held upright. She can also use the touch screen on the computer, but she needs help with sitting. Jillian is dependent for mobility and all other functional activities.

QUESTIONS

1. List five factors that might result in increased tone for Jillian while she is engaged in functional activities while seated.
2. From the information you have so far, what might be the goals of seating for Jillian?
3. Describe the ideal position for Jillian to promote function while sitting in the chair.
4. A chest strap and lap belt are used to help Jillian maintain a functional position. Under what conditions would these components be considered restraints? Describe an effective care plan to ensure proper use of these components while Jillian is engaged in educational activities.

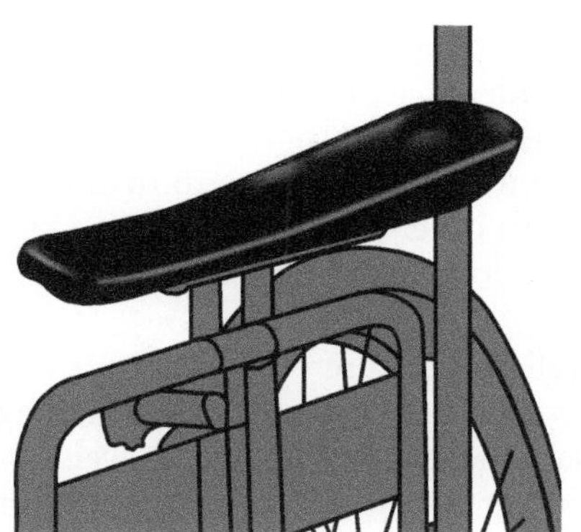

Figure 4-14 Arm trough. (Courtesy Otto Bock, www.ottobockus.com/products/r_wheel.htm.)

PRINCIPLES OF SEATING FOR TISSUE INTEGRITY

A second major goal of seating interventions is pressure management. The emphasis in this area is to manage sitting pressure and maintain the skin in a healthy condition so that pressure ulcers are prevented. A **pressure ulcer** is a lesion that develops as a result of unrelieved pressure to an area that results in damage to underlying tissue.[5] Pressure ulcers usually occur over bony prominences, with the sacrum, coccyx, ischial tuberosities, trochanters, external malleoli, and heels being the areas most commonly affected. These lesions have also been referred to as decubitus ulcers, bed sores, pressure sores, and dermal ulcers. Because pressure is the major factor influencing the development of these lesions, it is recommended that the term pressure ulcer be used to describe them.[39]

Much research has been conducted attempting to determine the various factors that contribute to the development of pressure ulcers and to identify tools and strategies for preventing their occurrence. However, it is difficult to isolate all the variables that affect individuals as they go through their daily lives and then to make substantive conclusions for a population as a whole on the basis of this research. Each person must be considered individually, and a comprehensive program of risk assessment and prevention must be developed to address his or her needs. The rehabilitation assistant needs to be aware of the role of seating, as well as all the other variables, to lower the risk of pressure ulcers.

Incidence and Costs of Pressure Ulcers

Individuals who remain in bed for prolonged periods of time or who use a wheelchair and have limited ability to reposition themselves are at risk for development of pressure ulcers. In particular, individuals with spinal cord injury are at a high risk because they lack sensation and have limited movement below the level of the spinal cord lesion. It is estimated that approximately one third of individuals with spinal cord injury will encounter some type of tissue breakdown during their lifetimes and that approximately 25% of the health care costs associated with the consequences of a spinal cord injury are related to a pressure.[25] Other populations with a high incidence of pressure ulcers include individuals with hemiplegia caused by stroke, multiple sclerosis, or cancer; the elderly; those who have dementia; individuals who have had a femoral fracture; and anyone in a wheelchair who is unable to weight shift independently.

The incidence of pressure ulcers varies across settings. Woodbury and Houghton (2004)[56] found the following incidence rates in Canadian settings: acute care hospital, 25.1%; non-acute facilities such as rehabilitation centers and long term care, 29.9%; mixed health care (acute and non-acute), 22.1%; and community, 15.1%. It is estimated that the cost of treating a single pressure ulcer ranges from $500.00 to $50,000 USD, depending on severity.[43]

In addition to the costs for health care, there are social costs, which have a greater effect on the client and their family.[26] Krouskop et al. (1983) identify these costs as including: (1) time lost from work, which affects the person and his or her family: (2) time lost from school; (3) time away from family, which can affect the person's social development; and (4) loss of personal independence and productivity, which results in decreased self-esteem and self-worth.[26]

Origins of Pressure Ulcers

Many factors contribute to the development of pressure ulcers; these are shown in Figure 4-15. External forces applied to a localized area are considered to be the primary cause. With application of external pressure, the normal flow of blood and oxygen to tissue in that area is reduced. If this situation continues over a long time, changes occur in the tissue cells, and these changes eventually lead to death of the cells. Recent literature suggests that pressure ulcers actually start as a deep tissue injury, developing from muscles out to the surface, rather than the other way around.[17] Individuals who have limited movement and lie in bed or sit in a wheelchair for prolonged periods generate compression forces that

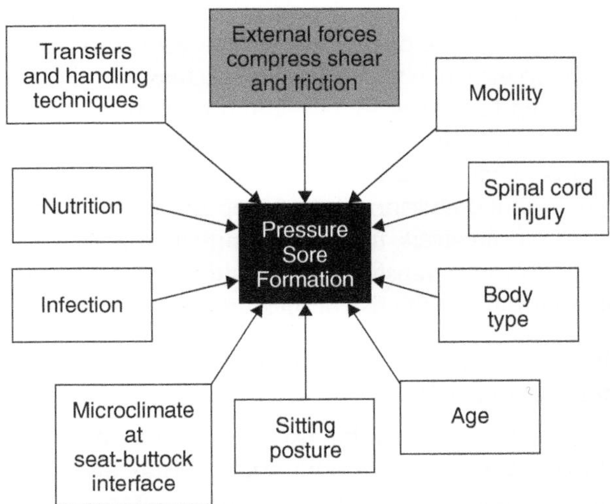

Figure 4-15 Factors that contribute to pressure ulcer development.

reduce the blood supply to the tissues and make them prone to pressure ulcers. Pressure ulcers are most common over weight-bearing, bony prominences because the force at these sites is greater than at other locations covered by subcutaneous tissue.

The amount and duration of pressure sustained are important variables related to the formation of pressure ulcers. Gefen (2009) conducted a review of the evidence on the amount of time required for a pressure ulcer to form from clinical, animal model, and engineering models.[17] He concluded that under sustained high pressure, deep-tissue changes that might ultimately lead to a pressure ulcer were detected in the first hour. Load on the tissue was higher in sitting than in lying, although the time to development of a pressure ulcer was not studied in the sitting position. This information should be considered with caution as newer pressure redistribution technologies were not used in the studies reviewed, so their effect on minimizing the risk of pressure ulcer formation is not known.[17]

Recall the discussion of force earlier in this chapter. The direction and type of force are important elements in understanding how position in sitting and movement during sitting or transferring to other surfaces affect pressure ulcer development. Compression forces are perpendicular to the plane of the body. These are key forces in the development of pressure ulcers in individuals with limited ability to reposition themselves over time. Parallel (or shear) forces play a significant role in the formation of pressure ulcers as well. Shear forces are generated when two surfaces move across each other in opposite directions; these occur, for example, when an individual slides his hips forward in a wheelchair and assumes a sacral sitting posture. In this situation, the superficial structures meet more resistance to movement because they are in contact with the support surfaces of the wheelchair. The deeper structures are more mobile and move forward with the body movement. The resulting position change between these structures may stretch blood vessels, which over time, may become blocked, leading to damage of the deep tissues.

Friction, the force between two surfaces at rest or in motion, is another component of shear and the development of pressure ulcers. Friction leads to injury and ulceration of the surface of the skin. A typical friction injury to the skin occurs when the client moves across a rough surface such as bedding. Moisture, heat, and properties of materials, such as clothing, can increase frictional forces. Friction and these other forces should be considered when transferring the client or assisting them to reposition in the chair. It is vital that caregivers, including family members, are educating on proper transfer and repositioning techniques in order to minimize the risk of pressure ulcer development.

Other Factors That Contribute to Pressure Ulcer Development

Some individuals can be exposed to the mechanical forces of pressure and shear without pressure ulcers developing, whereas others have very little tolerance to these mechanisms. Although compression and shear forces are typically considered to be the chief causes of pressure ulcers, there are several other factors that contribute to skin breakdown and cause some individuals to be more susceptible than others.

Mobility

Moving to relieve pressure over an area is how the body typically responds to prevent tissue damage. Persons without disabilities make side-to-side weight oscillations several times per minute while sitting.[54] Normally, pain signals from nerve endings signal the need to change position. There are two situations when a person does not move in response to body signals to shift position: lack of sensation to detect pain signals and lack of muscle power or control to respond to them. Individuals who have sustained a spinal cord injury or a congenital condition such as spina bifida are included in group that lacks sensation.[10] The latter group is much more diverse and includes individuals who have no or limited movement due neuromuscular or musculoskeletal conditions or frailty. Mobility may also be limited by the client's personal preferences; for example, a client may wish to remain in his wheelchair for much of the day and refuse to be transferred to another support surface (e.g., a bed). In these situations, technology solutions such as cushions, discussed below, or tilt wheelchairs, discussed in Chapter 12, may assist the client to remain in his chair for a prolonged time.

A risk evaluation is important for individuals who have the potential to develop a pressure ulcer. Two commonly used scales that assess these factors are the Norton Scale[40] and the Braden Scale.[3] Box 4-6 shows the components of each of these scales.

BOX 4-6 Common Scales for Assessing Risk of Pressure Ulcer Formation

BRADEN SCALE[3]

Components

- Sensory Perception
- Moisture
- Activity
- Mobility
- Nutrition
- Friction and Shear

First four items scored on a 1–4 scale, last item on 1–3 scale, with higher numbers denoting lower risk. Score of less than or equal to 9 suggests a very high risk.[6]

NORTON SCALE[40]

Components

- Physical Condition
- Mental Condition
- Activity
- Mobility
- Incontinence

Items scored on a 1–4 scale, with a lower number suggesting a higher risk.

Spinal Cord Injury

As discussed previously, loss of sensation and limitations in mobility put individuals with spinal cord injury at great risk for development of pressure ulcers. In addition, some researchers speculate that other changes in the body that result from the denervation caused by the spinal cord injury increase a person's susceptibility to pressure ulcers. There is evidence of a loss of muscle mass following spinal cord injury.[27]

Body Type

The body type of the individual has some effect on pressure distribution. A thin person has less subcutaneous fat to act as padding, and therefore forces per unit area of the skin are increased. However, obese clients may be more susceptible to pressure ulcers since their higher body weight exerts greater pressure on bony prominences when they are sitting.[17] Further, it may be more difficult for the overweight individual to perform pressure relief exercises. Caregivers may also have more difficulty moving an overweight individual, which may make shearing and friction forces a greater possibility.

Nutrition

Inadequate nutrition is often associated with weight loss and muscular atrophy, both of which reduce the amount of tissue between the seat surface and the bony prominences. Inadequate dietary intake, which results in anemia, decreased protein levels, and vitamin insufficiency, is linked with greater risk for pressure ulcer development.[12,15,46] Poor nutrition also affects the normal integrity of the tissue[57] and has been linked not only to pressure ulcer development but also to delayed healing. An increased intake of protein and calories is recommended as part of best practices to enhance healing pressure ulcers.[12,15,46]

Infection

Acute infection may also contribute to pressure ulcer formation.[44] Fever caused by infection increases the metabolic rate, which increases the demand for oxygen, which in turn endangers areas that are ischemic. Second, severe infection can also affect the nutritional balance of the body. Finally, localized bacteria increase the demand on metabolism in the localized area.

Age

As people age, the skin loses some of its elasticity and muscles atrophy, which increases vulnerability to friction or shearing. Vascular and neurological diseases associated with aging (e.g., diabetes or renal disease) affect the circulation and may also increase an individual's susceptibility to skin breakdown. Frail older adults may also have poor nutrition and limited ability to move, which will put them at further risk for pressure ulcer development.

Sitting Posture

Posture and deformity can affect the pressure distribution of the seat/buttock interface and seat/back interface. These situations may contribute to skin breakdown. Two specific postures that pose a risk for pressure ulcer formation are pelvic obliquity and sacral sitting. Pelvic obliquity, which was discussed in detail in a previous section, results in increased pressure and shear under the affected lower ischial tuberosity and the posterior aspect of the lower greater trochanter.[21,58,59] The loss of lumbar lordosis when sitting is another risk factor. This position occurs as a result of limited hip mobility for flexion or decreased spinal mobility for extension.[58] Consequently, a sacral sitting posture is typically assumed, which results in significant amounts of pressure being placed on the sacrococcygeal region.

Microclimate at the Seat/Buttock Interface

The microclimate between the body and the seating surface is a critical factor that is often overlooked. The temperature of the skin and the presence of moisture both affect the formation of pressure ulcers. Moisture, from perspiration or incontinence, also increases the risk of skin breakdown for a number of reasons. Wet skin is weaker than dry skin and therefore more likely to incur damage as a result of compression and friction.[44,57] Additionally, moisture increases the potential for bacterial growth and infection. Keeping the skin clean and dry is important for these reasons.

Transfers and Handling Techniques

Abrasions or ulcerations can be caused by hitting objects (such as wheelchair leg rests or armrests) or sliding across a surface during transfers. Whether the individual transfers independently or has someone providing assistance, care should be taken to prevent abrasions. The same holds true for mobility in bed. Pulling an individual across the bed sheets can cause abrasions or ulcerations from the friction. Caregivers should be reminded to lift an individual to move him or her in bed instead of sliding the individual across the bedding.

The development of pressure ulcers is a complex process, and there is still much to be learned about the exact mechanisms involved. Identifying factors that predispose an individual to pressure ulcers will help in developing a comprehensive pressure ulcer prevention program. A program for preventing pressure ulcers should include (1) a wheelchair and seating prescription for pressure redistribution, postural alignment, and stability; (2) a pressure redistribution program; (3) dietary instruction and adequate nutrition; (4) instruction in proper transferring and lifting techniques; and (5) maintenance of good personal hygiene and skin care.[32,44,46,57] The development and implementation of the prevention program should be considered a continuing team effort involving the consumer, his or her therapists, the rehabilitation assistant, and healthcare personnel. The rehabilitation assistant is frequently responsible for posting the prevention program in the client's room and communicating it with caregivers and staff.

CASE STUDY – LOUISA

Louisa is 82 years old and has multiple age-related impairments, including rheumatoid arthritis, osteoporosis, dementia, and macular degeneration. Because of these impairments, she is quite frail and not very mobile. She frequently indicates that she is in pain. Louisa lives in a long-term care facility. She uses a standard walker for short distances, such as from her bed to the bathroom located in her room. She spends most of her day sitting in wheelchair with a foam seat and contoured back. Staff members often find her sitting slumped in the chair. She propels the wheelchair using her feet. Staff must encourage her to eat at most meals. She is on a high-calorie diet but does not have much appetite. She is able to transfer with minimal assistance but requires physical assistance for dressing, toileting, and bathing. You are a rehabilitation assistant in this facility.

QUESTIONS

1. Which of the pressure ulcer formation risk factors discussed previously do you think are most important to consider? Why?
2. What are the key features of a care plan to minimize the influence of the risk factors you identified above?
3. What key points of information would you include in an educational program for Louisa's family members who regularly assist her with her daily activities?

Pressure Measurement

Attempts to measure force are important to understanding the mechanisms that promote the development of pressure ulcers and to guide clinical decisions regarding seating technology with a goal of redistributing pressure. In the clinic, pressure mapping systems are the primary means of quantifying pressure. These systems quantify pressure at the buttock/seat interface, allowing a comparison among various cushions. The output of these systems is a pressure map that shows pressure distribution at the buttock/seat interface. These maps are analyzed to identify areas of concentrated high pressure, areas where the pressure increases rapidly, and asymmetries in the client's sitting position. Many commercial pressure measurement systems are available. These technologies are constantly improving, but there are concerns about the consistency of the measurements and the lack of agreement concerning best practices for a pressure measurement protocol.

The three most common pressure mapping systems are the Force Sensing Array, F-Scan (Tekscan) and Xsensor (Xsensor Technology Corporation).* Each of these systems uses a flexible matrix of pressure sensors that provide a map of the distribution of pressure at the interface between the seat cushion or back and the client's body. These sensors are arranged in a grid pattern on the pressure mat. The output from each of these systems is generally similar but measurements taken with different systems cannot be compared directly. All the systems provide a visual output (Figure 4-16) that allows a quick inspection of the pressure distribution. The visual output may show pressure distribution with a color display or as peaks and depressions. The actual pressure value for each cell can be displayed as well. The system provides data on peak and average pressure, number of sensors activated, minimum and maximum pressure, and the location of the center of pressure. The breadth of information that these systems provide is both useful and a distraction. Although data showing peak and mean pressure seem easy to interpret, there is little consensus on what is desired pressure at the seat/buttock interface.

The protocol used to obtain and interpret pressure measurements is an important consideration. Work is ongoing to identify a protocol that is generally accepted and used by clinicians globally. Consistency of the setup of the equipment and cushions to be evaluated, an initial check of the equipment, length of recording time, palpation of bony prominences, and documentation will foster more confidence in the conclusions that are made when making comparisons among pressure mapping results across different cushions.[51] Swaine (2006) suggests that interpretation of the results should be based on peak pressure, the area of the client's buttocks that are in contact with the pressure mat, and any asymmetries of pressure distribution. Swaine's work provides a useful basis

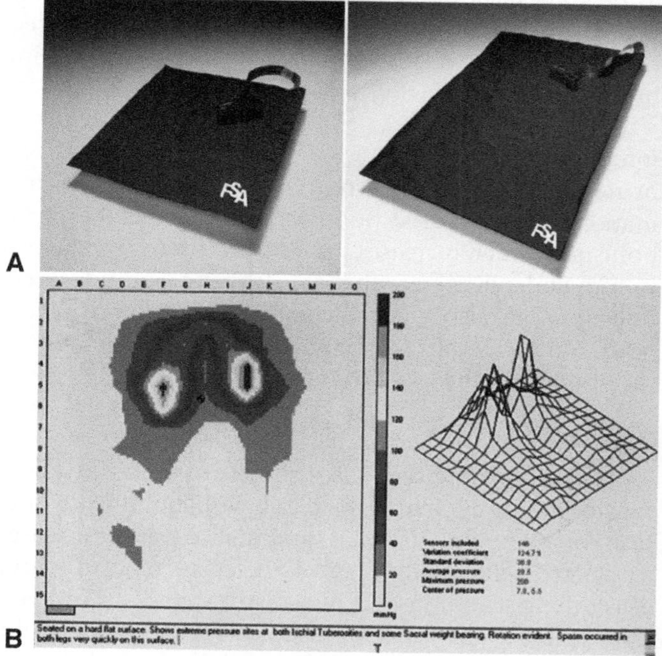

Figure 4-16 Pressure measurement system. **A,** Map with an array of sensors. **B,** Sample display of an individual's pressure distribution profile. (Courtesy www.pressuremapping.com.)

*Vista Medical: www.pressuremapping.com; Tekscan: www.tekscan.com; Xsensor Technology Corporation: www.xsensor.com

for clinicians using pressure mapping as a component of an evaluation to determine the optimal cushion for their clients' needs.[51]

PRINCIPLES OF SEATING FOR COMFORT

This section considers seating and technologies that address seated comfort. There are three distinct populations who can benefit from seating technologies for comfort: (1) wheelchair users who have sitting discomfort and pain (e.g., individuals with post-polio syndrome, amyotrophic lateral sclerosis, and multiple sclerosis), (2) the elderly, and (3) individuals with low back pain. Discomfort in seating can lead to a decreased ability to participate in activities of daily living. In cases of severe discomfort, the individual may be limited to bed rest or time on a mat for some or all of the day, further limiting their ability to engage in desired activities of daily living. There are unique technologies for each of these populations, but the commonality is that they enhance comfort in the seated position.

The current technological approaches to meeting the seating comfort needs of individuals are not nearly as effective as the approaches in the other two categories of need (postural control and tissue integrity). There are a number of reasons for this. One is that equipment that is deemed necessary for comfort typically is not paid for by third-party funding sources because it is not considered a medical necessity. Another reason is that there is very little agreement among researchers on how to define and assess comfort and discomfort.[23] Although much research has been done to identify reliable means to assess comfort, it is a difficult variable to objectively measure because it can be highly subjective and involve multiple factors. A cushion that is described as comfortable by one individual may feel uncomfortable to another. The challenge with measuring comfort has two effects: (1) it is difficult to make an objective determination between seating systems as to which promotes the greatest level of comfort, particularly when the client cannot express their opinion; and (2) outcomes of seating intervention for comfort are difficult to quantify, which makes it difficult to demonstrate the need to fund these technologies, on both an individual and system basis.

Principles related to seating for comfort are not as well defined as those for pressure redistribution and postural control. Discomfort is experienced by those individuals who are not sitting in a well-supported position or who do not have adequate pressure distribution. While healthcare professionals often view postural control or pressure redistribution as the primary reasons for seating system modification, the client most often indicates pain as their reason for seeking changes to their system.[33]

Comfort can be increased by proper positioning, as described in the section on seating for postural control. Here it is important to determine if the client is well supported by the seating system so she doesn't need to use extra effort to maintain an upright and midline position. Monitor the client for fatigue over the course of the day. Ensure that both upper and lower extremities and the head are well supported. When belts, laptrays, sub-ASIS bars, or other straps are used, monitor the client's reaction to them over time and ensure that they are properly adjusted throughout the day.

TECHNOLOGIES FOR SEATING AND POSITIONING MANAGEMENT

There is considerable overlap between the technologies used to address goals related to the seating needs of postural control, tissue integrity, and comfort. Further, many clients require seating that addresses two or more of these needs. Seating technologies in general will be discussed, with identification of their specific application to these goals where appropriate. This section is divided into two components: the design and the construction of the seating system and the properties of the materials used to construct it. The client should be allowed a trial period of use of the system because comfort and functional issues will become evident with use of the system over time. The length of time for a trial period should provide the opportunity for the client to sit in the system for different lengths of time and to engage in a variety of activities in a number of different environments. It is important to include both week and weekend days during the trial in order to capture the client's typical range of activities.

Design and Construction of Seating Systems

The design of the seating system refers to the degree of contouring present in the seat and back and the degree of adjustability that is present in the components. These technologies range from systems that are relatively flat, without any contouring to match the shape of the body segments they support (planar), to custom-contoured systems that are constructed to match as closely as possible the body contours of the user. Prefabricated technologies are available so that the ATP no longer needs to construct the components in the seating system.

Planar

Planar technologies are flat surfaces that support the body only where they easily come in contact with the body, such as at bony prominences. In general, they are appropriate for individuals who require minimal support. Other positioning components can be added to this basic structure if additional support is required. Planar foam cushions, as shown in Figure 4-17, are designed from flat blocks of foam. These foams vary by thickness (up to 4 inches) and density. Cushions are made from a single block of foam or a combination of foams of different thickness and density.[22] For example, a piece of

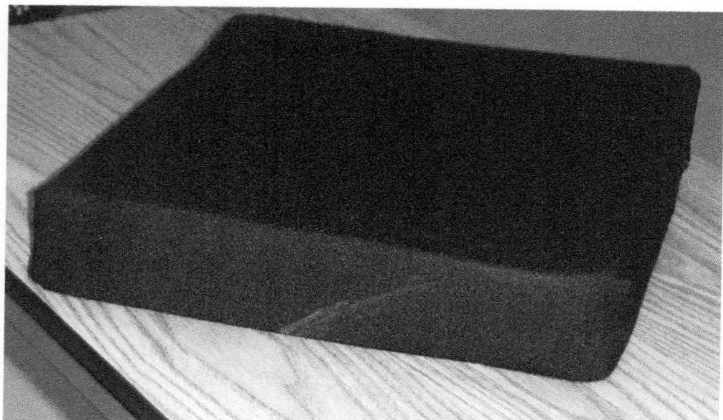

Figure 4-17 Planar foam cushion.

dense foam, 1 to 2 inches thick, might be used as the bottom layer to provide a stable base. A thinner piece of foam placed on top of this layer provides for pressure redistribution. Planar foams can be adapted by cutting out (e.g., under the ischial tuberosities) or building up areas as necessary for pressure distribution or postural management.

Prefabricated

Prefabricated planar components are made in standard sizes to fit a wide range of individuals. The back and seat surfaces are generally plywood or molded plastic pieces to which foam has been attached. Lateral supports and an abductor for pelvic and hip support can be attached with hardware to the basic seat, and lateral supports for trunk stability can be attached to the back section (Figure 4-18).* The seat and back are attached to the wheelchair frame with interfacing hardware once the upholstery has been removed. Much of the hardware that interfaces the various components can be adjusted for angle, width, and depth. The advantage of having adjustable components is that they allow the system to be modified for growth or postural changes.

Custom Fabricated

Custom-fabricated planar systems are made of similar materials and design as prefabricated systems, but the dimensions of the seating surface and components are customized to fit the individual. These systems can be fabricated on site directly with the consumer, or specifications of the consumer's measurements can be sent to a manufacturer for fabrication. The density of the foam pieces can also be selected to accommodate the needs of the individual. Lateral supports, headrests, and other components are added to the basic foam and plywood (or plastic) structure. This approach can be highly labor intensive and is being replaced at many wheelchair vendor facilities as a result of the advent of a large array of off-the-shelf technologies.

*Adaptive Engineering Lab, Inc., *www.aelseating.com*

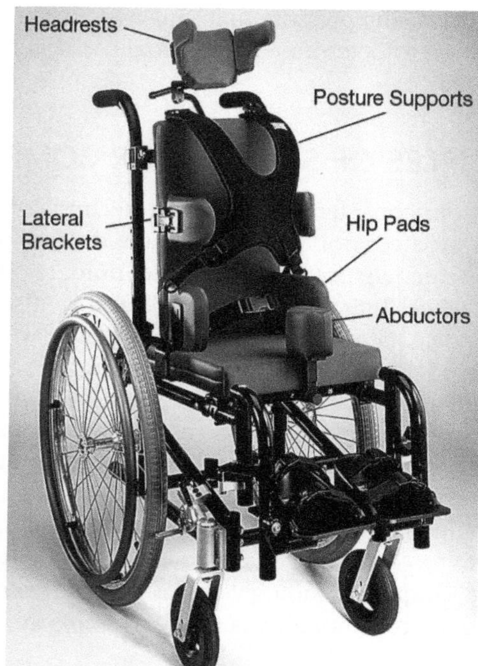

Figure 4-18 Planar seating system with positioning components. (Courtesy Adaptive Engineering Lab, Inc., www.aelseating.com.)

Standard Contoured Modules

Contoured technologies are useful for individuals with moderate seating and positioning needs for postural management or who are at low risk for pressure ulcer development. These technologies use curved surfaces that more closely match the shape of the human body. They provide greater contact with the user's body and thereby provide increased support and control. Many styles of contoured cushions are available that provide a cost-effective means of support for a wide range of individual sizes and abilities. The Matrix is one example of a standard contoured cushion (Figure 4-19).*

Custom Contoured

The cushion that provides the greatest amount of body contact and therefore the most support is one that has been shaped, or custom contoured, to the individual's body. These cushions are much more costly to make and take longer to obtain. The need for these cushions is diminishing as the number of standard contoured cushions increases. A number of technologies are available to achieve a custom-contoured system. One example is shown in Figure 4-20. These types of systems differ primarily in terms of the fabrication techniques used and whether the fabrication is completed on-site or in a central location. The advantages offered by a custom contoured system may be outweighed by the disadvantages, which include the following: (1) transfers to and from the system are more difficult; (2) the system is static and

*Invacare, *www.invacare.ca*

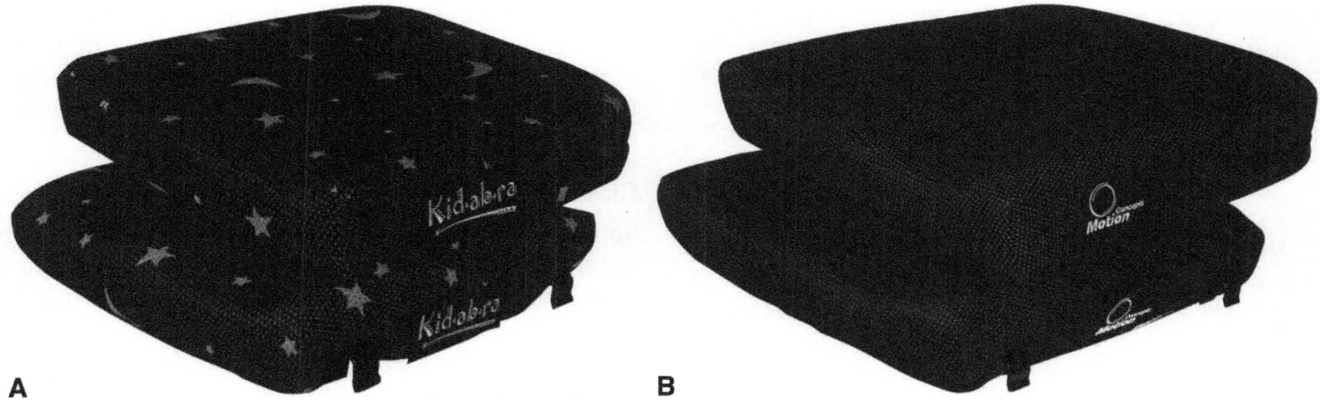

Figure 4-19 Matrix cushion. **A,** Child's version. **B,** Adult version. (Courtesy of Invacare Corp., www.invacare.ca.)

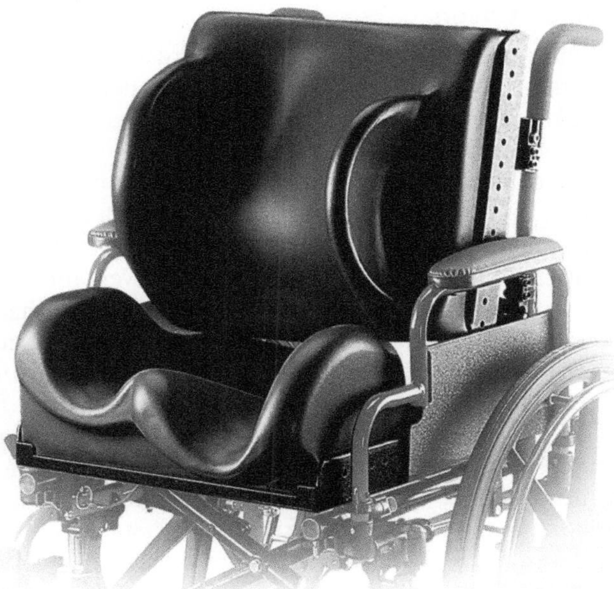

Figure 4-20 Custom-contoured seating system. (Courtesy Invacare Corp., www.invacare.com.)

has no dynamic properties, thus limiting the individual to one fixed position; and (3) there is limited ability within the system to allow for growth of the individual. Box 4-7 summarizes the variety of custom contoured support systems.

Prefabricated Adjustable Backs

Prefabricated adjustable backs have become available in recent years. These products provide a large degree of adjustability that can be accomplished in the clinical setting. The Infinity Back is an example of an adjustable back. The ATP can make adjustments on the basis of an optimal seated position determined by a mat assessment. These backs allow the clinician to adjust the back's height and depth, as well as the width, back angle, and placement of the laterals. Some of these systems allow the ATP to create a biplanar back in which the upper and lower segments of the back are set at different angles. This configuration is often used to provide specific postural control. Although the pivot point can be placed at any spinal level, when

BOX 4-7 Examples of Custom Contour Technologies

FOAM IN PLACE

- Client sits in position of comfort and function in frame with flexible covering.
- Covering is shaped to conform to the client's body contours.
- Foam is added, which expands to match the client's shape.
- Client is transferred from the frame.
- Foam hardens over several hours.
- Once the foam has hardened, further contouring is done by hand.
- When a satisfactory fit is achieved, the foam is covered, attached to a firm base, and mounted on the client's wheelchair.
- This type of contour cushion can be made on-site.

VACUUM CONSOLIDATION

- Client sits in a position of comfort and function on a latex bag filled with beads, which is placed either on their wheelchair or on a fitting chair.
- The bag is then contoured to match the shape of the client.
- A vacuum is used to draw air out of the bag, consolidating the beads.
- The cushion is then made by making a negative and then a positive mold.
- This type of cushion is either made on-site or sent to a commercial manufacturer.

SEATING SIMULATORS

- Client sits in a position of comfort and function in a simulator chair.
- The simulator chair can be adjusted in many ways (e.g., seat depth, width, seat-to-back angle).
- The chair has multiple mechanical plungers, arranged in a matrix, that are positioned to simulate the contours of the client's body.
- A baseline measurement is made of the position of the chair and the plungers without the client seated in it.
- A second measurement is made once the client is properly positioned, the chair adjusted, and the plungers set.

(Continued)

BOX 4-7 Examples of Custom Contour Technologies—cont'd

SEATING SIMULATORS—cont'd

- The difference in these two measures defines the configuration of the seat or back cushion.
- This information, along with any other information regarding foam density, type of foam, and accessories such as laterals or strapping systems, is sent to a commercial manufacturer who constructs the cushion.
- The Shape Sensor system by Invacare (http://www.invacare.com) is an example of this technology.

placed at the level of the posterior superior iliac spine, it can assist with control of the pelvis. Studies have investigated the effect of pelvic stability on function,[35,45] but there have been no clinical studies that have evaluated the effect of this particular back configuration on postural control and, subsequently, function.

PROPERTIES OF MATERIALS USED TO CONSTRUCT SEATING SYSTEMS

Sprigle (1992)[48] identifies and describes five properties of cushion materials: (1) density, (2) stiffness, (3) resilience, (4) dampening, and (5) envelopment. These properties determine how different cushions provide support and how the cushion changes with use.

Density of a material is the ratio of its weight to its volume. A greater density generally means a more durable material, but not always. Low-density materials will fatigue faster than high-density ones under the same loading conditions. **Stiffness** of a material describes how much it gives under load. In a cushion, this is the distance that the person sinks into the cushion. Soft materials may bottom out, leaving the user to sit on the hard base of the cushion. Failure to compress can lead to a loss of contact between the cushion and the user, leading to higher seating pressures and tissue breakdown. **Sliding resistance** is a cushion property related to friction. A cushion with high resistance limits how much the user slides, helping to support upright posture, but consequently makes transfers more difficult.

Resilience is the ability of a material to recover its shape after a load is removed or to adjust to a load as it is applied. Short-term resilience is the immediate recovery of original shape when a load is altered, such as when someone shifts weight on a seat cushion. Long-term resilience is the overnight recovery of a cushion that has been loaded and then unloaded. **Dampening** is the ability of the cushion to soften on impact; it is best observed by dropping a relatively heavy object on the material. If the object sinks into the material, then dampening is occurring. If it bounces off, or if the material does not react to the object, then the material is poorly dampened. This is the "shock absorber" feature of cushion materials and is important in minimizing the transmission of forces from the ground to the individual as they travel over rough surfaces or obstacles. **Envelopment** is the degree to which the person sinks into the cushion and the degree to which the cushion surrounds the buttocks. Good envelopment promotes stability and helps reduce peak pressures. **Recovery** refers to the degree to which a cushion returns to its preloaded state when a load is removed.

Classification of Cushion Technologies

Sprigle, Press, and Davis (2001)[50] describe uniform terminology for classification of the material used to construct wheelchair cushions. They described the following categories of cushions: (1) made from cellular materials, (2) containing fluid, and (3) other constructions. Table 4-1 summarizes the different types of cushion materials, their advantages, and disadvantages[48,50,52]

Cushion Covers

Selection of a cover for a seat or back cushion can be as important as the determination of the material used to make the cushion, because an improper cover can negate some of the benefits of that material. The cover selected should conform integrally to the cushion's contours, particularly in contour systems. It should not interfere with the envelopment properties of the cushion nor add to shearing and friction. A cover that is too tight will prevent the client from sinking into the contours of the cushion. One that is too large will wrinkle, creating additional pressure points.

Cushion cover fabrics vary in their response to moisture. Attention to the condition of the cover is required for clients who are incontinent, perspire excessively, or use their cushion outdoors where it might become wet. Most cushions will be used in hot, humid conditions for at least part of the year, so perspiration is an issue even when incontinence is not a concern. Many technical fabrics, blending Lycra and polyester, wick moisture away from the body. This is an important consideration when prevention of pressure ulcers is a goal. Some covers combine two fabrics, one to wick moisture away from the user and another to prevent moisture from seeping through to the cushion below. The cushion cover should be removable and able to be cleaned.

TECHNOLOGIES THAT INCREASE COMFORT FOR OLDER ADULTS

As individuals age, mobility is often reduced as a result of acute illnesses or trauma, such as stroke, hip fracture, or progressive conditions such as arthritis. Similarly, seniors become frailer with age, becoming more easily fatigued. The amount of time spent sitting or lying increases. In addition, changes in skin elasticity and distribution of adipose tissue raise their vulnerability to pressure ulcers. The goal of seating in this category depends on the individual's needs and skills, as it does for the other categories. Just as there is a range of needs for the elderly population, there is also a range of seating technologies. Seating technologies for the aging population can be matched to the individual's level of functional mobility, whether it is (1) ambulatory; (2) mobile, nonambulatory; or (3) dependent mobile.[16]

TABLE 4-1 Classification of Cushion Technologies*

CUSHIONS MADE FROM CELLULAR TECHNOLOGIES			
Type	Description	Advantages	Disadvantages
Foam	1. Most common material used to make seat back cushions 2. Come in variety of thicknesses and densities	1. Inexpensive 2. Lightweight 3. Compress with weight so have good envelopment	1. Foam that is too soft will "bottom out" so that the client is in contact with the underlying support structure 2. Tendency to trap heat 3. Prone to deterioration with moisture and light 4. Lose resilience over time
Open cell foams	Foams with interconnected, perforated cells that allow airflow (e.g., polyurethane and latex)	1. Open cell foams allow better ventilation 2. Less dense than closed cell foams so they weigh less	1. Absorb moisture, making them difficult to clean 2. Tend to break down quicker than other foams
Closed cell foams	Composed of individual cells encased in a membrane (e.g., ethafoam)	1. Lightweight 2. Easy to shape 3. Provide a good base for other, softer foams	1. Tend to be rigid so don't provide much envelopment, which provides less postural stability 2. Will break down with moisture and heat 3. Airflow is restricted to provide less ventilation
Viscoelastic foam or matrix (Figure 4-21) Examples: Sunmate, T-foam, and Tempur-med	1. Originally developed for space travel 2. Very dense foam that is distinguished by its ability to retain its shape for a length of time 3. Sometimes called "memory foam" 4. Available in different densities	1. Accommodate slowly to a constant load 2. Have "memory" that delays their return to their original shape 3. Provide good envelopment, which provides a stable base for posture 4. Good thermal properties (conduct heat away from the body)	1. Degree of envelopment can increase the sliding resistance 2. Resilience and dampening are variable depending on the density
Flexible matrix (Figure 4-22) Example: Stimulite cushion from Supracor	1. Honeycomb structure composed of thermoplastic material 2. Arranged in layers of interconnected open cells that flex when pressure is applied 3. Available in both planar and contoured versions	1. Conform to user's body providing pressure redistribution 2. Open cells allow airflow for ventilation, limiting accumulation of moisture from sweat or urine 3. Good resiliency	Less envelopment than viscoelastic products

(Continued)

TABLE 4-1 Classification of Cushion Technologies*—cont'd

Type	Description	Advantages	Disadvantages
CUSHIONS CONTAINING FLUID			
Air-Filled (Figure 4-23) Example: ROHO	1. Consists of a sealed receptacle that holds air 2. May be a single compartment or, more commonly, have multiple compartments	1. Good long-term and short-term resilience 2. Pressure distribution properties tend to be good, but dependent on maintenance 3. Many models allow the cushion to be inflated to different degrees, providing pressure redistribution as needed 4. Lightweight materials do not deteriorate over time	1. Must be properly inflated: over-inflation results in poor postural stability and lack of envelopment under-inflation results in "bottoming out" of the cushion 2. Users with poor sensation may not detect inadequate inflation 3. High maintenance, prone to tears and punctures plus need to monitor inflation level
Viscoelastic fluid (Figures 4-24 and 4-25) Examples: Jay cushions, Action cushions	1. Viscosity refers to the degree to which fluid molecules move across each other: low viscose fluids move easily (e.g., water) 2. Most cushion materials in this category have high viscosity	1. Good dampening and thermal properties 2. Provide a stable base	1. Poor envelopment, and poor short- and long-term resilience 2. Affected by temperature—will freeze in cold weather 3. Fluid will shift allowing user to sit on hard surface 4. Require kneading to ensure uniform distribution of the gel

Type	Description	Advantages	Disadvantages
OTHER CONSTRUCTION			
Hybrid cushions (Figure 4-26) Examples: Examples: Otto Bock Cloud, Jay Cushions, Invacare Infinity Cushions	1. Combination of materials described in other categories 2. Most common is closed-cell foam base with membrane that contains gel, viscous fluid, or air on top or inserted into a cutout	1. Good envelopment, thermal properties and pressure redistribution 2. Good postural support	1. Weight varies depending on material 2. Maintenance varies depending on material and configuration of components

* Data from Sprigle S: The match game, *Team Rehabil Rep* 3:20–21, 1992; Sprigle S, Press L, Davis K: Development of uniform terminology and procedures to describe wheelchair cushion characteristics, *J Rehabil Res Dev* 38:449–461, 2001; Tang S: Seat cushions. In Webster JG, editor: *Prevention of pressure sores*, Bristol, United Kingdom, 1991, IOP Publishing.

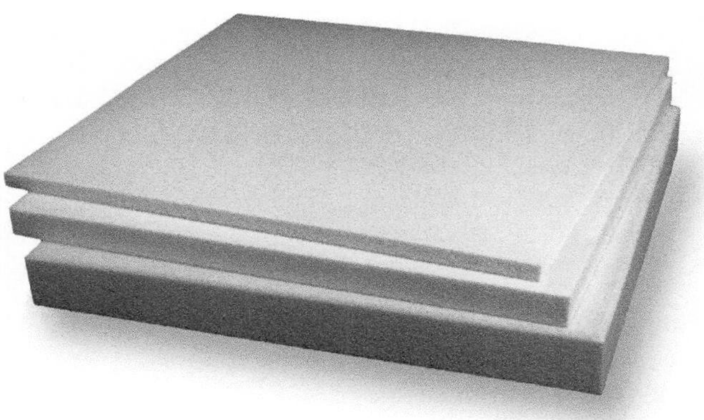

Figure 4-21 Examples of Viscoelastic foams, Sunmate foam. (Courtesy Sunmate, www.sunmatecushions.com.)

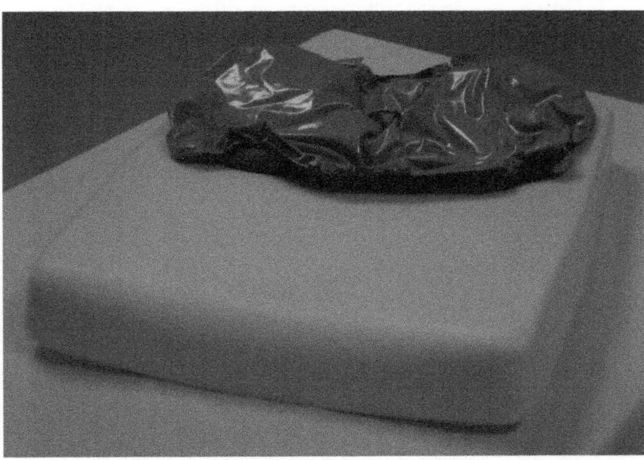

Figure 4-24 Example of viscoelastic fluid cushion, J Extreme. (Courtesy J. Polgar.)

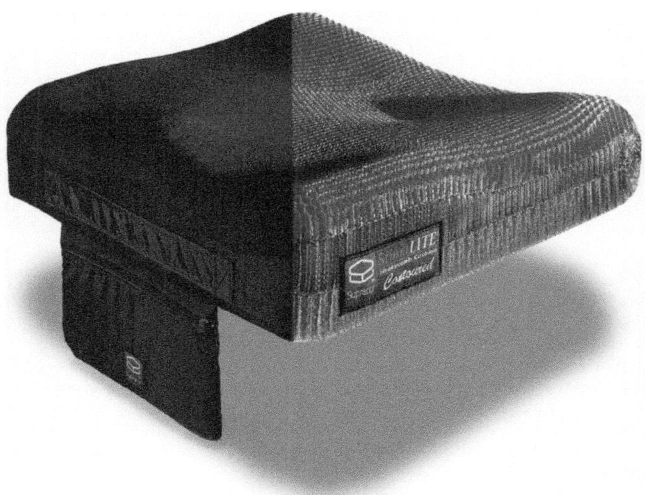

Figure 4-22 Flexible matrix technology, Stimulite cushion. (Courtesy of Supracor Inc., www.supracor.com.)

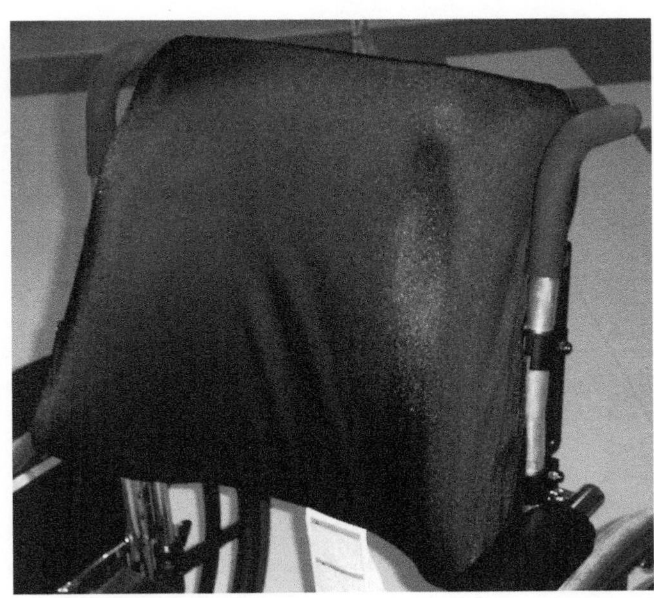

Figure 4-25 Jay back system.

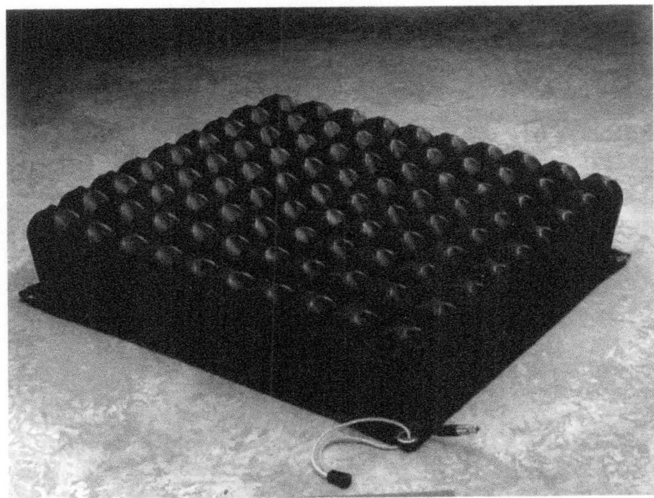

Figure 4-23 The ROHO High Profile air-filled cushion. (Courtesy J. Polgar.)

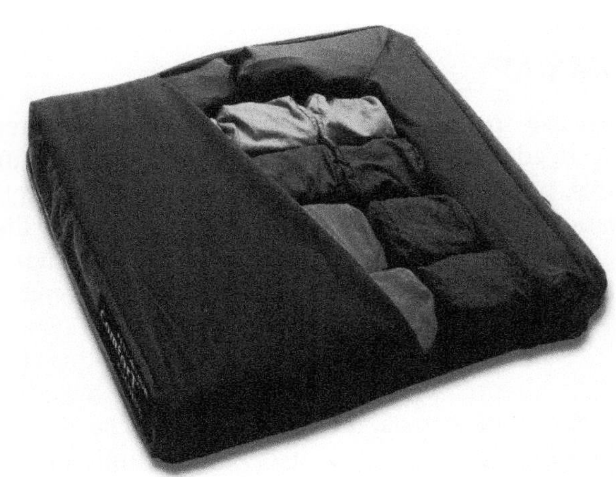

Figure 4-26 Example of a hybrid cushion. (Courtesy of Otto Bock, www.ottobock.com.)

CASE STUDY – CARLOS, MARIE, AND LUCAS

Carlos is an occupational therapy assistant who works in a long-term care facility. An occupational therapist routinely visits the facility and, as part of her consultation, assesses the residents' seating and mobility needs and makes recommendations for wheelchairs and seating devices. Two residents have recently received their new devices and Carlos has been asked to properly position them in their new chairs and seating systems. These devices were provided for the following reasons:

(1) Marie is a 74-year-old woman who sustained a right-sided cerebral vascular accident (stroke) 14 months ago. She has little return of function on the left side of her body, with high tone in her left lower extremity and flaccid tone in the upper extremity. She requires support to maintain a functional sitting position.

(2) Lucas is 69 years old and has had Type 2 diabetes for 15 years. He has a unilateral above-knee amputation on the right side. He is obese, requiring bariatric equipment. He is prone to developing pressure ulcers on his buttocks.

QUESTIONS

1. Describe Carlos' role with each client (a) on receipt of their seating equipment and (b) on a regular, daily basis.
2. What is the primary purpose of seating for Marie?
3. Describe an optimal seating position for Marie.
4. What type of seat cushion do you think would be most beneficial for Marie? What does Carlos need to consider in the regular use and maintenance of this cushion?
5. What is the primary purpose of seating for Lucas?
6. Family members think that a pillow under Lucas' buttocks will reduce the risk of a pressure ulcer. What information should Carlos provide to them about the factors that contribute to the development of a pressure ulcer? What information should he provide them about strategies to minimize the risk of development of pressure ulcers, specific to seating practice?

SUMMARY

Proper use and maintenance of a seating system meets many needs of the user, including effective postural control, pressure redistribution, and comfort. The rehabilitation assistant, occupational and physical therapy team, and family members require information on daily setup and care and long-term maintenance. Box 4-8 provides a tip sheet that summarizes use and care of seating systems that were discussed in this chapter. This chapter provides information on the role of the rehabilitation assistant in assessment of seating and positioning needs. Further, it describes different technologies and principles of positioning for clients of different ages and needs.

BOX 4-8 Tip Sheet: Use and Care of Seating System Components

PRIOR TO ASSISTING THE USER TO TRANSFER INTO THE WHEELCHAIR

- Ensure that the seating system components are properly installed on the chair.
- Make sure that the components are properly oriented—front to back and top and bottom. Sitting on a contoured cushion that is installed backwards is really uncomfortable. Front and back, top and bottom should be marked on each cushion.
- Ensure that all components are properly secured to the chair:
  - Brackets securely fastened
  - Velcro properly attached and still functional
- Check the cover to ensure that it is secure, doesn't have any "wrinkles" in it, and is clean and dry.
- Ensure that peripherals such as headrests are adjusted to the correct height.

ASSISTING THE USER TO BE COMFORTABLY SEATED IN THE WHEELCHAIR

- Help client to sit as symmetrically as possible.
- Ensure there are no wrinkles in the clothing and that the clothing is properly adjusted for comfort and to reduce the likelihood of undue pressure.
- Ensure that all controls (e.g., the joystick) are within the user's reach.
- Check that adjustable features of the wheelchair (e.g., armrests, footrests) are properly positioned.
- Ensure that the wheelchair "restraint system" is secure and in the proper position (e.g., across the lap, not the abdomen, and not causing pressure under the arms).

MAINTENANCE OF THE WHEELCHAIR SEATING SYSTEM

- Air-filled cushions should be properly inflated according to instructions from the ATP; periodically check for leaks in these cushions.
- Ensure that the gel in flowing gel cushions is evenly distributed so the user is not sitting on the base of the seat.
- Cover should be clean and dry.
- Periodically check foam or other materials to ensure that they are still functioning and providing the necessary support for the user.

SPECIAL CONSIDERATIONS

- Gel-filled cushions are affected by temperature so do not expose them to extremes of heat or cold.
- Protect air-filled cushions from punctures by keeping them away from sharp objects.
- Moisture hastens breakdown of foams, so extra care needs to be taken to limit their exposure to moisture (keep waterproof cover clean and replace as needed).
- Be aware that anything placed on top of the cushion (e.g., incontinence pad or sling from transfer aid) will change how the cushion functions in terms of pressure redistribution and support. Whenever possible, avoid putting anything on top of the cushion.

STUDY QUESTIONS

1. Describe the three primary goals of seating intervention.
2. What are the key elements of a mat assessment? Describe each of these.
3. Describe the influence of the physical, sociocultural, and institutional contexts on the design of a seating system.
4. Describe four components of a care plan for restraint use. Describe three alternate strategies to use of restraints.
5. What are the three types of force? Why are they relevant to seating and positioning?
6. Describe the basic premises underlying seating intervention for postural control.
7. Why is the pelvis the starting point when seating for postural control? Describe the major approaches used to obtain alignment and control of the pelvis.
8. List three methods used to support the trunk in postural control seating systems, and describe when each method is indicated.
9. Describe how the head can be positioned posteriorly, anteriorly, and laterally. What factors lead to the use of each of these?
10. What is the major cause of pressure ulcer development? What are other factors that contribute to the development of pressure ulcers?
11. What is a flexible matrix cushion material? What advantages does it have over other approaches?
12. How do viscoelastic, fluid-filled, and foam cushions differ? List an advantage and disadvantage of each.
13. What are the primary populations for whom comfort is the major goal in developing a seating system?
14. Identify the reasons why there are limited technologies available for populations for whom comfort is the major goal.

REFERENCES

1. Bergen AF, Presperin J, Tallman T: *Positioning for function: the wheelchair and other assistive technologies*, Valhalla, NY, 1990, Valhalla Rehabilitation Publications.
2. Bergen AF, Presperin J, Tallman T: Planning intervention, *Team Rehabil Rep* 3:38–41, 1992.
3. Bergstrom N, et al: The Braden Scale for Predicting Pressure Sore Risk, *Nurs Res* 36(4):205–210, 1987.
4. Bertenthal B, Von Hofsten C: Eye, head and trunk control: the foundation for manual development, *Neurosci Biobehav Rev* 22(4):515–520, 1998.
5. Bouten CV, et al: The etiology of pressure ulcers: skin deep or muscle bound? *Arch Phys Med Rehabil* 84(4):616–619, 2003.
6. Braden B: Risk assessment in pressure ulcer prevention. In Krasner D, Rodeheaver G, Sibbald RG, editors: *Chronic wound care: a clinical sourcebook for healthcare professionals*, ed 3, Wayne, PA, 2001, HMP Communications.
7. Buck S: *More than 4 wheels: applying clinical practice to seating, mobility and assistive technology*, Milton, ON, 2009, Therapy NOW! Inc.
8. Cailliet R: *Scoliosis: Diagnosis and management*, Philadelphia, 1975, FA Davis.
9. Centers for Medicare and Medicaid Services (42 CFR 483.13 (a)).
10. Chen Y, DeVivo MJ, Jackson AB: Pressure ulcer prevalence in people with spinal cord injury: age-period-duration effects, *Arch Phys Med Rehabil* 86(6):1208–1213, 2005.
11. Collins LG, Haines C, Perkel RL: Restraining devices for patients in acute and long-term care facilities, *Am Fam Physician* 79(4):254–256, 2009.
12. Consortium for Spinal Cord Medicine: *Pressure ulcer prevention and treatment following spinal cord injury: A clinical practice guideline for healthcare professionals*, 2000 United States Government, Paralyzed Veterans of America.
13. Cook AM, Miller Polgar J: *Cook and Hussey's assistive technologies: principles and practice*, St. Louis, Mo, 2008, Mosby.
14. Dunk N, Callaghan J: Gender-based differences in postural responses to seated exposures, *Clin Biomech* 20(10):1101–1110, 2005.
15. Ferguson M, Cook A, Rimmasch H, et al: Pressure ulcers among patients admitted to home care, *J Am Geriatr Soc* 48:1042–1047, 2000.
16. Fernie G, Letts RM: Seating the elderly. In Letts RM, editor: *Principles of seating the disabled*, Boca Raton, FL, 1991, CRC Press.
17. Gefen A: How much time does it take to get a pressure ulcer? Integrated evidence from human, animal, and in vitro studies, *Ostomy Wound Manage* 54, 2009. Downloaded from http://www.o-wm.com/. January 17, 2011.
18. Geyer MJ, et al: Wheelchair seating: a state of the science report, *Assist Technol* 15(2):120–128, 2003.
19. Hadders-Algra M, Brogren E, Forssberg H: Development of postural control—Differences between ventral and dorsal muscles? *Neurosci Biobehav Rev* 22(4):501–506, 1998.
20. Hadders-Algra M, et al: Development of postural adjustments during reaching in infants with CP, *Dev Med Child Neurol* 41(11):766–776, 1999.
21. Hobson DA: Contributions of posture and deformity to the body-seat interface variables of a person with spinal cord injury. In *Proceedings of the Fifth International Seating Symposium* Memphis, TN, 1989, pp 153–171.
22. Hobson DA: Seating and mobility for the severely disabled. In Smith RV, Leslie JH, editors: *Rehabilitation engineering*, Boca Raton, FL, 1990, CRC Press.
23. Hobson DA, Crane B: *State of the science white paper on wheelchair seating comfort*, February 2001. www.rercwm.pitt.edu/RERCWM_PDF/SoSreport.pdf, May 15, 2001. Accessed March 16, 2005.
24. Kangas KM: Creating mobility within mobility systems, *Rehab Manag* 13(5):58–60, 62, 2000. http://www.rehabpub.com/trehab/672000/3.asp. Accessed October 11, 2006.
25. Krause JS, et al: An exploratory study of pressure ulcers after spinal cord injury: relationship to protective behaviors and risk factors, *Arch Phys Med Rehabil* 82(1):107–113, 2001.
26. Krouskop TA, et al: The effectiveness of preventive management in reducing the occurrence of pressure sores, *J Rehabil Res Dev* 20:74–83, 1983.
27. Lander-Ganz E, Engelberg S, Scheinowitz M, et al: Pressure–time cell death threshold for albino rat skeletal muscles as related to pressure sore biomechanics, *J Biomech* 39(14):2725–2732, 2006.
28. Law M, et al: *Canadian Occupational Performance Measure*, ed 3, Toronto, 1997, CAOT Publications ACE.
29. Letts RM, editor: *Principles of seating the disabled*, Boca Raton, Fla, 1991, CRC Press.

30. Low J, Reed D: *Basic biomechanics explained*, Oxford, 1996, Butterworth Heinemann.
31. Mayall JK, Desharnais G: *Positioning in a wheelchair: a guide for professional caregivers of the disabled adult*, Thorofare, NJ, 1995, SLACK.
32. McDonald H: Preventing pressure ulcers, *Rehab Manag* 14(6):40, 42–46, 2001.
33. Miller WC, Miller F, Trenholm K, et al: Development and preliminary assessment of measurement properties of the seating identification tool (SIT), *Clin Rehabil* 18(3): 317–325, 2004.
34. Miller WC, Mortenson B, Garden J: The WhOM: A client specific outcome measure of wheelchair intervention. In *Proceedings of the Twenty-Second International Seating Symposium*, Vancouver, BC, March, 2006, pp 65–68.
35. Miller Polgar J, et al: Comparison of occupational performance between two methods of pelvic stabilization. In *Proceedings of the Tri-Joint Congress*, Toronto, ON, June, 2000.
36. Miller Polgar J: The myth of neutral technology. In Oishi MMK, Mitchell IM, Van der Loos HFM, editors: *Design and use of assistive technology: social, technical, ethical, and economic challenges*, New York, 2010, Springer.
37. Mills T, et al: Development and consumer validation of the Functional Evaluation in a Wheelchair (FEW) instrument, *Disabil Rehabil* 24:38–46, 2002.
38. Mortenson B, Miller WC, Miller Polgar J: Measuring wheelchair intervention outcomes: development of the Wheelchair Outcome Measure, *Dis Rehabil Assist Technol* 2(5):275–285, 2007.
39. National Pressure Ulcer Advisory Panel: *Statement on pressure ulcer prevention*, 1992. www.npuap.org/positn1.htm, June 15, 2001. Accessed October 10, 2006.
40. Norton D, McLaren R, Exton-Smith AN: *An investigation of geriatric nursing problems in hospital*, London, 1975, Churchill Livingstone (Original work published in 1962).
41. Louise-Bender PT, Kim J, Weiner B: The shaping of individual meanings assigned to AT: a review of personal factors, *Disabil Rehabil* 24:5–20, 2002.
42. Parkinson MB, Chaffin DB, Reed MP: Center of pressure excursion capability in performance of seated lateral-reaching tasks, *Clin Biomech* 21(1):26–32, 2006.
43. Pompeo M: The role of "wound burden" in determining costs associated with wound care, *Ostomy Wound Manage* 47(3):65–71, 2001.
44. Registered Nurses Association of Ontario (RNAO): *Risk assessment and prevention of pressure ulcers (revised)*, Toronto, ON, 2005, RNAO.
45. Rigby P, et al: Effects of a wheelchair-mounted rigid pelvic stabilizer on caregiver assistance for children, *Assist Technol* 13(1):2–11, 2001.
46. Royal College of Nursing (RCN): *Pressure ulcer assessment and prevention*, London, UK, 2000, RCN.
47. Savelsbergh GJP, Van der Kamp J: The effect of body orientation to gravity on early infant reaching, *J Exp Child Psychol* 58(3):510–528, 1994.
48. Sprigle S: The match game, *Team Rehabil Rep* 3:20–21, 1992.
49. Sprigle S: Effects of forces and the selection of support surfaces, *Top Geriatr Rehabil* 16(2):47–62, 2000.
50. Sprigle S, Press L, Davis K: Development of uniform terminology and procedures to describe wheelchair cushion characteristics, *J Rehabil Res Dev* 38(4):449–461, 2001.
51. Swaine J: Seeing the difference, Accessed October 31, *Rehab Manag*, 2006. www.rehabpub/features/112003/4.asp.
52. Tang S: Seat cushions. In Webster JG, editor: *Prevention of pressure sores: engineering and clinical aspects*, Bristol, United Kingdom, 1991, IOP Publishing.
53. Tilly J, Reed D: *Falls, wandering and physical restraints: interventions for residents living with dementia in nursing homes*, Chicago, 2006, Alzheimer's Association.
54. Tredwell S, Roxborough L: Cerebral palsy seating. In Letts RM, editor: *Principles of seating the disabled*, Boca Raton, FL, 1991, CRC Press.
55. Trefler E, Hobson DA, Taylor SJ: *Seating and mobility for persons with physical disabilities*, Tucson, 1993, Therapy Skill Builders.
56. Woodbury G, Houghton P: Prevalence of pressure ulcers in Canadian healthcare settings, *Ostomy Wound Manage* 50(10):22–38, 2004.
57. Wound Ostomy and Continence Nurses Society (WOCN: *Guidelines for preventing and management of pressure ulcers*, Glenview, IL, 2003, WOCN.
58. Zacharkow D: *Wheelchair posture and pressure sores*, Springfield, IL, 1984, Charles C Thomas.
59. Zacharkow D: *Posture, sitting, standing, chair design and exercise*, Springfield, IL, 1988, Charles C Thomas.

CHAPTER 5

Making the Connection: User Inputs for Assistive Technologies

CHAPTER OUTLINE

LEARNING OBJECTIVES

Upon completing this chapter, you will be able to do the following:

1. Describe the elements of the human/technology interface and its role within the assistive technology component of the HAAT model
2. Describe the ways that various anatomic sites can be used to control assistive technologies
3. Identify and define the basic selection methods
4. Describe the means by which the user's physical control can be enhanced
5. Discuss the outcomes that can be achieved through implementation of a motor training program and how technology can be used to improve motor response

KEY TERMS

Abbreviation Expansion
Acceptance Time
Automatic Scanning
Circular Scanning
Coded Access
Control Interface
Control Sites
Direct Selection
Directed Scanning
Group-Item Scanning
Human Technology Interface
Indirect Selection
Inverse Scanning
Linear Scan
Rotary Scanning
Row-Column Scanning
Scanning
Selection Methods
Selection Set
Step Scanning
Word Completion
Word Prediction

The human/technology interface is a major part of the assistive technology component of the Human Activity Assistive Technology (HAAT) model (see Figure 2-5). Bailey (1996)[3] defines an interface as "the boundary shared by interacting components in a system" (p 173) in which "the essence of this interaction is communication or the exchange of information back and forth across the boundary." The **human/technology interface** is the boundary between the human and the assistive technology, across which information is exchanged. In practice, the human/technology interface describes the way in which the human controls the device.

If the individual has good fine motor control, she may use a keyboard and/or mouse to control a computer or assistive technology device. This control would also let her drive a powered wheelchair using a joystick. If another individual has poor fine motor control, it may be necessary to find alternative ways for him to control assistive technologies or mainstream devices, such as computers or cell phones, by using gross motor movements.

In this chapter we discuss the possible movements that can be used to control an assistive or mainstream technology electronic device, and the most common ways of accommodating for lack of motor control.

ANATOMIC SITES FOR CONTROL OF ASSISTIVE TECHNOLOGIES

The *Human/Technology Interface* (HTI) for assistive technologies described by the HAAT model has two major components: the human and the technology (see Figure 2-5).

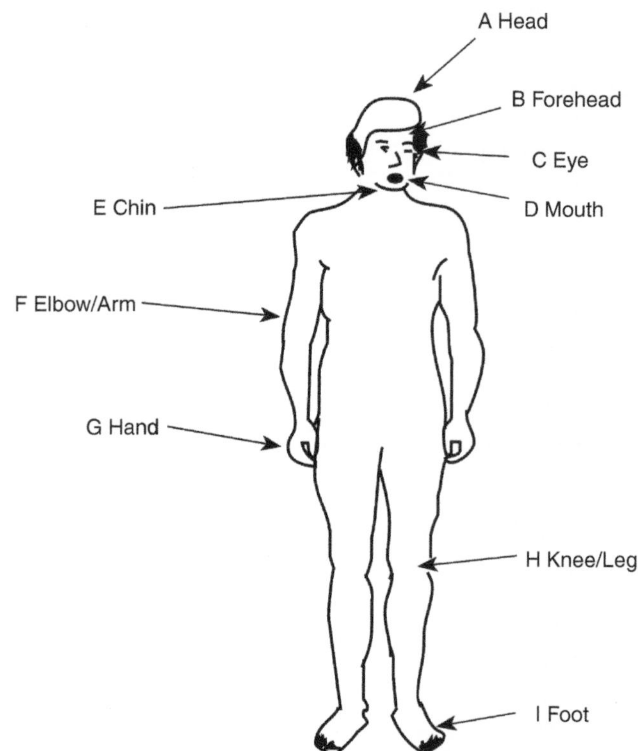

Figure 5-1 Anatomical sites commonly used for control of assistive technologies. (From Webster JW, Cook AM, Tompkins WJ, Vanderheiden GC: *Electronic Devices for Rehabilitation,* New York, 1985, John Wiley and Sons, p 207.)

The human capabilities that are required to use the **control interface** (e.g., keyboard or joystick) are described in this section.

Figure 5-1 shows the body sites that can be used to control a device. These are called **control sites**. Control sites include hand or finger, arm, head, eye, leg, foot, and mouth (for switches based on respiration or phonation). Each control site is capable of performing a variety of movements or actions. When the interaction between a person with a disability and an assistive device involves relatively fine control (e.g., using a keyboard), the hand and fingers are the preferred control sites because they are typically used for manipulative tasks. Even if hand control is limited, there are control interfaces that can accommodate for limitations in fine motor control. It is also possible to improve the existing function by using control enhancers (described later in this chapter).

If fine motor control limitations prevent hand use, then the use of the head as a control site is preferred. Using pointers of various types (e.g., a head pointer) as control enhancers, it is possible to obtain relatively precise control using head movements such as tilting side to side, horizontal rotation, and linear forward and backward movement. Very few functional movements are purely horizontal, vertical, or rotational.

If both hand and head control are poor, then control interfaces—generally switches—can be used to detect movements of the shoulder, elbow, forearm, hand, or finger. The use of the arm or leg is less desirable for precise tasks because these represent naturally gross movements controlled by large muscle groups, and therefore they are less desirable for manipulative functions such as keyboard use. Shoulder movements include elevation, flexion, extension, abduction (away from the body), and adduction (toward the body). The movements of the elbow are flexion and extension. The movements of the forearm consist of pronation (turning the palm down) and supination (turning the palm up). The wrist can flex or extend or move from side to side (radial deviation or ulnar deviation). The fingers can individually flex and extend, or together perform a grasp and release movement. The thumb can flex and extend, abduct and adduct, and oppose each of the fingers. Each of these types of movements can be detected by an appropriate control interface.

Another control site is foot movement. For fine manipulative tasks, the foot is less desirable than the hand or head because visual monitoring can be difficult and the foot is generally not as finely controlled as the hand. However, some individuals are able to develop fine control of the foot for typing (Figure 5-2). Control movements used in the lower extremities include raising and lowering of the leg at the hip (e.g., hip abduction and adduction), knee flexion and extension, foot plantar flexion (toes point down) or dorsiflexion (toes point up), and foot inversion or eversion (rotary movements, similar to pronation and supination). Switches of various types can be controlled by these movements.

Finally, respiratory air flow can be detected and used as a control site by sip (inhaling) or puff (exhaling) switches. *Phonation* may produce sounds (including whistling) or speech. There are control interfaces that can detect sound, and speech recognition can also be used as a control interface. Tongue movements can also be used for control.

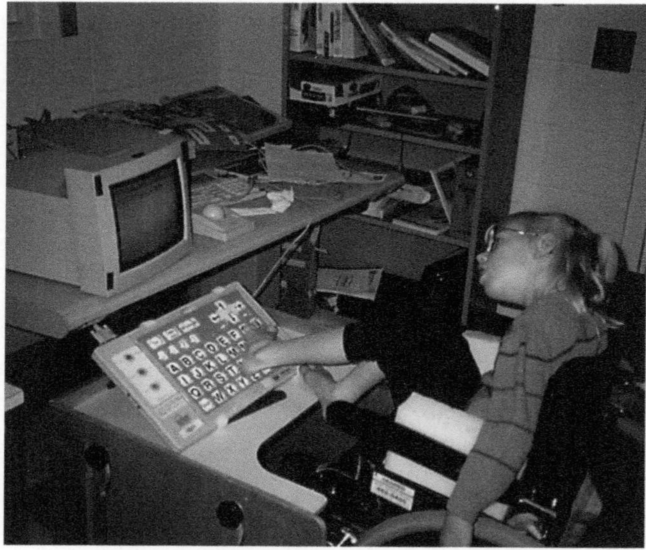

Figure 5-2 Child using her foot to control an expanded keyboard.

CASE STUDY – COMPARATIVE EVALUATION

Max is an 18-year-old male who has cerebral palsy. He lives in a residential facility and attends a work program through United Cerebral Palsy. Max has been referred to ABC Assistive Technology Center for a communication device. He currently communicates with others using a manual communication board and eye blinks for "yes" and "no."

Through evaluation of Max's range and resolution, it has been determined that his best control sites are his right hand and his head. However, he does not have fine enough control at either site to use direct selection. You decide to perform comparative interface testing using a tread switch with his hand and a lever switch at the side of his head. Data collected during the comparative testing phase of the evaluation show that Max is more accurate and faster activating the switch with his head (versus his hand). However, Max has indicated a preference for using his hand instead of his head.

QUESTIONS

1. Given Max's limited verbal communication, how would you gather information from him regarding his opinion on the hand and the head switches?
2. What type of subjective information would you want to gather from Max regarding his use of and preference for each of these two switches?
3. Your data indicates that Max is faster and more accurate using the head switch. However, Max has indicated to you that he prefers the hand switch. What would your recommendation be and why?

CONNECTING THE USER TO THE TECHNOLOGY

There are three technology elements of the human/technology interface that contribute to the operation of a device: the control interface, the selection set, and the selection method. These three elements are interrelated, and careful attention must be given to each element to have an effective human/technology interface.

Control Interface

The **control interface** is the hardware by which the human in our assistive technology system operates or controls a device. It is sometimes also referred to as an *input device*. Examples of control interfaces include a keyboard, one or more switches, a touch screen or touch pad, a mouse, and a joystick.

When the control interface is activated by the user, information is sent via a signal to the *processor*. The processor interprets the information and generates two signals that are converted (1) into feedback to any display that is being used and (2) into an activity output, depending on the functions of the assistive technology system. For example, the power wheelchair (Chapter 12) joystick is typically setup so that the signal for the UP input is transformed into forward movement of the wheelchair, DOWN into reverse movement, LEFT into movement to the left, and RIGHT into movement to the right. That same joystick can be used to control a television set (Chapter 14) in which the same four movements of UP, DOWN, LEFT, and RIGHT control television volume up, volume down, channel up, and channel down. The *selection set* must include an element corresponding to each function of the device.

Selection Set

Each control interface allows the user to choose one or more items that provide input to the assistive technology device or control its operation in some way. The group of items available from which choices are made is called the **selection set.**[11] For example if a person wants to use a power wheelchair, the selection set might be forward, back, left, right, and stop. For typing on a computer with a special control interface, the selection set would be the entire computer keyboard. Selection sets can be represented by traditional orthography (e.g., written letters, words, and sentences), symbols used to represent ideas, computer screen icons, line drawings, or pictures. The modalities in which the selection set is presented can be visual (e.g., letters on the keyboard or icons on the screen), tactile (e.g., Braille), or auditory (e.g., spoken choices in auditory scanning).

The size, modality, and type of selection set chosen are based on the user's needs and the desired *activity output* (see Figure 2-5). Activity outputs in the HAAT model include communication (replacing or augmenting speech or writing), mobility, manipulation (e.g., things we would normally do with our hands and arms) and cognition (assisting with mental activities). An electronic aid to daily living (EADL) (Chapter 14) or a power wheelchair (Chapter 12) typically have fewer choices in the selection set than an augmentative communication device (Chapter 11) or computer (this chapter). The size of the selection set may also vary according to the user's skills and age. For example, an individual who spells and has good physical control has the skills to use the selection set of a standard keyboard, which consists of all the letters and function keys. Another individual who is working on developing language and communication skills may have a selection set consisting of only two picture symbol choices displayed on a lap tray.

Selection Methods: Direct and Indirect Selection

There are two basic **selection methods** that an individual with a disability can use to make selections with a control interface: direct selection and indirect selection. Direct selection methods generally have one interface for each selection that can be made. For example, each letter on a keyboard has a separate key. Indirect selection methods include scanning, directed scanning, and coded access.

Direct selection allows the individual to use the control interface to randomly choose any item in the selection set. The person indicates her choice by using voice, finger, hand, eye, or other body movement. In this method of selection the user identifies a target and goes directly to it.[15] At any one time, all the elements of the selection set are equally available for selecting. Typing on a keyboard or picking a flower from the garden is direct selection. Direct selection is the most difficult method physically because it requires refined, controlled movements. Because there is an immediate, direct result from the selection made, it is more intuitive and easy to understand and the cognitive demands are not great. Figure 5-3 shows the input that is made using direct selection to obtain the letter *S*. The various types of control interfaces that allow the individual to use direct selection are described later in this chapter.

When an individual's physical control does not support direct selection, indirect selection methods are considered. **Indirect selection** involves intermediary steps in order to make a selection. The most common indirect selection methods are scanning, directed scanning, and coded access. Most electronic assistive technology devices can be accessed by more than one type of control interface and selection method. The selection set on most devices also can be varied to match the user's needs. From a manufacturing perspective, the versatility of a device allows it to be applicable to a wider population, which helps to contain the cost of the device and makes it possible to adapt to changing user needs and skills.

Scanning

With **scanning**, the selection set is presented on a display and each item in the selection set is sequentially lighted and/or indicated by sound or speech. When the particular element that the individual wishes to choose is presented, the user activates a control interface to select that item. The control interface used for scanning is typically a single switch or an array of two or more switches. Depending on the needs of the user, scanning can vary in format (i.e., the type of symbols and the way they are presented). The way that the control interface signal is used to make the selection can also vary. Scanning requires good visual tracking skills, a high degree of attention, and the ability to sequence. The advantage of scanning is that it requires very little motor control to make a selection.

Because scanning is inherently slow, there have been a number of approaches used to make it more efficient and faster for the user.[5] The major method for improving scanning efficiency is to use techniques that are efficient in that they allow the user to select groups of entries (e.g., letters) as opposed to entering them singly. Approaches that do this are called rate enhancement and they are discussed later in this chapter.

Directed Scanning

Directed scanning is a hybrid approach in which the user activates the control interface to select the direction of the scan, vertically or horizontally. There is typically one switch for each direction of movement. This is often four directions, but it can be as many as eight. The user first selects the direction in which he wishes to scan. The cursor continues to move in the selected direction by the user holding the switch down. When the switch is released, the cursor stops and the user either waits for an **acceptance time** interval or hits an additional switch. The selected item is sent to the device.

A joystick or an array of switches (two to eight switches) is the control interface used with directed scanning. Figure 5-4 gives an example of the input required to select the letter *S* using directed scanning with a four-position joystick. Directed scanning requires more steps than direct selection but fewer steps than single-switch scanning. The user needs to be able to activate and hold the control interface and to release it at the appropriate time. If the individual can produce the movements required to use this method, the outcome is faster entry of the desired selections into the device.

Selection Techniques for Scanning

The action required by the user to activate the control interface to make a selection during scanning and directed scanning usually can be varied to accommodate the user's skills. Table 5-1 lists the three scanning techniques and the level of motor skill required by each technique. This table is helpful in matching the scanning technique to the

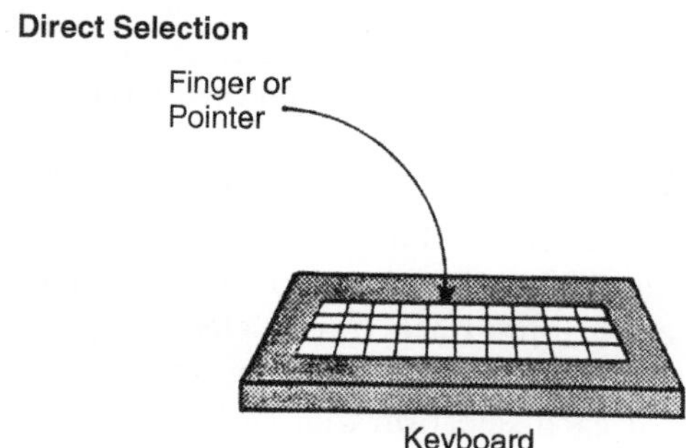

Input	Output
Press S	S

Figure 5-3 This figure shows the input required to obtain the letter *S* using direct selection. (From Smith RO: Technological approaches to performance enhancement. In Christiansen C, Baum C, editors: *Occupational therapy: overcoming human performance deficits*, Thorofare, N.J., 1991, Slack.)

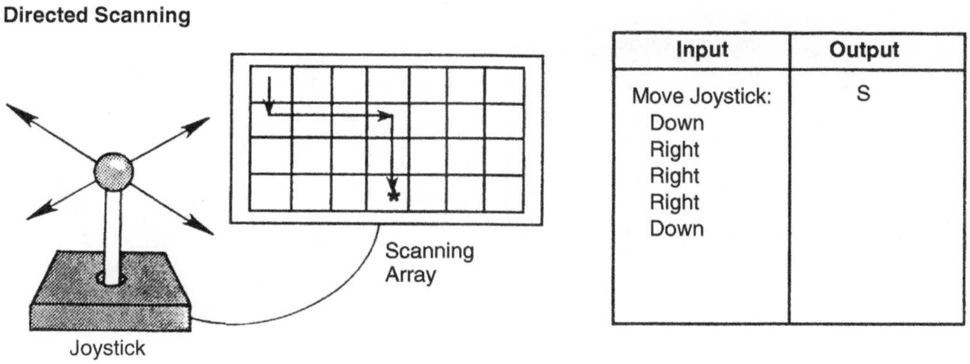

Directed Scanning

Input	Output
Move Joystick: Down Right Right Right Down	S

Scanning Array

Joystick

Figure 5-4 Directed scanning showing the input required to select the letter S. The user selects the direction of the scan and the items in the selection set are scanned sequentially by the device. When the desired item is reached, the user makes the selection. (From Smith RO: Technological approaches to performance enhancement. In Christiansen C, Baum C, editors: *Occupational therapy: overcoming human performance deficits,* Thorofare, N.J., 1991, Slack.)

TABLE 5-1 Importance of Techniques for Scanning and Directed Scanning

	Automatic Scanning	Step Scanning	Inverse Scanning
Wait	High	Low	Medium
Activate	High	Medium	Low
Hold	Low	Low	High
Release	Low	Medium	High
Motor Failure	Low	High	Low
Sensory/Cognitive Vigilance	High	Low	High

Modified from Beukelman D, Mirenda P: *Augmentative and alternative communication,* ed 3, Baltimore, 2005, Paul H Brookes, p 184.

user's skills. For example, some techniques depend more on the ability to react quickly to activate a switch. Others require vigilance and the ability to wait until a choice appears. Still others require the user to hold a switch until the choice appears and then release.

Automatic scanning sequentially presents items that the user may choose. The rate of presentation (scan rate) can be set and adjusted according to how fast the user can respond. When the desired selection is presented, the user selects the choice by activating the control interface and stopping the scan. Automatic scanning requires a high degree of motor skill by the user to wait for the desired selection and then to activate the control interface in the given time frame. It also requires a high degree of sensory and cognitive vigilance for attending to and tracking the cursor on the display.

In **step scanning**, the user activates the control interface once for each item to move through the choices in the selection set. When the user comes to the desired choice, there are two possibilities for selecting it. Either an additional control interface is used to give a signal to select that choice or an acceptance time is used. Step scanning allows the user to control the speed at which the items are presented. The ability to wait is not required for the scan, but it may be for the acceptance of the selection. The ability to activate the control interface repeatedly, however, is important for step scanning. Motor fatigue can be high because of repeated control interface activation.

Inverse scanning is initiated by the individual activating and holding the control interface closed. As long as the control interface is held down, the items are scanned. When the desired choice appears, the individual releases the control interface to make the selection. Inverse scanning requires holding the control interface and releasing it at the proper time. Inverse scanning may be easier for some people than automatic scanning, which requires activation of the control interface within a specified time frame. For individuals who require lots of time to initiate and follow through with movement, inverse scanning can be helpful. Like automatic scanning, motor fatigue is reduced over step scanning because of fewer control interface-activations; however, sensory and cognitive fatigue are higher because of the vigilance required to attend to the display.

Selection Formats for Scanning

There are a number of formats in which the items in the selection set can be presented to the user for selection in scanning (Box 5-1). In a **linear scan** format, as shown in Figure 5-5, the items in the selection set are presented in a vertical or horizontal line and scanned one at a time until the desired selection is highlighted and selected by the user. **Circular scanning** (or, **rotary scanning**) (Figure 5-6) presents the items in a circle and scans them one at a time. Because of the slowness inherent in both these types of scanning, Vanderheiden and Lloyd (1986) recommend that the array be limited to 15 choices.[16]

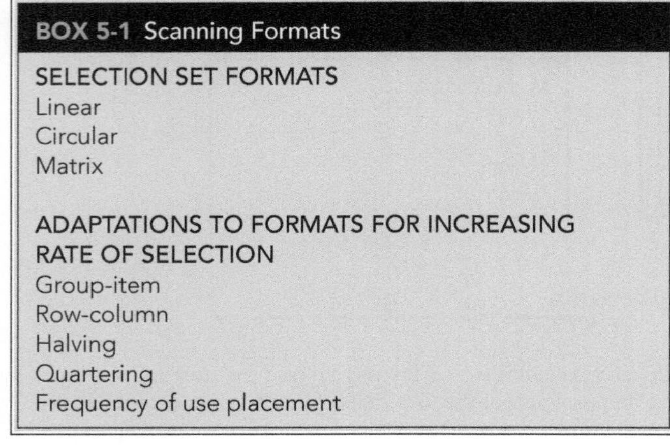

BOX 5-1 Scanning Formats

SELECTION SET FORMATS
Linear
Circular
Matrix

ADAPTATIONS TO FORMATS FOR INCREASING RATE OF SELECTION
Group-item
Row-column
Halving
Quartering
Frequency of use placement

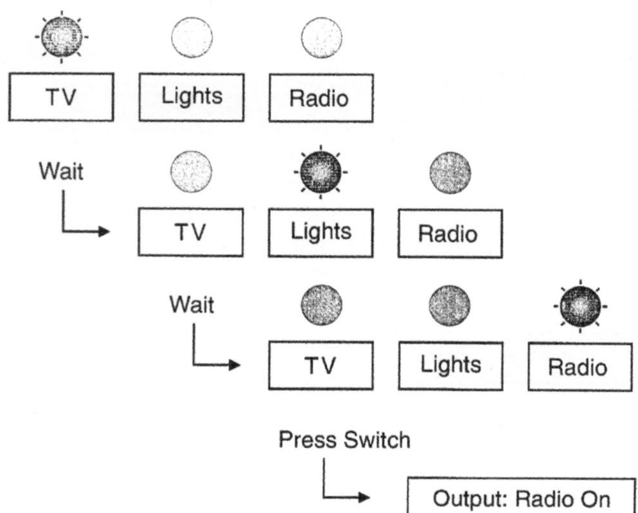

Figure 5-5 In linear scanning, choices are presented vertically or horizontally one at a time.

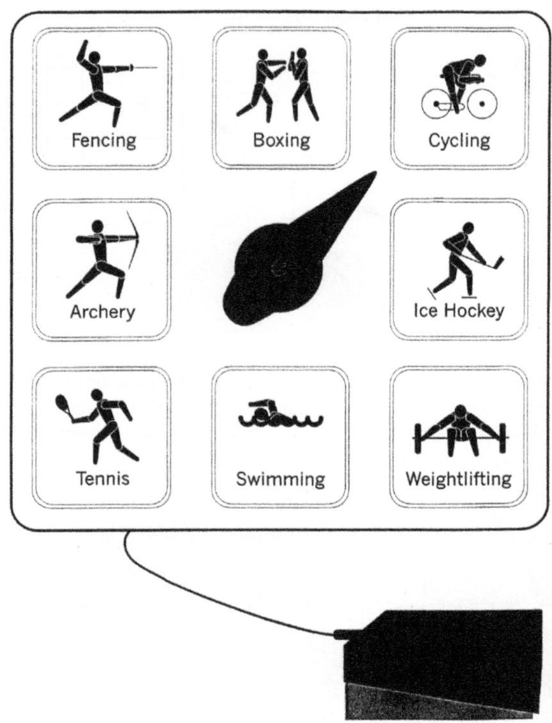

Figure 5-6 In rotary scanning, choices are presented one at a time in a circle.

To increase the rate of selection during scanning, **group-item scanning** can replace the singular-item scan. In this case there are several items in a group and the groups are sequentially scanned as a whole. The individual first selects the group that has the desired element. Once the group has been selected, the individual items in that group are scanned until the desired item is reached. When there are a large number of items, a *matrix* scan can be used. In this type of scanning the *group* is a row of items and the *items* are located in columns; this is called **row-column scanning**. In row-column scanning there may be several rows of items and each complete row is highlighted sequentially. The row with the desired item is selected; then each column in that row lights up until the desired item is selected. Figure 5-7 shows the input required using a single switch with row-column scanning to produce the letter S.

There are other ways that scanning formats can be adapted to increase the user's rate of selection. *Halving* is a group-item approach in which the total array is divided in halves. Each half is scanned until the user selects the

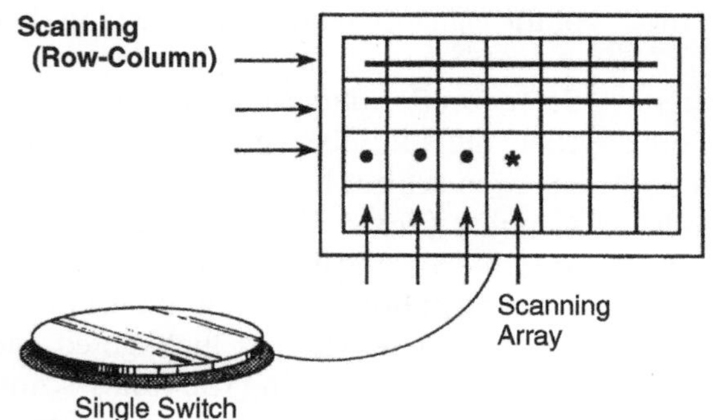

Input	Output
Press Switch Wait Wait Press Switch Wait Wait Wait Press Switch	S

Figure 5-7 Row-column scanning showing the input required for selecting the letter S. The rows are first scanned and the user selects the row with the desired item. Then each item in that row is scanned until the desired item is selected. (From Smith RO: Technological approaches to performance enhancement. In Christiansen C, Baum C, editors: *Occupational therapy: overcoming human performance deficits,* Thorofare, N.J., 1991, Slack.)

desired half. The scanning then proceeds in a row-column format as described above until the desired item is reached. This same concept can be used in a *quartering format,* in which the array is divided into fourths.

Another method used to increase rate of selection is to place the selection set elements in the scanning array according to their frequency of use. For example, if letters are being used as the selection set, placement of *E, T, A, O, N,* and *I* (the most frequently used letters) in the upper left positions of the scanning array results in an increase in rate of selection of about 35%.[16] The application of these principles to augmentative communication is discussed in Chapter 11.

Coded Access

Another form of indirect selection is **coded access**, in which the individual uses a distinct sequence of movements to input a code for each item in the selection set. Like the other two methods of indirect selection, intermediate steps are required for making a selection. The control interface used is a single switch or an array of switches configured to match the code. Morse code is one example of coded access, wherein the selection set is the alphabet but an intermediate step is necessary in order to obtain a letter. Each letter in the alphabet has a code consisting of short (dot) or long (dash) entries. The required sequence of movements for obtaining the letter *C* is dash, dot, dash, dot. Figure 5-8 shows the steps required for obtaining the letter *C* using two-switch Morse code.

In single-switch Morse code the system is configured so that a quick activation and release of the switch results in a dot and holding the switch closed for a longer period before releasing it results in a dash. Letter boundaries are distinguished by a slightly longer pause than between dots and dashes within one letter. As long as the user holds one of the switches it continues to send dots or dashes. In two-switch Morse code, one switch is configured to represent a dot and the other switch a dash. This can make the entry of codes much faster, but it requires motor control sufficient to activate and release a switch quickly enough to avoid extraneous dots or dashes to be entered. The rate at which dots or dashes are repeated is usually adjustable. The computer automatically interprets the code as a letter or other character and treats it as if it had been typed.

Input	Morse Code	Output
Press Switch 1	—	
Press Switch 2	•	
Press Switch 1	—	
Press Switch 2	•	C

Figure 5-8 The input required for selecting the letter *C* by using Morse code.

The user must enter a series of long or short switch presses to access a letter or other keyboard entry (e.g., space bar, number, or special symbol such as $ or #). Morse code was developed to be very efficient by assigning the most frequently used letters the shortest codes, (e.g., *E* is one dot, *T* is one dash). Figure 5-9 shows the symbols for international Morse code. This efficiency can be useful in written or conversational communication. In addition, Morse code does not require that a selection set

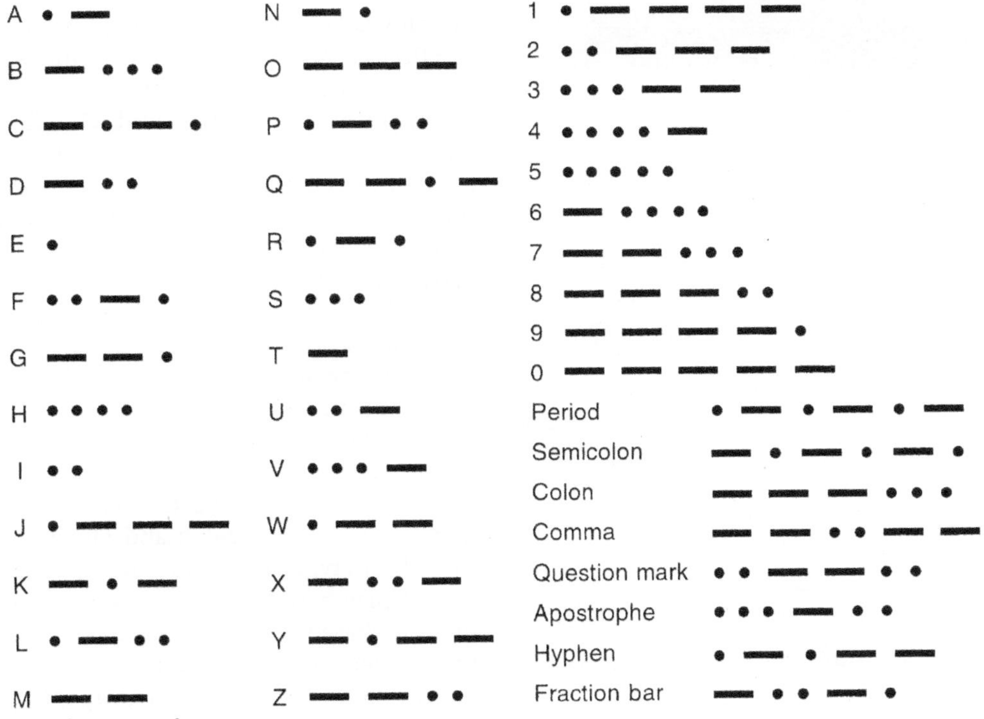

Figure 5-9 International Morse code.

be displayed as in scanning. The codes are usually memorized, although visual displays, diagrams, or charts can be used to aid in recalling the codes (see Figure 5-10).

Like scanning, coded access requires less physical skill than direct selection. The advantage of coded access over scanning, however, is that the timing of the input is under the control of the user and is not dependent on the device. For example, in coded access the user decides how long a dot and dash lasts and how long to hold the switch to generate each one for Morse code, but in scanning she has to wait for the correct choice to be presented, because the device controls the timing. The disadvantage of coded access, however, is that it takes more cognitive skill, especially memory and sequencing, than direct selection.

Because codes are typically memory based, they do not require a selection display (a set of characters on the screen) as is needed for an on-screen keyboard or scanning array. This method allows the entire screen to be used for the application software being run. It can also be used by people who have visual impairments. Original Morse code (letters and numbers only) did not include other computer items such as the ESC or RETURN keys; or characters such as punctuation; or symbols such as "\," "/," "@," "#," "$," or "%." The absence of standardized codes for anything other than alphanumeric characters has resulted in different assistive technology Morse code systems having different codes for these characters. Examples of codes developed for computer use by several different manufacturers are listed in Table 5-2. Note that in some cases the codes for the same characters are different for the three systems and in other cases they are the same. Once the set of codes is learned and the motor patterns developed, it is very difficult to change to a new set of codes; therefore, changing from one system to another can be both time consuming and frustrating for the consumer.

TABLE 5-2 Nonstandardized Morse Codes Used for Computer Access

Character	Kenx*	Darci Too†
ESC	- - -.	..-..
ENTER	.-.-	.-.-
DELETE	..- -..	-..-.
TAB	-.-..-	-.- -.
.	.-.-.-	.-.-.-
!	.-..-	.-..- -
$	.-.-.	-...-.
SPACE	..- -	..- -
,	- -..- -	- -..- -
"	-.- -	- -.- -
(	..- -.	...- -.
)	..-.-	-.. - -.
UP ARROW	- -.- -	- ---..
DOWN ARROW	- -..-	------
LEFT ARROW	- - - -	-----.
RIGHT ARROW	..-..-	- -.-.-.
SHIFT	....-.	..-.-

Note: Standard alphanumeric Morse code characters are shown in Chapter 7.

* Kenx: The product is now available from Able Net http://www.ablenetinc.com/

† Darci Too for Windows-based computers: WesTest Engineering, Bountiful, Utah.

RATE ENHANCEMENT

Rate enhancement refers to all approaches that result in the number of characters generated being greater than the number of selections the individual makes. For example, using "ASAP[space]" for "As soon as possible [space]" saves 16 keystrokes. Because an increased level of efficiency is obtained, the user has to make fewer entries and the overall rate is increased. Rate enhancement goals and approaches differ for direct selection and scanning. In direct selection the goal is to reduce the number of keystrokes while increasing the amount of information selected with each keystroke. In scanning the goal is to optimize the scanning array to reduce the time required to make a desired selection. Specific approaches are discussed later in this section. Rate enhancement is used for many electronic assistive technology applications, including augmentative communication (Chapter 11), computer access (this chapter), and cell phone access and electronic aids to daily living (Chapter 14). Many mainstream software applications employ some form of rate enhancement, also called input acceleration. For example, users of email will be familiar with the list of options that appear after a few letters of an address are typed. These represent the email addresses that the program has "learned" from previous entries. This application had its origin in assistive technology word prediction applications. Similar functionality is present in many cell phones.

Effective rate enhancement requires that the motor tasks become automatic.[4] Motor patterns become more automatic as they are practiced. One familiar motor pattern is that of entering a commonly used phone number. Sometimes we can't actually remember the digits of the number, but we can enter it just by the stored motor pattern. As the skills improve, motor and cognitive tasks become more automatic and the user becomes an "expert." As Blackstone (1990)[4] points out, once these motor patterns are established, even small changes in the task may result in dramatic *decreases* in rate. This effect on efficiency is why it is important to keep menu items or selection set items in the same place even as new items are added.

Rate enhancement techniques fall into two broad categories: (1) encoding techniques and (2) prediction techniques. Vanderheiden and Lloyd (1986) distinguish three basic types of codes: memory based, chart based, and display based.[16] These are compared in Table 5-3. A memory-based technique requires that both the user and his partner know the codes by memory or that the user has the codes memorized for entry into his device. Chart-based techniques are those that have an index of the codes and their corresponding vocabulary items. This can

TABLE 5-3 Modes (Memory, Chart, Display) of Presentation of Codes to the User

Type	Memory-Based	Chart-Based	Display-Based
Memory required	Recall	Recognition	Recognition
Advantages	Can be used by those with visual limitations	Can be seen by both user and partner	Can be updated (dynamic display) giving many stored items
Disadvantages	Limited to 200–300 items for most people	Must have chart in visual field, chart can become separated from device	Requires attention to display, can slow down text selection because of split attention

be a simple paper list attached to an electronic device or a chart on the wall (e.g., two eye blinks = "call nurse"; three eye blinks = "please turn me"; eyes up = "yes"; eyes down = "no"). Figure 5-10 illustrates both a chart-based and display-based approach for Morse code.[16] In each device, two switches are used. The right switch produces dots and the left one produces dashes.

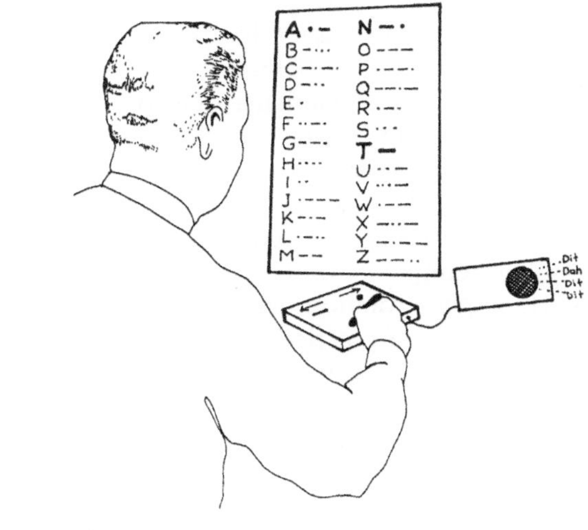

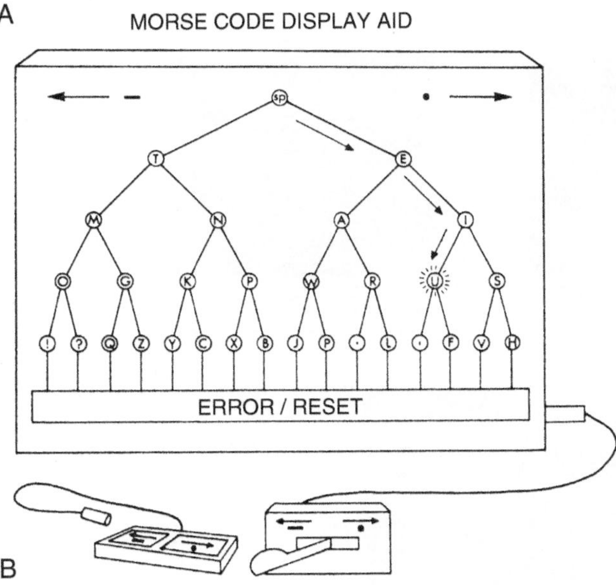

Figure 5-10 Encoding systems may be either **(A)** chart based or **(B)** display based. (From Blackstone S: *Augmentative communication,* Rockville, Md., 1986, American Speech Language Hearing Association.)

Word prediction or **word completion** approaches employ a window on the screen that displays an ordered list of the most likely words based on the letters entered. In word completion, the user selects the desired word, if any, by entering its code (e.g., a number listed next to the word) or by continuing to enter letters if the desired word is not displayed (Figure 5-11). (See Case Study – Word Prediction Vocabularies.) Word prediction devices offer a menu of words based on the previous words entered (e.g., "*computer*" leads to a list of the words "software," "system," "program," and "keyboard"). The most important advantage of this approach is that the user needs only recognition memory, not recall. It also eliminates the need for memorizing codes. Word prediction (or completion) approaches require that the user re-direct their gaze from the input (keyboard keys or scanning array) to a list of words after each entry to check for the presence of the desired word, which can reduce the item selection rate compared to letter-by-letter typing. This reduction in selection rate is due to "cognitive or perceptual load" that can offset the benefits achieved in keystroke savings and can result in an overall decrease in text generation rate.[7] There are also cognitive demands placed on the user by the way in which the rate enhancement is implemented.

CASE STUDY – WORD PREDICTION VOCABULARIES

Assume that one college student is taking a course in assistive technologies and another student is taking a course in world religions. If both students have word completion/prediction systems, compare the word lists you might expect to be used for writing homework assignments for each course. Would most words be the same or would they be different for the two applications? How would the word lists vary in (1) an adaptive system, and (2) a nonadaptive system? What words would you start with as a basic vocabulary in each case?

If the word lists are placed on the screen at the point in the document where the typed letters appear, then the user does not need to redirect his gaze to check the word list while typing. This approach can result in significantly fewer control interface activations in scanning. One application of this approach, called Smart Lists™*, can be used with either keyboard or scanning entry. Smart Keys™† is

(Continued)

CASE STUDY – WORD PREDICTION VOCABULARIES—cont'd

similar to the Minspeak icon prediction (see Chapter 11). After each entry only the keys that contain a prediction based on that entry are left on the on-screen keyboard, which can make scanning significantly faster since only the relevant keys need to be scanned.

Predictive approaches may be fixed or adaptive. Fixed types have a stored word list based on frequency of use that never changes. This method is anticipated and consistent for the user, and can help in the development of motor and cognitive patterns for retrieval. Adaptive vocabularies change the ordering of words in the dictionary list by keeping track of the words used by the person. The words are always listed in frequency-of-use order customized to the individual user and are more directly matched to the user's needs and recent usage.

Current technologies may include combinations of abbreviation expansion and word prediction. **Abbreviation expansion** is a technique in which a shortened form of a word or phrase (the abbreviation) stands for the entire word or phrase (the expansion). The abbreviations are automatically expanded by the device into the desired word or phrase. Abbreviations are more direct, since the user can merely enter the code and immediately get the desired word, and they allow complete phrases and sentences. Predictions are easier to use because they do not require memorization of codes. These two techniques are actually very similar for fixed predictive systems. For example, in Figure 5-11, the entry for "thinking" is the sequence *thi4* (keystroke *t-h-i* followed by the number *4* when the word selection pops up).

*Applied Human Factors, Helotes, TX, www.ahf-net.com

†Applied Human Factors, Helotes, TX, www.ahf-net.com

DEVELOPMENT OF SKILLS FOR THE USE OF CONTROL INTERFACES

Assistive technology provides many individuals who have physical disabilities with their first opportunity to perform a motor act to access communication, mobility, and environmental control. Without these technological options individuals with severe physical disabilities had few or no opportunities to utilize their existing motor movement. For this reason, there are many instances in which an individual may have a control site and the ability to activate a single switch, but the ability to activate this control interface is not consistent enough to justify the purchase of an assistive device such as a wheelchair, computer, or augmentative communication system. The intervention then becomes one of improving the individual's motor control so they will be able to reliably activate the control interface.

Training and Practice to Develop Motor Control

When an individual has limited upper extremity fine motor control, it is necessary to use alternative anatomic sites such as head movement or gross arm, hand, or leg movements. The efficient use of a control interface requires the equivalent of fine motor control regardless of the anatomic site. Because these alternative sites have not been used for fine motor control, a combination of training and practice is required to develop the necessary skills. For example, in order to be effective at activating a switch by head rotation, an individual will need to develop skills through practice. What is initially chosen as the best control site and method for an individual may not necessarily remain constant over time.

An individual may have the prerequisite motor skills to use a specific anatomic site, but lacks sufficient skill to control the recommended control interface. She will

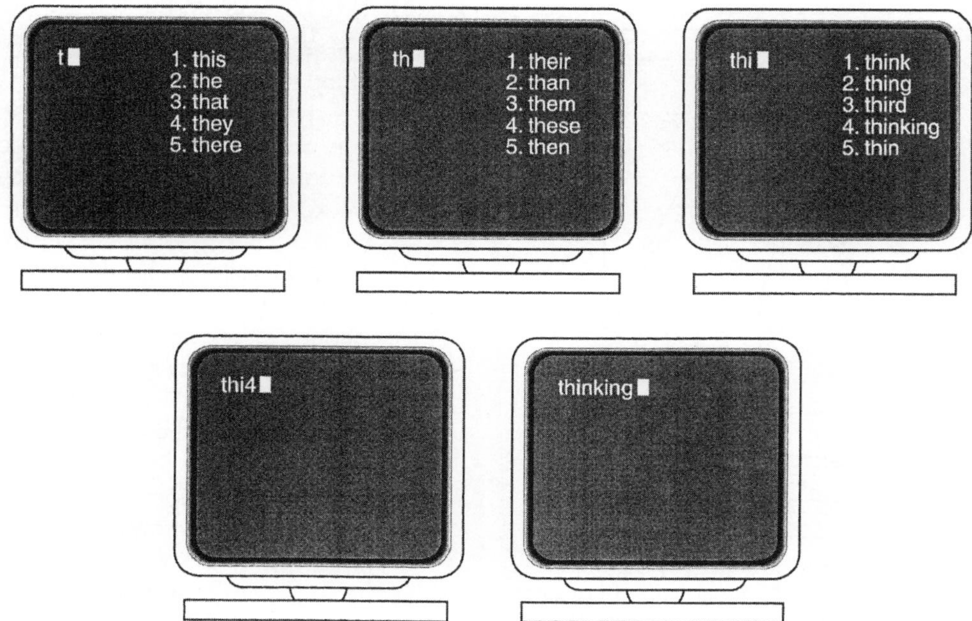

Figure 5-11 Word completion systems present a series of choices based on previous letters entered.

require training to refine her skills. Refining these motor skills may result in an increased rate of input, fewer errors, or increased endurance for using the control. For example, a person may be able to select directly but needs training to learn to use a specific keyboard layout to reduce fatigue or increase speed.

Refinement of motor skills for mouse use, especially if an anatomic site other than the hand and fingers is used, will also require training and practice. There are many software programs available that have been developed to gradually improve a person's ability to use a mouse or an alternative pointing device (see Chapter 7). These programs include activities for developing targeting skills and mastering point-and-click and click-and-drag skills. Use of mechanical and electronic pointers worn on the head typically require substantial training to gradually build the consumer's tolerance and effectiveness in using the control enhancer (see Chapter 6). Similarly, strengthening of the person's existing neck, facial, and oral musculature and a gradual development of tolerance for the mouth stick should take place before having him perform tasks such as writing or typing. Playing simple board games, painting, or batting a balloon are examples of activities that can be used to develop skills for mouth stick or head pointer use. Many games can also be adapted so that a person using a light pointer practices using the interface through play activities.

The developmental of motor skills for the operation of one or more control interfaces can also have carryover into more general motor skill development. Three outcomes can be achieved by a motor training and practice program: (1) the individual can broaden his repertoire of motor capabilities and the number and type of inputs that can be accessed; (2) the individual can refine the motor skills she has in using an interface to increase speed, endurance, or accuracy; and (3) the individual who lacks the motor skill to use any interface functionally can develop these skills.

CASE STUDY – MRS. BENNETT

Mrs. Bennett is a patient at the skilled nursing facility where you work as a rehab assistant (OTA or PTA). She sustained a stroke and has recently been transferred to your facility. In order to get her involved in using her right side, you have been asked to develop a motor training program that will engage her in using a joystick. How would you proceed?

Kangas (1988)[10] recommends that practitioners encourage users to develop a repertoire of control methods, so that they broaden the potential number of devices they can access. For example, if a child who previously used a single switch becomes proficient in the use of a joystick, both these control options can be maintained through different activities. The joystick can be used to play computer games or activate a communication device, and the single switch can still be used to turn on some music. Similar to the concepts presented by Kangas is the *parallel interventions model*,[2,15] which proposes that the individual use an initial switch for accessing a device while simultaneously participating in a motor training program to maximize his ability to operate control interfaces. Broadening the person's repertoire allows access to a greater number of devices and may allow the user to lessen her reliance on assistive technology. For example, after a period of training, the user may be able to progress from using a single switch to a switch array or from an expanded keyboard to a standard keyboard.

Developing Scanning Skills

In Table 5-4 we list four steps that can be used to develop motor skill sufficient for scanning control of an assistive device (e.g., a communication device, computer access, or an electronic aid to daily living). The steps in Table 5-4 are only strategies intended to meet short-term objectives. The long-term goal is participation in an activity using assistive technology. Research on scanning has resulted in useful information regarding training and practice (Box 5-2).

Scanning requires cognitive skills that are not intuitive, especially for a person with significant motor limitations. The cognitive skills required are causality, ability to wait, vigilance to the task to be ready when the desired choice is presented, and reaction time to respond quickly enough to select the desired item. If an individual has difficulty with scanning, it can be challenging to determine if the difficulty is due to motor limitations or cognitive understanding of the task. Therefore the systematic

TABLE 5-4 Sequential Steps in Motor Training for Switch Use

Goal	Tools Used to Accomplish Goal
1. Time-independent switch use to develop cause and effect	Appliances (fan, blender) Battery-operated toys/radio Software that produces a result whenever the switch is pressed
2. Time-dependent switch use to develop switch use at the right time	Software that requires a response at a specific time to obtain a graphic or sound result
3. Switch within specified window to develop multichoice scanning	Software requiring a response in a "time window"
4. Symbolic choice making	Simple scanning communication device Software allowing time-dependent choice making that has a symbolic label and communicative output

BOX 5-2 Research on Scanning

Piché and Reichle (1991)[14] identified these steps for teaching scanning in either manual (i.e., "no-tech") or technologically assisted systems:

- Selecting a signaling response
- Learning to use the signaling response conditionally (i.e., to indicate an item)
- Learning to use the signaling response with a larger array of items
- Learning to use the signaling response in different types of arrays (e.g., vertical, horizontal, row/column, or circular)

Jones and Stewart (2004)[9] surveyed 56 OTs and SLPs who were experienced in teaching scanning to determine how they carried out this training. This study yielded four themes:

- The process of training scanning is progressive and parallel.
- Clients must be considered on an individual basis when developing a training program. Training scanning is inextricably linked to functional goals.
- It is important to train both the child and the primary care givers using a collaborative approach.

They also found that:

- Parallel training was often used, with the OT using scanning games on the computer and other activities and with the SLP developing scanning skill on an AAC device. This is especially true when a new mode or device was added to an existing, effective mode.
- A general progression from linear to row column takes place by using branching arrays.
- OTs were involved in all phases of scanning training, with the SLPs being more involved in later stages.

Adapted from Dowden P & Cook AM: Choosing effective selection techniques for beginning communicators. In Reichle J, Beukelman D, Light J, editors: *Exemplary practices for beginning communicators,* Baltimore, 2002, Paul H Brookes (pp 395–432).

BOX 5-3 Tips for Preparing a Learner for Motor Skill Development

Before engaging the learner in early scanning activities, make sure that:

- there is at least one comfortable position for an engaging activity
- an appropriate control site and switch have been identified for learner's motor control
- the switch is well-positioned and stable
- movement to activate the switch is easy for the learner
- the learner's switch activation is nearly 100% accurate upon stimulus/cue without scanning
- the scanning method matches the learner's motor patterns (see Table 5-1)
- the initial scan speed is 1.5 times the learner's reaction time[12]
- the learner is not rewarded for inappropriate activations (e.g., during stimulus)
- there are empty spaces (foils) in the scanning array in addition to targets
- the scanning pattern is simple: either linear or circular
- the presentation of the options is highly salient to the learner[13]
- the cue/stimulus should be in the same modality as the selection set items (e.g., for visual scanning, the cue should be visual, for auditory scanning, the stimulus should be audible)
- use natural cues and prompts rather than unnatural ones such as "Hit the switch now"
- for visual scanning, be sure the learner is able to look at the display continuously
- the feedback upon selection is salient and reinforcing[13]

Adapted from Dowden P, Cook AM: Choosing effective selection techniques for beginning communicators. In Reichle J, Beukelman D, Light J, editors: *Exemplary practices for beginning communicators,* Baltimore, 2002, Paul H Brookes (pp 395–432).

approach (see Table 5-4) starts with evaluating *cause and effect* and providing training at that level as needed. Cause and effect refers to the ability of the individual to understand that he can control things in his environment and can make something happen. It encompasses the prerequisite skills of attention and object permanence. The individual must be able to attend to and be aware of his environment and the permanence of objects in that environment. Information can be gathered on the individual's ability to understand cause and effect through the use of a single switch.

Some tips for preparing for this type of training are shown in Box 5-3. At the first step in Table 5-4, the goal related to assistive technology use is for the individual to be able to activate the switch at any given time and associate the switch activation with a result. The individual is asked to use a control site to activate a single switch that is connected to some type of reinforcer. The OTA or PTA can provide initial information on what the individual enjoys and finds reinforcing. Objects that can be adapted for switch input and that may be of interest include battery-operated toys, a radio, a blender, or a fan. The child shown in Figure 5-12 is using a switch with a battery-operated toy as the reinforcer. Typically the individual who is aware that she has generated an effect will show some type of response, such as smiling, crying, or looking toward the reinforcer. Computer software programs that provide interesting graphics, animation, and auditory feedback each time the switch is activated can be used as an alternative type of reinforcement. Individuals of all age groups find the programs enjoyable.

At the second step in Table 5-4, the goal is for the individual to activate his switch consistently at a specific time. Vigilance, the ability to wait, and the ability to activate the switch at the correct time are important at this step. With some computer games the individual needs to activate the switch for an object to move or to carry out an action such as shooting a basket, hitting a target, and so

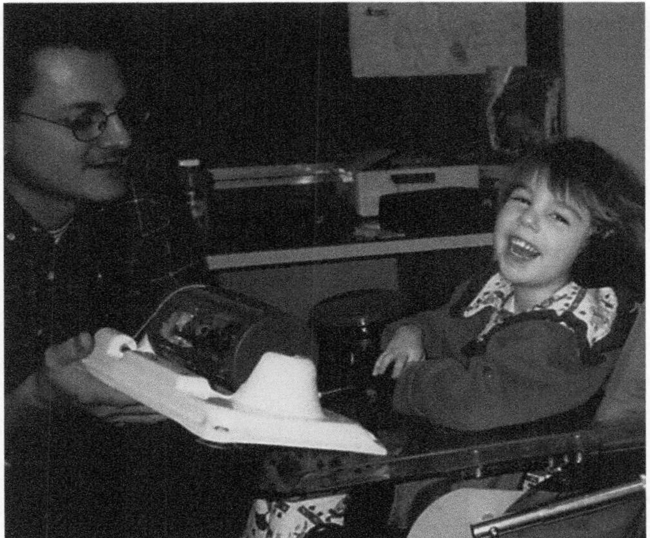

Figure 5-12 Child using a single switch with a battery-operated toy as a reinforcer.

BOX 5-4 Tips for Teaching Scanning

The following tips can be used while teaching early switch control to emerging communicators:

- Cues to the AAC user should always be natural environmental cues; for example, silence in the middle of a song. Using explicit commands such as saying "Hit the switch" will keep the learner dependent on that prompt and impede learning.
- The learner must not repeatedly or continuously activate the switch in anticipation of the right moment. This would prevent him/her from learning to wait for the right moment (and later from using a cursor in scanning).
- It is unfair to expect communicative use of the switch/selection method before ensuring that the individual has reliable control (operational competence) over the interface itself.

From Dowden P, Cook AM: Choosing effective selection techniques for beginning communicators. In Reichle J, Beukelman D, Light J, editors: *Exemplary practices for beginning communicators*, Baltimore, 2002, Paul H Brookes (pp 395–432).

on. With some programs, as long as the individual successfully activates the switch, the movement of objects on the screen speeds up.

Linda Burkhart* has many suggestions for computer-based and non–computer-based activities that can be used for motor training. One suggestion for a non–computer-based activity is to use a battery-operated toy fireman that climbs a ladder as long as the switch is activated. To make this a time-dependent activity, a picture of a reinforcer is attached somewhere along the ladder, and the individual is asked to release the switch to stop the fireman at that picture to receive the reinforcement.

The third step of the scanning training program adds a "time window" and the individual is asked to use the switch to choose from two or more options. The skills involved at this stage include vigilance, waiting, and reaction time as in step two. The additional required skill is the understanding that a choice is only available during a "window" in which the item to be selected is highlighted. Toys, appliances, and computer software programs can also be used at this stage.

The goal is to gradually increase the number of choices from which the individual is to select. The increase in the number of choices is important if scanning is to be used for communication or environmental control. One approach is to highlight locations on the screen in sequence. When the switch is hit on a highlighted item, the program provides an interesting result. In some programs the highlighted areas can be limited so that only one is correct, which helps the consumer develop scanning selection skills in the absence of language-based tasks.

The final training phase shown in Table 5-4 is intended to add communicative intent to the task. At this stage the cognitive skill of symbolic representation is added to the choice making. Development of the individual's language skills may have been taking place in parallel with the motor skills training (Box 5-4), and this linguistic step may follow naturally. The amount of training required for successful use is also generally greater for children who have disabilities than it is for typically developing children or adults. A summary of research that is relevant to the development of motor skills for assistive technology use is shown in Box 5-5.

Selection of symbol systems is discussed in Chapter 11. Through this phase the individual makes the transition from object manipulation (environmental control) to concept manipulation (communication). Greater resources are available at this stage to convey needs, wants, and other information. Simple scanning communication devices or multiple choice computer programs can also be used for further skill development as a precursor to a scanning communication device.

*See also: www.lburkhart.com

SUMMARY

In this chapter we have defined the elements of the human/technology interface and their relationship to the other components of the assistive technology. The elements of the human/technology interface include the control interface, the selection method, and the selection set. The selection set encompasses the items in the array from which the user can choose. There are two basic methods by which the user makes selections: direct selection or indirect selection. Indirect selection encompasses a subset of selection methods known as scanning, directed scanning, and coded access. Each selection method applies to a different set of consumer skills. The development of motor and cognitive skills for scanning requires a thoughtful and well-designed approach.

BOX 5-5 Research on Developing Motor Skills for Assistive Technology Use

1. Jagacinski and Monk (1985)[8] evaluated the use of joysticks and head pointers by young non-disabled adults. The task involved moving from a center point to one of eight lighted targets as fast as possible. The skill in using these devices for this task was acquired with some difficulty over many trials. Based on a criterion of less than 3% improvement in speed over 4 consecutive days, proficient joystick use required 6 to 18 days and head pointer use required 7 to 29 days of practice for young non-disabled, highly motor-skilled participants.
2. Jones and Stewart (2004)[9] surveyed 56 occupational therapists (OTs) and Speech Language Pathologists (SLPs) experienced in teaching scanning to determine how they carried out this training. They indicated that:
   - The time taken to achieve reliable results varies widely among children.
   - Most children received parallel training from an OT using scanning games on the computer while developing scanning skills on a communication device.
   - OTs were involved in all phases of scanning training, with the SLPs being more involved in later stages.
3. Angelo (2000)[1] reported 9 essential elements of a single switch assessment as identified by experienced occupational therapists: reliability of movement, volitional nature of movement, safety, easily performed movement, use of activities in which learners participate regularly, efficiency of movement, previous successful movements, ability to perform a timed response within a time frame, and time required between switch activations is appropriate to the child's reaction/response time.
4. Cook and Polgar (2008)[5] found that speed of response and accuracy of response are often used to compare control interfaces. *Speed of response* is a time-based measurement that is related to reaction time. *Accuracy of response* is often based on moving to the correct position, and it is therefore a spatial measurement. The standard of performance for accuracy is usually the number of correct responses out of the total number of trials. For novice users, speed of response and accuracy are generally inversely proportional to each other.
5. Cress and French (1994)[6] found that skill development varies greatly across different input devices (touch screen, trackball, mouse, locking trackball, and keyboard):
   - Three groups: adults without disabilities, typically developing children between 2.5 and 5.0 years, and children with intellectual disabilities (mental age 2.5 to 5.0).
   - Adults without disabilities mastered all of the devices without training.
   - About 50% of typically developing children were able to master all devices except the locking trackball without training.
   - After training, 80% of the typically developing children mastered all devices. The trackball was the easiest to master.
   - Children with intellectual disabilities averaged between 0% and 46% mastery (depending on the device) without training, and less than 75% mastery with training. The locking trackball was significantly more difficult to master than the other devices.
   - Adults were able to use the devices faster than the children, and the typically developing children used most devices slower than the children with intellectual disabilities (which was probably related to the greater chronological age of the children with intellectual disabilities).
   - Performance by typically developing children was related to age and gross motor abilities.
   - Performance of children with intellectual disabilities was also related to pattern analysis skills, and the individual input devices showed distinctly different relationships to cognitive and motor development than for the typically developing children.
   - Selection of control interfaces for a given individual depends on cognitive and motor requirements presented by a particular interface as well as the skills of the individual in these areas.
   - Extrapolation from successful use by adults without disabilities or typically developing children to children with disabilities is not appropriate.

From Dowden P, Cook AM: Choosing effective selection techniques for beginning communicators. In Reichle J, Beukelman D, Light J, editors: *Exemplary practices for beginning communicators*, Baltimore, 2002, Paul H Brookes (pp 395–432).

STUDY QUESTIONS

1. Define the elements of the human/technology interface and how they are related to the processor and the output.
2. What are the major anatomic sites that are used for control of assistive technologies?
3. Describe the available movements for each anatomic site.
4. What is the order of preference in considering alternative anatomic sites? Why is this order used?
5. What are the major challenges for a person using head control for a fine motor task such as typing?
6. What is a selection set?
7. What is a control interface?
8. What are the two basic selection methods used with control interfaces?
9. What are the scanning formats that can be used to accelerate scanning?
10. What is "directed scanning"? Why is it useful?
11. Why is coded access an indirect selection method? What is the selection set for Morse code?
12. Examine Table 5-2. Which Morse codes listed in the nonstandard section are the same for both example systems? Why do you think these particular codes happen to be the same, given that there are no standards? Why do you think that the other codes are different for different systems?

13. Describe the three different selection techniques used with scanning and directed scanning. Which one provides the user with more control, and why?
14. What are the relative advantages and disadvantages of the three common scanning methods? Select a client profile that would benefit from each type.
15. Describe distributed and integrated control. What are the advantages and disadvantages of each?
16. What are the cognitive skills necessary to use scanning?
17. What do we mean by the "processor" in an assistive technology system? What does it do?
18. What does "rate enhancement" mean? What are the two main types?
19. What memory skills does a person need to use word prediction or word completion?
20. What is "abbreviation expansion"? What cognitive skills are required to use it?
21. What outcomes can be achieved through the implementation of training programs for development of motor skills?
22. Describe the steps taken in a training program to develop motor control.
23. Why is it recommended that a selection skill (e.g., scanning) be developed with games or other activities before the person uses it for a functional task?
24. Assume that you are asked to train a person to use scanning. How would your approach differ for:
    a. A 60-year-old man who has recently sustained a stroke
    b. A five-year-old child with cerebral palsy
    c. A 45-year-old woman with multiple sclerosis
25. If you are the person tasked with making a new system work with an individual, how would you determine if the selection system was the correct one for that person?

REFERENCES

1. Angelo J: Factors affecting the use of a single switch with assistive technology devices, *J Rehabil Res Dev* 37(5):591–598, 2000.
2. Angelo J, Smith RO: The critical role of occupational therapy in augmentative communication services. In American Occupational Therapy Association, editors: *Technology review '89: perspectives on occupational therapy practice,* Rockville, Md, 1989, pp 49–53.
3. Bailey RW: *Human performance engineering,* ed 2, Upper Saddle River, NJ, 1996, Prentice Hall.
4. Blackstone S: The role of rate in communication, *Augment Commun News* 3(5):1–3, 1990.
5. Cook AM, Polgar JM: *Cook and Hussey's assistive technologies: principles and practice*, St. Louis, 2008, Mosby.
6. Cress CJ, French GJ: The relationship between cognitive load measurements and estimates of computer input control skills, *Assist Technol* 6(1):54–66, 1994.
7. Hortsman HM, Levine SP, Jaros LA: Effect of word prediction features on user performance, *Augment Altern Commun* 12:155–168, 1996.
8. Jagacinski RJ, Monk DL: Fitts' Law in two dimensions with hand and head movements, *J Mot Behav* 17(1):77–95, 1985.
9. Jones J, Stewart H: A description of how three occupational therapists train children in using the scanning access technique, *Aust Occup Ther J* 51(3):155–165, 2004.
10. Kangas K: Assessment and training of methods of access and optimal control sites, *Assist Device News* 5(1):1988.
11. Lee KS, Thomas DJ: *Control of computer-based technology for people with physical disabilities: an assessment manual,* Toronto, 1990, University of Toronto Press.
12. Lesher GW, Higginbotham J, Moulton BJ: *Techniques for automatically updating scanning delays, Annual Conference on Rehabilitation Technology (RESNA)*, Orlando, FL, 2000, RESNA Press.
13. McCarthy J, Light J, Drager K, et al: Re-designing scanning to reduce learning demands: the performance of typically developing 2-year-olds, *Augment Altern Commun* 22(4): 269–283, 2006.
14. Piché L, Reichle J: Teaching scanning selection techniques. In Reichle J, York J, Sigafoos J, editors: *Implementing augmentative and alternative communication: strategies for learners with severe disabilities*, Baltimore, 1991, Paul H Brookes, pp 257–274.
15. Smith RO: Technological approaches to performance enhancement. In Christiansen C, Baum C, editors: *Occupational therapy overcoming human performance deficits*, Thorofare, NJ, 1991, Slack.
16. Vanderheiden GC, Lloyd LL: Communication systems and their components. In Blackstone S, Bruskin D, editors: *Augmentative communication: an introduction*, Rockville, Md, 1986, American Speech Language and Hearing Association.

CHAPTER 6

Control Interfaces for Assistive Technologies

CHAPTER OUTLINE

LEARNING OBJECTIVES

Upon completing this chapter, you will be able to do the following:

1. Describe the elements of the human/technology interface and its role within the assistive technology component of the HAAT model
2. Describe the characteristics of control interfaces
3. Discuss a framework for control interface evaluation
4. Identify technologies for direct selection
5. Identify technologies for indirect selection

KEY TERMS

Acceptance Time
Activation Characteristics
Concept Keyboards
Control Enhancers
Control Interface
Distributed Controls
Integrated Control
On-Screen Keyboards
Sensory Characteristics
Spatial Characteristics

The user of an assistive device activates a **control interface** to provide an input to operate the device (e.g., turn it on, make a selection, or make it talk). Control interfaces come in many different sizes and shapes. The user's needs and activities dictate the type of control interface that is chosen. The user's needs are those elements of their motor, sensory, and cognitive abilities that influence the successful use of a control interface. User's activities include a variety of tasks such as turning on a light using an enlarged light switch, or accessing a portable communication system using a single switch. In order for the person to know that they have successfully activated the device, it is necessary for there to be feedback from the device to the person. This usually takes place through a visual or auditory display or both. These displays are considered a component of the human/technology interface. Alternative displays for people with visual or auditory impairments are discussed in Chapters 8 and 9, respectively.

This chapter begins with a discussion of the characteristics that make control interfaces useful for particular individuals. Options for control interfaces for both direct and indirect selection are described with an emphasis on how to make their use successful.

CHARACTERISTICS OF CONTROL INTERFACES

Control interfaces differ according to their spatial, sensory, and activation characteristics.[4,8] Consideration of these characteristics can be helpful when working to optimize the effectiveness of a particular device for an individual. The important factors are the placement and size of the control interface (which we call spatial characteristics), how the person uses the control interface to make a selection (**activation characteristics**), and what feedback is obtained as a result of the person using it (sensory characteristics). These characteristics and their use in control interface assessment and recommendation is discussed in detail by Cook and Polgar (2008).[8]

Spatial Characteristics

The **spatial characteristics** of a control interface are (1) its overall physical size (dimensions), shape, and weight; (2) the number of available targets contained within the control interface (e.g., a keyboard has over 100 targets while a joystick may have only 4); (3) the size of each target; and (4) the spacing between targets.

The target size and spacing should be matched to the individual's fine and gross motor skills. Targets that are large and spaced far apart are useful for individuals with good range of motion but limited fine motor control (e.g., someone with a coordination disorder or a tremor). Small, closely spaced targets are useful for individuals with limited range of motion, muscle weakness, and accurate fine motor control (e.g., someone with arthritis). For example, a single control interface has one target, and the target size is the dimension (height and width) of the control interface (see Figure 6-10, *A*, for example). Typically, a single control interface can accommodate an individual who has limitations in range of motion and limited fine motor control. Control interface arrays (including joysticks) have two to five switches, each representing a different target and a different result when activated. The user's range of motion required to access a switch array needs to be larger than for a single switch, but it can still be relatively small, depending on the spacing between the switches. The user's fine motor control needs to be more refined than that required for a single control interface and less refined than that for a keyboard.

A contracted keyboard has keys (targets) of small size in close proximity to each other. Its overall size is also small. The keys on these keyboards range in size from 0.5 to 1.5 cm, and they require relatively fine resolution from the user. The requirement for the user's range is moderate (less than 15 cm in both horizontal and vertical directions). Standard or commonly used keyboards require moderate range and relatively fine resolution of the user. Expanded keyboards have large overall size and enlarged target size, requiring relatively large range and fine resolution. Control interface arrays and keyboards can have from 2 to more than 100 targets.

Activation and Deactivation Characteristics

There are many characteristics related to the activation of the control interface.[8] The effort expended and the amount of movement required to activate the control interface are important to consider when evaluating how effective a control interface is for an individual or when troubleshooting a situation that is not working well. Deactivation or the release of a control interface may be different than activation and also needs to be considered. While the choice of a control interface for a given individual will be part of the team assessment, the rehabilitation assistant (e.g., OTA, PTA) will often be the one interacting with the user on a regular basis. This frequency will allow the rehabilitation assistant to see if the person is able to use the device easily or if some adjustments are needed.

Control interfaces can be activated by a variety of methods that are shown in Table 6-1. The first column identifies the three ways the user can send a signal to the control interface (i.e., movement, respiration, and phonation); the middle column shows how each of these signals is detected by the control interface; and the column on the far right provides examples of each type of control interface.

TABLE 6-1 Method of Activation

Signal Sent, User Action (What the Body Does)	Signal Detected	Examples
1. Movement (eye, head, tongue, arms, legs)	1a. Mechanical switch: activation by the application of a force	1a. Joystick, keyboard, tread switch
	1b. Electromagnetic switch: activation by the receipt of electromagnetic energy such as light or radio waves	1b. Light pointer, light detector, remote radio transmitter
	1c. Electrical switch: activation by detection of electrical signals from the surface of the body	1c. EMG, EOG,* capacitive, or contact switch
	1d. Proximity switch: activation by a movement close to the detector but without contact	1d. Heat-sensitive switches
2. Respiration (inhalation-expiration)	2. Pneumatic switch: activation by detection of respiratory airflow or pressure	2. Puff and sip
3. Phonation	3. Sound or voice switch: activation by the detection of articulated sounds or speech	3. Sound switch, whistle switch, speech recognition

*EMG: Electromyographic; EOG: electroculographic.

Movements by the user can be detected by the control interface in three basic ways. Mechanical control interfaces detect a bodily movement that generates a force. This mode of activation represents the largest category of control interfaces. Most control interfaces, keyboard keys, joysticks, and other controls (e.g., mouse or trackball) that require movement or force for activation fall into this category. Electromagnetic control interfaces do not require contact from the user's body for activation. They detect movement at a distance through either light or radio frequency (RF) energy. Examples include head-mounted light sources and detectors and the transmitters used with EADLs (Electronic Aids for Daily Living) for remote control (similar to garage door openers). Electrical control interfaces are sensitive to electric currents generated by the body. One type, called a capacitive switch, detects static electricity on the surface of the body. This is similar to the game children play when they attempt to shock someone with static electricity. A common example of this type of interface is seen in some elevator buttons. The control interface requires no force, making them useful to individuals who have muscle weakness. Other electrical control interfaces use electrodes attached to the skin to detect the electromyographic (EMG) signal associated with muscle contraction. Electrodes placed near the eyes can measure eye movements and generate an electroculographic (EOG) signal based on them. Proximity control interfaces detect movement, without coming into contact with the body.

The second type of body-generated signal shown in Table 6-1 is respiration. The signal detected is either airflow or air pressure. The use of this type of control interface, generally called a sip-and-puff switch, requires that the user be able to place and maintain her lips around a tube and produce good control of airflow.

In order to activate a control interface the individual must exert some effort. The effort required varies from zero for touch switches upward to a relatively large amount for some mechanical switches. For a switch requiring physical movement, effort is the force required to activate the switch.

For an individual using a light pointer to choose from an array of different items, the effort required is sufficient head movement to aim the light beam at one item and move between items, and enough postural stability to hold the light beam on the desired item. Electrical interfaces require a range of effort from zero (for a capacitive switch) to relatively high for muscle force activation of an EMG.

The activation effort of pneumatic control interfaces is the amount of exhalation or inhalation required for activation, which can be either how hard (pressure) or how fast (flow) air is exhaled or inhaled. For example, some power-wheelchair processors use a system in which a hard puff (large effort and high pressure generated) is forward, a soft puff (small effort and low pressure generated) is a right turn, a hard sip is reverse, and a soft sip is a left turn. The difference in these control signals is based primarily on effort generated. Phonation signals also have a level of effort related (at the simplest control interface level) to volume or loudness.

There is also a force required to release, or deactivate, some control interfaces. Muscle contraction is necessary to remove, or release, the body part from the interface. Weiss (1990)[17] measured both activation and deactivation forces for several mechanical switches and found that force was required to release the control interface in all cases, but the deactivation force was approximately one third to one half that required for activation.

Sensory Characteristics

The auditory, somatosensory, and visual feedback produced during the activation of the control interface comprises its **sensory characteristics**. Some control interfaces provide auditory feedback in the form of a click when activated. For example, keyboards that use mechanical switches for each key usually click when pressed, thus providing auditory feedback. Other keyboards have a smooth membrane surface that does not provide any natural auditory feedback. Often a tone is emitted to let the user know that a selection has been made.

When the interface is within the consumer's visual field, visual data are obtained through observation of the placement and the movement of the control interface. For some individuals the type of visual data will mean the difference between successful and unsuccessful use of a control interface. For example, someone who has difficulty attending to objects in the environment may be more attentive to a control interface that is large and brightly colored.

The eye is sensitive to colors in the visual spectrum (from violet to red), but the eye is not equally sensitive to all colors in this range. If the eye is fixed and not allowed to rotate, the limits of color vision are 60 degrees to each side of the midline. Within this range, the response of the retina to colors is not equal for all wavelengths (colors). Figure 6-1 illustrates that blue objects are visible over the

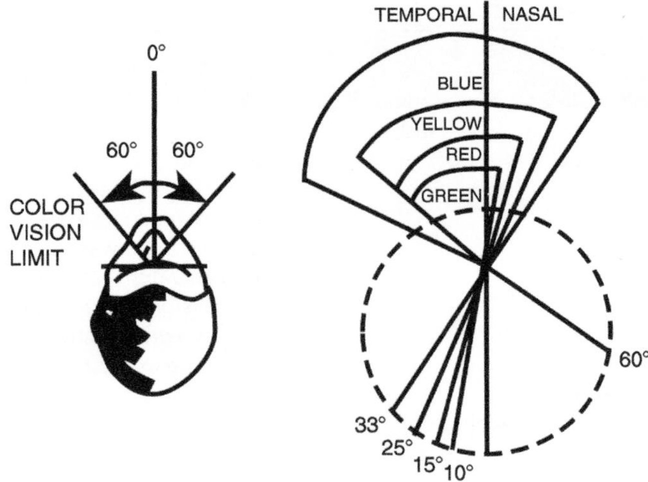

Figure 6-1 Color response of the eye differs with visual angle. (Modified from Woodson W. and Conover D. *Human engineering guide for equipment designers*, Berkeley, 1964, University of California Press.)

entire 60-degree range, whereas yellow, red, and green are recognizable only at points closer to the fixed (center) point of vision. This limitation on color sensitivity has a practical implication when working with individuals who rely on peripheral vision or who have difficulties in moving their eyes to track objects. If a target (e.g., a switch) is green or red, its position may limit the person's ability to see the object. We can increase the visibility of the switch by using blue or yellow.

Somatosensory feedback is the tactile, kinesthetic, or proprioceptive input sensed on activation of the control interface. For example, the texture or "feel" of the activation surface provides tactile data. The position in space of the body part and its movement when the user activates the control interface provides proprioceptive feedback. Many mechanical control interfaces require movement and force for activation. The displacement of the control interface provides kinesthetic (movement) feedback, as well as tactile and proprioceptive feedback that are beneficial to the user. If there is not much movement, as with a membrane keyboard or touch screen, the sensory feedback is less and the individual may press harder than necessary, thinking that more force is needed to activate the keys. This extra, sustained force may result in errors, since many keyboards will repeat entries if a key is pressed for more than a second or two.*

Control interfaces that require more effort typically provide more sensory feedback. Likewise, switches that require very little effort provide very little sensory feedback. For example, a contact switch that is activated by an electric charge from the body (i.e., requiring only touch) does not provide the user with any somatosensory or auditory feedback. Many mechanical switches provide abundant feedback through the feel (tactile), an observable movement of the mechanism (visual), and an audible click (auditory).

IS IT WORKING? EVALUATING THE EFFECTIVENESS OF A CONTROL INTERFACE

Selecting a control interface for an individual is a complex process.[8] Once a control interface is selected and implemented for an individual, its effectiveness must be evaluated on an ongoing basis. The evaluation of effectiveness may be at the time of initial use or at any point where a change has occurred. The desired change in control method may be due to the individual (e.g., a degenerative condition that makes use a particular control interface difficult). Alternatively, the change may be required due to a change in technology. For example, a new wheelchair may be acquired and the control interfaces will have to be mounted to the new wheelchair and set up for the user, or the new wheelchair may use a different control interface to operate it. A new device to be controlled (e.g. a more advanced augmentative communication system) may be introduced, requiring changes in the control interface. Finally, the consumer may be experiencing difficulties (poor accuracy, excessive fatigue) using the control interface for the desired activities. In all of these cases, reevaluation of effectiveness is required.

Evaluating the effectiveness of a control interface that has been selected and installed can be challenging because of the large number of factors that can be involved. Figure 6-2 shows a systematic approach to evaluation of how well a control interface is working for an individual consumer. The process includes observation of the consumer carrying out the desired tasks. The range of possible tasks for which a control interface might be used includes controlling a power wheelchair (Chapter 12), making choices with an Electronic Aid to Daily Living (EADL; Chapter 14), using an augmentative communication system (Chapter 11) or cognitive assistive technologies (Chapter 10), or providing input to a computer as we discuss later in this chapter.

When observing the consumer carry out the desired activity, it is important to note whether the speed and accuracy of selection are sufficient to accomplish the desired task and whether the effort expended results in fatigue during routine use. In general, accuracy is more important than speed. If indirect selection is being used, then accuracy is measured by whether the switch (or switches) can be pressed on command. If direct selection is being used with a keyboard, then accuracy involves not only hitting a key on a keyboard or a location on a touch screen, but also hitting the correct key or screen location. A consumer using an adapted mouse input could be asked to move the mouse pointer to a specific screen location and carry out other mouse functions such as click, double click, or dragging an icon to a new location. A user controlling a power wheelchair with a joystick may be asked to drive the wheelchair to a specific location or to turn in a specific direction.

Because they provide daily care and interact on a regular basis with individuals using assistive technologies, rehabilitation assistants (e.g., OTAs, PTAs) are often responsible for evaluating the effectiveness of a control interface. The first step is to ensure that the individual is properly positioned. The chosen anatomic site must be free to move as much as possible without restriction (e.g., from a head rest, wheelchair arm, or other constraint). The next step is to be sure that the control interface is placed in a position where the consumer can easily activate it without losing body position or exerting undue physical effort.

Once the individual and the control are properly positioned, it is possible to determine how accurately the consumer is using the control interface. In order to determine if the task was completed accurately, the observer must know what the consumer was trying to accomplish. The observer should direct the consumer to make specific

*This can be adjusted on most computers and many assistive devices. See Chapter 7.

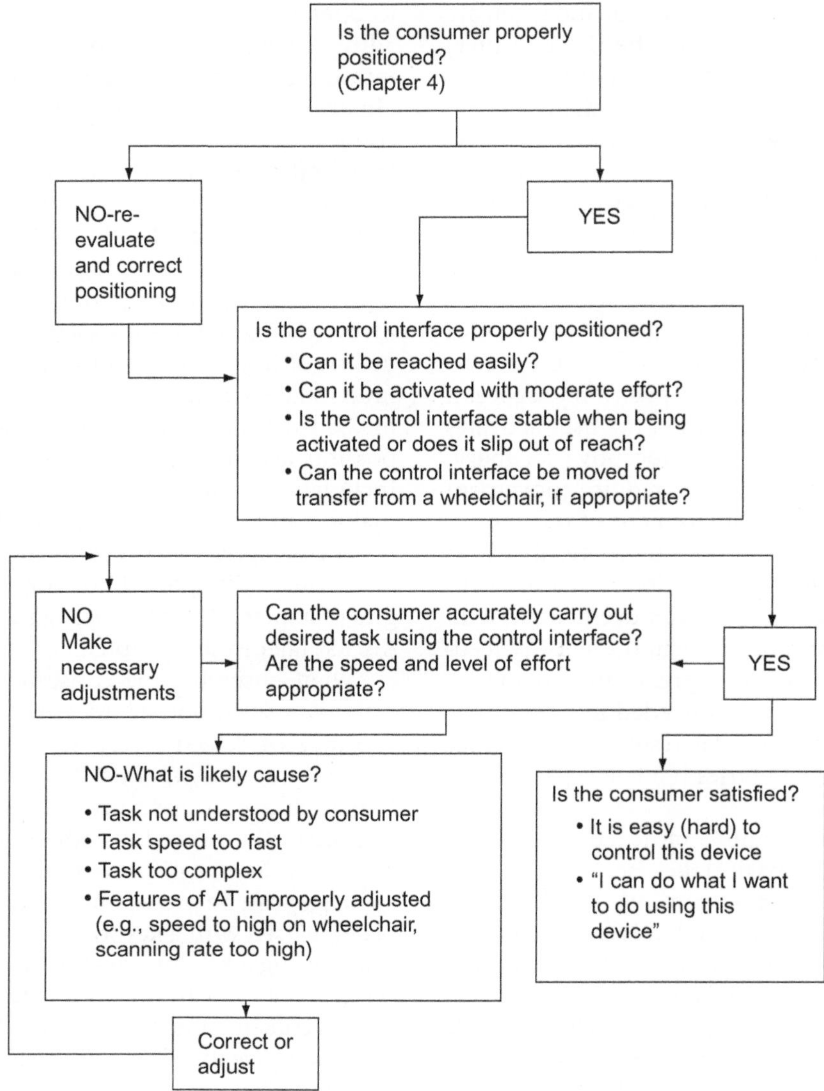

Figure 6-2 Evaluation of the effectiveness of a control interface in use.

selections using the control interface, keeping track of how long it takes to complete each task, how accurately it is done, and how much effort it requires.

Any limitations in accuracy or speed or high levels of fatigue require changes in the system. This may mean repositioning a control interface to make it easier to activate, choosing a control interface that requires less force or range of motion to activate it, or looking for an entire new control interface–anatomic site combination that is less fatiguing. It is also important to note the consumer's evaluation of how successful the control interface–anatomic site combination is in meeting his or her needs.

ENHANCING CONTROL: PROPER POSITIONING AND ARM SUPPORTS

Control enhancers are aids and strategies that enhance or extend the physical control (range and resolution) a person has available to use a control interface. In some cases a person's control may be enhanced to the extent that he can select directly. In other cases control enhancers can minimize fatigue. Control enhancers include strategies such as varying the position or the characteristics of the control interface and devices such as mouthsticks, head and hand pointers, and arm supports.

The person and the control interface should both be positioned to maximize function. The importance of proper positioning to maximize an individual's function is discussed in Chapter 4. A person's position should be observed as he or she uses a device to be sure that activation of the control interface does not result in an undesirable change in body position. If inadequate positioning appears to be affecting the person's ability to control an interface, it should be addressed. The position of the control interface can also affect the person's ability to activate it, and changing the height or the angle of the control interface even slightly may dramatically improve the person's control ability.

Features that enhance control are sometimes incorporated into the interface. For example, some joysticks have a feature, called tremor dampening, that allows adjustment of the joystick for people who have tremors. Tremor-dampening joysticks are able to distinguish between tremors, which are faster and smaller in amplitude, and intentional movements, which are slower and larger. The joystick is adjusted so that the tremors are disregarded and only intentional movements are detected. This adjustment enhances the ability of an individual who might otherwise be unable to operate a joystick to control a power wheelchair. A similar feature, called FilterKeys, is employed in Windows. When the FilterKeys feature is activated in Windows, brief keystrokes are ignored and the delay is lengthened before a key repeats itself when pressed for an extended period of time.

Head Pointers, Hand Pointers, and Mouthsticks

For individuals who lack functional movement in their arms and hands, a mouthstick or head pointer (Figure 6-3) can be used with head and neck movement to access a keyboard or perform other types of direct selection tasks (e.g., dialing a telephone number or turning pages in a book). A mechanical head pointer is a rod with a rubber tip that is attached to a head band. The individual can use the end of the head pointer to depress keys. Besides being able to move the head vertically and horizontally, the individual must have the ability to move the head forward to depress keys.

There are also light pointers that can be worn on the head or held in the hand to control devices. One advantage of head-controlled light pointers is that it is not necessary for the user to move the head forward or backward. Light pointers are described in greater detail in the section on pointing interfaces.

Hand pointers (Figure 6-4, *B*) can be grasped with a gross hand grip. These devices include a projection with a rubber tip that can be used to press keys. These are sometimes referred to as typing aids. A pointing aid may help an individual who has the gross motor ability to move her arm and hand around a keyboard but has difficulty extending and isolating a finger to depress a key. There are commercially available aids that can be strapped onto the hand to assist in pointing, such as the typing aid shown in Figure 6-4, *B*. In some cases it is necessary to custom fabricate a pointing aid in order for it to fit the consumer's hand appropriately. These custom-fabricated aids can range from complex hand splints to simple tools, such as a pencil with an enlarged eraser.

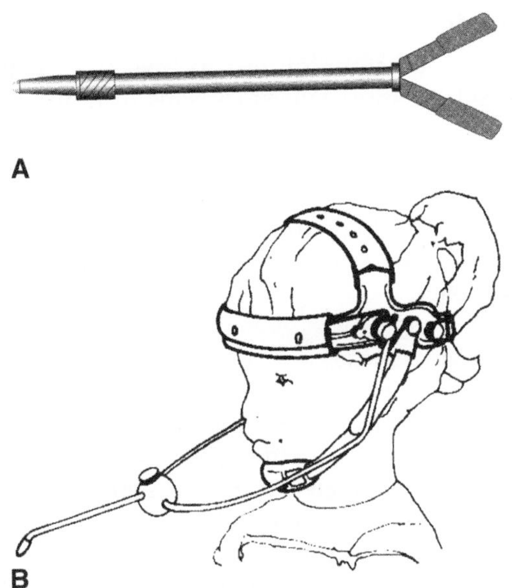

Figure 6-3 Control enhancers. **A**, Mouthstick. **B**, Head pointer.

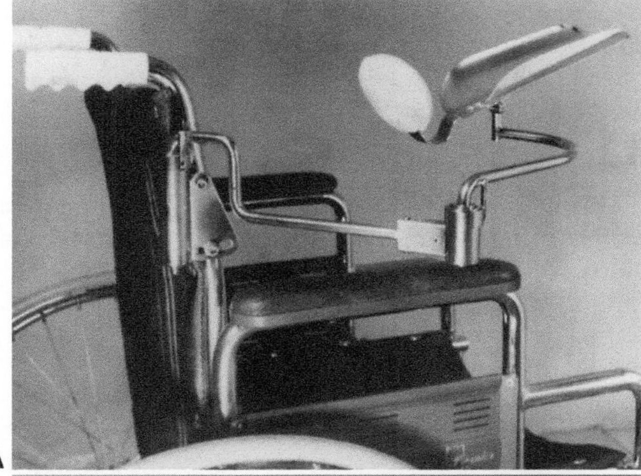

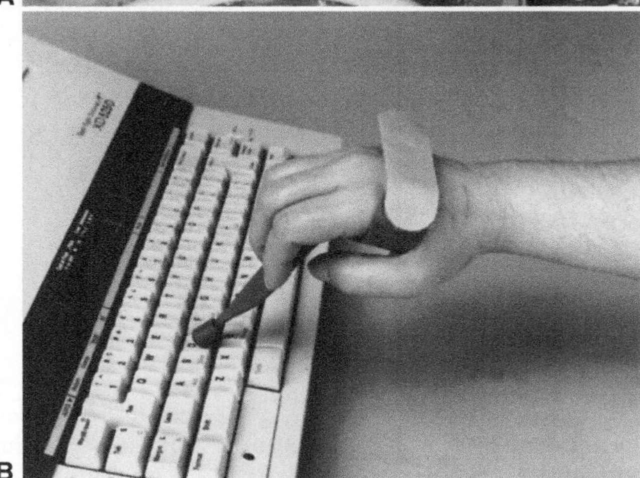

Figure 6-4 Control enhancers. **A**, Mobile arm support used to enhance the control in the upper extremity for accessing a control interface. **B**, Typing aid used to enhance a person's ability to point and access a keyboard. (Courtesy Sammons Preston Co., Bolingbrook, Ill)

Mouthsticks are often used by individuals with quadriplegia as a result of a spinal cord injury. A mouthstick consists of a pointer attached to a mouthpiece. The user grips the mouthpiece between his teeth and moves his head to manipulate control interfaces or other objects. The shaft of the mouthstick can be made from a wooden dowel, a piece of plastic, or aluminum. In some cases, interchangeable tips for different functions (e.g., painting, writing, or typing) can be inserted into the distal end of the shaft. The mouthpiece can be a standard U shape that is gripped between the teeth or a custom-made insert. Mouthsticks are also available from several suppliers.* Use of a mouthstick requires good oral-motor control; later in this chapter we discuss training to develop these skills.

Mobile Arm Supports

Individuals who have weakness in the arm may not have enough strength to access the full range of a keyboard adequately. A mobile arm support (Figure 6-4, *A*), which props the arm and assists in arm movements by eliminating some of the effects of gravity, may then allow the individual to access a keyboard.

Positioning the Keyboard for Use

In all situations it is necessary to address the position and placement of the control interface so that it is optimally accessed by the user. Most keyboards are connected with a cable to the computer, which allows some latitude in positioning them so they are accessible. Keyboards can be placed on stands that raise them (e.g., for mouthstick use) or easels that tilt them (e.g., for easier hand access or foot access). Some keyboards (e.g., contracted keyboards) can be mounted to wheelchairs.

CONTROL INTERFACES FOR DIRECT SELECTION

Direct selection is generally preferable to indirect selection because it is faster and more efficient. For that reason it is often worth the effort to work with direct selection approaches, if possible, before trying scanning or encoded access. Control interfaces for direct selection include various types of keyboards, pointing interfaces, speech recognition, and eye gaze. While the hands are preferred because of the inherent fine motor control, many individuals use foot or head control for direct selection, and automatic speech recognition allows a "hands free" approach to directly selecting items.

Several direct selection approaches utilize **on-screen keyboards** that employ a video image of the keyboard on the video screen, together with a cursor (see Figure 7-1, A). The user makes choices by moving the cursor to the desired key and selecting it (e.g., by clicking). A variety of mouse pointing methods or scanning can be used to position the cursor and make a selection (see Chapter 7).

The critical questions presented in Box 6-1 can assist in determining the effectiveness of a keyboard for a specific individual. Affirmative responses to all seven questions indicate that the control interface is meeting the consumer's needs. A negative answer to any one or more questions will direct the rehabilitation assistant's attention to the area or areas needing attention.

In some situations, speed is of primary importance (e.g., in a work setting). In general, speed and accuracy are in opposition. That is, as speed increases, accuracy decreases. In some cases, the consumer may make selections so slowly and deliberately to be accurate that the use of the control interface under investigation becomes impractical. For example, if it takes several seconds to select a key, this rate may be equivalent to the use of scanning to make a selection. Because scanning takes much less physical effort, it should then be considered as an alternative to direct selection. The criterion for accuracy is somewhat subjective and subject to clinical judgment. We recommend that a goal of at least three out of four selections (75%) be established as a minimum for determining the effectiveness of a particular interface.

If the answer to any of the questions in Box 6-1 is determined to be "no," then the use of a less limiting keyboard, a control enhancer, or modifications to the keyboard should be considered. For example, if a standard keyboard cannot be used because of a targeting problem, we may consider the following: (1) an enlarged keyboard with larger targets (less limiting), (2) a keyguard (modification), or (3) a typing aid (a control enhancer).

BOX 6-1 Critical Questions for Evaluating Keyboard Use

1. Can the consumer reach all the keys on the keyboard?
2. Are the size, spacing, and sensory feedback of the keys appropriate?
3. Is the consumer's speed of input adequate for the task?
4. Does the consumer target keys with approximately 75% accuracy?
5. Is the consumer able to simultaneously hold down a modifier key and select another key?
6. Is the consumer able to control the duration for which a key must be pressed before it repeats itself?
7. Does the consumer effectively use the standard keyboard layout?

Keyboards

For written communication, a keyboard is typically considered the most efficient means of inputting information. The standard keyboard is the first choice for computer access. However, many individuals with disabilities are unable to use a standard keyboard. Fortunately, there are a number of alternatives. Table 6-2 provides examples of some commercially available alternatives to the standard keyboard.

Standard Keyboards

Some individuals may have difficulty writing because of fatigue or minimally impaired motor control. A standard keyboard on a computer may be all that is needed to allow them to complete writing tasks effectively. Because it is readily available, the standard keyboard is the most desirable interface for direct selection for text entry. The standard keyboard typically has a full alphanumeric array consisting of letters; numbers; punctuation symbols;

* For example: http://www.orthobionics.com/rehab1/pointers/64.htm

TABLE 6-2 Alternative Keyboards for Direct Selection

Category	Description	Device Name/Manufacturer
Expanded keyboards	Generally membrane keyboards that have enlarged target areas, often programmable so that key size can be customized; useful for individuals with good range and poor resolution; also useful for individuals with limited cognitive/language skills or visual impairment.	IntelliKeys (IntelliTools); USB King Keyboard (TASH, Inc.); Expanded Keyboard (Able Net, Inc.); Big Keys Plus (Inclusive Technologies); Expanded Keyboard (Maltron)
Contracted keyboards	Miniature, full-function keyboards, typically with membrane overlay; useful for individuals with limited range of motion and good resolution.	USB Mini Keyboard (TASH, Inc.); Mini Keyboard (Able Net, Inc.); The Magic Wand Keyboard (In Touch Systems)
Touch screens/touch tablets	Activated by either breaking a very thin light beam or by a capacitive array that detects the electrical charge on the finger; the electrode array used to detect where the finger or pointer is touching is transparent; touch screen can be placed over the face of a monitor.	Touch Window (RiverDeep); MagicTouch (Laureate Learning Systems, Inc.)
TongueTouch Keypad	Battery-operated, radio frequency–transmitting device with nine pressure-sensitive keys activated by tongue; universal controller processes information sent from keypad to receiver.	
Special-purpose keyboards	Keyboards on special-purpose devices, such as augmentative communication and environmental control devices; available keys may be much more limited in number or may be specific in function compared with standard keyboard.	See Chapter 11

Data from: RiverDeep, San Francisco, Calif. (http://rivapprod2.riverdeep.net/); Able Net, Inc., Minneapolis, MN, (http://www.ablenetinc.com/); Laureate Learning Systems, Inc., Winooski, Vt. (www.laureatelearning.com); IntelliTools, Frederick, CO (www.intellitools.com); Inclusive Technologies, (http://www.inclusive.co.uk/catalogue/index.html); In Touch Systems, Spring Valley, N.Y. (www.magicwandkeyboard.com); Maltron-USA (http://www.maltron-usa.com/expanded.htm); TASH, Inc., Ajax, Ontario, Canada, or Richmond, Va. (www.tashinc.com).

special characters such as "\," "/," "@," "#," "$," and "%"; and special keys (e.g., END, DEL, SHIFT, CONTROL, and ALT). Key size and spacing and the amount of distance the keys travel vary depending on the type and manufacturer of the keyboard. Small keyboards are now readily available on the consumer market.

To keep the overall size down, laptop computers in particular have smaller keyboards. In many cases the laptop keyboard is flat, as opposed to the tiered key rows on a full-size keyboard. This can be more difficult for some individuals.

Ergonomic Keyboards

The term repetitive strain injury (RSI) encompasses several musculoskeletal disorders that develop as a result of sustained, repetitive movements.[5] Carpal tunnel syndrome is the most common RSI. Standard keyboards place the hands in an unnatural position with the forearms pronated and the wrists extended and ulnarly deviated. This position causes strain on the tendons and nerves. Numerous alternatives to the standard keyboard have been developed in attempts to reduce this strain on the wrist and hands. These alternatives range from minor rearranging of the keys to major redesign of the keyboard shape and configuration.

Ergonomic keyboards attempt to reduce the strain placed on the hands and wrists during the repetitive motion of keying by putting the forearms, wrists, and hands in a neutral position, which is more natural and more comfortable for the typist. There are three basic ways in which the standard keyboard has been redesigned. The first and most common type of ergonomic keyboard is the fixed-split keyboard (e.g., Figure 6-5, *A*). The difference between these keyboards and standard keyboards is that the keys are spaced farther apart and the keyboard is curved, so that the hands are placed in a more neutral position. Many of these keyboards have a built-in wrist rest to support the wrists while typing.

The second basic type of ergonomic keyboard is the adjustable-split keyboard (Figure 6-5, *B*). This type also splits the keyboard layout into two parts. A mechanism on the keyboard allows one or both sides of the keyboard to be adjusted horizontally and vertically, from 0 to 30 degrees, to the position where it is most comfortable.

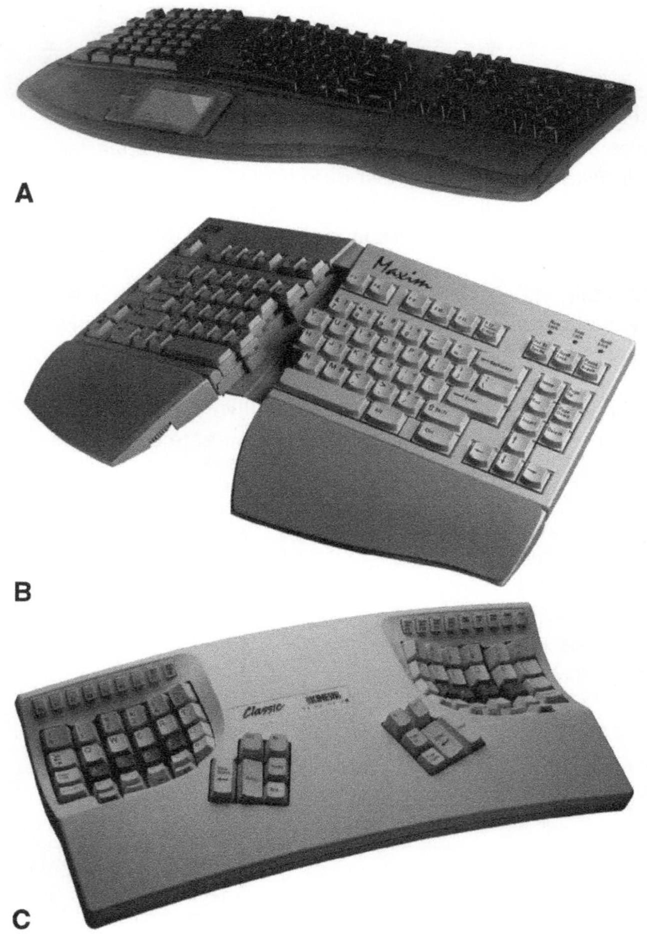

Figure 6-5 Ergonomic keyboards. **A,** Tru-Form Keyboard. **B,** Maxim Adjustable Keyboard. **C,** Contoured Keyboard. (**A,** Courtesy Adesso Inc., www.adessoinc.com; **B** and **C,** Courtesy Kinesis Corporation, www.kinesis-ergo.com.)

A user who does not need to look at the keyboard may be able to take advantage of this range of adjustment. However, for those individuals who need to see the keyboard, adjusting the angle too far may make it difficult to see the keys.

The third type of ergonomic keyboard uses a concave keywell design (Figure 6-5, *C*) in which the keys are arranged in a well. The principle behind this design is that finger excursion is reduced by having the keys arranged at the same distance from each of the finger joints.[2]

Manufacturers of ergonomic keyboards claim that their keyboards reduce the strain placed on the wrists and hands. However, the effectiveness of the use of ergonomic keyboards in reducing symptoms of RSI has not been demonstrated in controlled studies. For this reason, it is advised that ergonomic keyboards not be recommended for the purpose of preventing RSI.[2,16] Situations in which an ergonomic keyboard may be recommended for a consumer include (1) meeting the needs of the consumer with physical limitations (e.g., limits in range of motion) and (2) when the consumer finds the ergonomic keyboard more comfortable to use than a standard keyboard. The most critical factor to consider when selecting a keyboard is the user's level of comfort with the different keyboards .[2]

Expanded Keyboards

Individuals who do not have sufficient control to target the keys on a standard keyboard but still have adequate control to select directly may be able to use an expanded keyboard. Expanded keyboards are generally membrane-type keyboards that have enlarged target areas from which the individual can select directly (Figure 6-6, *A*). The minimal size of the target areas on an expanded keyboard is 1 inch square. If the person still has difficulty targeting this size of key, the expanded keyboard can be customized by grouping keys together to form larger keys. In this way the keyboard can be redesigned to match the skills of the user.

Expanded keyboards vary in overall size and can be chosen depending on the size of the selection set needed by the individual and the key size the individual is able to target accurately. IntelliKeys* has a large surface area that can be configured for a variety of key sizes and shapes. It comes with several standard keyboard overlays, such as the one shown in Figure 6-6, *B*. This overlay is an example of a layout that has been configured with different sizes and different shapes of keys on the same keyboard. The IntelliKeys can also be customized to match specific applications by using the companion Overlay Maker software.

* www.intellitools.com/

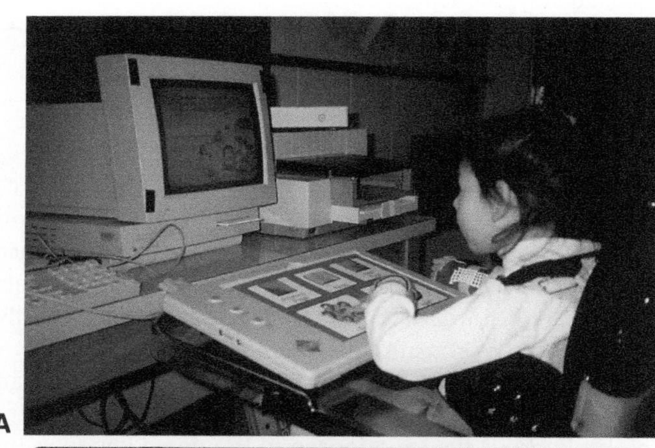

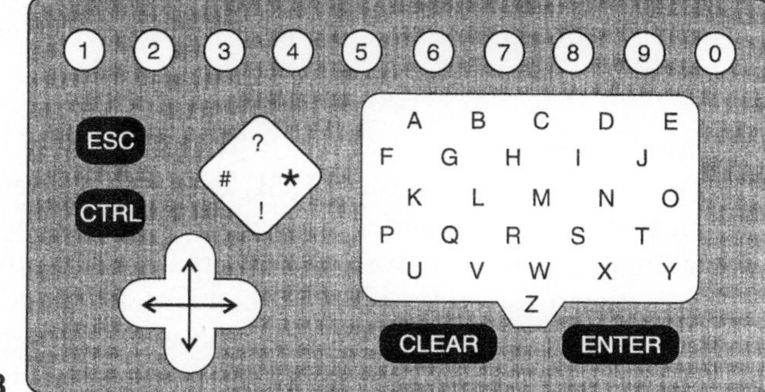

Figure 6-6 **A,** Consumer using an expanded keyboard with thumb. **B,** Expanded keyboard showing configuration with different sizes and shapes of keys on the same keyboard.

The keys can be labeled with letters, words, symbols, or pictures. Because they can be customized, expanded keyboards are also useful with individuals who have a cognitive or visual impairment. Examples of expanded keyboards are shown in Table 6-2.

Contracted Keyboards

Some individuals may have sufficient resolution but lack the range of motion to reach all the keys on a standard keyboard. In this situation a contracted, or mini, keyboard may be the solution. These keyboards use either raised keys or a membrane surface. For computer use, contracted keyboards must meet the requirement that all keys of the standard keyboard be represented, which is accomplished by using additional modifier keys. Figure 6-7 shows a consumer being evaluated on using a mouthstick with the USB Mini keyboard. This keyboard is approximately 7.25 × 4.2 inches in overall size, with the size of each key approximately one half inch on a side. Several of the keys have multiple functions, depending on which modifier key is pressed first. The functions corresponding to various modifiers can be colored to match the modifier key. The selection set (the alphabet) in Figure 6-7 is not placed in the QWERTY format typical of standard keyboards. The letter placement is based on a "frequency of use" system in which the letters most commonly used in the English language are placed toward the center, with the less commonly used letters placed in the outer edges of the keyboard. This arrangement is used to minimize the distance that the person has to move in order to make selections when typing. This approach makes sense because contracted keyboards are typically used when the individual's range of motion is restricted. Because of the small key size and closeness of the keys, the user of a contracted keyboard must have good fine motor control and visual scanning abilities. Persons using contracted keyboards type with a single digit, a handheld typing stick, or a mouthstick.

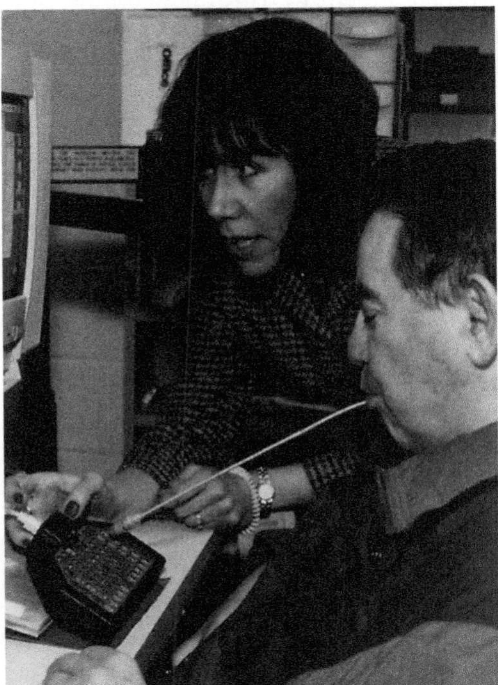

Figure 6-7 Consumer being evaluated using the WinMini Keyboard and a mouthstick.

Special-Purpose Keyboards

Keyboards are also used on special-purpose devices, such as augmentative communication and environmental control devices. In these cases the available keys may be much more limited in number or they may be very specific in function compared with the standard keyboard. For example, in some augmentative communication devices (see Chapter 11) the keyboards have membrane keys and are restricted to a relative small number of key (e.g., a total of from 4 to 32 keys). These keys are not assigned any specific character or function when manufactured but can be programmed to represent just about anything the user would like. Other devices come with certain keys that have been designated to be specific functions. For example, a key may be designated "SPEAK," and pressing it will cause whatever was entered to be spoken. In all these cases, however, the keyboard provides the same function: direct selection input from the user to the processor.

Touch Screens and Touch Tablets: Laptops, Pad Devices, and Smart Phones

The smart phone, pad devices, and other mainstream technologies use touch screens as do a number of augmentative communication devices (Chapter 11) and Electronic Aids to Daily Living (Chapter 14). The advantage of touch screens for children is that the child can directly touch a picture or symbol and have the device carry out a task. Touch screens are also useful for older adults who have limited experience with a computer and who find it difficult to use a mouse. The selection set varies with the application program being used.

Other mainstream devices (e.g., touch pads, cell phones) have a flat screen that uses an image of the keys for text entry. This type of keyboard provides very little feedback and can be difficult for users who have fine motor limitations. Cell phones have even smaller keys or require fine motor control for touch screen access.

For people who have disabilities, there are possible benefits of smart phone technologies, but special considerations must be taken into account to make the phone accessible. People who have upper extremity motor limitations may require alternatives for input because small mobile keyboards may be unusable. For people with sensory limitations the size, contrast, and spacing of display items may be limiting. For individuals with cognitive limitations, the complexity of operating systems and multimedia websites may prevent or severely limit use. General issues for all people with disabilities are the compatibility of mainstream technologies and websites with assistive technologies such as SGDs.

There are four features of cell phone technology that affect access for people with disabilities: (1) increased processing power, (2) ease of downloading applications into the phone, (3) wireless connection to a worldwide network, (4) low cost and easily obtained by persons with disabilities since these features are built into standard cell phones.[10] Open source code refers to an operating system that is freely available to anyone. This is the feature that has led to the plethora of "apps"—applications for a wide variety of purposes that can be downloaded in a Smart phone or pad device. This means that new applications can be developed by many individuals without having to rely on the original owner of the software to integrate them. Commercially available cell phones have increasing diversity of software for tasks such as text-to-speech output, voice recognition, and many other applications for particular activities or tasks. Typical tasks include business (banking and financial planning), entertainment (music, games, books, and magazines), self care (fitness), travel (flight and hotel booking), and many more. There are also many apps being developed to meet the needs of person with disabilities.

Concept Keyboards for Users with Cognitive Limitations

Concept keyboards replace the letters and numbers of the keyboard with pictures, symbols, or words that represent the concepts being used or taught. When the user presses on the picture, the correct character is sent to the computer to create the desired effect. As an example, a child who is having difficulty with basic arithmetic and monetary concepts may be more successful using a concept keyboard in which each key displayed is a coin of a particular denomination, rather than the coin's value (number) or name (letters). The child can push on the coin and have that number of cents entered into the program. A simple program that asks the child to make change could be used to encourage the child to develop subtraction skills while also learning the value of specific coins. This approach is more motivating for some children because it is easier for them to press on a key labeled with a quarter than to enter "2" and "5."

Very simple programs may require only two keys. For example, the SPACE key can move a cursor to different matching choices and the ENTER key can select the desired one. This concept can be used to match shapes or numbers or to control any two-choice task. It functions as a keyboard, even though only two keys are used.

Another approach to concept keyboards is the use of specially designed software together with special-input keyboards. These systems do not require the use of a special input interface because they plug directly into either a serial, parallel, or USB port. The software also comes with overlays for the keyboard. For example, a program to teach language concepts can be implemented by placing pictures of the concepts on specific keys and having the child generate words by pressing the correct key, causing the concept to be spoken and the picture to be repeated on the screen. When the child plays with the objects described, she learns to label her actions as well as the objects. Concept keyboards provide a direct relationship between the task and the child's action. For example, by using a picture of the body as the "keyboard" and each body part as a "key," a child can touch the body part when the program instructs him to do so. When he does, the program can repeat the body part name and cause it to be moved on the screen. The Intellikeys* keyboard is often used as a concept keyboard.

There are also commercial emulation programs that reduce the complexity of the Windows environment for users who have cognitive disabilities. The Voyager suite of programs from Saltillo allows individuals with cognitive disabilities to launch programs, communicate via email, and browse the web. The entire suite operates with pictures rather than words to present the user with choices, thereby removing the necessity for the user to be able to read or write. Receiving e-mail is accomplished by using text-to-speech to provide an auditory output. The user sends e-mail by selecting a set of pictures that enable the send function, selecting the recipient by picture or name, and then following prompts to record a message and send it. Assistive technologies for persons with cognitive limitations are discussed in more detail in Chapter 10.

Eye-Controlled Systems

Often consumers use directions of eye gaze as their only means of indicating. Manual eye-controlled communication systems have been in use for a long time. In manual systems the user communicates "yes" or "no" through eye blinks or uses the eyes to point to letters on an alphabet board to spell utterances. This manual form of using eye movement as a means of input can be automated by electronically detecting the user's eye movements as a control interface for direct selection.

There are currently two basic types of eye-controlled systems. One type employs an infrared video camera mounted adjacent to a computer display. An infrared beam from the camera is shined on the person's eye and then reflected by the retina. The camera picks up this reflection of the individual's eye as he looks at the on-screen keyboard appearing on the computer monitor. Special processing software in the computer analyzes the images coming into the camera from the eyes and determines where on the screen and for how long the person is looking. The user makes a selection by looking at it for a specified period, which can be adjusted according to the user's needs. The EyeGaze System,† Quick Glance,‡ and Tobii§ are examples of two eye-controlled systems of

* Cambium Learning Group, Inc., Dallas, Texas (www.cambiumlearning-technologies.com/)

† LC Technologies, Inc., www.eyegaze.com

‡ Eye Tech Digital Systems, www.eyetechds.com/assistive-technology

§ Tobii Technology, www.tobii.com

this type. The operating principles generally require that the user of the technology be capable of maintaining a stable head position (preferably in midline) and that they are able to focus their point of regard on the target for a sufficient period of time. Smooth vertical and horizontal eye movements throughout the majority of the range of motion are also required.

Eye-controlled systems can be beneficial for individuals who have little or no movement in their limbs and who may also have limited speech (e.g., someone who has had a brain stem stroke, has amyotrophic lateral sclerosis [ALS], or has high-level quadriplegia). Some disadvantages of eye-controlled systems are that sunlight, bright incandescent lighting, and contact lenses may interfere with system tracking. The cost of such systems is still rather high in comparison with other input methods. For some individuals, however, it may be the only reliable means of voluntary movement for controlling an assistive device.

Pointing Interfaces

Because direct selection involves choosing from an array of items, we can think of mouse use or other pointing as direct selection. When using a graphic user interface (icons on a screen), the mouse is moved to the icon of choice and is then clicked or double clicked to open or run the chosen file or program. This is direct selection. See Chapter 7 for a discussion of various approaches to mouse emulation. There are also alternative pointing interfaces that can replace the mouse, such as a trackball, a head sensor, a continuous joystick, or the use of the arrow keys on the keypad (called MouseKeys). Box 6-2 identifies the critical questions to consider when assessing an individual for using any type of pointing interface.

To make a selection on the screen using a pointing device, it is necessary to direct the pointer to the desired item on the screen (the target) and stay fixed on the target while executing the action needed to make a selection (e.g., clicking or double clicking, or clicking and holding to drag the item). These all imply that the targeted selection is accurate. The person may be able to get to a target area on the screen, but the size of the target may affect her ability to maintain that position while selecting it. Any location on the screen can be a target and these can be of different sizes. Depending on the software program, the size of the target may be fixed or it may be possible to modify the size to meet the user's needs.

The user can employ one of two techniques to make a selection. The first method is called an **acceptance time** selection. In this technique the user pauses at the selection for a predetermined time period (which is adjustable). At the end of the acceptance time period, the device automatically executes whatever function was selected (click, etc.). The other approach is called manual selection. In this technique, the user activates a separate control interface to let the device know that the selection has been made. The second approach provides more control for the user, but it also requires additional user motor control to activate the acceptance control interface.

BOX 6-2 Critical Questions for Evaluating Use of Electronic Pointing Interfaces

1. Can the consumer use the pointing interface to reach all the targets on the screen?
2. Is the size and spacing of the screen targets appropriate?
3. Is the consumer able to complete the action needed to make a selection and perform other mouse functions required by the application software (i.e., click, drag, and double-click)?
4. Is the sensory feedback provided by the control interface and the user display adequate?
5. Does the consumer use the keyboard layout effectively?

CASE STUDY – EVALUATION AND SELECTION OF A POINTING INTERFACE

David is a 21-year-old male who has muscular dystrophy. He would like to be able to access the family computer for educational and recreational purposes. David would like to play computer-based games and use drawing programs that typically require using a mouse. He lacks movement in his four extremities, with the exception of wrist and finger movement. He is able to reach with each hand from within 3 inches of his body to 8 inches out from his body. With his right hand he can reach approximately 5.5 inches to the right of midline and with his left hand he can reach 3 inches to the left of midline. He cannot cross midline with either hand.

David tried a contracted keyboard, and he was able to point to keys in a restricted range near the middle of the keyboard. He was unable to access other areas of the keyboard without assistance for repositioning of his arms. He was able to move a continuous joystick in all four directions and use it with the on-screen keyboard software, but this was difficult for him. A trackball was also used with the on-screen keyboard software to determine whether David could use it. He could easily use the trackball as a pointing device to point to the keys shown on the screen. Using a drawing program and the trackball, he was able to direct the cursor to various parts of the screen with enough precision to draw lines and shapes. However, he was unable to both hold the trackball in place with the cursor on the desired selection and simultaneously press the button on the trackball with the same hand to make his selection. The acceptance time selection technique was shown to him, and he was able to easily use this technique.

(Continued)

CASE STUDY – EVALUATION AND SELECTION OF A POINTING INTERFACE—cont'd

QUESTIONS

1. From the data given, would you recommend a contracted keyboard for David?
2. From the information given, what would be the optimal control interface for David? Is there other information you would like to find out regarding David's needs and skills that might influence your recommendation?
3. What other software will David need to operate the recommended control interface?

Pointing interfaces vary in terms of the tactile and proprioceptive feedback they provide, which may affect the user's performance. Using a pointing interface also requires a significant amount of coordination between the body site executing the movement of the cursor and the eyes following the cursor on the screen and locating the targets. It is important to determine whether the layout of the items on the screen (the selection set) is beneficial or detrimental to the user's performance. For example, it may be easier for the user to see one part of the screen than another. It may also be more difficult to move the pointer to some parts of the screen because of motor control limitations. It is possible to rearrange the elements on the screen, to reposition the pointing device, and to change the size of the elements on the screen to compensate for these problems. The selection set and its layout will vary depending on the pointing interface and the software being used. It is important to know whether the layout of the selection set can be modified for a particular pointing interface and what type of modifications will benefit the user.

Light Pointers

A visible light beam may be used as a pointing interface for direct selection. In a simple form the light can be pointed at objects in a room or at letters on a piece of paper. The effectiveness of the light pointer is directly related to how bright and focused it is, and this in turn affects its size and weight. Light pointers are most commonly attached to a band worn on the head, but they can also be held in the hand. Highly focused light sources such as laser pens may cause damage if they are shined directly into the eye (Box 6-3).[15]

Modifications to Keyboards and Pointing Interfaces

There are several problems that may be experienced by individuals with a physical disability in using any of the control interfaces just described. If a consumer is having difficulty using a particular control interface, there are three paths to pursue. A control enhancer may resolve the difficulty (e.g., when the user has limited range for accessing the interface). Modification of the interface being evaluated is another alternative, and trying an interface that requires less motor control is the third approach. Before introducing an interface that requires less motor control, modification of the method being evaluated should be considered. Table 6-3 lists the areas of need for which modification of a control interface may be beneficial and approaches that can be used. Each of these difficulties in using a keyboard can be addressed by either hardware or software modifications.

BOX 6-3 Tips on Safe Use of Laser Light as a Head Pointer

Laser light sources (including laser pens) are a source of highly focused light of high intensity. Because they are focused, the energy is all concentrated on a small area—including the retina if the light is shined in the eye of another person. Lasers are grouped into 5 classes: I (<0.01 mw), II (0.01 to 1 mw), IIIa (1 mw to 5 mw), IIIB (1 mw to 0.5 w) and IV (>0.5 w).[13] Salamo and Jakobs (1996)[15] recommend an exposure of less that 0.0004 milliwatts (0.4 microwatts) for 1 second as the limit for safe continuous exposure as might occur in a classroom. Only class I lasers meet this criteria and they are so dim as to not be visible in a brightly lit classroom. Laser pointers are at least Class II. Because of the continuous use, the possible limitation of protective reflexes that protect non-disabled individuals from exposure to Class I lasers, and the uncontrolled environment, the classroom, caution should be exercised when using laser pointers for choice making and pointing?

CASE STUDY – LARRY

Larry was 25 when he sustained a traumatic brain injury (TBI) in a car accident. That was two years ago. He attends a day program where you work. He wants to get a job, but all the jobs that he can do require him to use a computer. Unfortunately his intention tremor makes it difficult for him to type.

What types of keyboard modifications would you suggest that Larry try? Why did you choose them?

Keyboard Layouts

The QWERTY keyboard layout (Figure 6-8, *A*), the one most familiar to people, was originally designed more than 100 years ago to slow down 10-finger typists using a manual typewriter so the keys would not jam. The QWERTY layout requires much excursion of the fingers and assumes that two hands with 10 fingers will be used. With an increasing number of individuals using computers, there has been a substantial increase in repetitive strain injuries to the hand. Redefining the layout of the characters on the keyboard can reduce the amount of finger movements required by the user to access the keys and may reduce fatigue and the likelihood of an individual's incurring a repetitive strain injury.

TABLE 6-3 Modifications to Keyboards and Pointing Interfaces

Need Addressed	Approach
User's speed not adequate for task prediction software*	Modify keyboard layout, macros, rate enhancement software, word completion/prediction
User has problems making accurate selections	Keyguard, template, shield, delayed acceptance*
User has difficulty holding down the modifier key while pressing another key	Mechanical latch, software latch*
User cannot release key before it starts to repeat	Keyguard, careful selection of keyboard characteristics, software to disable key repeat function*

*Software modifications are discussed in Chapter 8.

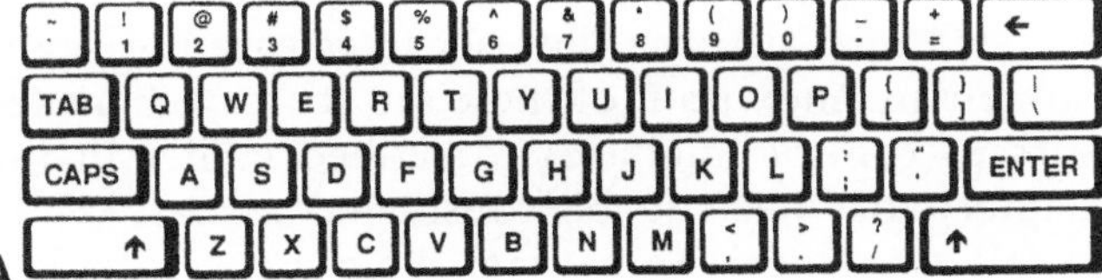

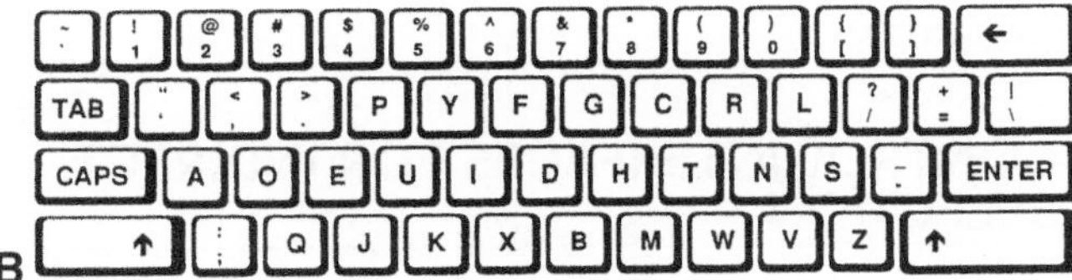

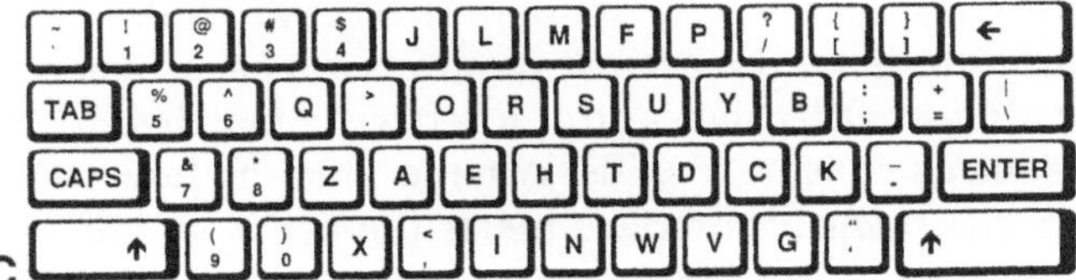

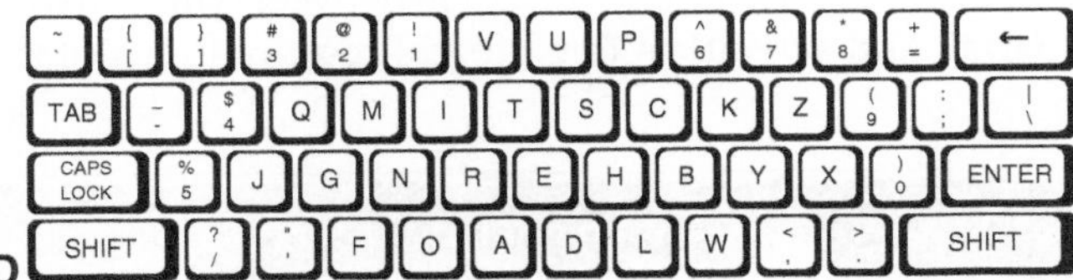

Figure 6-8 **A,** Standard QWERTY layout. Dvorak keyboard layouts: **B,** two-hand layout; **C,** one-hand layout, right hand; **D,** Chubon keyboard layout for a typist who uses a single digit or a typing stick.

Alternative keyboard layout designs have been developed to accelerate typing speed when an individual is using only one hand or a mouthstick or another alternative access device. The definition of the keyboard layout on computer keyboards is determined by software in the computer and the keys are labeled with the corresponding characters. The keyboard hardware (other than labeling of the keys) is not modified with any of the alternative keyboard layouts.

The Dvorak keyboard layout was designed in the 1930s to reduce fatigue and increase speed by placing letters that are most frequently used on the home row of the keyboard. On the left side of the home row are all the vowels. Five of the most used consonants are on the right side of the home row. There are three Dvorak keyboard layouts: one for two-handed typists (Figure 6-8, *B*), one for right hand-only typists (Figure 6-8, *C*), and one for left hand-only typists (similar to that shown for right hand-only typists but flipped). Information on how to redefine the computer keyboard as a Dvorak layout can be found at this Web site: web.mit.edu/jcb/www/Dvorak/index.html.

The Chubon keyboard is a layout pattern that was designed to be used by the single-digit or typing-stick typist.[7] In this layout (Figure 6-8, *D*) the letters in the English language that are used most frequently are arranged near each other in the center. This layout also places letters that are most frequently used together (e.g., *r* and *e*) in close proximity, which reduces the amount of movement required by the user for entering text and helps to increase the rate of input. For individuals who use a mouthstick or typing stick, an alternative keyboard layout that reduces the amount of travel to keys can significantly increase efficiency.

Another alternative keyboard layout is an alphabetical array. Often individuals who are nonverbal and have been using a manual communication board to spell have learned to use an array in which the letters are placed in alphabetical order. They are very familiar with this arrangement and may be very efficient in selecting characters. For these individuals, it often does not make sense to have them learn a completely new letter arrangement. In this case the keyboard can be redefined to have an alphabetical arrangement by using software.

When selecting a keyboard pattern, several factors need to be considered. The first factor to consider is whether the user is already familiar with one particular keyboard layout. If this is the case, it is important to keep in mind that the time needed for retraining to use a new keyboard pattern is estimated at 90 to 100 hours.[2] Another factor to consider is whether the keyboard is shared with other individuals. It is possible to have the computer keyboard defined to use two keyboard patterns (e.g., QWERTY and Dvorak) and to label the keys so that the standard keys are not obscured (e.g., via a clear overlay with the new key labels on them, so when placed over the standard keys the original labels are still visible). However, this modification can be confusing to all typists. There are little data to support the claims that alternative keyboard patterns increase speed or reduce injury. Selecting an alternative keyboard, like other technologies, depends on the needs and skills of the user and which layout she feels most comfortable and efficient using.

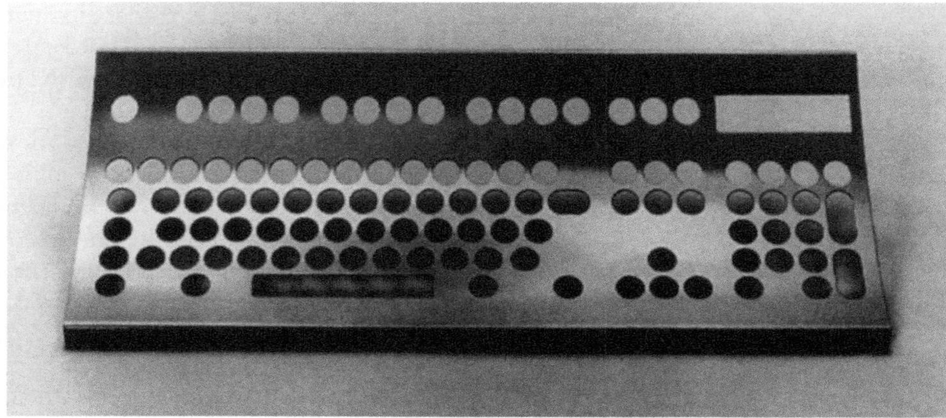

Figure 6-9 Keyguard. (Courtesy TASH, Inc., Ajax, Ontario, Canada.)

Keyguards, Shields, and Templates

Some people may be able to select individual keys directly, but they may occasionally miss the desired key and enter the wrong key. For individuals who have difficulty in accurately targeting and activating keys, a keyguard (Figure 6-9) placed over the keyboard helps by isolating each key and guiding the person's movement. A keyguard is also useful for individuals who have extraneous movements each time they bring their hand off the keyboard in their attempt to target a new key. Instead of moving away from the keyboard to make the next selection, the person can rest his hand on top of the keyguard without activating any keys and make relatively isolated, controlled (and thus faster) selections. Although keyguards have been shown to increase the user's accuracy, speed is typically compromised.[15] In nearly all situations a clear keyguard is preferred, so that there is minimal obstruction of the labels on the keys. Still, the position of the keyboard with a keyguard needs to be assessed to ensure that the key labels are not being obstructed from the user's view. Keyguards are commercially available for the common computer keyboards. In situations where an individual using a special terminal in a work setting would benefit from a keyguard, a custom keyguard can be fabricated out of clear plastic.

Similar to the use of a keyguard is the use of a shield on the keyboard to block out certain keys. This modification is typically done with children who are just beginning to use computers and are using software programs that only require the use of a few select keys. To guide the child to the correct keys and increase her chances of success with the program, a shield is placed over the keys that are not being used.

Technologies for Reducing Accidental Entries

Many keyboards produce multiple entries of characters by prolonged pressing of the key called key repeat. Although this feature is useful to nondisabled users (e.g., to obtain multiple spaces or underlines), it can present a problem for persons with disabilities who may not be able to release the key fast enough to prevent double entries. There are a number of ways this can be avoided. Certain types of keyboards and their sensitivities may increase or decrease double entries, and auditory feedback (e.g., a beep) when a key is activated may also cue the user to release the key in a timely manner. Both of these are sensory characteristics of control interfaces (described earlier in this chapter) that need to be considered as part of the overall assessment. Sometimes the presence of a keyguard helps to diminish the double entries. If the double entries remain a problem, FilterKeys can be used (see Table 7-1).

CONTROL INTERFACES FOR INDIRECT SELECTION

Indirect methods of selection use a single control interface or an array of control interfaces and require that the consumer be able to carry out a certain set of skills. Box 6-4 shows the critical questions to pose when evaluating whether the control interface is matched to the required consumer skills. When evaluating how well a specific control interface meets the needs of the consumer, it is first necessary to determine whether the user can activate the control interface, which determines whether there is a match between the sensory, spatial, and activation (e.g., force) requirements of the

BOX 6-4 Critical Questions for Evaluating Single Switch and Switch Array Use

1. Can the consumer activate the switch?
2. Can the consumer wait for the appropriate selection?
3. Can the consumer activate the switch at the right time?
4. Can the consumer maintain switch activation (hold)?
5. Can the consumer release on command?
6. Can the consumer repeatedly carry out the steps necessary for selection?

control interface and the physical and sensory skills of the user. If activation is possible, it is necessary to look at other skills related to the way the control interface is to be used for indirect selection. The first of these is whether the consumer can wait for the desired selection to be presented. This task requires that the consumer have sensory skills for awareness of the selections being presented. Depending on the consumer's sensory abilities, selections can be presented visually or auditorily. An inability to wait can result from problems with central processing or motor control. If the consumer is having difficulty waiting, it is important to determine the underlying cause (i.e., sensory, central processing, or motor). The cause is not always easy to determine, but asking questions such as those shown in Table 6-4 can help to identify the problem(s) and modify the task.

The consumer must also be able to reliably activate the control interface at the right time (i.e., when the desired selection is presented). This is a function of reaction time, visual tracking, and vigilance. Difficulties with any one of these individually or in any combination can lead to difficulties in selecting a target during scanning.

Another critical condition is that the consumer be able to hold a control interface in its closed position for the time it takes the signal from the control interface to register. This time is a variable of the control interface and may differ from control interface to control interface. In addition, applications such as Morse code input, inverse scanning, and wheelchair mobility require the user to hold the control interface closed. Within each of these applications, the length of this hold time varies. For example, for the person using one-switch Morse code, the hold time varies from shorter to longer depending on the input signal (dot or dash). For power wheelchair control, the control interface (joystick) is held down until the user wants the chair to stop. Frustration, embarrassment, and possibly serious injury can result if the user cannot carry out precise holding of the control interface. If the consumer is having difficulty activating or holding the control interface, the control interface itself may require too much force or displacement for activation, or the sensory feedback it provides may be inadequate. If this is the case, having the consumer experiment with control interfaces that are more matched to her needs (i.e., physical effort, sensory feedback, and task to be performed) is recommended. If there is a problem even activating the control interface, or if the consumer fatigues after several activations, try one that requires less activation force. If the consumer keeps pressing on the control after it has activated, then the sensory feedback may not be enough to signal successful activation. Try a control interface that provides more feedback (e.g., a clicking sound).

Releasing the control interface in a timely manner is also important. Difficulty in releasing the control interface can cause inadvertent selections. It is easier for some individuals to activate and hold the control interface than to release it. Many assistive technologies allow choice of automatic, inverse, or step scanning. Finally, it should be determined whether the consumer is able to carry out these sets of skills repeatedly.

The OTA or PTA can evaluate the effectiveness of a control interface by using simple technology such as a tape recorder or battery-operated toy as an output when the control interface is activated. If the consumer's skills are adequate to use the control interface on command to control a simple output, then asking them to hold the switch and to release it at a particular time will show how successfully they might use the control interface for more functional tasks. If one body control site doesn't work for the person after practice and training, it may be necessary to consider a different anatomic site or a different control interface. Using the critical questions to evaluate each pairing (control site and interface) will help the OTA or PTA to evaluate how well things are working for the consumer.

TABLE 6-4 Troubleshooting Consumer Difficulties with Waiting for a Cursor During Scanning

Possible cause	Considerations
Range of motion	Can the consumer easily reach the control to activate it?
Visual	Can the consumer see the target? Move the target in the visual field and ask the consumer to indicate when he or she sees it.
Motor control	Can the consumer activate the switch if a target is not present?

Types of Single Switches

There are numerous single control interfaces (switches) that are commercially available. It is also possible to custom fabricate switches, but there are a number of reasons why this option is not advised. Although it may seem less expensive to purchase only the materials to make a switch, when you factor in the time it takes to make the control interface, the cost involved increases significantly. In addition, custom-made switches are not as durable as commercially available switches and will not hold up over time.

When evaluating the effectiveness of a control interface for an individual, it is important to consider the spatial, activation-deactivation, and sensory characteristics discussed earlier. Single switches come in many different sizes and shapes and have diverse force and sensory requirements. It is critical that the consumer has the opportunity to try out any switch being considered for a control interface. Table 6-5 summarizes the types of single-control interfaces and gives a sampling of control interfaces that are commercially available based on the categories shown in Table 6-1.

TABLE 6-5 Examples of Single-Switch Interfaces

Category	Description	Switch Name/Manufacturer
Mechanical switches	Activated by the application of a force; generic names of switches include paddle, plate, button, lever, and membrane	Pal Pads, Taction Pads (Adaptivation Corp.); Big Buddy Button, Microlight Switch, Grasp, and Trigger Switches (TASH); Big Red and Jelly Bean Switches (AbleNet Inc.); Lever, Leaf, and Tread Switches (ZYGO Industries); Dual-rocking, P and Wobble Switches (Prentke Romich Co.); Access and Finger Access (Saltillo); FlexAble, Rocking Action, and Plate Switches (AMDi)
Electromagnetic switches	Activated by the receipt of electromagnetic energy such as light or radio waves	Fiber Optic Sensor, (ASL); Proximity Switches (AMDi); SCATIR (Tash); Infrared/sound/touch switches (Words +)
Electrical control switches	Activated by detection of electrical signals from the surface of the body	D-Box Standalone EMG Switch (Emerge Medical); Brainfingers 9Cyberlink (Adaptivation Corp.)
Proximity switches	Activated by a movement close to the detector, but without actual contact	ASL 204 and 208, Proximity Switch (Adaptive Switch Laboratories, Inc.); Untouchable Buddy (Tash Inc.)
Pneumatic switches	Activated by detection of respiratory airflow or pressure	Pneumatic Switch (Adaptivation); LifeBreath Switch and Sip and Puff Switch (Toys for Special Children); ASL 308 Pneumatic Switch (Adaptive Switch Laboratories); PRC Pneumatic Switch Model PS-2 (Prentke Romich Co.); Pneumatic Switch Model CM-3 (ZYGO Industries); Wireless Integrated Sip/Puff Switch (Madentec)
Phonation switches	Activated by sound or speech	Voice Activated and Sound Activated Switches (Enabling Devices); Infrared/Sound/Touch Switch (Words +)

Data from Ablenet Inc., Minneapolis, Minn. (www.ablenetinc.com); Adaptive Switch Laboratories, Inc., Spicewood, Tex., www.asl-inc.com; Adaptivation Co., Sioux Falls, S.D. (www.adaptivation.com); AMDi, Hicksville, N.Y. (http://www.amdi.net/index.htm), Emerge Medical, Atlanta, Ga. (http://www.emergemedical.com/); Madentec Limited, Edmonton, Alberta, Canada (www.madentec.com); Prentke Romich, Wooster, Ohio (www.prentrom.com); Saltillo (http://www.saltillo.com/),TASH, Ajax, Ontario, Canada or Richmond, Va. (www.tashinc.com); Enabling Devices—Toys for Special Children, Hastings-on-Hudson, N.Y. (www.enablingdevices.com); Words + Inc., (www.words-plus.com); ZYGO, Portland, Ore. (www.zygo-usa.com).

Mechanical Control Interfaces

Mechanical control interfaces are the most commonly used type of single switch, and they can be of various shapes and sizes. Paddle switches (Figure 6-10, *A*) have movement in one direction. On some types of paddle switches the sensitivity can be adjusted according to the user's needs. Wobble (Figure 6-10, *B*) and leaf (Figure 6-10, *C*) switches have a 2- to 4-inch shaft that can be activated by the user in two directions. The wobble switch makes an audible click when activated but the leaf switch does not, making the wobble switch more desirable when the switch is out of the user's visual range, such as during head activation. Lever switches (Figure 6-10, *D*) are similar to wobble switches with the exception that they can only be activated in one direction. This type of switch usually has a round, padded area at the end of a shaft and produces an audible click, which also makes it desirable for activation by the head.

There are also various types of button switches that come in different sizes, from a large, round switch such as the "Big Red" switch, to a small button switch that can be held between the thumb and the index finger, such as the "Cap" switch. Membrane switches consist of a very thin pad, which requires some degree of force to activate. These pads are available in various sizes, from as small as 2 inches × 3 inches to as large as 3 inches × 5 inches. The advantage of these membrane pads are that they are flexible, can be paired with an object (by being directly attached to it), and can be used to teach the user to make a direct connection between the object and the switch. The main disadvantage of membrane control interfaces is that they provide poor tactile feedback, which can lead to extra activations or failure to apply enough force to activate the control interface. All these control interfaces are activated by body movement that produces a force upon the control interface. They are considered passive control interfaces because they do not require any outside power source. Mercury switches can be activated by a change in position such as lifting an arm or finger or tilting the head, which removes the need to activate a mechanical control interface.

Proximity Switches

There are also control interfaces that are activated with body movement but do not require force or even contact with the control interface. These are referred to

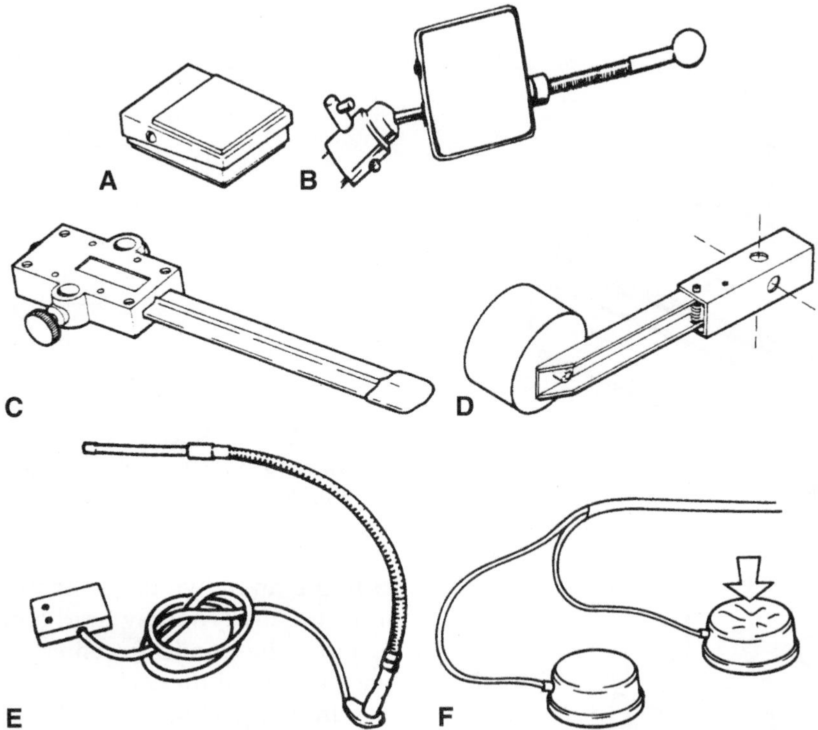

Figure 6-10 Examples of single switches. **A,** Paddle switch. **B,** Wobble switch. **C,** Leaf switch. **D,** Lever switch. **E,** Puff-and-sip switch. **F,** Pillow switch. (**A, C,** and **D,** Courtesy ZYGO Industries, Portland. **B, E,** and **F** from Bergen AF, Presperin J, Tallman T: *Positioning for function: wheelchairs and other assistive technologies,* Valhalla, NY, 1990, Valhalla Rehabilitation Publications.)

as proximity switches. The switch is activated when it detects an object within its range. The activation range of these types of switches varies from nearly touching the switch to 3 feet away and usually is adjustable. The switches in this series utilize different technologies, ranging from photoelectric to fiber optic, to detect the movement. These switches are active, meaning they require an outside power source, such as a battery, to operate.

Pneumatic Control Interfaces

Pneumatic switches are activated by detection of respiratory airflow or pressure and include puff-and-sip and pillow switches. Puff-and-sip switches (Figure 6-10, *E*) are activated by the individual's blowing air into the switch or sucking air out of it. The individual can send varying degrees of air pressure to the switch, which then provides different commands to the processor. Pillow switches (Figure 6-10, *F*) respond to air pressure when squeezed (such as with a hand bulb).

Switch Arrays, Discrete Joysticks, and Chord Keyboards

Control interfaces are commercially available in preconfigured switch arrays (from two to eight), and any of the single switches we have discussed earlier can be used to design a custom array to meet the needs of the consumer. These offer the advantages of multiple signals while retaining the requirement of low resolution typical of single switches.

Paddle switches are often used in switch arrays when two to five input signals are desirable. A type of paddle switch that provides dual input from one control is called a rocker switch (Figure 6-11, *A*). A rocker switch is like a seesaw and does exactly what it says: it rocks from side to side around a fulcrum. This design allows the user to maintain contact with the switch and perform a rotating movement with the control site to activate each side. This type of dual-switch array is often used for Morse code input, with one side signaling dots and the other side dashes. The Slot Switch (Figure 6-11, *B*) is one example of a commercially available paddle switch array that is already configured. The switches in this array are mounted on a base piece that has dividers between the control interfaces. The purpose of the dividers is to help the user isolate the appropriate switch. This array is typically used with the hands or feet by someone who has gross motor skills and a fairly large range of motion. The isolation of each switch helps when the user may not be able to locate the switch visually. There are other switch arrays that are mounted and activated using the head. Switch arrays are often used for power wheelchair control; we discuss them in greater detail in Chapter 12.

At the other extreme, in terms of size, is the Penta switch array. This array consists of five switches, each approximately a quarter inch in diameter. Its overall size is 2 inches in diameter, and it is small enough so that it can be held in the palm of the hand and be activated by the thumb.

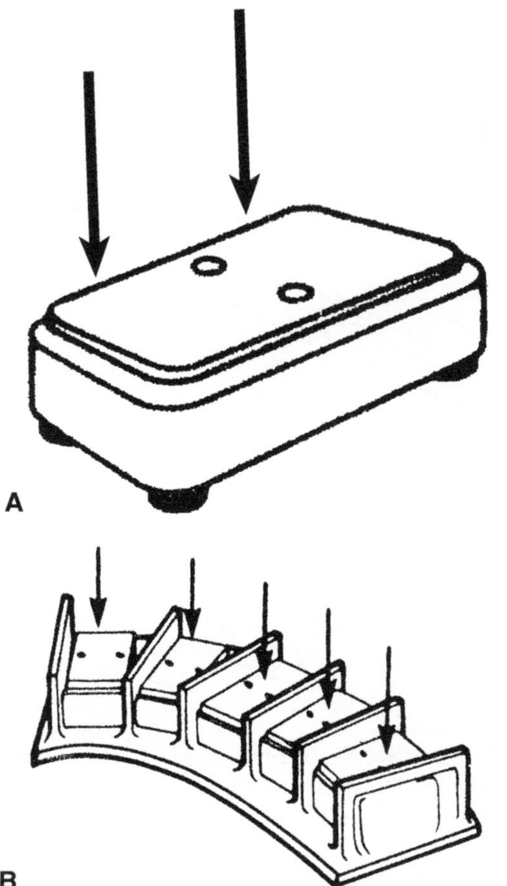

Figure 6-11 Examples of switch arrays. **A,** Dual rocker switch. **B,** Slot switch. (**A** from Webster JG et al, editors: *Electronic devices for rehabilitation,* New York, 1985, John Wiley and Sons; **B,** Courtesy ZYGO Industries, Portland, Ore.)

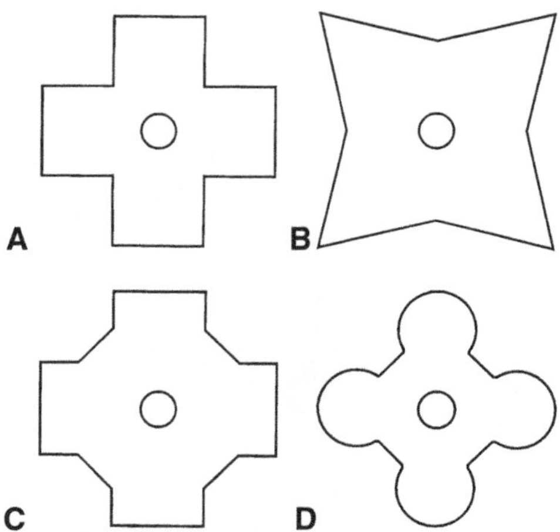

Figure 6-12 A–D, Four different shapes of joystick templates to maximize user's skills.

A discrete joystick is also considered an array of switches. It consists of four or five control interface input signals (UP, DOWN, LEFT, RIGHT, and ENTER) that are either open or closed (off or on), with nothing in between. To close the switched joystick the control handle is moved in the direction of one of the switches. Switched joysticks require limited range but moderate resolution by the user. They are available with a variety of displacements, forces, and handles to accommodate different grasping abilities of the user. If there is a maximum of five items (e.g., directions of a power wheelchair) in the selection set, the joystick functions as an interface for direct selection. When the selection set is more than five, indirect selection is required using directed scanning. Using the joystick with this method, the individual selects the direction and the device determines the speed of cursor movement.

Control-Enhancing Joystick Templates

A template used on a joystick to guide the individual's movement is akin to the use of a keyguard for a keyboard. The template has four channels that guide the movement of the joystick. The shape of the channel may vary depending on the template, and can be a factor in the individual's ability to control the joystick. For example, an individual using the cross-shaped template in Figure 6-12, *A,* may need a more precise movement to move the joystick to enter the desired channel, but once in one of these channels, the user will be able to stay in easily. However, if the template is like the one in 6-12, *B,* it will be easy for the individual to enter one of the channels but difficult to stay. A compromise solution is to use a template similar to the one shown in Figure 6-12, *C.* In this case, because the entrance to each arm of the cross has been widened, it is easier to move in each direction. Because the end of the slot in each direction retains the cross shape, it is easier to keep the joystick in one direction. We can also improve the performance of the star template (Figure 6-12, *B*) by restricting the travel at the end of the channel once the movement has been made in a direction. This change is shown in Figure 6-12, *D.* For some individuals, the use and type of joystick template means the difference between success or failure in the operation of a power wheelchair (Table 6-6).

Mounting the Control Interface for Use

It is also necessary to mount single switches, joysticks, and switch arrays in a convenient location. The most common mounting locations are attachments to a table, a desk, a wheelchair lap tray, or to the person's body. There are commercially available mounting systems for table and wheelchair mounting. Some mounting requirements are more challenging than others. For example, it is generally more difficult to position a joystick for foot or chin use than it is to place it for hand use.

There are flexible and fixed mounting systems. Flexible mounting systems (Figure 6-13) can be adjusted and placed in various positions, which is advantageous in settings where more than one person needs a control interface mounting. Costs can be controlled by using the same mounting system at different times for several people. This type of mounting system is also advantageous for individuals who require changes in the position of their

TABLE 6-6 Control Enhancers and Technique Modifications

CONTROL ENHANCERS: Devices or equipment to extend or enhance motor control for direct selection (or for indirect selection where indicated by the *).

Postural Supports	At Hands/Arms	At Head
Lap tray*	Finger splint/pointer	Mouthstick
Arm rests*	Universal cuff with typing stick	Head pointer
Hip belt*	Wrist strap pointer	Head light
Chest straps*	Mobile arm supports*	Head mouse
Lateral supports*	Hand brace*	Head rest*
Abductor/adductor	Hand splint*	

TECHNIQUE MODIFICATIONS: Changes to the selection technique to reduce the demands for direct selection (or for indirect selection as indicated by the *).

Selection Set Design	Interface Adjustments	Additional Aids
Target size*	Acceptance time*	Keyguards
Spacing*	Delay until repeat*	Templates*
Array shape*	Repeat rate*	Shields*
Angle*	Cursor speed*	Hand rest*
Height*	Sensitivity*	
Order of items	Activation feedback*	

From Dowden P, Cook AM: Choosing effective selection techniques for beginning communicators. In Reichle J., Beukelman D., and Light J., editors: *Exemplary practices for beginning communicators*, (pp 395–432), Baltimore, 2002, Paul H. Brookes.

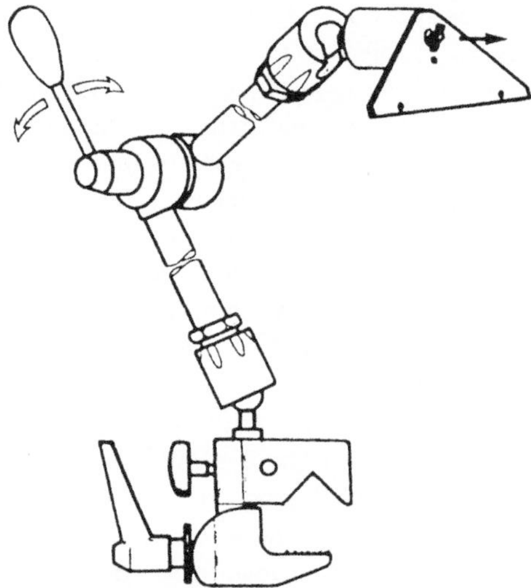

Figure 6-13 Flexible mounting system. (Courtesy ZYGO Industries, Portland, Ore.)

control interface because of fluctuating skill or need. The disadvantage of flexible mounting systems is that the position for the control interface must be determined each time it is put in place. Sometimes even a slight fluctuation in the position of the control interface can make a significant difference in the individual's ability to access it. Therefore, it is important to know the correct position of the switch to maximize ease of use. The switch needs to be placed in the correct position each time the individual is set up to use the device. The rehabilitation assistant is likely the one who will notice whether the position needs to be changed or not. Other mounting systems are fixed and are designed for use of a specific control site and control interface. The advantage of this approach is that the mounting system is not as likely to move or change position and require adjustment.

Switches are occasionally attached to the individual by straps. Attachment to the body has the major advantage of not being as affected by the person's change in body position. If a control interface is mounted to the wheelchair and the person shifts his position even slightly, the control interface may no longer be reachable or the new position may make it difficult to generate enough force to activate the control interface. One again, it is the OTA or PTA who is most likely to notice whether the switch is still in the best position for use.

The majority of control interfaces have a cable that connects them to the device being used. However, there are wireless keyboards, pointing interfaces, and switches. There are also separate wireless links that can be used with most control interfaces. Table 7-4 lists a number of wireless switch interfaces. These links consist of a transmitter that is plugged into the control interface and a receiver that plugs into the device. When the control interface is pressed, the signal is transmitted to the receiver and the device. The control interface is not physically connected to the device. Wireless control interfaces communicate with the processor via infrared signals such as those used with television remote controls. The obvious advantages of a remote control interface are that there is one less wire for the user to become entangled in and that it looks better. It can also be advantageous to have a wireless control interface when the interface is mounted on the person's wheelchair. This arrangement allows the person to move to or away from the device being used without having to connect or disconnect the interface. In many situations the person with a disability needs a personal attendant to assist with connecting the cable of the interface to the computer. The use of a remote control interface allows the person to come and go independently, so an attendant is not needed for this task.

Multiple versus Integrated Control Interfaces

Although generally an individual's "best" available control site is used, in some cases more than one control site must be identified. This situation most often occurs when one person uses several types of assistive technologies. For example, head control may be used for augmentative communication and foot control for a powered wheelchair. In other cases, such as with some neuromuscular disabilities (e.g., amyotrophic lateral sclerosis), multiple sites need to be identified because of progressive paralysis. The course of this progression can vary from months to years. The variation in ability to use effectors over the course of the disease makes it necessary to find flexible control interfaces that can be used with multiple control sites or to find separate control interfaces for several sites initially (see Chapters 4 and 7). Another reason for having multiple switch sites is fatigue during the day. Sometimes people need to switch to another control because the first is fatiguing and they can't sustain its use over the course of the activity or the day.

A long-standing goal of rehabilitation engineers and other rehabilitation therapy professionals is the integration of systems for augmentative and alternative communication (AAC), power mobility, environmental control, and computer access.[3,6] One of the major reasons for this emphasis is to allow the use, called **integrated control**, of the same control interface for several applications. Integration of controls can free the individual from multiple controls and can reduce the jumble of electronic devices surrounding the person.

It is possible to operate several devices by controlling just one of them (e.g., an augmentative communication system (Chapter 11), power wheelchair (Chapter 12), or environmental control system (Chapter 14). The main or controlling device is generally only capable of operating one single function device at a time, and the user designates the mode in which he or she would like to function. For example, there are several power wheelchairs with processors that allow the consumer to use one interface, such as a joystick, to control many functions. By selecting the drive mode, the person uses the joystick to propel the wheelchair in all directions. The person can exit the wheelchair drive mode, select the mode designated for environmental control, and turn the lights on and off in the house.

CASE STUDY – EVALUATION AND SELECTION OF SWITCHES

Mrs. Antonelli is a 30-year-old woman who has spastic quadriplegia as a result of meningitis at age 10. She lives with her husband and 2-year-old daughter. Mrs. Antonelli was referred for an evaluation for an augmentative communication system for conversation and writing. She has limited functional speech and communicates primarily by finger spelling with her left hand. Her husband interprets the finger spelling, but many others with whom Mrs. Antonelli would like to communicate do not understand her finger spelling. She independently uses a powered wheelchair that she controls by a joystick with her left hand.

Mrs. Antonelli showed limited range using either hand, and her resolution seemed fair; therefore, her ability to use keyboards was assessed using a contracted keyboard with each hand. She copied words with a great deal of effort and was less than 50% accurate.

Because Mrs. Antonelli uses a switched joystick to control her powered wheelchair, a switched joystick was tried with an electronic communication device in a directed scanning mode. Mrs. Antonelli used her left hand with the joystick in approximately the same position as her wheelchair joystick. She was able to move this joystick in all four directions. However, when asked to hold and release the joystick on a specific target, Mrs. Antonelli had difficulty. She was able to do this, but it required significant effort and several attempts to successfully select the desired target.

The pad switch,* a pneumatic switch, and a rocker switch† were then tried to evaluate the potential for Mrs. Antonelli to use coded access. The switches were positioned one at a time on the right wheelchair armrest and used with her right hand. Both a single-switch approach, in which a short switch hit produces a dot and a long switch hit produces a dash, and a dual-switch approach (one side produces dots and the other dashes) were tried. Mrs. Antonelli had difficulty with the one-switch mode because she was unable to consistently hold the switch for the appropriate length of time. In the two-switch mode, Mrs. Antonelli was able to move easily between the two parts of the rocker switch to generate dots and dashes. Mrs. Antonelli pressed one side of this switch with her index finger and one side with her middle finger. Mrs. Antonelli felt that the single switches were more difficult to operate than the rocker switch. Mrs. Antonelli also indicated a preference for the dual switch over the joystick for communication. She wanted to continue using her left hand to operate the joystick on her powered wheelchair and use her right hand for Morse code input into her communication device. Mrs. Antonelli acquired the communication system and, with a period of training, she quickly memorized the Morse code and her rate of input became rapid.

* TASH, Inc., Ajax, Ontario, Canada
† Prentke Romich Co., Wooster, Ohio

TABLE 6-7 Guidelines for Using Integrated Controls[11,12]

Integrated Controls Should Be Used When:	Integrated Controls May Not Be Useful When:
(1) the person has one single reliable control site; (2) the optimal control interface for each assistive device is the same; (3) speed, accuracy, ease of use, or endurance increases with the use of a single interface; (4) the person or his family prefers integrated controls for aesthetic, performance, or other subjective reasons.	(1) performance on one or more assistive devices is severely compromised by integrating control; (2) an individual wishes to operate an assistive device from a position other than from a power wheelchair; (3) physical, cognitive, or visual/perceptual limitations preclude integrating; (4) it is the individual's preference to use separate controls; (5) external factors such as cost or technical limitations preclude the use of integrated controls.

BOX 6-5 What the Research Tells Us About Integrated Controls

Consumer satisfaction with integrated controls:

- Reported that the majority of respondents indicated they were either very satisfied or satisfied with their integrated control device.
- An increase in independence and the ability to control other equipment such as televisions and computers were reasons the respondents gave for being satisfied with their integrated control devices.[1]

Ding et al (2003)[9] reviewed applications of integrated controls in power mobility, augmentative communication, electronic aids to daily living, and computer access. Linnman (1996) also describes the Multiple Master Multiple Slave (M3S) protocol for interfacing assistive technologies.[14] This protocol is an open network standard for interconnecting electronic rehabilitation devices for power mobility (Chapter 12), electronic aids to daily living and robotics (Chapter 14), and augmentative communication (Chapter 11). The M3S standard also includes safety features that allow rapid shutdown of electronic controls (especially wheelchair and robotics) if a failure occurs. It also provides a framework for assistive technology interfaces that makes them more compatible and more easily combined into integrated controls.

There is an inherent value in the simplification that can result from integration of control over separate functions; however, there are also many situations in which separate control interfaces (called **distributed controls**) and devices for each of the functions are warranted. Before deciding whether to use an integrated control or distributed controls, the implications of each method for the consumer should be carefully considered. Pros and cons of using integrated controls are listed in Table 6-7. Research in integrated controls is described in Box 6-5.

In some cases the consumer may have only one body site that she can control, and she may also have limited range and resolution of this control site. Trying to position more than one control interface for use by this site could be difficult, and using the same control interface for multiple functions would be easier and more effective. The optimal way for the consumer to operate each assistive device can be important. Assume that the consumer needs to control both a power wheelchair and an AAC device. If the consumer can easily control a joystick, that would be the optimal control interface for the power wheelchair. If this is also the easiest control interface for the consumer to use for controlling an AAC device, it would stand to reason that using an integrated control (the joystick) to operate both devices would be beneficial. However, if this person is able to use direct selection with an expanded keyboard for controlling an AAC device, the keyboard would be the optimal control interface for AAC. Integrating the control interfaces by using the joystick for both functions would not make sense in this situation.

In the example of Mrs. Antonelli (see Case Study), it was easy for her to control her power wheelchair using the joystick with her left hand. However, this method was not the easiest method for her to use to operate the communication device. She had the option, however, of using another body site, and it turned out that the "best" way for her to access the communication device was by using a dual rocker control interface with her right hand. If the controls had been integrated and she was to use the joystick for both power mobility and AAC, her activity output for communication would have been significantly compromised. The decision was made to use distributed controls, and her performance in communication was much improved.

SUMMARY

In this chapter we have defined the technology elements of the human/technology interface and their relationship to the other components of the assistive technology. Control interfaces can be characterized by their sensory, spatial, and activation-deactivation features. Understanding these characteristics can help the rehabilitation therapy practitioner/ATP sort through the maze of control interfaces. This chapter also described a framework that provides the rehabilitation therapy practitioner/ATP with a systematic process for matching the interface to the needs and skills of consumers. Critical questions were identified that relate to the user's skills needed to control particular types of interfaces. Addressing these questions during the evaluation can facilitate the selection of an appropriate control interface for the consumer.

STUDY QUESTIONS

1. What is the function of the control interface? Describe the difference between a discrete and a continuous input with examples for each.
2. Define the elements of the human/technology interface and how they are related to the processor and the output.
3. What factors are important when evaluating whether a control interface is working for an individual?
4. What are the somatosensory characteristics of control interfaces that need to be considered when evaluating the usefulness of a control interface for a consumer?
5. List two disabilities or conditions that might lead to the need for enhanced sensory feedback from a control interface.
6. What are the two factors that determine the spatial characteristics of a control interface?
7. Compare the user profile for a standard, an ergonomic, an expanded, and a contracted keyboard.
8. What is the major purpose of an ergonomic keyboard?
9. What are the two most common approaches to detecting eye position and movement for use as a control interface?
10. What are the major types of single switches in terms of how they are activated by the consumer?
11. What is point of gaze, and why is it a potential limitation in eye-tracking systems?
12. List three types of modifications to keyboards and pointing devices, and give an example of the problems that each solves.
13. Review the description of control interface flexibility in the section on characteristics of control interfaces. Pick three control interfaces described in the text, including one that is very flexible, one that is moderately flexible, and one that is not flexible. Justify your choices.
14. What are the steps you would use to determine is a control interface is working well for an individual consumer?
15. Describe distributed and integrated control. What are the advantages and disadvantages of each?
16. What are the major considerations in determining whether a control interface is mounted correctly for a consumer?
17. What kinds of problems can be caused by poor mounting?
18. What are the two types of mounting systems for control interfaces?
19. What role does proper positioning play in successful use of a control interface?

REFERENCES

1. Angelo J, Trefler E: A survey of persons who use integrated control devices, *Assist Technol* 10(2):77–83, 1998.
2. Anson DK: *Alternative computer access: a guide to selection,* Philadelphia, 1997, FA Davis.
3. Barker MR: *Integrating assistive technology: communication, computers, control and seating and mobility systems.* Presented at Demystifying Technology Workshop, Sacramento, CA, 1991, CSUS Assistive Device Center.
4. Barker MR, Cook AM: A systematic approach to evaluating clients' physical ability for control of assistive devices. In *Proc 4th Ann Conf Rehabil Eng,* June 1981, pp 287–289.
5. Bear-Lehman J: Orthopedic conditions. In Trombly CA, editor: *Occupational therapy for physical dysfunction,* ed 4, Baltimore, MD, 1995, Williams and Wilkins.
6. Caves K, et al: The use of integrated controls for mobility, communication and computer access. In *Proc 14th RESNA Conf,* June 1991, pp 166–167.
7. Chubon RA, Hester MR: An enhanced standard computer keyboard system for single-finger and typing-stick typing, *J Rehabil Res Dev* 25(4):17–24, 1988.
8. Cook AM, Polgar JM: *Cook and Hussey's assistive technologies: principles and practice,* St Louis, 2008, Mosby.
9. Ding D, et al: Integrated control and related technology of assistive devices, *Assist Technol* 15(2):89–97, 2003.
10. Fruchterman JR: in the palm of your hand: a vision of the future of technology for people with visual impairments, *J Vis Impair Blindness* 97(10):585–591, 2003.
11. Guerette PJ, Nakai RJ: Access to assistive technology: a comparison of integrated and distributed control, *Technol Dis* 5(1):63–73, 1996.
12. Guerette P, Sumi E: Integrating control of multiple assistive devices: a retrospective review, *Assist Technol* 6(1):67–76, 1994.
13. Hyman WA, Miller GE, Neigut JS: Laser diodes for head pointing and environmental control. In *Proc RESNA Conf,* 1992, pp 377–379.
14. Linnman S: M3S: The local network for electric wheelchairs and rehabilitation equipment, *IEEE Trans Rehabil Eng* 4(3):188–192, 1996.
15. Salamo GJ, Jakobs T: Laser pointers: are they safe for use by children? *Augment Altern Commun* 12(1):47–51, 1996.
16. Tessler FN: *The Apple adjustable keyboard,* November 1993, MACWORLD.
17. Weiss PL: Mechanical characteristics of micro-switches adapted for the physically disabled, *J Biomed Eng* 12(5): 398–402, 1990.

CHAPTER 7

Computer Access – Augmenting the Keyboard and Mouse

KEY TERMS

Control Interface
Continuous Input
Digital Recording
Emulation
Graphical User Interface (GUI)
Mouse
Multitasking
On-Screen Keyboard
Speech Synthesis
Text-To-Speech Programs
USB port

CHAPTER OUTLINE

LEARNING OBJECTIVES

Upon completing this chapter, you will be able to do the following:

1. Describe the computer-user interface
2. List the major components of a computer system and give the function of each
3. Describe the major approaches to keyboard and mouse emulation
4. Describe the major issues facing people with disabilities who want to use mainstream technologies
5. Describe the major approaches to electronic speech generation used in assistive technologies

In the United States, many computer adaptations are mandated by the legislation described in Chapter 1 (e.g., PL 508). The best approach to adapting a computer for use by individuals with physical limitations is to begin with the simplest modifications designed for the most minimal of physical limitations on the part of the user. If the minimal adaptation is not sufficient for a given user, then more complex adaptations can be evaluated.

No matter how complex the adaptation, the goal is always to make sure that: (1) all of the functions of the computer are available to the user who has a disability; and (2) all application software that runs on the unmodified computer runs on the adapted computer. All the keyboard keys, including modifier (e.g., shift, control, alt) and special function keys, and all the mouse functions, such as point, click, and drag, must be available on the adapted input system. If a program (e.g., word processor) works with the standard computer, then it should work with the adaptations that are provided for the individual with a disability.

KEYBOARDS – TYPICAL AND UNIQUE

On-screen Keyboards

On-screen keyboards have a selection set on the screen that resembles a physical keyboard (Figure 7-1, *B*). In order to enter a character or select a function, the user of the on-screen keyboard positions the cursor inside the desired "key" or icon on the screen. Movement of the cursor can be by mouse, trackball, joystick, control interface array, head-controlled mouse, or touch screens. Once the cursor is located inside the targeted screen item, the user makes the selection by tapping on the screen, activating another **control interface**, or by holding the cursor on the choice until it is accepted by the device. This is often referred to as acceptance time or *dwell time*.

Many on-screen keyboards allow changes in the keyboard arrangement, size of the on-screen keys, and location of the keyboard on the screen. Some on-screen keyboards also include other characteristics such as a word prediction feature that displays frequently used

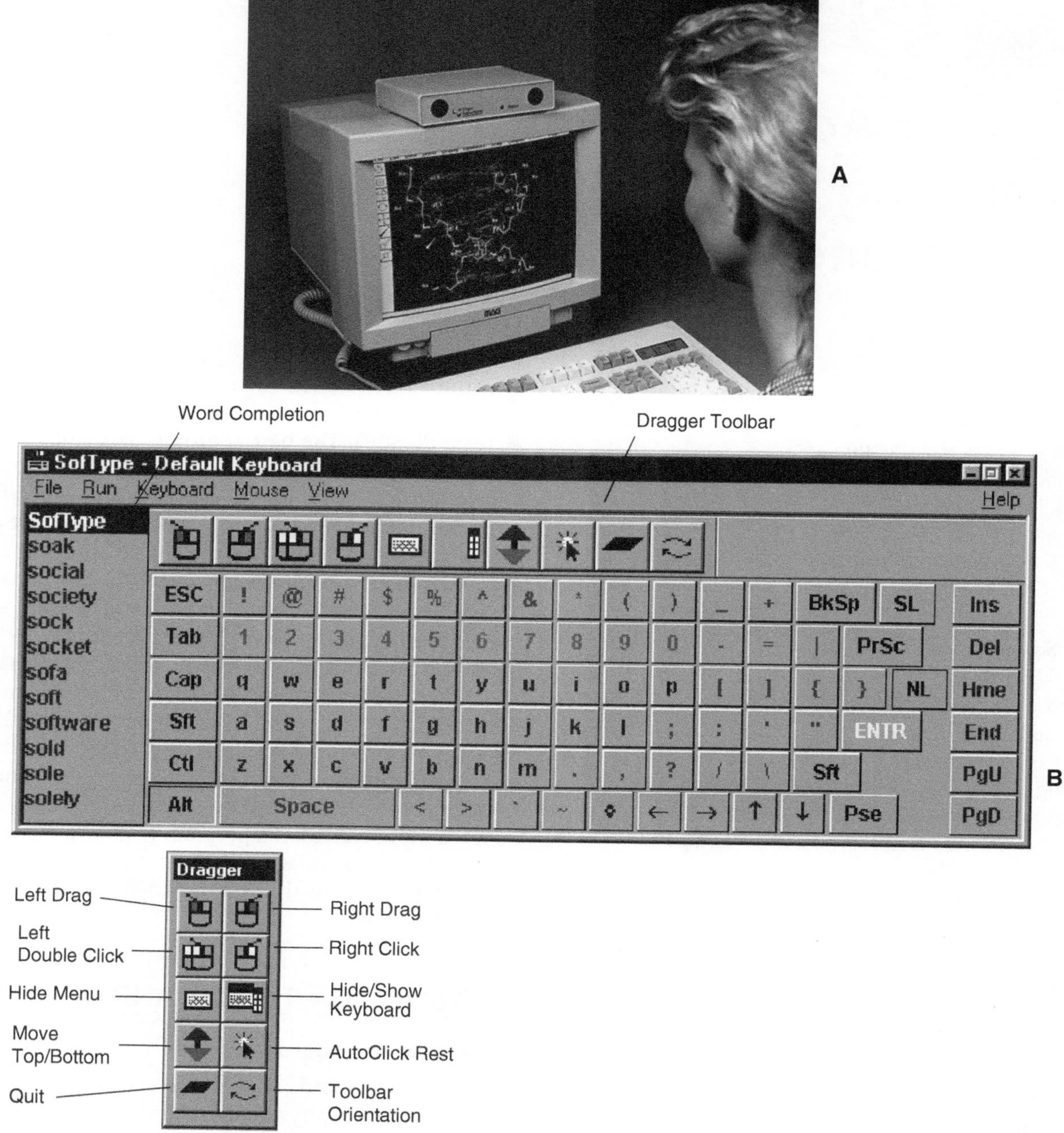

Figure 7-1 **A,** Head-controlled mouse. **B,** An example of an on-screen keyboard screen for Microsoft Windows. (Courtesy Origin Instruments Corporation, www.orin.com.)

words as the first few characters of a word are typed. Other adjustments intended to make use easier and more efficient include horizontal and vertical cursor movement speed control, keyboard layouts, and location of the keyboard image on the screen (e.g., top or bottom, depending on the type of application program that is running). Touch screens that provide feedback (i.e., a sound when you activate a key or a change of color to indicate a key has been activated) are often helpful for people with cognitive impairment or for those who are just learning to use these kinds of devices. Also, the ability to increase the visual contrast and magnification and to change colors can be useful. For example, it can be easier to understand the information on the screen if the color is appropriate for what the image represents (e.g., blue for water).

On-screen keyboards may also be used with single- or multiple-switch scanning formats. When the on-screen keyboard is used for typing it may occupy up to half of the screen, with the rest of the screen being used to display the program being used (e.g., word processing or email).

For individuals who have limited motor capabilities, one or more of the scanning techniques and formats described earlier in Chapter 5 may be used. Switches are connected to the computer using USB switch connectors described later in this chapter. Once a scanning selection is made, the device responds if it had been directly selected.

Built-in Software Adaptations to the Standard Keyboard

Persons with disabilities often have difficulty pressing more than one key at a time because they are single-finger typists. They may also have accidental key activation due to poor fine motor control. Software adaptations for these and other problems are shown in Table 7-1. These software adaptations are built into Windows[i] and Apple Macintosh™* operating systems. The software adaptations can be adjusted for an individual user through the control panel. Accessibility for the Macintosh includes those features shown in Table 7-1. When StickyKeys is used, the modifier keys are converted to sequential rather than simultaneous use. This means that instead of having to press the shift key and another key at the same time, the user can press the shift key and then press another key, and the second key will be shifted. StickyKeys allows either a single finger or a head pointer or a toe to be used to access all the functions on standard keyboards. FilterKeys and other designations such as BounceKeys, SlowKeys, and RepeatKeys are options designed to avoid double entries due to holding a key too long or accidentally hitting a key multiple times due to lack of fine motor control. Both Windows and Macintosh operating systems all provide many options to make the keyboard and mouse faster and easier to use. In both cases the operating system leads the user through choices based on a description of the need.

[i] Microsoft accessibility website: http://www.microsoft.com/enable/products/windowsxp/default.aspx

TABLE 7-1 Minimal Adaptations to the Standard Keyboard and Mouse*

Need Addressed	Software Approach
Modifier key cannot be used at same time as another key	StickyKeys†
User cannot release key before it starts to repeat	FilterKeys†
User accidentally hits wrong keys	SlowKeys,† BounceKeys,† FilterKeys†
User cannot manipulate mouse	MouseKeys†
User wants to use augmentative communication device as input	SerialKeys† in Windows XP or an alternative (like AAC Keys)
Keyboard is difficult	Touch Screen (Windows) Ulti-Touch (MacBook)
User cannot access keyboard (Windows Vista)	On-screen keyboard (Windows XP and Macintosh) Built-in ASR (Windows and Macintosh Vista)

*Universal Access in Macintosh operating system, Apple Computer, Cupertino, Calif.; Accessibility Options in Windows XP, Microsoft Corp., Seattle, Wash.

†Software modifications developed at the Trace Center, University of Wisconsin, Madison. These are included as before-market modifications to the Macintosh operating system or Windows in some personal computers and are available as after-market versions in others. The function of each program is as follows:

StickyKeys: user can press modifier key, then press second key without holding both down simultaneously.

SlowKeys: a delay can be added before the character selected by hitting a key is entered into the computer; this means that the user can release an incorrect key before it is entered.

BounceKeys: prevents double characters from being entered if the user bounces on the key when pressing and releasing.

FilterKeys: the combination of SlowKeys, BounceKeys, and RepeatKeys in Microsoft Windows.

MouseKeys: substitutes arrow keys for mouse movements.

SerialKeys: allowing any serial input to replace mouse and keyboard, this function has largely been replaced by USB standard devices.

Touchscreen: with a touch-screen monitor, uses finger on screen to move icons, point, resize windows, play media, and pan and zoom.

Multi-touch: can use gestures on the track pad to control input, pinch, swipe, or rotate gestures (similar to iPOD touch and iPhone).

Both Windows and Macintosh have built-in on-screen keyboards. Two modes of entry are available when an on-screen key is highlighted by mouse cursor movement: clicking and dwelling. In the latter the user keeps the mouse pointer on an on-screen key for an adjustable, preset time and the key is entered. The on-screen feature also allows entry by scanning. An area of the screen can be designed as a "hot key" with text, graphics, or control functions (such as opening a file or running a program) stored at that location. When the hot spot is selected by pressing, scanning, tapping, or other means, the stored text or function is entered into the computer. An auditory click or flashing icon or other feedback may be provided to indicate selection of a hot spot. Limited automatic speech recognition capability is also included in Windows, Macintosh, and several smart phone operating systems.†

Automatic Speech Recognition as an Alternative Keyboard

Automatic speech recognition (ASR) technology can be used for computer access by allowing the user to speak the names of keys or key words and have these spoken utterances interpreted by the computer as if they had been typed. This approach is appealing because human speech is so rapid and voice control is so natural. ASR systems that are extremely reliable, flexible, and easy to use are available for use as full-function keyboard and mouse emulation. For example, if a word processing program is being run, then control functions such as *delete, move,* and *print,* as well as the most common vocabulary items the person normally uses (e.g., a greeting and ending for a business letter, and other similar vocabulary items) can be used. If the user changes to a spreadsheet program, he can use vocabulary that contains items specific to that application.

* Apple accessibility website: http://www.apple.com/accessibility/

†For example, Android: http://developer.android.com/resources/articles/speech-input.html

CASE STUDY – EVALUATION AND SELECTION OF SPEECH RECOGNITION

Marilyn Abraham is a 44-year-old woman who has been diagnosed as having reflex sympathetic dystrophy (RSD) of both wrists. Apparently caused by vasospasm and vasodilation, RSD is a reaction to pain after an injury[16] (Kasch, Poole, and Hedl, 1998). It results in edema; shiny, blotchy skin; and pain. Ms. Abraham is a secretary in a large state office, which she shares with other co-workers. She uses the computer for much of the day. The RSD ensued in her right wrist as a result of the repetitive motion she uses in performing her job. After this injury she received retraining to transfer her hand dominance to her left hand, and the Dvorak one-handed keyboard layout was recommended (see Figure 6–8). Subsequently she broke her left wrist in a motor vehicle accident, which also resulted in RSD. She is able to type or use the mouse for only 10 minutes before her hands and forearms swell. Ms. Abraham has tried different positions and adaptations when typing. For example, she used a pointer held by a cuff in her palm to type so that her forearm remained in a neutral position. This still resulted in swelling and pain. She also experiences neck pain when using the keyboard.

Ms. Abraham first tried using a trackball with her hand and the on-screen keyboard. After using the trackball for a short time, Ms. Abraham found that it also caused pain. Ms. Abraham next tried using her right foot with an expanded keyboard and then a trackball. There were concerns about the utility of both these approaches because of potential neck strain from looking down and the possibility that the repeated movement of her ankle to input characters using the trackball might lead to repetitive motion problems with her foot.

Next Ms. Abraham tried a head-controlled interface that was worn on a band and attached to her head. She used this interface with an on-screen keyboard and acceptance time to make a selection. She was able to control this interface without difficulty but thought that after a period of use her neck would become tired.

QUESTIONS

1. What other switches could you try with Ms. Abraham?
2. If you evaluate automatic speech recognition for Ms. Abraham, what issues will you need to take into consideration?

Two basic types of ASR systems exist. With a *speaker-dependent system,* the user trains the system to recognize his voice by producing several samples of the same utterance. The method in which the training is handled varies among systems. The system analyzes these samples so that it can recognize variations in the user's speech and generate a computer input (e.g., enter a given letter, a string of letters, or a control key such as "return") corresponding to what was spoken. Even after the system has been trained using several speech samples, there likely will be times when the system does not recognize the user's speech and does not produce a response. Recognition accuracy is steadily increasing as advances are made in the computer algorithms used for analysis. Rates can be greater than 90% for general input and nearly 100% for isolated word applications (e.g., command and control, database, or spreadsheet). Speaker-dependent systems can be further divided into continuous and discrete categories.

Speaker-independent systems recognize speech patterns of different individuals without needing training.[14] These systems are developed using samples of speech from hundreds of people and information provided by phonologists on the various pronunciations of words.[6] The tradeoff with this type of total-recognition system is that the vocabulary set is small. In assistive technology applications, speaker-independent systems are primarily used for environmental control (Chapter 14) and power mobility (Chapter 12).

Speech recognition can be used for computer access, wheelchair control, and EADLs. The systems shown in Table 7-2 allow the consumer to use his speech to enter text directly into a computer application program. Recognition of control words used in word processors, such as "save file," is also trained. System vocabulary is also growing rapidly. Early systems had recognition vocabularies (the list of words the system can recognize when spoken) in the 1000 to 5000 range. Current systems have vocabularies of 50,000 words or more. The faster speech rate, larger vocabularies, and continuous recognition all place significant demands on the speed and memory of the host computer. Continuous speech recognition systems require large amounts of memory and high-speed computers. As the cost of this added computer functionality continues to decline, these additional requirements will be less important. However, ASR systems do require more computer resources than other alternative input methods.[3]

TABLE 7-2 Types of Automatic Speech Recognition

Category	Description	AT Application
Speaker-dependent systems	Recognition depends on the system's learning the user's speech patterns and building a user vocabulary.	Used for general mainstream technology access. Computers, smart phones, pad computers
Speaker-independent systems	The operation is similar to continuous speech recognition systems, but there is no training required. Generally limited to small, application-specific vocabularies.	Used in special-purpose assistive devices for environmental control or robotic control (see Chapter 14) and wheelchair control (see Chapter 12).

There are other acoustic or audio issues that are important in ASR as well. Foremost of these is the microphone. Anson (1997)[4] discusses considerations in the choice of a microphone for ASR. Although the microphones supplied with ASR systems are satisfactory for use by nondisabled users, they are not adequate when the user has limited breath support, special positioning requirements, or low-volume speech. Most ASR systems use a standard headset microphone. Individuals who have disabilities may not be able to don and doff such microphones independently, and therefore desk-mounted types are often used. Current ASR systems do not require separate hardware to be installed in the computer, and they utilize commonly available sound cards.[3]

Electronic Aids to Daily Living (EADLs) may also utilize speech recognition to access their functions (see Chapter 14). In such devices the individual can instruct the system to turn lights on and off or perform other functions using her voice. She can train the system to execute these commands with just about any sound, letter, or word.

The questions listed in Box 7-1 can be used to determine the usefulness of speech recognition for a given consumer. The key for success in using speech-activated systems is that the user be able to produce a *consistent* vocalization or verbalization. Differences in speech production are found not only among individual speakers, but also within the same speaker. Variability in the user's speech can cause problems with recognition. For this reason, this type of control interface may not be effective for individuals who have dysarthria. Individuals who have had a spinal cord injury and have no functional use of the upper extremities yet have good speech control are potential candidates for a speech recognition system. It is important when considering a speech recognition system to determine whether the user's voice pitch, articulation, and loudness change or fatigue over time. Other noises or voices in the area where the speech-activated system is being used can also confuse the system, resulting in either an incorrect selection or the system having difficulty registering any selection and causing the user to repeat the vocalization several times.

BOX 7-1 Critical Questions for Evaluating Use of Speech Recognition Interface

1. Can the client consistently utter all the sounds necessary to access the speech recognition system?
2. Is the recognition vocabulary adequate?
3. Is the client's voice articulation, pitch, and loudness consistent enough for accurate selection?
4. Is there likely to be background noise in the client's context that will interfere with the speech recognition system?
5. Would an alternative template or vocabulary be beneficial?

MOUSE

The standard computer **mouse** is intended to be gripped by the user's hand and moved across a flat surface. Successful use of the mouse requires sufficient vision to see the pointer and the icons on the screen and adequate eye-hand coordination to allow the user to cause the pointer to go to the desired icon or text by moving the mouse. Once the pointer is located at the desired element the user must click, double click, or click and hold to drag the element. These can be difficult for someone who has fine motor control limitations. There are several adjustments built into computers that can help match a user's needs to the mouse functions by changing the speed of mouse movement, changing the time allowed for clicking, etc.

The mouse is ideally suited for functions such as drawing, moving around in a document, or moving a block of text. The mouse can be a useful tool for individuals with disabilities who cannot otherwise draw using a pen or pencil. However, mouse use requires a high degree of eye-hand coordination and motor coordination and a certain amount of range of motion. Standard computer mice are available in many different shapes and sizes. If a consumer is having difficulty using the mouse that came with the computer, the solution may be as simple as finding a mouse that fits his hand better.

The standard mouse requires a great deal of motor control and many individuals with disabilities find that the use of a standard computer mouse is difficult or impossible. Another option is to try a different control site for mouse use. If the consumer has better control of his feet than his hands, his foot can be used with a foot-controlled mouse such as the No Hands Mouse.* There are also alternatives to mouse use that are easier for many persons with disabilities. Any control interface that can imitate the two-dimensional movement (up/down, left/right) of the mouse can be made to appear like a mouse to the computer. Table 7-3 lists the major alternatives to mouse input, as well as sample technologies. Examples of several of these approaches are shown in Figure 7-2.

Touch Screen Mouse Emulation

Many mainstream devices such as tablet computers, pad computers, and smart phones have touch screens that allow mouse-like control. The screen elements (text or icons) can be moved by touching and dragging them with finger movements that scroll through choices, open and close files, and expand and contract the number of displayed elements. Selection, the equivalent of clicking or double clicking a mouse button, is done by tapping the text entry or icon. Scrolling to new screens or new items within a file is done by swiping the finger across the screen from side to side or up and down.

*http://www.footmouse.com/nohands.php

TABLE 7-3 Alternative Electronic Pointing Interfaces

Category	Description	Device Name/Manufacturer
Keypad mouse	Mouse movement is replaced by keys that move the mouse cursor in horizontal, vertical, and diagonal directions. One or more keys perform the functions of the mouse button (click, double-click, drag).	Included with Windows and Mac OS.
Trackball	Looks like an inverted mouse; a ball is mounted on a stationary base. Included on the base are one or more buttons that provide the functions of the standard mouse buttons. The base and hand remain stationary and the fingers move the ball. Requires minimal range of motion and less eye-hand coordination.	Big Track, n-Abler (Inclusive Technology); EasiTrax (Inclusive Technology); Trackman Marble Plus (Logitech); EasyBall (Microsoft); Roller Trackball (Traxsys Computer Products).
Continuous input joysticks	Joysticks (continuous input and switched) are used as direct selection interfaces for powered mobility. For computer use, movements are similar to wheelchair control; easy to relate cursor movement (direction, speed, and distance) to joystick movement.	Jouse (Compusult Limited); Roller Joystick II (Traxsys Computer Products); EasiTrax (Inclusive Technology); all manufacturers of powered wheelchairs have their own joystick, which is supplied with wheelchair.
Head-controlled mouse	An interface controlled through head movement; the user wears a sensor on the head, which is detected by a unit on the computer. Movement of the head is translated into cursor movement on the screen.	Origin Instruments; Able Net http://www.ablenetinc.com/, also available in some speech generating devices.

Data from Adaptivation, Sioux Falls, SD (www.adaptivation.com); Compusult Limited, P.O. Box 1000, Mount Pearl, Newfoundland (http://www.jouse.com/jouse2/home); Logitech, Fremont, CA (www.logitech.com); Inclusive Technology (http://www.inclusive.co.uk/hardware/mouse-alternatives); Microsoft, Redmond, WA (www.microsoft.com); Origin Instruments, Grand Prairie, TX (www.orin.com); Traxsys Computer Products (http://www.traxsys.com/AssistiveTechnology/tabid/1087/Default.aspx); Prentke Romich Co., Wooster, OH (www.prentrom.com).

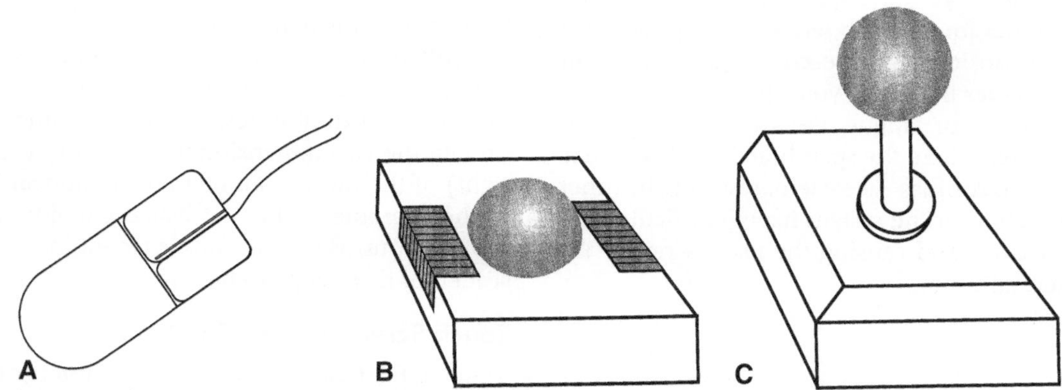

Figure 7-2 Pointing interfaces. **A,** Standard computer mouse. **B,** Trackball. **C,** Proportional joystick.

Keypad Mouse

For those individuals who are able to use a standard keyboard but have difficulty using a standard mouse, the first alternative to evaluate is the keypad mouse. A numeric keypad is embedded in most standard computer keyboards. MouseKeys, included in the Accessibility Options (Table 7-1) for Windows and in the Macintosh operating systems allows use of the keypad to simulate mouse movement. When the NUM LOCK key is engaged, each key on the numeric keypad functions as the number to which it is assigned (1 to 9). When the NUM LOCK key is disengaged and MouseKeys is running, these keys can perform the same functions as a mouse. There is an option in the control panel that will reverse these functions of the NUM LOCK key (i.e., MouseKeys will be active when the NUM LOCK key is engaged). The "5" key serves as a mouse click, and the surrounding number keys move the mouse in vertical, horizontal, or diagonal directions. This software interprets the keys as mouse input when MouseKeys is active and interprets them as arrow keys when it is not active. MouseKeys allows adjustment of the mouse speed (distance the cursor moves with each arrow key press) and acceleration (the rate at which the cursor moves).

There are also keypad mice that are external to the standard keyboard. The advantage of external keypads is that they can be placed in any position in the workspace. The disadvantage is that they take up more space on the work surface. External keypad mice are also available with expanded keypads and enlarged keys, with up to 1.5-inch square keys. When a trackball, joystick, or other hardware alternative is substituted for the mouse, it is necessary to accommodate the mouse button functions including clicking (rapid press and release), double-clicking, and dragging (holding the button while moving the mouse). Software adaptations replace these mouse button functions by selecting which mouse button function is required and then implementing that function when the user pauses on the selection.

Trackball

A trackball is a device that looks like an inverted mouse. There is either a ball or a small handle that is mounted on a stationary base. On some laptop computers, the trackball is a little stick in the middle of the keyboard. Included on the base are one or more buttons that provide the functions of the standard mouse buttons. The ball is rotated by moving the hand or finger across it, causing the cursor to move on the screen. The trackball is often helpful for people with disabilities that make using the mouse difficult because the trackball base and hand remain stationary and the fingers move the ball. Trackball use requires less range of motion than the standard mouse and is easier for some disabled users. It is also possible to use the trackball easily with other body sites such as a chin or foot. On most trackballs the user can latch the mouse button, which allows single-finger or mouthstick users to perform "click and drag" functions without having to hold down a button while simultaneously moving the mouse. This capability is also available as an option in the Windows control panel. Trackballs are available in a variety of sizes, shapes, and configurations.

Some trackballs have large softball-sized balls, and there are also very small trackballs that fit in the palm of the hand and require very little fine motor movement. If a consumer is having difficulty using one type of trackball, it may be useful to have her try a different type. Sometimes this can be done at a local computer store that has different models available for demonstration.

Continuous Input Joysticks

A joystick provides four directions of control and is thus ideally suited for use as another alternative to the mouse. There are two types of joysticks: proportional (**continuous input**) and control interfaced (discrete). A proportional joystick has continuous signals, so that any movement of the control handle in one direction results in an immediate response. Moving the joystick further causes the cursor to move faster. Proportional joysticks are most commonly used with power wheelchairs. The farther the wheelchair joystick moves away from the starting point, the faster the wheelchair goes. The proportional joystick is also more likely to be used as a mouse substitute, since the direction and rate of cursor movement can be controlled by the user. The Jouse* is a joystick-operated mouse that is controlled with the chin or mouth. Mouse button activations can be made using a sip-and-puff control interface that is built into the joystick. Just like the proportional joystick used for wheelchair control, the joystick used for a mouse substitute will cause the mouse pointer to move faster the farther away it gets from the center position. The joystick is always referenced to a center point that doesn't change. This is a major difference from mouse and trackball use. A mouse always causes the cursor to move relative to its current position, and there is no absolute reference point as there is with a joystick. This difference in reference point can cause difficulties for the consumer when first using the joystick. The user must spend some time learning how to use this control interface in order for it to be an effective alternative to the mouse.[4]

Head-Controlled Mouse Emulators

For individuals who lack the hand or foot movement to operate a mouse or joystick, there are alternative pointing interfaces that are controlled using head movement.[12] In general, head-controlled mouse systems operate by using a tracking unit that senses and measures head position relative to a fixed reference point. This reference point is the center of the screen for the cursor. As the head moves away from this point in any direction, the cursor is moved on the screen. Most of the systems currently available have a wireless connection, which allows the user to move around more freely. Several devices require only an adhesive reflective dot to be placed on the user's face (usually the forehead).†

Head-controlled mouse emulators are intended for individuals who lack upper extremity movement and who can accurately control head movement. For example, persons with high-level spinal cord injuries who cannot use any limb often find these head pointers to be rapid and easy to use. On the other hand, individuals who have random head movement or who do not have trunk alignment with the vertical axis of the video screen often have significantly more trouble using this type of input device.[10]

In one common commercial approach, the user wears an adhesive reflective dot that is attached either to the forehead or to a pair of glasses (Figure 7-1, *A*). A sensor on the tracking

---

* http://www.jouse.com/

†Tracker Pro, Madentec Ltd, Edmonton, AB, Canada (www.madentec.com) and Head Mouse Extreme, Origin Instruments, Grand Prairie, Tex., (www.orin.com)

BOX 7-2 What the Research Tells Us: Head-Pointing Mouse

Movement times for non-disabled individuals are greater for head-controlled cursor systems than for a conventional mouse. Movement times are also greater for small versus large targets and for far versus near targets in both healthy individuals and those with cerebral palsy.[23]

Users with high-level spinal cord injuries and those with cerebral palsy were evaluated for five currently available mouse alternatives based on head-tracking. SCI users had a preference for the Headmaster, but each of the devices was seen to have some advantages. Variable performance was reported for participants with cerebral palsy, even when using identical interfaces.[22]

For individuals with CP, direct target acquisition is a faster method than scanning.[2]

Three different technologies (infrared with a reflective dot,* ultrasound,† and gyroscopic‡) were compared in use by six non-disabled subjects. Each of the three approaches was fastest for 1/3 of the subjects and all were equally accurate. The preferred device was the Tracker 2000. While results for a person with disabilities would likely differ, this study did indicate that all head pointing technologies can yield fast and accurate results.[5]

Individuals with cerebral palsy may be able to utilize head-controlled cursor systems if they are given sufficient practice time with gradual reduction of target size as skill increases.[10]

Comparison of non-disabled university students' use of a head-controlled mouse§ and an expanded keyboard used as a key-pad mouse‖ showed that the time to capture a target decreased with practice for both devices, but the head pointer resulted in faster performance. Reaction time and the time to acquire a target based on the distance from the starting point was less for the head pointing device.[9]

Decreasing the sensitivity (the amount the cursor moves for a given head movement) improves accuracy.[18]

A head pointer built into a communication device¶ was shown to be less accurate than an external head pointer.** Varying the light conditions affects performance of infrared head pointers.[13]

*Tracker 2000, Madentec, Ltd, Edmonton, AB, Canada (www.madentec.com)
†HeadMaster, Prentke Romich, Wooster, Ohio (www.prentrom.com)
‡Tracer, Boost Technologies (www.boosttechnology.com)
§Tracker 2000, Able Net, Inc., Edmonton, AB, Canada (www.madentec.com)
‖Cambium Learning Group, Inc., Dallas, Texas (www.cambiumlearningtechnologies.com/)
¶Tracker Inside
**Tracker Pro, Abe Net, Inc., Edmonton, AB, Canada (www.madentec.com) and Head Mouse Extreme, Origin Instruments, Grand Prairie, Texas (www.orin.com)

unit attached to the computer detects the movement of the reflection from the dot, and therefore detects head movement. This movement is translated into a signal that the computer interprets as if it were sent by a mouse. When the user moves her head the cursor on the screen moves. Both vertical and horizontal movements are detected.

For mouse-related pointing tasks the head-controlled interface is a direct replacement. Clicking, double-clicking, and clicking and holding are done by using either an acceptance (or dwell) time (which can be adjusted to meet the user's needs) or a separate switch. In a later section we describe software programs that can be used to replace the switch for drag and click functions. For typing, the head-controlled interface must be used with an on-screen keyboard program (e.g., the type shown in Figure 7-1, *B*). Research related to head pointing is shown in Box 7-2.

CONNECTING AN EXTERNAL CONTROL INTERFACE TO THE COMPUTER

The control interface must have a way of connecting to the computer so that alternative approaches can be substituted for the keyboard and/or mouse. Examples are specially adapted mouse inputs and expanded or contracted keyboards. Each key on the standard keyboard has a code that is sent to the computer when that key is pressed. If another control interface or different keyboard is to be used as an alternative input device, pressing a control interface or key must generate the same coded information that the computer expects from a mouse or keyboard. This requires that we add a *decoder* between the control interface and the computer.[4] The term *keyboard or mouse emulator* is often used to describe devices that provide this decoding function. The emulator is just an alternative device that is made to function like a keyboard or mouse. The emulator often includes both direct and indirect selection methods as well as a variety of other features.

With the development of the USB standard, particularly the Human Interface Device (USB HID) component, nearly all of the functions previously developed requiring a special purpose emulator can now be accomplished through the USB interface.[21] The decoding previously carried out by the emulator is built into the control interface (particularly keyboards) and supplied to the computer through the **USB port**. An additional advantage of the USB port is that it supplies power to the external device from the computer, which eliminates the necessity for an external power source for USB input devices and is especially valuable for assistive technology applications that are based on portable computers. Additional software may need to be loaded into the computer to allow customization of the control interface selection setup (discussed later in this chapter).

There are challenges involved in utilizing the USB HID standard, and these can result in incompatibilities between assistive technology (AT) devices and between the AT device and the host computer.[26] The existing USB HID standard provides definitions for common human input devices such as keyboards, mouse pointers, joysticks, and game pads. However, it does not currently have a definition specifically for assistive technology input devices. So, AT products must still emulate one of the defined devices (such as a keyboard or mouse) to provide the specialized input. There are no general standards defined to do this for assistive technology developers to follow, which has resulted in different manufacturers using the USB HID in different ways. The lack of general standards results in some incompatibilities between AT products and confusion for the end users. In order to address this issue, the Accessibility Interoperability Alliance (AIA) has been formed by a group of leading information technology (IT) and assistive technology (AT) companies, content providers, and other key engineering organizations. Their goal is to create and harmonize standards for accessible technology.*

USB Switch Connectors

There are many switch connectors available for connecting single or multiple switches to the computer. Table 7-4 lists some of these together with their characteristics.

* http://www.atia.org/i4a/pages/index.cfm?pageid=3743

TABLE 7-4 USB Switch Interfaces

Switch interface	Features	Comments
AbleNet* Mouse Interface 5	Emulates mouse movements, 5 switch inputs.	Replaces mouse cursor movement and button press.
AbleNet† Mouse Mover USB	Emulates all mouse functions, 6 switch inputs.	Includes click, double-click, and drag.
Crick‡ USB Switch Box	4 switch inputs.	Works with Crick software; automatically detects which application and downloads setups.
Don Johnston§ Switch Interface Pro6 (USB)	5 switch inputs, 4 built-in scanning arrays for a variety of educational programs.	No software needed, supports Clicker 5 software. Scanning arrays: Row 1: Up arrow, down arrow, left arrow, right arrow, Click, Right Click, Double Click, Space, Enter. Row 2: Space, Enter, Tab, Shift Tab. Row 3: Click, 1, 2, 3, 0, Backspace. Row 4: Click, F3, F5, F7, F9.
Inclusive Technologies‖ Simple Switch Box	2 switch inputs, defined as [SPACE] and [ENTER].	Works with any programs requiring these two keys.
QuizWorks¶ Wireless Switch Interface	Receiver plugs into the USB port, up to five switches plug into transmitter that can be mounted wherever the switches are.	Switch inputs can be configured on the receiver, no software required.
Sensory Software International** JoyBox, USB	12 switch inputs for all mouse functions.	Works with Grid software or switch functions can be configured to be any key with Switch Driver (both from Sensory Software).
Sensory Software International†† Radio Switch or when tangling is an issue Widgit software	Receiver plugs into the USB port, two switches plug into transmitter that can be mounted wherever the switches are (e.g., on a wheelchair).	No drivers are needed for Grid, Clicker, or Widgit software. Switch functions can be configured to be any key with Switch Driver (from Sensory Software).
Madentec‡‡ IntelliSwitch	2 built-in switches, 5 switch inputs, wireless, scan to hot spots on the screen.	Works with Discover on-screen keyboards, IntelliKeys software.
PRC§§ USB Switch Interface Box	This has 6 single switch inputs.	Works with the WiViK onscreen keyboards, emulates all mouse functions with dual switch control interface.

*www.ablenetinc.com/
†www.ablenetinc.com/
‡www.cricksoft.com/
§www.donjohnston.com/
‖www.inclusive.co.uk/
¶www.quizworks.com/
**www.sensorysoftware.com/
††www.sensorysoftware.com/
‡‡www.madentec.com
§§www.prentrom.com

Some of these emulate both mouses and keyboards and some only one of them. Some require special software and others have hardware that can be customized. Some of the connectors are wireless, giving more freedom of movement and reducing the tangle of wires that often surrounds a person using adapted computer access.

Customizing the Emulator – The Use of "Setups"

Emulators have a general set of characteristics that allow the computer to be altered for a given application and a specific person with a disability. Some or all of these general characteristics are included in commercially available emulators. The characteristics of an emulator are customized for an individual application and user through a *setup*, a concept that originated with the Adaptive Firmware Card (AFC) for the Apple II series of computers.[24] As shown in Box 7-3, a setup consists of three basic elements: (1) an input method, (2) overlays, and (3) a set of options. Different manufacturers may use different names for these three elements, but their function is comparable across manufacturers. The features of the setup may be implemented in hardware (electronic circuits) or software (a program) or both. Setups are also usually stored in memory within the emulator hardware (e.g., an alternative keyboard) or in memory on the computer. This capacity allows different setups to be available for different users of a computer (e.g., in a classroom setting); they can be loaded into the computer or the emulator as needed. As shown in Box 7-3, the setup is used with an *application* program. The application program is just the task that the computer is to do. It could be word processing, email, social networking, or playing a video game. It could also be an educational program or software to aid rehabilitation, such as cognitive retraining software. Many application programs can use a generic setup with a few features. Others benefit from more customization. The concept of setup also applies to customization of augmentative communication systems (see Chapter 11).

Several examples of setups that may be used with different application programs are shown in Figure 7-3. The setup shown in Figure 7-3, *A*, is intended to be used for text entry in a business environment. The on-screen keyboard could be used with any pointing device by someone who has difficulty using the keyboard. For a single-control interface user, the setup includes an overlay on the screen for use as a scanning array with special characters included, as shown in Figure 7-3, *B*.

BOX 7-3 Major Features of Commonly Used Emulators

A SETUP CONSISTS OF THE FOLLOWING THREE PARTS

1. *Input method*
   Keyboard:
   - Assisted
   - Contracted
   - Expanded
   - Virtual
   - Normal

   Morse code:
   - One switch
   - Two switch

   ASCII:
   - Parallel
   - Serial

   Scanning:
   - Linear or row-column
   - Auto, inverse, or step
   - Single, dual, four, or five switch
   - Switched joystick

   Proportional:
   - Mouse
   - Trackball
   - Joystick
2. *Overlay: All three of the following may be the same or they may be different:*
   - User: the selection set arrangement from which the user chooses
   - Computer: the character or string of characters sent to the application program when the user chooses
   - Speech: synthetic speech used as a prompt to the user or as feedback when a selection is made
3. *Options:*
   - Abbreviations: text-based codes
   - Autocaps: CAP and 2 spaces after a period, exclamation point, or question mark
   - Key repeat rate
   - Levels: like a shift, can be many levels on one setup; equivalent in scanning is branching
   - Macros: codes can include control characters and functions
   - Mouse emulation: move, drag, click, and tab
   - Multitasking: can interrupt one mode for another
   - Predictive entry: previous characters determine user overlay
   - Rate: how fast or slow the user can input to the emulator
   - Screen selection display location: where on the screen the user overlay appears
   - Slowdown of programs

APPLICATION PROGRAM OR DISK

The business, education, or recreational program being used

	Method	Overlay	Options	Application
A	Virtual keyboard	User: QWERTY Layout Computer: Same Speech: No	Speed of mouse • •	Business, productivity software (word processing, spreadsheet, etc.)
B	Single-switch scanning	User: ETA Array Computer: Same Speech: No	Rate • •	
C	Expanded keyboard	User: ⟹ STOP Computer: Arrow, Return Speech: "This one," "Next one"	Speech Slowdown • •	Early education matching task with arrow and return
D	Single-switch scanning	User: ---> OK Computer: Arrow, Return Speech: "This one," "Next one"	Rate Speech Slowdown	

Figure 7-3 An emulator setup consists of three parts: input method, overlay, and options. **A** to **D**, Four examples of setups for different consumers and different applications are shown. ETA is the scanning array with the most frequent letters at the beginning of the array.

CASE STUDY – MR. COHEN

You work in an adult residential faculty. Mr. Cohen, a resident who sustained a closed head injury about two years ago, is expecting a visit from his son Bill, who lives out of town. Bill arrives with an iPad and the greeting, "This is just what dad needs to keep up with the world via the Internet!" Bill hasn't seen his father for a few months, and he also is not familiar with Mr. Cohen's program.

1. What questions would you ask Bill to start the process of evaluating the usefulness of the iPad for Mr. Cohen?
2. What would you ask Mr. Cohen to do to see if the device might actually meet one of his needs?
3. How would you address Bill's concerns for his father if you reach the conclusion that Mr. Cohen can't use the iPad?

For both Figure 7-3, *A* and 7-3, *B*, the application software can be a word processor, a spreadsheet, a database, or email. The major function is the entry of text characters, and the setup includes several options to make this process more efficient. Auto capitalization automatically enters one space and latches the shift function following sentence-ending punctuation (i.e., a period, question mark, or exclamation point). Abbreviations allow a few characters to be used as a code for a longer word or phrase. The user of the emulator stores both the sequences of characters and their corresponding abbreviations. When the abbreviation (code) is entered, the emulator automatically expands it into the whole stored word or phrase. For example, typing the two letters *MN* (for "my name") followed by an abbreviation key would result in the user's name and address being entered into a letter or email. Word completion or prediction may also be included as an option. The setup also includes *macros,* which are codes similar to abbreviations. The macros differ, however, in that they are often used to control application program functions. For example, assume that the user is entering data into a spreadsheet and wants to add a row. This task usually involves several mouse movements and clicking. The macro could accomplish all of these tasks with a single scanning array or on-screen keyboard location selection.

A second setup, shown in Figure 7-3, *C* and *D*, is for a young child who is using any of a wide range of software programs that require selection of an answer by matching a cursor (pointer) location with the correct item. The task may be to match numbers, letters, shapes, words, or pictures. Often the software requires that one key (e.g., RIGHT ARROW) be used to move the cursor and another key (e.g., ENTER) to select the one that the student believes is correct. Two setups are shown in Figure 7-3 for this application. In this case the user and computer overlays are different, and we also have included a speech overlay. Because the user is not likely to have learned to read yet, we use the speech overlay to help identify the choices to be made. We also use speech as a reinforcer when the choice is made, which is shown as a second speech overlay ("This one," "Next One") in Figure 7-3, *C* and *D*. The setup in Figure 7-3, *C*, is for use with an expanded keyboard that has a visual overlay that utilizes symbols. An example with four arrows is shown in Figure 7-4.

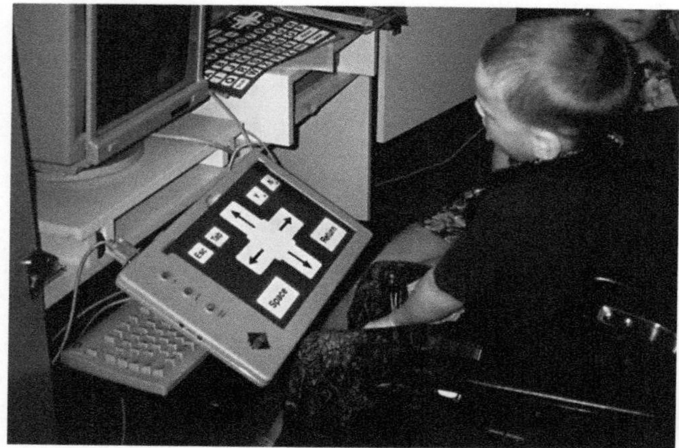

Figure 7-4 An overlay for cursor-controlling movement using arrows. This is being used with an expanded keyboard and an educational software program.

The overlay in Figure 7-3, *D*, uses scanning on the screen to make the choices. If we are restricted to text characters, we can generate an arrow with two dashes and the greater than (>) sign and use "OK" as the label for "this is the one I want" (the student's choice). For both these setups we use the speech, scanning rate, and program slowdown options. However, for the second setup (scanning) we also include an option that allows us to place the scanning array on any line of the display monitor. This option is important because the scan line can hide part of the program if it is in a fixed location.

Many USB-based emulators allow other features, such as mouse **emulation** and the use of macro instructions and **multitasking**. Mouse emulation substitutes a set of keys, a scanning array, or Morse code characters for mouse functions (similar to MouseKeys, Table 7-1). Macros can be used to return the mouse cursor to a specific location based on stored information. This function can save time when scanning is the mode used for mouse emulation. All these features can be incorporated into a setup that can be loaded when it is necessary or desirable to use the mouse.

All current commercially available devices utilize the USB standard for providing adapted input, and all are designed for either or both of the Windows-based and Macintosh computers. All adapted input devices have a hardware component, and some have software that may be used for operation and/or customization. All also have provisions for attachment of control interfaces (alternative keyboards, control interfaces, etc.). Some of these systems may also require a software program to be loaded into the host computer. This software may be used as part of the emulation process, and it also supports specialized setups for the adapted input device to be used with specific software programs. Box 7-4 lists the key steps in developing a setup for an individual. Remember that many standard setups are available for popular programs.

BOX 7-4 Tips for Creating a Setup

1. Determine the desired actions that you want the computer to carry out when a selection set element is chosen.
2. Determine the number of available motor actions from the user (i.e., a keyboard vs. a single or dual switch or mouse).
3. Determine the way in which you will present the choices to the user (e.g., graphics, words, or pictures).
4. Determine what happens when a selection is made by the user:
   a. Is there auditory feedback (e.g., "good job" or the name of the object selected)?
   b. Is there visual feedback (e.g., flashing image or change in the screen content such as a letter typed or a selection made in a program)?
   c. What does the computer do when the choice is made (e.g., run a program, turn the page of a story, etc.)?

General Purpose Emulators

The first general purpose keyboard emulator to be widely available was the Adaptive Firmware Card (AFC). The original version of this device was intended for use in the Apple II+ computer.[24] The features incorporated in the AFC are still fundamental to most current emulators. In a very real sense, virtually all the basic capabilities have their origins in the AFC. The major advances in emulator design have been the result of advances in the host computer, rather than fundamental insights into the process of keyboard and mouse emulation. Emulators also utilize built-in synthetic speech feedback in "talking setups" that allow the user to receive auditory as well as visual prompting and feedback. This is useful for young children who may not be able to read, for visually impaired individuals, and as an added input modality for persons with learning disabilities.

DiscoverPro* is an emulator designed for the Windows operating system. Envoy† is designed for the Macintosh OS X operating system. Both of these devices work with a number of alternative input devices including IntelliKeys,‡ IntelliSwitch,§ and head pointers such as TrackerPro‖ or HeadMouse.¶ Either system can be enabled at startup (when the power is turned on) or activated by clicking on the Discover or Envoy icon once the computer has booted. Some of the most useful features of Discover and Envoy are those that are specifically aimed at the **graphical user interface (GUI)**. It is possible with either system,

* Able Net (http://www.ablenetinc.com/)
† Able Net (http://www.ablenetinc.com/)
‡ Cambium Learning Group, Inc., Dallas, Texas (http://www.cambium-learningtechnologies.com/)
§ Cambium Learning Group, Inc., Dallas, Texas (http://www.cambium-learningtechnologies.com/)
‖ Able Net (http://www.ablenetinc.com/)
¶ Origin Instruments, Grand Prairie, Texas (www.orin.com)

for example, to set tabs on the screen where the mouse is to point, and then store the tab as a code (or macro). When the code is entered (using any of the basic selection methods and control interfaces), the mouse carries out the movement stored. By saving a series of mouse movements, it is possible to move to a menu, open it, select a specific entry, and then double-click (to start execution), all with one command. This not only saves many mouse movements, but it also avoids errors during tedious and complex movements. If a particular target software application has keyboard-equivalent commands to perform its functions, those can also be issued directly by Discover. Discover also provides row-column scanning with visually enhanced scanning arrays and audible cues, making it useful for people with multiple disabilities (such as blindness and motor impairments). Other useful features include digitized speech, on-screen keyboards, "invisible" setups (for issuing commands without an on-screen keyboard appearing), and development and printing of keyboard overlays for use with expanded keyboards. DiscoverScreen* is a software-only on-screen keyboard application that can be used with head pointing via the TrackerPro† or HeadMouse.‡ It can also be used with any mouse-like pointing device. There are a number of setups for the most common applications that come with DiscoverPro, Envoy, and DiscoverScreen.

The DARCI USB§ supports Morse code alternative input through the USB port. Morse code can be entered with one, two, or three switches. Input to the computer is through any USB port. Both a hardware component for attaching the external device to the computer and software to accept that input are included. No additional software is required, but the MouseKeys accessibility feature must be activated for use.

Using Scanning to Substitute for a Keyboard or Mouse

The **mouse** is used to select items by moving a pointer across the screen and then stopping on the desired target. Once the pointer is on the selected item, it can be dragged, opened by double clicking, or selected by single clicking. For consumers who only have enough motor control for a single or dual switch, there are several general approaches to scanning for emulation of these mouse functions.[7] One approach is Cartesian scanning in which pressing a switch causes a line to move slowly down the screen intersecting various on-screen icons. A second switch press causes a pointer or vertical line to move across the screen. When the pointer or vertical line is located over the desired screen icon, a third switch press selects that icon as though the mouse button had been pressed. This function is similar to matrix-type row-column scanning except that the scan is continuous rather than moving discretely between choices. A second approach is similar except that the movement of the lines is in discrete steps rather than continuous. This is easier for some users to follow and gives them a specific target time during which they must hit the switch. This method more closely approximates typical row column scanning.

A third approach is rotational scanning, which involves two steps: pointing toward a target, and then moving the mouse pointer toward the target. When the user activates the control interface once, a scan line is drawn from the center to the right-hand side of the computer screen. This scan line rotates about the center at a continuous speed counter-clockwise around the screen like a radar display. When the line intersects an on-screen target, the user activates the control interface a second time to stop the rotational scanning. This line remains visible and a second perpendicular line begins scanning outward from the center. When this line intersects the desired target, the user hits the control interface a third time to make the selection.

Commercial programs allow the user to select what mouse button function (click to select, double-click to open and run the application, or drag to move) is activated with the third control interface press. In some cases the selected function is implemented only after an acceptance time. If an additional control interface press occurs before the acceptance time (less than a second, typically) the selection is cancelled, which allows for error correction before an entry is made. Scan times, scanning line width, dwell time before rest or selection, and other characteristics are adjustable on most commercial products.

Another approach to mouse emulation is the creation of on-screen "hot spots" in software applications. These are scanned sequentially. This approach optimizes the scan to only those parts of the screen that are active during an application. For example, in a child's reading program the hot spots could be characters that speak during a story. The hot spot locations can be defined by the user (or more typically a supporter of the user). Many setups are available for popular programs and are stored for a particular application. A variety of approaches (e.g., automatic, inverse, and step) can be used to scan the hot spots with one or two switches. Several commercial products provide for mouse functions during scanning.* An example is shown in Figure 7-1, *A*. In general, these programs allow the user to select the mouse function following the selection of a target using any of the scanning or hot spot approaches described here. A more generic approach is one in which all interface objects in Windows™ are scanned as hot spots until the scan is stopped by control interface activation.† This action begins the next sequence (e.g., scanning down a list of choices in an opened menu).

* Able Net (http://www.ablenetinc.com/)
† Able Net (http://www.ablenetinc.com/)
‡ Origin Instruments, Grand Prairie, Texas (www.orin.com)
§ WesTest Engineering, Farmington, Utah (www.westest.com/)

* Dragger™, Origin Instruments, Grand Prairie, Texas, (www.orin.com); ScanBuddy™, Applied Human Factors, Helotes, Texas (www.ahf-net.com)
† WIVIK, also WiVik, (http://www.wivik.com/)

The basic operating system allows the speed of mouse movement, the trail left by the mouse, and other features to be adjusted. For individuals with severe motor impairments, the built-in adjustment of mouse speed, cursor size, etc., are not sufficient to allow use of the mouse or other pointing device. There are commercial products that extend the range of these adjustments and add other features such as wrapping the cursor around the screen when it reaches one side (i.e., when the cursor hits the right edge of the screen, it appears again on the left side).* Research relating to the use of scanning for mouse emulation is summarized in Box 7-5.

* For example, PointSmart, Infogrip, Ventura, Calif. (www.infogrip.com/)

BOX 7-5 Research about Scanning for Mouse Emulation

WHAT THE RESEARCH TELLS US ABOUT SCANNING FOR MOUSE EMULATION

- **Scanning methods:** two types of Cartesian scanning, rotational scanning, and a hybrid approach that scans quadrants of the screen and then scans within the quadrant.*
- **Participants:** Individuals who had cerebral palsy or a related condition.
- **Methods:** The subjects were given an opportunity to practice with each of the four techniques prior to using them in a controlled exercise. The length of practice required varied widely among the subjects.
- **Results:**
  - Accuracy (number of correct targets selected) was variable.
  - About half of the subjects had very similar results for all four methods. For the other half there was more variability among the methods with the hybrid approach generating the most errors.
  - Three types of errors occurred: hitting too early (before the cursor reached the desired target), hitting too late, and double control interface hits in quick succession (perseveration), which cancelled the entry.
  - Selection times for the two Cartesian and hybrid approaches were very similar. Selection times for the rotational approach were more than twice as long as the other three methods.
  - The majority of users favored the discrete Cartesian approach. Cartesian continuous was chosen as the favorite by a second group. None chose rotational scanning as the preferred method.
- **Conclusions:** While not directly applicable to clinical applications due to the use of a simplified scanning program for data collection, these results do point out the value of practice and the difficulties in using a rotational approach.

From Blackstein-Alder S, Shein F, Quntal J, and Weiss PL: Mouse manipulation through single control interface scanning, *Assist Technol* 16:28–42, 2004.

*For example, ScanBuddy™, Applied Human Factors, Helotes, Tex. (www.ahf-net.com)

COMMUNICATION DEVICES AS ALTERNATIVE COMPUTER INPUTS

Augmentative communication devices (Chapter 11) can also be used as computer input devices. There are two ways in which this is typically accomplished. Increasingly, AAC devices are developed around general purpose computers. In this case the communication device includes an operating system, generally Windows.* Due to funding peculiarities in the United States, these communication devices have two versions—one that is strictly for communication and one that gives access to the full Windows operating system. The dedicated versions limit user access to the computer built into the device. There are two models of devices in this category. The dedicated device is restricted to augmentative communication and is therefore fundable by Medicare in the United States (see Chapter 3). In this device, the user only has access to the hard drive directories that relate to communication, and all higher system-level directories are blocked. The open devices, which require the purchase of additional features, allow the user to access the entire hard drive of the device including the Windows operating system. When accessing the Windows environment, all of the special features of the communication software described in Chapter 11 (e.g., multiple selection methods, rate enhancement, text and character selection, and stored vocabulary pages customized for the user) are still available. Because the user of the communication device is familiar with these features, accessing Windows programs such as word processing, Internet browsing, or e-mail is easy and efficient without learning a new set of commands, rate enhancement techniques, or other features specific to computer access.

Other augmentative communication devices which are not built around a Windows operating environment generally provide computer access through a USB connection to the computer or a wireless infrared or Bluetooth link. This connection allows the communication device to send characters to the computer as if they were typed from the computer keyboard. As in the previous approach, this allows the user to have full access to the selection set and selection method, stored vocabulary, rate enhancement features, and any other customization features on the communication device while using the computer for word processing, e-mail, Internet browsing, or other applications.

ACCESSIBILITY FOR MOBILE DEVICES

Cell phone usage is pervasive throughout the world. In the United States it is estimated that 75% of adults have a cell phone.[15] For individuals with disabilities, the use of a cell phone can contribute to increased independence.

* For example, DynaVox V or Vmax (www.dynavoxtech.com); Prentke Romich, ECO-2 (www.prentrom.com), Words+ Conversa (www.words-plus.com/)

There are about 53 million consumers with disabilities in the United States.[25] This potential market for cell phones and other electronic technologies makes it important for these devices to be accessible to people with disabilities. In the United States there is an additional reason for cell phone manufacturers to be concerned about accessibility, and that is the Telecommunications Act of 1996. This act is designed to ensure that the 20% of United States citizens who have disabilities have equal access to cell phones and other telecommunications devices.[25] Individuals with a range of sensory and motor disabilities are included. Other countries, particularly in Europe and Asia, have similar legislation and policies to ensure access for people with disabilities.

Persons with disabilities are concerned about the complexity of current cell phones and have a desire for phones with basic features that are easily learned and can be accessed by individuals who have fine motor limitations.[25] In a study of people with a variety of sensory and motor disabilities, Kane et al. (2009)[15] found that most of the participants did not use a cell phone with accessibility features. The 24 participants described over 90 devices that they carried with them at least once a week. These devices included both high tech (cell phones and computers) and low tech (simple magnifiers) devices. Specific difficulties included using a phone while walking, using a phone in a crowded space, fatigue with prolonged usage, and device failure. The participants also identified strategies that helped them. Some installed accessibility software on their mobile devices, but not all of the cell phones had provisions for adding software. A number of participants, especially those who depended on their phone for geographic location or other security reasons, carried a second or third device as a backup. Cell phone use by persons with visual limitations is discussed in Chapter 8.

For persons with significant motor limitations it is necessary to customize the cell phone setup to allow independent access. Bryen and Pecunas (2004)[8] describe an application in which a cell phone was mounted to a wheelchair within range of a head pointer by an augmentative communication user. They describe specific issues such as protection from moisture, provision of continuous power from the wheelchair battery to ensure continued power with the unit on all the time, and the need for an external speaker and microphone to ensure that the synthesized speech from the communication device was clearly heard over the phone.

Individuals with spinal cord injuries have a slightly different set of problems, although physical access is still a major issue. Kane (2009)[15] describes the ideal cell phone for someone with a spinal cord injury.[17] Among the critical factors that he cites are: continuous power "on," since many "on/off" buttons are small and hard to activate; touch screen access that requires a flick of the finger, rather than continuous pressing of multiple keys; synchronizing with one or more email systems; a protective case since the unit may be dropped due to limited fine motor control; and a lanyard for retrieving the phone if it does drop. Less essential but useful is a Bluetooth earpiece, although it is important to find one that can be easily donned and doffed.

INTERNET USE BY PERSONS WITH PHYSICAL DISABILITIES

Many persons with physical disabilities who want to use the Internet require only an accessible computer, in contrast to individuals who have visual disabilities and also require carefully designed Web pages (see Chapter 8). People with disabilities have talked about Internet use as "leveling the playing field" because they can access the Internet and communicate with others through it in the same way as people who don't have a physical disability (Miller Polgar et al, 2009).[20] One participant commented that, "We are all given the exact same abilities in the digital environment...and when you are online, nobody knows you have a disability, so it [the disability] never really comes into it."[19]

The actual use by persons with physical disabilities has not been carefully studied in general, with the exception of people who have sustained a spinal cord injury (SCI).[11] A large group (516) of individuals with spinal cord injury from the 16 centers in the Model Spinal Cord Injury System (MSCIS) participated in a survey of Internet use. A smaller sample, derived from the larger group, also participated in an assessment of elements of the Health-Related Quality of Life (HRQOL) instrument. The rate of Internet access was 66%, compared to a rate of 43% in the general population. There were significant differences in access, however, based on race, employment status, income, education, and marital status. The most significant HRQOL impact on Internet usage was the pain interference parameter. Frequency of use varied widely from nonuse, to rare, to frequent. Most (81%) of the SCI respondents used the Internet at least weekly. Success in achieving desired outcomes from Internet use improved markedly from "infrequent" to "rare" use, but not from "rare" to "frequent." Primary uses were social (e-mail, chat rooms) and information seeking (health-related information, online shopping). A concern regarding Internet access is that it might reduce interpersonal contact and isolate people with disabilities from social interaction. This study indicated that the opposite was true, since the use of Internet contact reduced many of the barriers faced by people who have sustained spinal cord injuries (e.g., transportation, telephone use, and need for personal attendants for outside trips). With the increase in social media, people without disabilities are also using the Internet as their primary communication.

Vicente and López (2010)[27] investigated the differences between Internet users with and without disabilities in Spain. Affordability is an issue since people with disabilities have lower incomes, and they may also lack soft technologies (training and support). People with disabilities and elderly individuals have attitudes toward the Internet that can limit its usefulness to them. In general they have a lack of interest, low motivation, and anxiety about technology use. All of these factors are dependent on socio-economic background. Once online, certain factors of Internet use come into play. Digital skills decline with age and differ by gender. Enjoyment and perceived usefulness of functions such as e-banking and e-commerce are also lower for people with disabilities and the elderly than they are for the general population. In contrast to earlier studies, Vicente and López found that online patterns of use, when compared to users without disability, showed no difference.[27] Previous studies had indicated lower e-commerce, educational, information retrieval, and e-mail use for people with disabilities and the elderly. These considerations should be taken into account when working to establish mainstream technology use for people with disabilities or elderly individuals. This study indicates that the situation is changing and more people with disabilities and older individuals are increasingly finding the Internet to be both useful and accessible.

SPEECH OUTPUT

There are three major assistive technology applications that use speech: computer screen readers and print-material reading machines for persons who are blind (Chapter 8), voice output augmentative communication devices (Chapter 11), and alternative reading formats (i.e., auditory rather than visual language) for persons with cognitive disabilities (Chapter 10). The two types of speech output are digital recording and speech synthesis. They differ in the manner by which the speech is electronically produced. Table 7-5 lists the features and typical assistive technology applications for the two approaches.

Digital Recording

Digital recording stores human speech in electronic memory circuits similar to those used for audio music and speech recordings so it can be retrieved later. Even a few seconds of speech takes a great deal of memory. For example, 16 seconds of speech may take up to 1 megabyte (MB) of memory for storage. To make the storage more efficient, signal processing and speech compression are used. The major advantage of digital recording of speech is that it allows any voice to be easily stored in the device and played back. For example, if an AAC system (Chapter 11) using digital recording is being used by a young girl, we record the speech of a young girl and match the speech to the user. The main disadvantage is that all of the desired utterances must be prerecorded.

Speech Synthesis

Speech synthesis overcomes the major limitation of digitized speech by generating the speech electronically instead of recording a human voice. Using speech synthesis, any text that can be displayed on a screen or printed out can also be spoken. In order to produce synthesized speech, a computer program that simulates the human vocal system is used. Speech synthesizers can generate any word if the correct codes are sent to them in the correct order. **Text-to-speech programs** convert text characters into the codes required by the speech synthesizer. When these codes are received by the speech synthesizer, they are combined into spoken words. Aaron et al. (2005)[1] provide an excellent overview and tutorial on speech synthesis.

Audio Considerations

The quality of the amplifier and of any speech output system dramatically affects the intelligibility and quality of sound. Portable devices (e.g., augmentative communication systems) use low-power amplifiers and small, low-fidelity speakers. This technology can reduce the quality of the sound and therefore make it more difficult to understand. Greater fidelity is only achieved by more powerful amplifiers that require larger batteries and heavier, larger speakers. The most important rule that applies here is that "you don't get something for nothing"; higher quality in speech sound output is obtained only at the cost of increased weight and reduced portability.

TABLE 7-5 Types of Speech Output Used in Assistive Technologies

Types of Speech Output	Major Features	Typical Assistive Technology Applications
Digital recording	Uses actual voice and can easily be child, male, or female. Speech is limited to what is stored. Relatively low cost.	Augmentative communication.
Speech synthesis	Very high quality for single words or complete phrases. Intelligibility decreases for unlimited vocabulary with text-to-speech. Unlimited vocabulary with text-to-speech. Moderate intelligibility with letter-to-sound rules only. Highly intelligible with morphonemic rules. Cost depends on text-to-speech approach.	Speech output for EADLs. Augmentative communication. Screen readers for blind users. Speech output for users with learning disabilities. Speech output for phone communication for persons who are deaf.

SUMMARY

Mainstream technologies, primarily computer, cell phones (including smart phones), and pad computers are becoming more and more prevalent. These devices are very useful to many people. In order for them to be useful and effective for people with disabilities, they must be accessible. In this chapter we have discussed alternative ways to make these technologies accessible. Speech output is often used in assistive technology applications for individuals with low vision or blindness and those who have difficulty communicating by speech. The major ways that speech output is provided in assistive technologies have also been discussed.

STUDY QUESTIONS

1. What are the two major computer access goals for people with disabilities?
2. What are the features included in Universal Access and Windows Accessibility options?
3. What does emulation of the mouse or keyboard mean?
4. Explain the significance of having a USB HID specific to assistive technologies.
5. What is included in a "setup" used for computer access?
6. What is an on-screen keyboard?
7. What factors are important in making an on-screen keyboard effective for an individual's needs and skills?
8. List three means of selecting from on-screen keyboards.
9. What is the difference between speaker-independent and speaker-dependent automatic speech recognition systems (ASRs)?
10. How would you determine if an ASR is working well for your client?
11. There are acoustic or audio factors that might make an ASR system perform well or poorly. What are they?
12. There are several things about the way a computer mouse is used that can make it difficult for a person with a disability. Can you list three?
13. There are several adjustments built into computers that can help match a user's needs to the mouse functions. What are they?
14. What are the most common alternatives to a computer mouse? List at least one advantage and one disadvantage of each.
15. Why do you think a trackball might work better for a person with a disability than a standard mouse?
16. What is a Jouse, and why do you think it might work for some clients?
17. What is a head-controlled mouse emulator? What clinical factors and client characteristics are important in making them successful?
18. What is the most common way of connecting switches to a computer?
19. What are the two most common approaches to detecting eye position and movement for use as a control interface?
20. What are the major features of mainstream technologies (cell phones, smart phones, and pad computers) that can limit their usefulness to people who have disabilities?
21. What are the two basic methods used to provide speech output for assistive technologies?
22. What are the advantages and disadvantages of each of the speech output methods?
23. What does a text-to-speech program do?

REFERENCES

1. Aaron A, Eide E, Pitrelli JF: Conversational computers, *Sci Am* 292(6):64–69, 2005.
2. Angelo J, Deterding C, Weisman J: Comparing three head-pointing systems using a single subject design, *Assist Technol* 3(2):43–49, 1991.
3. Anson DK: Speech recognition technology, *OT Practice* 4(1):59–62, 1999.
4. Anson DK: *Alternative computer access: a guide to selection*, Philadelphia, 1997, FA Davis.
5. Anson D, Lawler G, Kissinger A, et al: A comparison of head pointer technologies. In *Proc 2003 RESNA Conf.* Retrieved June 28, 2005 from http://www.resna.org/ProfResources/Publications/Proceedings/2003/Papers/.
6. Baker JM: How to achieve recognition: a tutorial/status report on automatic speech recognition, *Speech Technol* 1(1):30–31, 36–43, 1981.
7. Blackstein-Alder S, Shein F, Quintal J, et al: Mouse manipulation through single switch scanning, *Assist Technol* 16: 28–42, 2004.
8. Bryen DN, Pecunas P: Augmentative and alternative communication and cell phone use: one off-the-shelf solution and some policy considerations, *Assist Technol* 16(1):11–17, 2004.
9. Capilouto GJ, Higginbotham DJ, McClenaghan B, et al: Performance investigation of a head-operated device and expanded membrane cursor keys in a target acquisition task, *Technol Disabil* 17:173–183, 2005.
10. Cook AM, Dobbs BM, Warren S, et al: Measuring target acquisition utilizing Madentec's Tracker system in individuals with cerebral palsy, *Technol Disabil* 17:155–163, 2005.
11. Drainoni ML, Houlihan B, Williams S, et al: Patterns of Internet use by persons with spinal cord injuries and relationship to health-related quality of life, *Arch Phys Med Rehabil* 85(11):1872–1879, 2004.
12. Evans DG, Drew R, Blenkhorn P: Controlling mouse pointer position using an infrared head-operated joystick, *IEEE Trans Rehabil Eng* 8(1):107–117, 2000.
13. Fitzgerald MM, Sposato B, Politano P, et al: Comparison of three head-controlled mouse emulators in three light conditions, *Augment Altern Commun* 25(1):32–41, 2009.
14. Gallant JA: Speech-recognition products, *EDN* 112–122, 1989.
15. Kane SK, Jayant C, Wobbrock JO, et al: Freedom to roam: A study of mobile device adoption and accessibility for people with visual and motor disabilities. In ASSETS '09, Pittsburgh, PA, USA, 2009, pp 115–122.
16. Kasch M, Poole SE, Hedl M: Acute hand injuries. In Early MB, editor: Physical dysfunction practice skills for the occupational therapy assistant, St. Louis, 1998, Mosby.
17. Larsen K: Computer Corner, PN, April 2009, pp 18–19.

18. LoPresti EF, Brienza DM, Angelo J: Head-operated computer controls: effect of control method on performance for subjects with and without disability, *Interact Comput* 14(4):359–377, 2002.
19. Miller Polgar J: The myth of neutral technology. In Oishi MMK, Mitchell IM, Van der Loos FHM, editors: *Design and use of assistive technology: social, technical, ethical and economic challenges*, Springer, NY, 2010, pp 17–23.
20. Miller Polgar J, Winter S, Howard S, et al: The meaning of assistive technology use. In *Proceedings of the 25th International Seating Symposium*, Orlando, FL, 2009, p 75.
21. Novak M, Olsen B: *Standards work involving the General Input Device Emulating Interface (GIDEI), SerialKeys, and the Universal Serial Bus (USB)*, University Wisconsin Trace Center, 2001. Retrieved from http://trace.wisc.edu/docs/gidei_usb/gidei-usb.html. August 15, 2005.
22. Phillips B, Lin A: Head-tracking technology for mouse control: a comparison project. In *Proceedings 2003 RESNA Conference*, 2003.
23. Radwin RR, Vanderheiden GC, Lin ML: A method for evaluating head-controlled computer input devices using Fitts' Law, *Hum Factors* 32(4):423–438, 1990.
24. Schwejda P, Vanderheiden G: Adaptive-firmware card for the Apple II, *Byte* 7(9):276–314, 1982.
25. Smith-Jackson TL, Nussbaum MA, Mooney AM: Accessible cell phone design: development and application of a needs analysis framework, *Disabil Rehabil* 25(10):549–560, 2003.
26. Vanderheiden G, Zimmermann G: State of the science: access to information technologies. In Winters JM, Robinson C, Simpson R, Vanderheiden G, editors: *Emerging and Accessible Telecommunications, Information and Healthcare Technologies*, Arlington, VA, 2002, RESNA Press, pp 152–184. Retrieved from http://trace.wisc.edu/docs/2002SOS-Report-IT/index.htm. August 20, 2005.
27. Vicente MR, López AJ: A multidimensional analysis of the disability digital divide: some evidence for Internet use, *Inform Soc* 26(1):48–64, 2010.

CHAPTER 8

Sensory Aids for Persons with Visual Impairments

CHAPTER OUTLINE

LEARNING OBJECTIVES

Upon completing this chapter, you will be able to do the following:

1. Describe the major approaches to sensory substitution, including the advantages and disadvantages of each
2. Describe the major causes of vision loss that can be aided by assistive technologies
3. Describe device use for reading and mobility by persons who have visual impairment
4. Describe how computer outputs are adapted for individuals with visual limitations
5. Describe the major approaches to Internet access for persons with visual impairments

KEY TERMS

Alternative Sensory System
Braille
Closed Circuit Television (CCTV)
Digital Audio-Based Information System (DAISY) Consortium
Digital Talking Books (DTBs)
Electronic Travel Aids (ETAs)
Environmental Interface
Graphical User Interface (GUI)
Human/Technology Interface
Information Processor
Internet
Magnification Aids
Mobility Aids
Optical Aids
Optical Character Recognition

Orientation and Mobility
Reading Aids
Refreshable Braille Display
Screen Readers
Scripts
User Agent
User Display
Video Magnifiers
Visual Accommodation
Windows

When an individual has a sensory impairment, their access to information via vision or hearing is restricted. Assistive technologies can provide assistance in the input of information via sensory systems. In this chapter we emphasize approaches that are used to aid or replace seeing. These include sensory aids that are intended for *general use* as well as assistive technologies that are used specifically for providing visual access to computers. Implications of sensory impairment or loss to daily activities and use of assistive technology are described in Chapter 3.

Individuals who have vision loss have a variety of needs that can be aided by assistive technologies. Stelmack et al (2003)[33] surveyed individuals with low vision to determine their major needs for assistive devices. Sixty-three activities in the categories of travel, food and shopping, communications, household tasks, self-care, recreation and socialization, and contrast were included in the survey. The participants were 149 individuals in the age range of 51–96 (mean 76). Two-thirds were male. The survey consisted of asking each participant if they could perform the activity independently or if they used a low-vision device, and whether they thought it was important to use a device to perform the activity independently. The highest-ranked items involved travel (finding a clear path, identifying landmarks, recognizing traffic signals, and stepping off a curb); self-care (applying make-up, shaving); reading (large print, signing checks, and finding food in kitchen); and recreation (watching television, recognizing persons close up). The needs identified in this study illustrate the range of applications of assistive technologies for people with visual impairments. In this chapter we discuss assistive devices designed to address this very broad range of needs. We begin this chapter by looking at the fundamental principles associated with sensory aids.

VISUAL FUNCTION

Visual function is measured by several parameters. Visual acuity is measured by determining the refractive index of the eye, and is usually reported in terms of the Snellen chart, in which letters are read from a fixed distance. The results are reported as the relative distance that a normal person would be able to read the letters that the person being tested is reading at 20 feet (6 meters). Three methods are used to report this score. In the United States and some other countries the score is reported as a fraction. A value of 20/20 means that the person's vision is normal. The metric equivalent is 6/6. In some countries a decimal is used in which 1.0 is normal. Better than normal would be 20/10, 6/3, and 2.0. The World Health Organization (WHO) definitions for levels of visual impairment based on visual acuity are shown in Table 8-1.

A visual impairment does not mean the individual has no ability to see. Frequently, persons with a visual impairment have some vision, but the level of impairment interferes with function. The Participation and Activity Limitation Survey (PALS)[25] defines low vision as difficulty seeing someone from a distance of 12 feet or difficulty reading a newspaper despite the use of corrective lenses. In other words, even with vision correction devices such as glasses, visual abilities are still limited, although the individual is able to see some things.

In the normal eye at rest, distant objects are focused on the retina. As the object is brought closer, the image falls in front of the retina unless the curvature of the lens is changed. **Visual accommodation** is the process by which the ciliary muscles change the curvature of the lens and hence the focal point of the eye. For a person

TABLE 8-1 Proposed Revision of Categories of Visual Impairment

	PRESENTING DISTANCE VISUAL ACUITY:	
Category	Worse Than:	Equal to or Better Than:
0 Mild or no visual impairment		6/18 3/10 (0.3) 20/70
1 Moderate visual impairment	6/18 3/10 (0.3) 20/70	6/60 1/10 (0.1) 20/200
2 Severe visual impairment	6/60 1/10 (0.1) 20/200	3/60 1/20 (0.05) 20/400
3 Blindness	3/60 1/20 (0.05) 20/400	1/60* 1/50 (0.02) 5/300 (20/1200)
4 Blindness	1/60* 1/50 (0.02) 5/300 (20/1200)	Light perception
5 Blindness	No light perception	
9	Undetermined or unspecified	

*Counts fingers
From World Health Organization, Cumulative Official Updates to the ICD-10 (pp 51–52), 2010, http://www.who.int/classifications/icd/Official_WHO_updates_combined_1996_2009VOL1.pdf

less than 20 years of age with normal visual accommodation, the eye is able to accommodate for an object located at about 10 cm. The ability to accommodate decreases as individuals age. For example, at age 50 years the eyes cannot accommodate to objects closer than approximately 30 cm. This situation leads to the prescription of reading glasses. Many types of disabilities affect accommodation; limitations in accommodation are referred to as *accommodative insufficiency*, which can be a significant factor when assistive technologies are used. For example, if a person is using a keyboard device with a visual display, the separation of these two system components may require constant accommodation as visual gaze is directed at the keyboard and then at the display and back to the keyboard. Appropriate placement of the keyboard and visual display can reduce the amount of accommodation that is required and can result in significantly improved overall system performance.

Another measure of visual function is visual field. With the head and eyes fixed on a central point, the normal range of peripheral vision in the right eye is 70 degrees to the left and 104 degrees to the right.[3] If the eyes are allowed to rotate but the head remains fixed, the range is 166 degrees to each side of the central point. The WHO standard states that "If the extent of the visual field is taken into account, patients with a visual field of the better eye no greater than 10° in radius around central fixation should be placed under category 3."[38] (See Table 8-1.)

In this chapter we use the term *low vision* to indicate that the individual is able to use her visual system for reading, but the standard size, contrast, and/or spacing are inadequate. We use the term *blind* to refer to individuals for whom the visual system does not provide a useful input channel for reading (including mainstream technologies such as computers or cell phones) and/or mobility.

COMMON VISUAL DISORDERS

There are many diseases of the eye that lead to low vision or blindness.[10] The low vision that results from some types of diseases can be aided by assistive technologies. In this chapter we focus on the most common of these diseases: age-related macular degeneration (ARMD), glaucoma cataracts, and diabetes-related vision loss.

Age-Related Macular Degeneration (ARMD)

ARMD is the most common cause of blindness in seniors in Western countries.[10] It occurs most frequently in individuals over 65, beginning in one eye and progressing gradually to both eyes. There are two types of ARMD: "dry" or atrophic and "wet" or endovascular. The dry form is much more common, but the wet form accounts for 80–90% of the cases of ARMD-related blindness. ARMD primarily affects the central vision, with the peripheral vision being preserved. As it progresses the size of the impaired central field gradually increases. A useful resource about ARMD, its treatment, and information for patients and families is the AMD alliance (http://www.amdalliance.org/en/home.html). Additional information and resources are available from the U.S. National Institutes of Health.*

Glaucoma

Glaucoma is a group of eye diseases that are caused by increased intraocular pressure that damages the optic nerve.[10] It is most common in individuals over 60. In contrast to ARMD, the affect on vision of glaucoma is loss of the peripheral visual field, with the central visual field retained. In early stages there are treatments that can prevent further vision loss.† As the disease progresses assistive technologies for low vision such as those discussed in this chapter can be helpful.

Cataracts

A cataract is a clouding of the lens of the eye that results in blurred vision.[10] The most common treatment is surgical replacement of the lens with an artificial lens. In some cases assistive technologies for low vision are useful if there is vision loss from cataracts or cataract surgery.‡

Diabetic Eye Disease

Individuals who have diabetes are also more likely to have eye diseases that can cause severe vision loss.[10] Diabetic-related eye disease may include: diabetic retinopathy, cataract, and glaucoma. Cataracts develop earlier in people who have diabetes, and a person with diabetes is nearly twice as likely to get glaucoma. Diabetic retinopathy is the most common type of eye disease that accompanies diabetes and is a leading cause of blindness.§ It is caused by changes in the blood vessels of the eye that affects the blood supply to the retina. The result is loss of parts of the visual field that are seen as black areas at random points.

Fundamental Approaches to Sensory Aids

If there are impairments in either visual sensing or perception, it is necessary to utilize sensory aids. Consideration of the nine levels of visual impairment shown in Table 8-1 is important when we apply these aids. If there is some visual function (e.g., levels 1 and 2 in Table 8-1) we can augment the input to make it useful to the person. For example, eyeglasses magnify (augment) the level of visual information. On the other hand, if there is more significant visual loss (levels 3, 4, and 5 in Table 8-1), then the sensory aid may need to provide information using an alternative sensory pathway. Either Braille (tactile pathway) or speech (auditory pathway) can be used for reading when vision is not functional because both are used to represent language. We describe both augmentation and replacement for visual information in this chapter.

---

* http://www.nei.nih.gov/health/maculardegen/armd_facts.asp#1a
† http://www.nei.nih.gov/health/glaucoma/glaucoma_facts.asp
‡ http://www.nei.nih.gov/health/cataract/cataract_facts.asp
§ http://www.nei.nih.gov/health/diabetic/retinopathy.asp

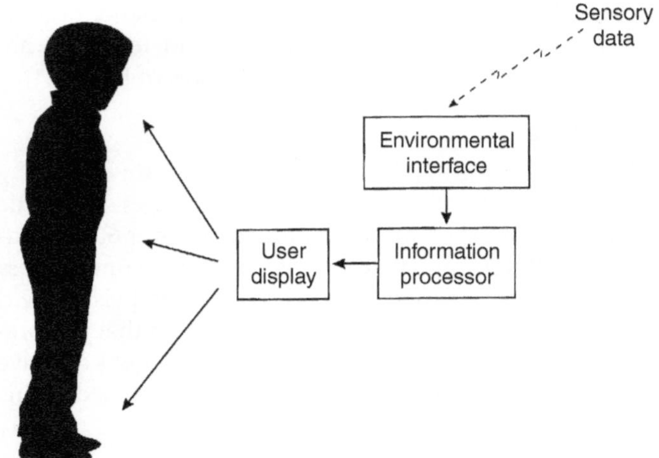

Figure 8-1 The major components of all sensory aids.

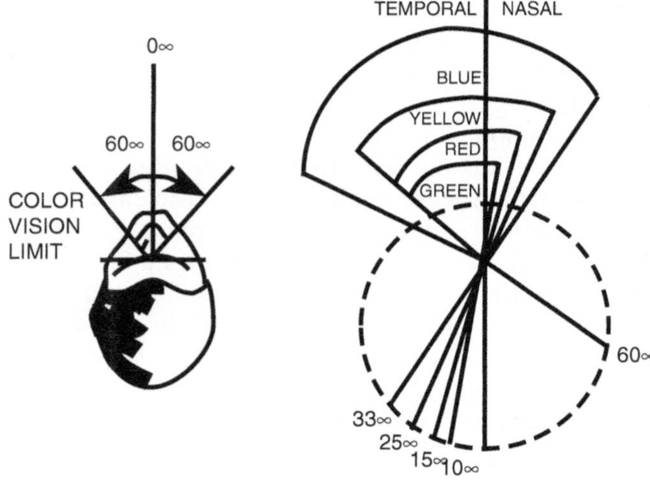

Figure 8-2 Color response of the eye differs with visual angle. (Modified from Woodson W, Conover D: *Human engineering guide for equipment designers*, Berkeley, 1964, University of California Press.)

Figure 8-1 shows the major components of a sensory aid based on the parts of the assistive technology component of the HAAT model (see Figure 2-5). The *environmental interface* for visual sensory aids is a camera that detects images that the human cannot obtain via her own sensory system. The environmental interface signal is fed to an **information processor** that either enlarges the sensory image or converts the visual information into a tactile or auditory form. The **human/technology interface** is a **user display,** which portrays the sensory information for the human user. For visual sensory aids the user display is either a visible display (e.g., a video screen), an auditory display (e.g., a speaker), or a tactile display (vibrating pins in the form of Braille cells).

Augmenting the Visual Pathway

Visual function depends on the size of the object being visualized (e.g., letters on a page, an object on the highway), the contrast between the object and the background, and the location within the visual field. When there is a limitation of visual acuity (size), contrast, or visual field, but there is still some capability remaining, assistive technologies can be used to compensate. We refer to these approaches to assisting visual function as *augmenting the exiting visual pathway*.

Low vision may be due to several types of limitations. The most common type of limitation is visual acuity. Eyeglasses are the most common type of aid used for visual acuity problems. When there are non-uniform refractive problems (i.e., astigmatism), an eyeglass lens can also be produced with compensation for this loss. In some cases eyeglasses are insufficient and further magnification is required. Some individuals have difficulty with particular combinations of background/foreground color combinations on electronic screens, in books, or in the environment. This is the second type of impairment, and it can be addressed by using filters or by varying contrast (e.g., black on white rather than white on black, or choosing different foreground/background colors) on a video or computer or cell phone display.

The *visual field* may be limited in several ways (see Figure 3-2). The most common approach to problems of this type is to use lenses that are designed to widen the field (e.g., prism glasses). Visual field and contrast overlap. For example, certain colors are seen best at specific parts of the visual field (Figure 8-2). This can be helpful in determining where to locate items and how to enhance them with specific colors to make them more visible. For example, objects that are red are seen more readily in the central visual field, and a red object may be more visible to a person with peripheral field loss. Conversely an object that is toward the blue part of the spectrum may be more visible for a person with central field loss and intact peripheral vision.

Use of Alternative Sensory Pathways

When the visual loss is very severe, an **alternative sensory system** is required. The use of Braille for reading by persons who are blind is an example of using tactile input as an alternative sensory pathway. There are fundamental differences in the way that the brain processes tactile, visual, and auditory information and these affect the ways in which sensory aids are implemented.

Tactile Substitution

The tactile system is used as the basis for many visual substitution systems. The tactile system functions best when there is both touch and movement. Kirman (1973)[19] provided the following example of the need for both movement and touch in the tactile system. The fingers are capable of distinguishing fine features such as those found on coins. However, it is very difficult to distinguish two denominations of coins merely by placing a hand on top of them without movement. In order to distinguish one denomination of coin from another, it is necessary to manipulate them in the hand. This movement of the coins provides temporal (time sequence) information that helps clarify the spatial information. When someone is reading by Braille, they move their hand across the Braille cells rather than merely placing it on top of the cells. This movement is necessary in order to gain all the possible information from the Braille cells.

In this classic paper Kirman[19] also described the difference between reading tactically in Braille and reading visually. Print on a page is organized spatially. We read by using saccadic eye movements, which jump from one group of letters to another. This allows the visual system to recognize shapes as letters, to assemble them into words, and to associate meaning with them. In contrast, a person reading with Braille moves his hand across the line of raised dots, obtaining both spatial (the organization of the six or eight Braille cells) and temporal (the moving pattern under his finger) information. If the sighted person were to use the method employed with Braille, the text would constantly move before her eyes, and this would result in a blurred image because the spatial information would be constantly changing. Thus movement interferes with the visual input of information. On the other hand, if the Braille user were to employ the approach used by the sighted reader, he would place his finger on a character, input the information, and then jump to the next character, losing the movement required by the tactile system and severely limiting the input of Braille information. Thus the visual and tactile methods of sensory input are very different, and we must take this into account when substituting one system for the other.

Tactile substitution is used very effectively for mobility. The most common approach is the long cane through which the user obtains information about the environment.

Auditory Substitution

The auditory system is temporally organized.[19] By this we mean that it is the time relationships in auditory signals that provide information. For example, it is the temporal sequence of sounds in speech that the auditory system uses to form words and derive meaning. The only widely successful auditory substitution for visual input has been speech.

Devices for visual mobility have employed auditory substitution with some success. This success is because mobility depends much more on gross cues (e.g., using tones that rise in frequency as objects get closer) than on precise spatial information, as in reading. In mobility the problem becomes one of identifying large objects as potential hazards.

READING AIDS FOR PERSONS WITH VISUAL IMPAIRMENTS

The major problems faced by persons with visual impairments are (1) access to printed reading material, (2) orientation and mobility (i.e., moving about safely and easily), and (3) access to computers, including the **Internet**. The term *reading* is used here to include access to all print material, including text, mathematics, and graphical representations (e.g., maps, pictures, drawings, and handwriting). As we discuss later, some types of reading have very specialized alternatives (e.g., talking compasses in lieu of maps, and talking bar code readers for medicines and food cans).

Magnification Aids

There are three factors related to visual system performance for reading: size, spacing, and contrast. Aids to assist people who have low-vision to read print material are generally referred to as **magnification aids**. Magnification may be vertical (size), or horizontal (spacing), or both. *Magnification* also includes assistive technologies that enhance contrast. There are three categories of magnification aids: (1) optical aids, (2) nonoptical aids, and (3) electronic aids.[31] Examples of these are listed in Box 8-1.

Assistive technologies can also be used to enhance visual cues for individuals who have low vision.[14] Color and contrast can be enhanced by using hues (i.e., using the named color such as red, blue, etc.), lightness (perceived intensity), and saturation (perceived differences in color). Griffin et al (2002)[14] provide the following guidelines for use in visual magnifiers, software, or Web site design for individuals with low vision: (1) use colors that differ as little as possible in lightness, (2) avoid colors from the ends of the spectrum, (3) avoid white or gray with any color of the same lightness, (4) avoid colors adjacent to each other in the color spectrum, and (5) avoid use of pastel colors. Spatial considerations are

BOX 8-1 Categories and Examples of Low-Vision Aids*

OPTICAL AIDS
Handheld magnifiers
Stand magnifiers
Field expanders
Telescopes

NONOPTICAL AIDS
Enlarged print
High-intensity lamps
Daily living aids
High-contrast objects

ELECTRONIC AIDS
Closed Circuit Televisions (CCTVs)
Portable CCTVs
Slide projectors
Opaque projectors
Microfiche readers

*Data from Servais SP, Visual aids. In Webster JG et al (eds): *Electronic devices for rehabilitation*, New York, 1985, John Wiley and Sons.

another consideration in enhancing visual access for children with low vision.[14] Space includes the size, patterns, outlines, and clarity of text and pictures. Optical magnifiers, software programs, and Web sites can address these features.

Optical Aids

More than 90% of all individuals who have visual impairments have some usable vision.[7] With the first type of magnification aid (optical aids) individuals with low vision may be able to see print, do work requiring fine detail, or increase the range of their visual fields. **Optical aids** directly affect the image that is presented to eye.

The simplest of optical aids is the handheld magnifier. These devices require little training, are lightweight and small (can fit in a pocket or purse), and are inexpensive. Some also have a built-in light to increase contrast, and others have several lenses that can be used alone or in combination, depending on the application. A selection of optical aids is shown in Figure 8-3. Sometimes it is difficult to hold a lens and carry out a task (e.g., a two-handed task such as embroidery). In other cases it may be difficult to hold a magnifier steady (e.g., for someone who has weak arms or a tremor). In these situations stand magnifiers, some of which have a built-in light, are useful. Some magnifiers are mounted on eyeglass frames to free both hands.

One approach to limitations of visual field is the use of field expanders. These are generally prisms or special lenses built into eyeglass frames. Magnification of the visual image (e.g., text) reduces the amount of information that is seen in the visual field when magnifying lenses are used. This effect can be seen on some automotive side mirrors that give an expanded field, but reduce the size of objects in that field. It is also the same effect observed when viewing a map on the computer screen. As you zoom out the field is expanded, but the image has less detail. The image is not reduced in size when prism lenses are used to expand the field.

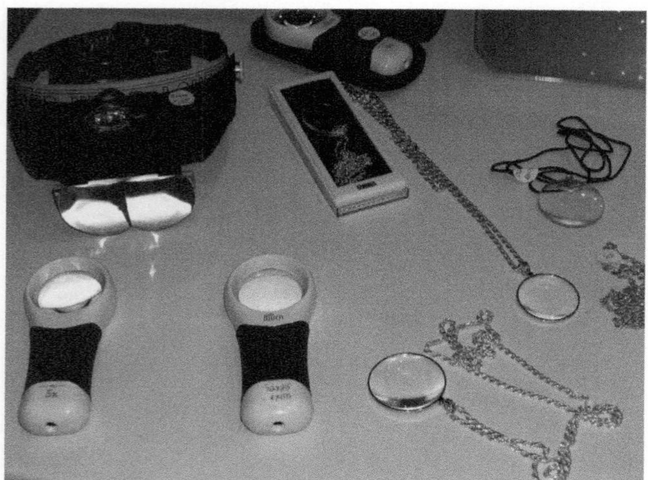

Figure 8-3 A selection of optical aids for low vision.

Telescopes assist with distance vision. These may be either worn on the head or held in the hand, and they may be monocular or binocular. They may be used, for example, by students who need to see a chalkboard or an adult who needs to monitor children playing outdoors. Telescopic aids provide an enlarged but narrowed visual field. Head-mounted units may be attached to eyeglass frames or have a separate frame. Head-mounted devices are particularly useful when long periods of wear are necessary, such as when watching television.

CASE STUDY – LIVING WITH GLAUCOMA

Karen is a 68-year-old woman with glaucoma. Her central vision is intact, but she is losing her peripheral vision. She has spent most of her time lately playing bridge, quilting, and reading. She would like to continue these activities as long as possible. What types of optical aids might help her continue with her recreational activities?

Nonoptical Aids

This approach to magnification is based on changes in the actual material that is to be read.[31] Common examples are large-print books or other materials such as menus, programs, and newspapers. High-intensity lamps can significantly increase contrast of reading materials, and high-contrast objects in the environment can aid in localization. For example, brightly colored furniture or dishes can help with visualization. A glass that stands out from a countertop is easier to find and fill with liquid. Attention to the contrast between the foreground and background can make visual objects such as signs, screens, and displays easier to view. High contrast (e.g., black on white, yellow on black) is easier to view than low contrast (e.g., red on blue). Nonoptical aids can be very useful under the right circumstances, but they are limited in application because they are specialized to one or a few tasks.

Electronic Aids

Optical approaches to magnification are fixed lenses, and this limits the amount of magnification and contrast enhancement that can be obtained. Electronic low-vision aids are called **video magnifiers**. These devices were originally based on **closed circuit television (CCTV)** systems and this terminology still used by some manufacturers. There are two primary advantages of video magnifiers: (1) the amount of magnification can be much more than for optical aids, and (2) the image can be manipulated and controlled. For example, brightness and contrast can be independently controlled. Most current video magnifiers are based on computers, so many of the common features of word processors such as searching a document or other text manipulation can be incorporated into the video magnifier. Image contrast can be dramatically affected by the use of color or reversed images (e.g., white type on black background).

The major components of a typical CCTV or video magnifier are a camera (environmental interface), a video display (user display), and a unit that controls the presentation of the image (information processor). Commercial devices are available with flat panel video displays. Many also allow connection to a standard television set for viewing. The material to be read is placed on a scanning table, which easily moves both left to right and forward and back to image different portions of the page or other objects being viewed (e.g., a prescription bottle, recipe, or photo of a grandchild). The scanning table can also be locked once the desired portion of the image is magnified.

When the text is enlarged, the relative position of the material on the page is lost, and a spotlight of high intensity is sometimes used to show the user which part of the page is being imaged. Using a split video screen, video magnifiers can be operated in conjunction with enlarged computer video displays to allow magnification of both computer data and the video image of standard print material. Other contexts in which video magnifiers are used are to complete job-related tasks, to access educational materials at all levels, and for recreational reading or hobbies such as sewing or painting.

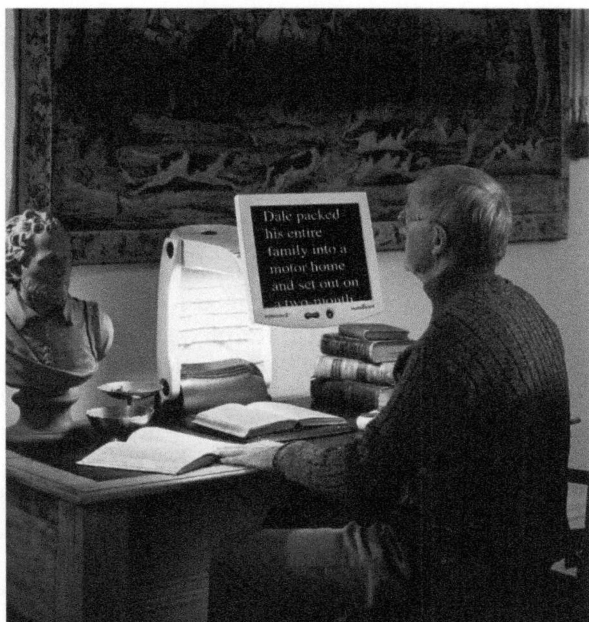
Dale packed
his entire
family into a
motor home
and set out on

Figure 8-4 A video magnifier in use. (Courtesy HumanWare, http://www.humanware.com/)

CASE STUDY – MANAGING ARMD

Marco is 65 and recently retired. He has ARMD and is losing his central vision. He wants to be as independent as possible in his daily life. This includes taking care of his own finances (including reading bills, writing checks, managing the family budget), doing minor maintenance on the family car (his wife now does the driving, but he still wants to check the oil level, measure the tire air pressure, etc., as he has always done. He has asked you for suggestions of assistive devices that might be helpful for him. What would you tell him? Consider all of the low vision aids discussed in this chapter.

An example of a video magnifier in use is shown in Figure 8-4. There is, however, a relatively wide range of features available in specific devices. The two broad categories of video magnifiers are desktop and portable. Size and spacing are controlled primarily by two factors in desktop units: (1) size of the video monitor (flat panels are smaller but more expensive), and (2) amount of enlargement provided by the electronics. Typical video monitors range in size from 17 to 22 inches, and maximal electronic magnification ranges from 45 to more than 80 times. There is a major tradeoff between monitor size and overall space required for the unit. Space requirements are often a significant limitation if a computer monitor, printer, and other office equipment must share space with the video magnifier. A split-screen system overcomes this space problem to a large degree. Video magnifiers often allow access not only to print material but also to the computer video screen. One such product is Topaz,* which allows the screen to be split into two. One half is used for video magnifier display of printed material and the other is used for enlarged computer output. This system also functions either as a computer screen magnifier only or as a video magnifier only. Other manufacturers have similar products. Most video magnifiers have simple controls for magnification (generally a rotating dial), contrast, and brightness. The controls are located directly under the video display for convenient access.

A major challenge for people using video magnifiers is navigation around text because it is often so enlarged that only a portion of a line or two of text is visible. This situation can result in missed words or difficulty in finding the beginning of the next line. One approach is to create a digital image of the page and then let the computer-based magnifier automatically scroll through the text.† Automatic reading can be one long row that scrolls across the screen, a column of text whose width is such that it all appears on the screen at once or one word at a time, with the user controlling the rate at which each word is displayed. Scrolling rate, magnification, and cursor movement around the text field are all adjustable and controllable by the user.

Contrast enhancement is generally provided by contrasting foreground and background colors. The video magnifier foreground and background contrast is adjustable and may be reversed (e.g., black letters on white or white letters on black). Color adds significant contrast enhancement because the user can choose alternative

* Freedom Scientific (www.freedomscientific.com)

† For example, myReader, HumanWare, Concord, Calif., (www.humanware.com)

background and foreground colors. Not all persons with visual impairments have the same color vision, and color vision varies with an individual's visual field. Having some control over the foreground-background color combination allows the display to be customized to the needs of the individual user. Some commercial video magnifiers include selection of contrast from a group of 20 or more preset foreground/background color combinations. Another advantage of color displays is that the original color of the print material can be retained. Maps with colored areas can be imaged; a preprinted form that calls for a signature "on the red line" shows the line as red, and so on. The major tradeoff with color monitors is that the image is not as sharp as the black and white image, especially at large magnifications. Most video magnifiers also have a black and white mode when a sharper image is required.

Fully *portable magnifiers* are designed to be carried with the user. The most significant differences between these portable units and desktop video magnifiers are size, weight, and battery power. Portable units weigh as little as 1–2 pounds and measure only about 9 × 3 inches for the display and 4 × 2 inches for the camera.* Some portable units have a handheld camera that is moved over the page and others have folding stands that can be set up to image a page, a whiteboard in a classroom, or other objects such as a medicine bottle.

Portable magnifying devices called *portable readers* include storage of text in digital form.† These devices have a built-in high resolution camera. The displayed image can be enlarged. Some portable devices are based on cell phone technology and others have a custom-designed computer and packaging. Using the built-in camera, these portable readers take a picture of text and magnify it for display on the built-in screen like other portable magnifiers (much like taking a picture with a digital camera). The image is then enlarged or converted to speech. The user can zoom in on a portion for greater magnification. Some devices also include a translation to auditory form via speech synthesis for users who are blind. Earphones provide privacy and avoid disturbing others. Stored data can be uploaded to a computer for further processing or conversion into MP3 or DAISY format.

Several portable video magnifiers connect to laptop computers for the image display.‡ Portable units consist of a camera and software to allow control over the video magnification. Maximal magnification varies from 3 to 64 times. Some units also allow the camera to be connected to a desktop video monitor or standard television set to display the video magnifier output, which allows it to be used in a portable or stationary mode, depending on the needs of the user. These cameras are extremely small (e.g., 2 inches × 2 inches × 4 inches, weighing 6 ounces). This flexibility is useful when greater magnification is needed for certain material (e.g., fine print), at certain times (e.g., at the end of the day, when fatigue is greater), and when the user must travel to different settings during the day. Portable video magnifiers are useful for students and in business applications where travel to various locations is important.

* For example, Pico, Telesensory Systems (www.telesensory.com); Smart View, HumanWare, Inc., Concord, Calif. (www.humanware.com); i-vu and RioCarrymate, Clarity (www.clarityusa.com/); and Magnilink, Vision Cue (www.visioncue.com/)

† For example, Intel Reader (http://www.careinnovations.com/Products/Reader/Default.aspx); KNFB Reader (http://www.knfbreader.com/products-mobile.php)

‡ For example, Smart View Graduate, HumanWare (www.humanware.com); and Pearl, Freedom Scientific (www.freedomscientific.com)

CASE STUDY – WORKING WITH PROGRESSIVE VISION LOSS

Stacy is a 45-year-old office worker who is gradually losing her sight due to diabetic retinopathy. She wants to continue working and needs to be able to use a computer, read paper documents, and perform clerical duties such as photocopying, making appointments, and setting up meetings. What kinds of assistive technologies would be helpful to her both now, while she still has some vision, and later, when her vision loss has progressed to the point of needing alternative means of access to visual material?

Braille as a Tactile Reading Substitute

The most widely used tactile substitution approach for persons with visual impairments is **Braille**. Each Braille character consists of a cell of either six or eight dots, as shown in Figure 8-5. Braille for written text uses 6 dots. The seventh and eighth dots are used to show cursor movement or to provide single-cell presentation of features such as upper and lower case alphabet, numbers, special symbols, and control characters such as ENTER. When text is directly translated into Braille letter-by-letter, it is referred to as *Grade 1*. There are also Braille codes for words (called *wordsigns*) and contractions (see examples in Figure 8-5). The use of these contractions significantly speeds up the rate of reading, and this type of Braille is called *Grade 2* or *Grade 3*, depending on the number of contractions used. Reading rates with Grade 2 Braille are about 104 words per minute (wpm).[29] Grade 1 reading rates are about 75% of Grade 2 rates.[22] Grade 3 Braille has more contractions and eliminates some vowels, and it is used primarily for taking notes.[29] Traditionally, Braille has been produced by embossing on heavy paper, and this method is still widely used. For persons who develop skill with it, Braille can be a fast and efficient method for accessing print materials.

Limitations of Printed Braille

Embossed Braille material is heavy and bulky, and each Braille page has significantly less information than a printed page of the same size. For example, a Braille version of a book would be about two and a half times bigger in Braille.[21] A second disadvantage is that the cost of producing Braille in an embossed form is high compared

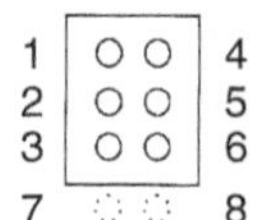

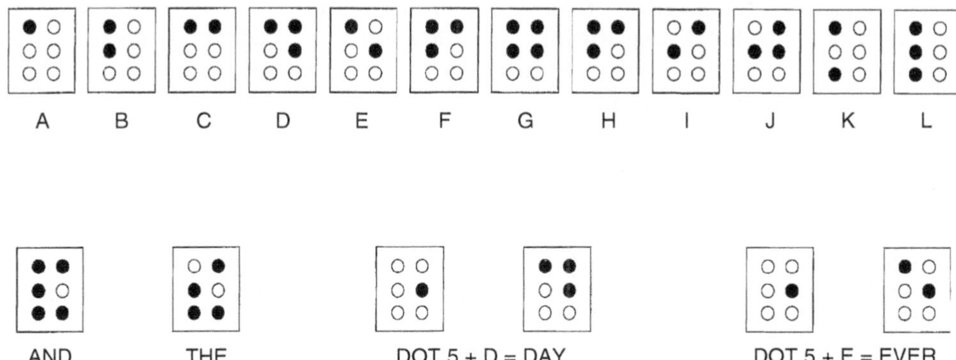

Figure 8-5 Examples of Braille letters, word signs, and contractions.

with print materials. For this reason, only a fraction of the total print literature is available in embossed Braille form. It is difficult to scan a Braille document to find a particular piece of text as is typically done with print material. Finally, Braille embossers do not allow corrections to be made.

Less than 10% of persons with severe visual impairment learn to use Braille. This is partially true because more than 65% of all persons who become blind do so after age 65,[23] and many of these cases are the result of diabetes, which also affects the tactile sense. This situation makes Braille less desirable than other alternatives such as talking books. Despite all these limitations, Braille is the modality of choice for many persons with severe visual impairment. The disadvantages of embossed paper can be overcome with a refreshable Braille display.

Refreshable Braille Displays

Because Braille is represented by a series of dots, a **refreshable Braille display**, shown in Figure 8-6, uses raised pins to represent the dots in a Braille cell rather than the traditional embossed paper. Stand-alone refreshable Braille displays are available from several manufacturers.* These refreshable displays are controlled by a computer, just like a printer or video display, which allows text information to be displayed in Braille as it would be in visible text. Because the text material is in electronic form, it can be edited, searches can be made, and copies of Braille material can be easily produced in electronic form. The refreshable Braille cell (or cell array) can also be used as the output mode for an automatic reading machine.

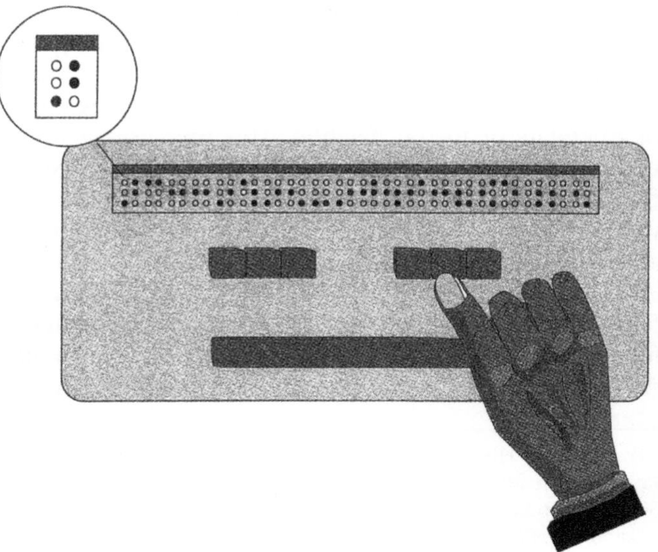

Figure 8-6 A set of refreshable Braille cells.

Some portable reading and note taking aids, discussed later in this chapter, also use refreshable Braille cells.

Each refreshable Braille cell has a set of small pins arranged in the shape of a standard Braille cell. The pins that correspond to the dot pattern for a letter or word sign are raised. Both Grade 1 and Grade 2 Braille can be presented on refreshable displays using software that converts text from ASCII format to Braille. Arrays of from 1 to 80 cells are available. Some Braille displays also include a Braille keyboard.*

Stationary refreshable Braille displays have arrays with multiple Braille cells that are connected to a computer

* For example, HumanWare, Concord, Calif. (www.humanware.com), Freedom Scientific, St. Petersburg, Fla. (www.freedomsci.com); ALVA BC640, Vision Cue, Portland, Ore. (http://www.visioncue.com/); and Baum (http://www.baum.de/en/products/brailledisplay/svario.php)

* For example, Braille Connect, HumanWare, Concord, Calif. (www.humanware.com); Focus 40, Freedom Scientific, St. Petersburg, Fla. (www.freedomsci.com), ALVA BC640, Vision Cue, Portland, Ore. (http://www.visioncue.com/)

through a USB interface. Typically the array sizes are 20, 40, or 80 cells.* These refreshable Braille arrays can be used as an alternative to the computer video display. Many refreshable Braille displays also have a wireless Bluetooth link to increase flexibility of use.

The ALVA† Braille terminals provide 44-, 70-, and 80-cell refreshable displays for desktop use and 23- and 44-cell displays for portable applications (battery operated). All versions have eight-dot Braille cells. All ALVA models also provide extra status cells that display the location of the system cursor, which line of text is displayed in Braille, which attributes are active, and the relationship of those attributes to the characters on the screen. This information can be monitored with the left hand while the right hand reads the text on the Braille display. USB and serial ports are available for data transfer. Text is provided in both Grade 1 and Grade 2 Braille.

Freedom Scientific‡ makes 40- and 80-cell Braille displays. The 40-cell unit includes a Braille keyboard. Both the 40- and 80-cell versions have navigation features accessible through a series of buttons on the display. Combinations of buttons are used to enter commands. Another product, the PAC Mate Omni™ portable Braille display is a 20- or 40-cell refreshable Braille display that functions as a portable computer. It can be connected to any computer through a USB port to synchronize email or calendars or to transfer files. This unit uses a seamless design between Braille cells that makes the display feel like paper. It works with most Windows-based software packages. HumanWare§ makes a series of refreshable Braille displays shown in Figure 8-7. The 40-cell and 24-cell Brailliant refreshable Braille displays are designed for use with a laptop or desktop computer, and are offered for both. The Brailliant 32, 64, and 80 are 8-dot Braille displays for desktop computers. All these models are configured for split-window display or as programmable status cells, and all include Bluetooth and USB connectivity. The latter features are accessed by clicking a sensor located above one of the Braille cells to instantly move the mouse pointer or cursor to a new location for editing. Grade 2 Braille translation is included on all models.

* For example, HumanWare, Concord, Calif. (www.humanware.com); Freedom Scientific, St. Petersburg, Fla. (www.freedomsci.com); ALVA Series, Vision Cue, Portland, Ore. (http://www.visioncue.com/)
† Vision Cue, Portland, Ore. (http://www.visioncue.com/)
‡ Freedom Scientific, St. Petersburg, Fla. (www.freedomsci.com)
§ HumanWare, Concord, Calif. (www.humanware.com)

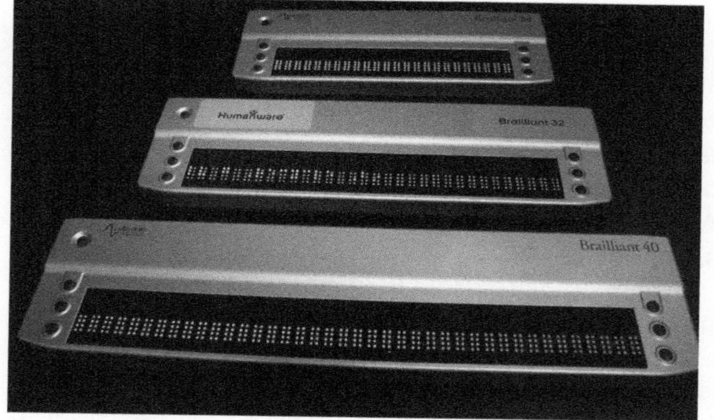

Figure 8-7 Refreshable Braille cells are available with a variable number of cells.

Speech as an Auditory Reading Substitute

Because reading is based on visual language, it is logical that auditory substitution for reading also uses language—that is, speech. Audio technology is the primary method for information storage and retrieval used by individuals who are blind.[30] Synthetic speech for reading systems designed for the blind is available in a variety of languages using the approaches described in Chapter 7.

Recorded Audio Material

The oldest and still the most prevalent use of auditory substitution for persons with visual impairment is recorded material. Current technology used in recorded audio material is CDs and digital recording (e.g., MP3 device format and downloadable files).* There are still sites that provide books on cassette tapes for those who do not have access to digital media. Special machines are needed for high-speed cassette playback. These are available from some libraries, including the National Library Service for the Blind (NLS).† The variable speed allows the listener to review material faster than it was originally spoken. With practice, it is possible to understand speech up to four times as fast as normal speaking rates. Some people use digital recording and playback to record lectures and then review the material in lieu of note taking. The common current digital formats are shown in Table 8-2.

The use of CDs allows a great deal of information to be placed on a single disk. One CD-ROM can store a large amount of data, and reproduction costs are low. The major advantages of CDs are greatly increased fidelity, resulting from greater frequency response, and indexing, which can be used to find a particular track. The use of digitized audio information allows voice recordings to be mixed with headings that allow easier searching of the text. Multimedia presentations are also commonplace with digitized audio information, allowing both visual and auditory presentation of information and thereby increasing the potential market and reducing price.

Audio displays are also being used for the presentation of mathematical information using computers and speech synthesizers and as a substitute for data presentation (e.g., tables and charts).[30] In this form a book can be loaded into a personal computer word processor and

* For example, Recording for the Blind and Dyslexic (www.rfbd.org); National Library Service for the Blind and Physically Handicapped, Library of Congress (http://www.loc.gov/nls/index.html). Recording and Playback Devices at National Federation of the Blind (http://secure.nfb.org/ecommerce/asp/default.asp)
† http://www.loc.gov/nls/index

TABLE 8-2 Audiobook Formats

Features and Functionality	Downloadable DAISY (AudioPlus)	DAISY CDs (AudioPlus)	WMA Downloadable (AudioAccess)
Requires separate purchase of specialized DAISY hardware and/or software	Yes	Yes	No
Compatible with MP3* players and Windows Media Player**	No	No	Yes
Download chapters or sections of a book	No	No	Yes
Enhanced (DAISY) navigation, bookmarking and variable speed control	Yes	Yes	No
Requires online access	Yes	No	Yes
Compatible with iOS Devices	Yes	No	No

- **Downloadable DAISY Books** provide instant access with enhanced navigation, bookmarking, and variable speed control. Play from Microsoft® Windows® compatible computer with RFB&D-enabled software or specialized DAISY players.
- **DAISY CDs** offer enhanced navigation and play on RFB&D-enabled specialized DAISY players.
- **Downloadable books in WMA** (Windows Media Audio) play on Microsoft Windows–based computers using Windows Media Player Version 10 or higher. These books can be synched to commercial MP3 players with DRM capabilities.

*MP3 players must have DRM (Digital Rights Management) capabilities to play encrypted content.
**Windows Media Player 10 or higher.
Courtesy Recording for the Blind and Dyslexic, http://www.learningally.org/

displayed on the screen. Because the data are digital, sophisticated search strategies can be used to find a particular item or place in the text. For persons with low vision or blindness, the availability of digital-based reading materials opens up many different options for obtaining access to print materials. For example, with an enlarged screen output, reading material on a CD can be accessed and presented to a person with low vision using a computer.

One of the challenges in any electronic format is standardization. Different countries have different recording formats for talking books on tape, and there are many formats for word processors in digital form. For this reason an international group, the **Digital Audio-Based Information System (DAISY) Consortium** (www.daisy.org) has developed an international standard for **digital talking books (DTBs)**.[18] This standard includes production, exchange, and use of DTBs. The DAISY standard is hardware platform and operating system independent, and it makes use of the Web accessibility standards developed by the World Wide Web Consortium (W3C). There are several on-line sources for books in the Daisy format.* These sites have thousands of titles including books for children and adults, textbooks, and newspapers. Many of the books are available in both Daisy and BRF Grade-II Braille format for printed books or for using refreshable Braille displays. Players for Daisy format CDs are available from several manufacturers.† A typical Daisy format reader is shown in Figure 8-8.

* For example, Benetech (www.bookshare.org); National Library Service, U.S. Library of Congress (www.loc.gov/nls); Recording for the Blind and Dyslexic (www.rfbd.org); Dolphin Audio Publishing, (http://www.yourdolphin.com/)
† For example, Telex, Burnsville, Minn. (www.telex.com), FSReader, Freedom Scientific, St. Petersburg, Fla. (www.freedomsci.com), EaseReader, Dolphin Audio Publishing (http://www.yourdolphin.com/); Victor, HumanWare, Concord, Calif. (www.humanware.com)

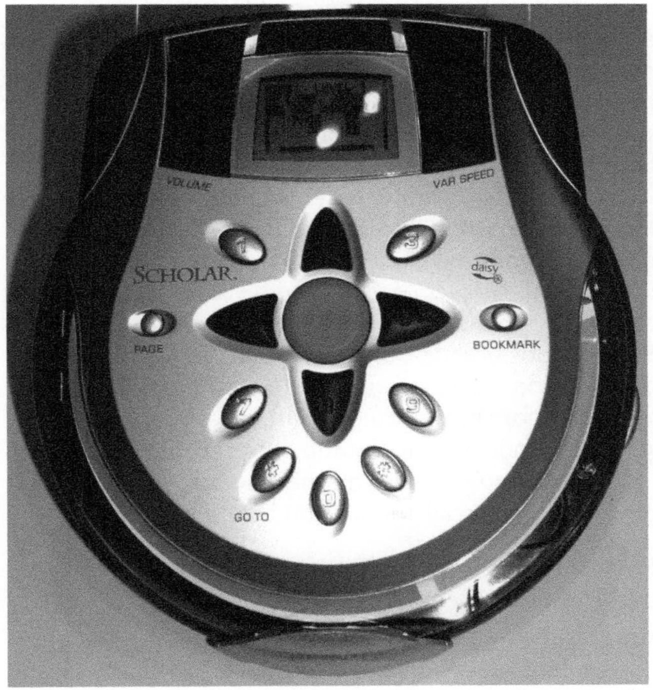

Figure 8-8 Typical DAISY reader.

Devices That Provide Automatic Reading of Text

The major components of an automatic reading machine are shown in Figure 8-9. Automatic reading involves scanning of a document, conversion of the printed material to computer data using an **optical character recognition** (OCR) program, and the translation of the computer data into either Braille or speech for the user (see Figure 8-9).* Most reading machines provide synthesized speech output, and some provide Braille or both Braille and speech.

* For example, ScannaR, HumanWare (www.humanware.com/)

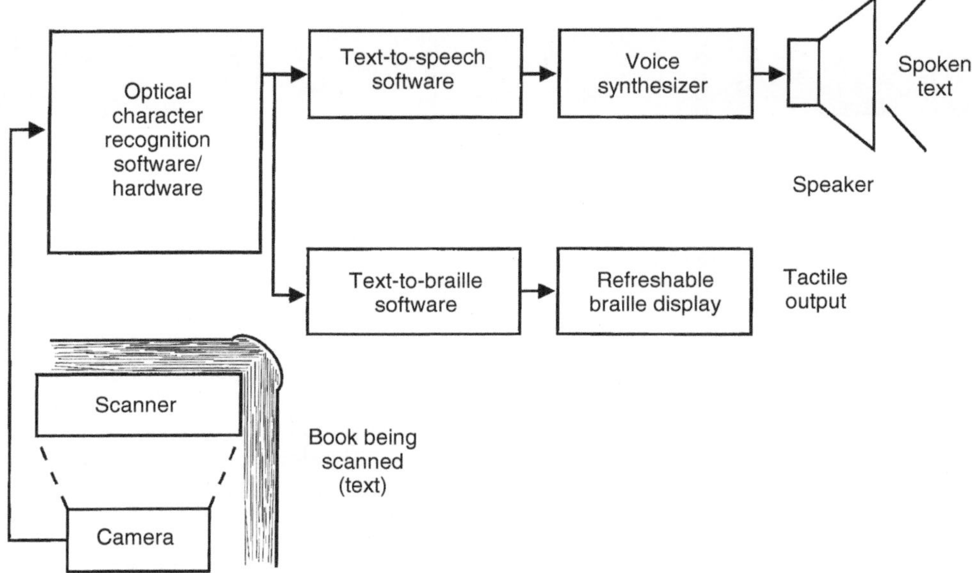

Figure 8-9 The major components of an automatic text reading machine for persons with total visual impairment.

Some automatic reading devices utilize standard computers with special software for information processing and output to a refreshable Braille display or speech synthesis program.* Stand-alone automatic reading machines offer simple one-button operation to scan a document and have it read.

Some desktop reading systems have scanners built into them.† These systems include a flatbed scanner, built-in computer, voice output, and a hard drive with room for up to 500,000 pages of text. In some cases DAISY reading capability for digital books (see following) is included. Scanned documents can be saved in MPS, WAV, DAISY, or plain-text format. Some units also provide multiple languages for spoken output. Other reading systems are software products that include optical character recognition and text-to-speech synthesis and are designed to use external commercial scanners and computers.‡

Portable Braille Note Takers and Personal Organizers

Many individuals who are blind use digital recording for note taking at meetings or in class. Others use portable note takers as stand-alone data managers or personal organizers. These units vary in size from a compact 4.5 inches square and about 1.5 inches thick to the size of a laptop computer (approximately 9 × 12 inches).* A typical model is pictured in Figure 8-10. Some models use a Braille keyboard for input and others use a standard QWERTY keyboard. The Braille keyboard has one key for each of the eight dots in a Braille cell. Additional keys are used for control, editing, and data management. Synthesized speech is available in all units with either a speaker or earphone output for the synthesized speech. Some models include a refreshable Grade 2 Braille display (from 8 to 32 Braille cells) either alone or paired with synthetic speech. The speech synthesizer and refreshable Braille display can also be used as outputs on the unit (replacing the output from the video monitor) or in conjunction with screen reader software on a PC. Additional

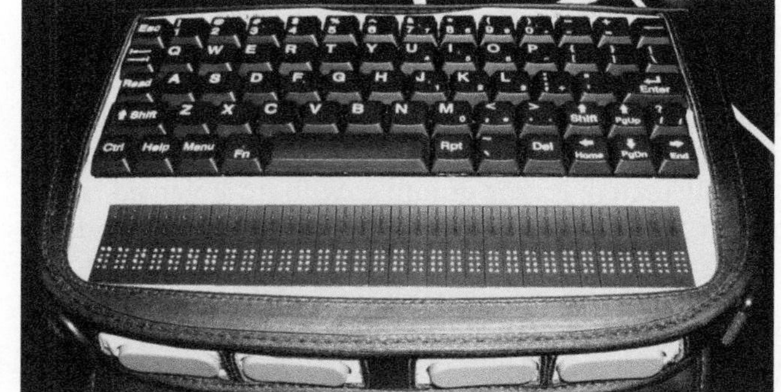

Figure 8-10 A personal organizer with Braille display and synthesized speech output.

* For example, Open Book, Freedom Scientific (www.freedomscientific.com/)

† For example, Ovation, Telesensory, Sunnyvale, Calif. (www.telesensory.com); Sara, Freedom Scientific, St. Petersburg, Fla. (www.freedomsci.com); Pulse Tech Book Reader (www.plustek.com); POET-Compact, Baum (www.baum.de/index-e.php); ScannaR, HumanWare, Concord, Calif. (www.humanware.com); Sophie, Handy Tech Elektronik GmbH (www.handytech.de/)

‡ For example, Open Book, Freedom Scientific, St. Petersburg, Fla. (www.freedomsci.com); Cicero, Dolphin Products (www.dolphincomputeraccess.com)

* For example, the; Braille Desk 2000, *Braillino*, Handy Tech Elektronik GmbH, Germany (www.handytech.de); Braille Note, HumanWare, Concord, Calif. (www.humanware.com); Aria, Sensory Tools, Robotron Proprietary Limited, St. Kilda, Australia (www.sensorytools.com/products.htm); PacMate, Freedom Scientific, St. Petersburg, Fla. (www.freedomsci.com)

outputs available on selected models include computer file transfer, Internet and e-mail access, and print. Some models also dial a telephone automatically from the data in the built-in address book.

Built-in programs vary somewhat among various note taker models. All include word processing for writing when away from a computer (e.g., while sitting by the pool or riding a bus to work), editing documents developed on a PC word processor, and taking notes in class or at meetings. Other programs built into specific models, in various combinations, include a calendar, address book, calculator, timer or watch, e-mail access, and Internet browser, all with full access through speech or Braille. Storage of data is in both computer memory and flash memory cards. Direct transfer of data from a PC to a portable reader or vice versa is available using a USB port. MP3 music players and Web access via Bluetooth or WiFi protocols are also available on many units. Some note takers can also be used as computer keyboards through the built-in USB port or can function as cell phones. Storage and manipulation of information may be in the form of Braille or print or both. Control features may be via additional keys with specific functions or via a speech output menu of choices.

CASE STUDY – BRAILLE NOTE TAKING IN SCHOOL

Jenny is an eighth-grade student. She uses many pieces of technology to assist her in being successful at school. She has been using a Braille 'n Speak since the fifth grade to take class notes, complete assignments, take tests, keep an assignment notebook, and maintain a personal phone and address book. Review the features of this device (www.freedomsci.com) and list those that are likely to benefit Jenny in each of these applications.

MAKING MAINSTREAM TECHNOLOGIES ACCESSIBLE FOR INDIVIDUALS WHO HAVE LOW VISION OR ARE BLIND

Graphical User Interface

The most commonly used method for inputting information into a computer and many other mainstream technologies such as smart phones and pad computers is through a **graphical user interface (GUI)**. The GUI has three distinguishing features: (1) pointer that is moved around the screen; (2) a menu of graphical images (icons) on the screen that can be selected to run a program, open a file, or branch to more choices; and (3) one or more **windows**, which provide a menu of choices. Movement of the pointer around the screen is caused by a mouse, keystrokes, trackball, head pointer, joystick, or finger on a touch-sensitive display. Any icon can be selected by clicking with a mouse, tapping with a finger, or other means. Dragging of icons, text, files, or other elements is also an important feature of the GUI. The graphical environment can save typing, reduce effort, and increase accuracy. The use of icons generally helps with recall and ease of use. The GUI allows the use of windows, which partition the screen into smaller screens, each showing a particular computer application that is running. A typical graphical user interface (GUI) is shown in Figure 8-11.

The GUI presents unique and difficult problems to the blind computer user because it uses an approach to video display that creates many more options for the portrayal of graphical information than just text. Many different graphical symbols can be created. These symbols are useful to sighted computer users because they can rely on "visual metaphors" (e.g., a trash can to represent deleted files).[5] The graphical labels used to portray these functions are referred to as *icons*. Another feature of the GUI is

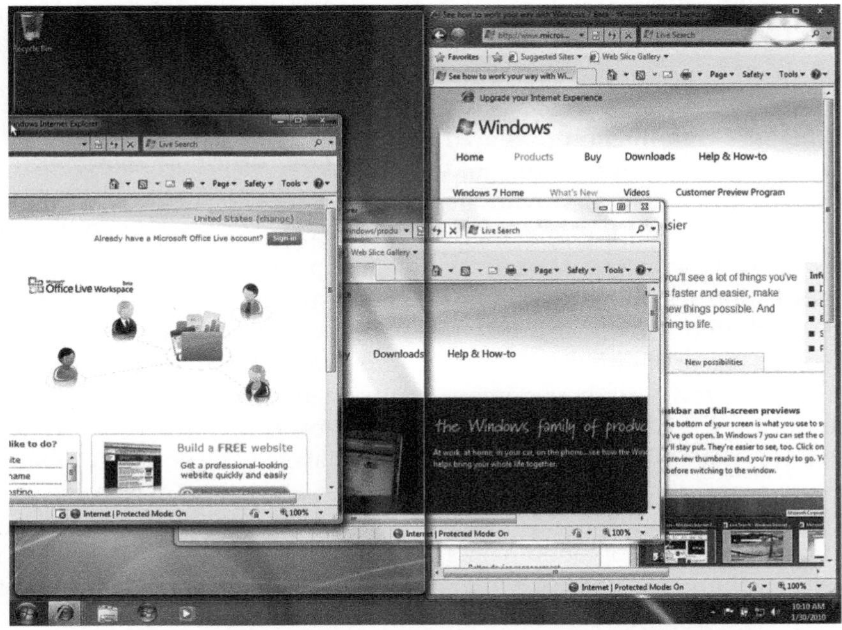

Figure 8-11 An example of a graphical user interface with several windows open for different applications. (Courtesy of Microsoft)

that it provides a specific, consistent layout of controls on the screen. These conventions aid the visual user (especially a novice) in accessing programs, since everything is consistent within an application and from one application program to another.

The GUI and the Blind Computer User

The GUI presents several problems to the blind user. First, the graphical characters are not easily portrayed in alternative modes. Text-to-speech programs and speech synthesizers are designed to convert text to speech output (see Chapter 7). However, they are not well suited to the representation of graphics, including the icons used in GUIs. However, most icons used in GUIs have text labels with them. One approach to adaptation is to intercept the label and send it to a text-to-speech voice synthesizer system. The label is then spoken when the icon is selected. Another major problem presented to blind users by GUIs is that screen location is important in using a GUI, which is not easily conveyed via alternative means. Visual information is spatially organized, and auditory information (including speech) is temporal (time based). It is difficult to convey the screen location of a pointer by speech alone. It is difficult to portray two dimensional spatial attributes using speech. An exception is a screen location that never changes. For example, some screen readers use speech to indicate the edges of the screen (e.g., right border, top of screen). A more significant problem is that the mouse pointer location on the screen is relative, rather than referenced to an absolute standard location, which means that the only information available to the computer is how far the mouse has moved and the direction of the movement. If there is no visual information available to the user, it is difficult to know where the mouse is pointing. Other challenges presented to the visually impaired user of a GUI include: the organization of the screen with elements spatially clustered visually; multitasking in which several windows are open simultaneously, with one possibly occluding another (i.e., visually displayed "on top" even though both windows are active); and graphical semantics (information portrayed through visual elements such as font size, colors, and style).[27] Another obstacle faced by individuals who are visually impaired is the use of graphical information in tables and graphs. Three primary issues are: the size of the table (i.e., providing information regarding the boundaries), overloading with speech information, and knowledge of current location of the cursor within the table.

Ratanasit and Moore (2005)[27] reviewed three primary types of non-speech sound cues used for representing visual icons used in GUIs: (1) auditory icons, (2) *earcons*, and (3) *hearcons*. Auditory icons are everyday sounds used to represent graphical objects. For example, a window might be represented by the sound of tapping on a glass window or a text box by the sound of a typewriter. The Screen Access Model and Windows™ sound libraries are used in some applications. Earcons are abstract auditory labels that do not necessarily have a semantic relationship to the object they represent. *Motives* are components of earcons such as rhythm (e.g., the length of a musical note or a Latin beat), pitch (e.g., a musical C vs A), timbre (e.g., sound of a type of instrument), and register (e.g., octaves on the musical scale). An example of an earcon is a musical note or string of notes played when a file, window, or program is opened or closed. Different musical instruments may be used to represent different actions, such as a trumpet representing opening a file and a drum representing closing. In evaluations by blind users, earcons associated with musical characteristics were more effective than those using unstructured sounds (i.e., sounds lacking rhythm, pitch, and other cues). Hearcons are either nature sounds or musical works or instruments. Hearcons are completed musical sounds such as those produced by a running river or birds or a musical work, whereas earcons are separate audio components. In an evaluation by visually impaired participants, hearcons did not sufficiently portray semantic relationships to be effective. Font types have been represented by male versus female synthesized voices for normal and hyperlink text or softer and louder sounds for normal versus bold font.

Various methods have been developed to represent this information auditorally.[27] Non-speech sounds are used to provide spatial relationships (e.g., a plucked violin string earcon might be used to represent the lines in a table or graph) and the text-based information contained in the table or graph is provided by synthesized speech. Another technique used is to associate higher pitches with larger numbers and lower pitches with smaller numbers in portraying trends and similar graphical data. Evaluation with visually impaired participants indicated greater success in using tables when non-speech cues were combined with speech-based information. Another graphical approach is to represent numerical values by pitch, as above, but use a different timbre (instrument sound) for each axis.

Access to Mobile Telephones for Individuals with Low Vision or Blindness

In Chapter 7 we discussed a study of people with a variety of sensory and motor disabilities by Kane et al (2009).[17] Participants in this study who had low vision or blindness reported several types of problems in accessing and using cell phones. Environmental lighting dramatically affected readability for people with low vision, and this was made worse by fatigue for a number of participants. The most common assistive devices were portable Braille note takers with phone capabilities. The relatively high cost of specialized assistive technologies led many participants to opt for standard devices even if the devices were less effective in meeting their needs. Some also mentioned that there was an inherent stigma in using an assistive device because it identified them as disabled whereas using a standard commercial device did not.

Cellular telephones have become more powerful with capabilities similar to personal computers. Fruchterman (2003)[9] describes four significant factors to assist people with disabilities, especially those with low vision or blindness: (1) standard cell phones have sufficient processing power for almost all the requirement of persons with visual impairments,* (2) software can be downloaded into these phones easily, (3) wireless connection to a worldwide network provides a wide range of information and services in a highly mobile way, and (4) many of these features are built into standard cell phones making the cost low and accessible by persons with disabilities. The cell phone industry has moved away from proprietary software to an open source approach, much like personal computers. This has lead to a greater diversity of software for tasks such as text-to-speech output, voice recognition, and optical character recognition in a variety of languages. Many applications for people with disabilities can be downloaded from the Internet. For example, downloading a DAISY reading program into a cell phone can provide access to digital libraries, and outputs in speech or enlarged visual displays allow access to standard text messaging.

Accessible cell phones with the capability of adding software for specific functions open up a range of options for people who have a visual impairment. These options include calendar/appointments, personal contact databases, note taking, multi-media messaging, and Web browsing. Many other possibilities exist as well; for example, with a built-in camera and network access a blind person could obtain a verbal description of a scene by linking to on-line volunteers who provide descriptions of images. Advances of this type will occur rapidly.

One reason for the optimism surrounding these types of advancement is the increasing application of universal design in information technology products.[34] Universal design principles (see Chapter 1) call for mainstream technologies to be accessible to a wide range of individuals with and without disabilities. Tobias (2003)[34] describes government regulations that underlie access in many countries and the challenges in implementing them. When mainstream technologies employ open source operating systems, network-based accommodations can be accessed by users without specially designed equipment. This can reduce cost and thereby increase availability. These applications include ATMs, cell phones, vending machines, and other systems that are encountered on a daily basis.[34]

The Royal National Institute of Blind People (RNIB) in Britain has developed a checklist for mobile phone accessibility (www.tiresias.org/research/guidelines/checklists/mobile_phones.htm). The checklist includes the major areas of the keypad and controls, the display, the physical characteristics (e.g., size, weight, ease of insertion of memory cards, etc.), operation (e.g., indicators for on/off, accessible controls and labels for menus and other functions), audio output, peripheral device compatibility, battery charging, and the documentation (e.g., clear instructions with alternate formats available). For each category of features, the checklist identifies those that apply to people with visual, hearing, cognitive, or physical impairments. The Tiresias website (www.tiresias.org) operated by RNIB provides many useful resources for persons with visual impairments who want to access cell phones. This site has both product information and user case studies that provide lots of practical advice for people with low vision in selecting and using a cell phone.

Another useful source of information for individuals with visual impairments who want to access PDAs and mobile phones is Code Factory (http://www.codefactory.es/en). The Code Factory develops accessible software applications for mobile phones. Their website includes a selection wizard to help individuals find specific products that will meet their needs based on the PDA or mobile phone that they intend to use. Products described include screen readers, screen magnifiers, GPS Navigation Aids, and a mobile DAISY player.

Accessibility features of the Apple iPad, iPhone, and iTouch are described on the Apple website (www.apple.com/accessibility). The standard or built-in features are a screen reader (Voice Over), screen magnifier (Zoom), and reverse (white on black) contrast. All of these features take advantage of the touch screen and the use of gestures (e.g., swipe or tap) to make a choice or to navigate around Web pages. There are also a number of third party hardware and software products that adapt the iPhone for people with disabilities. These are listed on the Apple accessibility website.

Computer Adaptations for Visual Impairments

Computer users generally receive output from a computer by looking at a visual display. In order to assist individuals who have visual limitations, it is necessary to understand how computer outputs can be adapted. Video displays are found in computers, personal digital assistants (PDAs), cell phones, and many other devices. Printed output is also commonly used in computer applications. Computers also provide auditory outputs in sound, music, or synthetic speech. These outputs are important to individuals who have visual impairments.

Standard visual computer outputs are often not usable by persons who have vision impairments. The degree of vision loss (as in Table 8-1) determines the amount and type of adaptation necessary for successful computer access. For individuals who are blind, we must use tactile or auditory pathways to provide input. Because low-vision and blindness needs are so different from each

* Popular applications-oriented operating systems include Android, http://market.android.com/; Apple's iOS, http://www.apple.com/ca/ipad/ios4/; and BlackBerry OS, http://us.blackberry.com/apps-software/blackberry6/

BOX 8-2 What the Research Tells Us: Computer Use by Visually Impaired Adults

- Computer use by individuals who are blind or have low vision is less compared to non-disabled individuals[12]
  - Less access to the Internet.
  - Are on-line less.
  - More likely to be on-line from work than at home.
- Effect of severity of impairment and existence of multiple impairments
  - Individuals under 65 have greater use and access than those over 65.
  - Important given the high prevalence of visual impairment in the population over 65.
  - People who are employed are more likely to use computers and the Internet, with same percentage as non-disabled population.
- Computer usage patterns of individuals who have visual impairments[11]
  - Focus groups at national conferences and subscribers to a technology and visual impairment publication.*
  - This sample represents the group of visually impaired individuals who use computers and the Internet, but it is not representative of the broader visually impaired community.
  - 50% had no useable vision, and the other 50% had variable amounts of vision.
  - 50% had been blind since birth, 85% had some university education, and 73% were employed.
  - Computer use allows access to employment and the creation of flexibility in finding work, including telecommuting.
  - Computer also allowed employed individuals to create a cultural identity by being successfully employed.
  - Computer use created access to information including newspapers and magazines as well as Web-based sources of information.
  - Respondents reported that it was rewarding to read for themselves using technology rather than have someone read to them.
  - Improvement in writing skill also occurred.
  - Major benefit of computer use is social connections made through the Internet that reduced feelings of isolation and loneliness: independently sending and receiving e-mail and participating in on-line discussions.
  - Concerns, which includes lack of training in use of adapted computers, training material in accessible form, and being shut out of the advances due to accessibility lags.
- Training availability (U.S. focused)[36]
  - Group training more common than individual training.
  - More demand than available opportunities.
  - Training for all major technology types.
  - Major challenge is keeping trainers up to date as technologies change.
- Quality of Training[37]
  - Positive comments: good overall quality of the training, greater self-confidence of the trainees following training, and (to a lesser extent) the quality of the trainers.
  - Negative comments: training was too short or too infrequent, too few computers were available for hands-on practice, training was not relevant to technology available on the job, the pace of training was too slow or too fast, material was presented at too basic a level, and there was too much variability in trainee experience that limited content that could be covered.
  - There is a need to stay abreast of technology changes.
- The amount and type (e.g., social networks, email, shopping, banking, etc.) of use of the Internet were not statistically related to either the perception of social support received or a sense of well being among individuals with visual impairments.[32]

Access World : Technology and People with Visual Impairments, American Foundation for the Blind, New York, http://www.afb.org/

other, we discuss them separately. Box 8-2 describes research related to computer use by individuals who have a visual impairment.

Access to Visual Computer Displays for Individuals with Low Vision

Magnifying software that enlarges a portion of the computer screen is the most common adaptation for people who have low vision. The unmagnified screen is called the *physical screen*. Screen magnifiers can enlarge the whole physical screen image or just one portion of the physical screen.[4] The enlarged portion of the screen is called the *magnification window*, and the size of text in this window is the *magnification*. The magnification varies from 2 to 36 times or more in current magnifier programs.

At any one time the user has access to only the portion of the physical screen that appears in the magnification window. The magnification program will follow a particular part of the screen referred to as the *focus* of the screen.[4] Typical foci are the location of the mouse pointer, the location of the text-entry cursor, a highlighted item (e.g., an item in a pull-down menu) or a currently active dialog box. Screen magnifiers automatically track the focus and enlarge the relevant portion of the screen, and the magnification window tracks any changes that occur on the physical screen. For example, if a navigation or control box is active, then the viewing window can highlight that box. If mouse movement occurs, then the magnification window can track the mouse cursor movement. If text is being entered, then the magnification window can follow the text entry cursor and highlight that portion of the physical screen.

Adaptations that allow persons with low vision to access the computer screen are available in several commercial forms. Lazzaro (1999)[20] describes several potential methods of achieving computer access. The simplest and least costly are built-in screen enlargement software programs provided by the computer manufacturer (Table 8-3). One system for the Macintosh OS X operating system is *Zoom*. This program allows for magnification from 2 to 40 times and has fast and easy text handling and graphics capabilities. There are options for the focus of the magnification, for contrast colors, for cursor size, and for the way in which the user can enable the magnification. More information is available on the Apple accessibility website www.apple.com/accessibility/macosx/. *Magnifier* (see Table 8-3) is a minimal function screen magnification program included in Windows (www.microsoft.com/enable/). It displays an enlarged portion of the screen (from 2 to 9 times magnification). Other *Magnifier* options include inverting (e.g., black background, white letters), changing the location of the magnification pane, and high-contrast modes. For individuals who need only the *High Contrast* option (available in the control panel "Accessibility Options" icon), there are many color combination options for text, background, windows, and other GUI features. None of these built-in options are intended to replace commercially available full-function screen magnifiers. The mouse pointer settings under the Windows "Mouse" control panel provide for changing the size, style, and color combination of all the pointers used during GUI interaction.

There are many screen magnification programs available for use with Windows (see www.microsoft.com/enable/ and click the "Products" tab) or Macintosh (see www.apple.com/accessibility/macosx/ and select "OS X solutions from third parties") operating systems.* These software programs offer wider ranges of magnification and have more features than built-in screen magnifiers. These programs generally offer access to Windows™ applications including spreadsheet and word processing, e-mail, and Internet browsers. Many can also run with a screen reader (speech output utility). In some cases the screen reader is bundled with the magnification software, and in other cases the screen magnifier speech output runs in conjunction with a separate screen reader. Magnification of up to 36 times or more is available. The various screen modes described above are available in most screen magnification software. These programs also allow tracking of the mouse pointer, location of keyboard entry, and text editing. The magnification window can be coupled with one or more of these to facilitate navigation for the user. All screen images (including windows, control buttons, and other window objects) are magnified. Automatic scrolling of the screen (left, right, up, down) is also available to make it easier to read long documents when they are magnified.

TABLE 8-3 Simple Adaptations for Visual Impairment*

Need Addressed	Software Approach**
User cannot see standard size text or graphics	Magnifier (M) Zoom (A)
User cannot see status of open windows, dialog boxes, etc.	Audio Description (M) ToggleKeys (M) Talking Alerts (A)
User requires greater contrast between foreground and background or greater size of characters on the screen	Magnifier or High Contrast color scheme (M) Zoom or High Contrast color scheme (A)
User requires speech output rather than visual output	Narrator (M) Voice Over (A)

*Software modifications developed at the Trace Center, University of Wisconsin, Madison. These are included as before-market modifications to Microsoft Windows and Apple OS X and iOS X operating systems, as well as some smart phones.
**M = Microsoft Windows, A = Apple OS X or iOS X.

CASE STUDY – COMPUTER ACCESS FOR LOW VISION

Cheryl is a college student. Her visual limitations prevent her from using the standard computer display. She has asked you to help her find a way for her to use the computer. The constraints on her situation are that she must use several different computers during the day: her own home computer, a laptop that she carries to class for note taking, and the computers in the student lab. What approach would you recommend for her? Would you recommend that she buy special hardware or software to meet her needs, or can she make use of features built into Windows? How would you evaluate the success of your solution for Cheryl?

Access to Computer Output for Individuals Who Are Blind

Individuals who are blind and want to access a computer will need to have an alternative to the video screen. The two primary options are to present information as either speech or Braille. Systems that provide speech or Braille output for blind users are called **screen readers**. A computer user who is blind should be able to access all the same graphics and text as a person who is sighted. Windows™ includes a basic function screen reader utility called *Narrator*† (see Table 8-3) that reads text that is

* For example, SuperNova from Dolphin, Computer Access, San Mateo, Calif. (http://www.yourdolphin.com/); MAGic from Freedom Scientific, St. Petersburg, Fla. (www.freedomsci.com); VIP and ezVIP from JBliss Imaging Systems, San Jose, Calif. (www.jbliss.com); Zoom Text, Zoom Text Express from AI Squared, Manchester Center, Vt. (www.aisquared.com); Galileo, Baum, Germany (www.baum.de/)
† www.microsoft.com/enable/

displayed on the screen. Audio description provides a speech description of videos played in Windows. *Toggle Keys* (see Table 8-3) generate a sound when the CAPS LOCK, NUM LOCK, or SCROLL LOCK key is pressed. The Apple Macintosh OS X operating system includes Voice Over.* This utility provides voice description of the screen as well as reading text. It also includes plug-and-play capability for many Braille displays. Talking Alerts automatically speak the contents of dialogs and alerts similarly to Toggle Keys.

A sighted computer user will often scan a screen for a specific piece of information or specific screen attributes (such as highlighted or underlined material or specific icons). For the user who is blind, duplicating this capability requires that the adapted output system include reading of text and descriptions of graphics. Screen readers also provide on-screen messages or prompts when the user is required to provide input during program operation. Graphic characters have text labels attached to them that can be read to the consumer.

Screen reader programs provide on-screen navigation assistance using keyboard commands. Examples of typical functions are movement to a particular point in the text, finding the mouse cursor position, providing a spoken description of an on-screen graphic or a special function key, and accessing help information.† Screen readers automatically read pop-up windows and dialog boxes to the user.[20] Options include speaking text in a document by line, sentence, or paragraph. Other features are also available; for example, Jaws for Windows‡ allows the user to read the prior, current, or next sentence or paragraph in all applications by using specified keystrokes (e.g., read prior sentence = ALT + UP ARROW; read next sentence = ALT + DOWN ARROW; read current sentence = ALT + NUM PAD). The user may use the standard Windows method of switching between applications (ALT + TAB). There are many other key combinations used in Jaws for navigating through text, tables, Web pages, and other documents. There are also special functions for individual programs such as those in Microsoft Office,§ Web browsers, and others.

All screen readers provide navigation; however, their specific keys and ways of organizing the functions vary. Some screen readers also provide a "window list" in which applications that are running appear in alphabetical order. This allows the user to switch between, close, or see the status of any active applications. This is a faster way to switch between applications when a user has many windows open, rather than moving the cursor to a pull-down menu or "close" box. SuperNova* is a screen reader designed to operate with the visible information on the screen. SuperNova recognizes objects by looking for distinct attributes, shapes, borders, highlights, etc. This is in contrast to using the standard labels of Windows, and it means that SuperNova is independent of whether an application has obeyed the rules of Windows programming. SuperNova recognizes objects by their final shape on the screen, rather than their Windows attributes. The advantage of this approach is that once set up for one application, all similar-looking applications will talk correctly without any adjustment to the settings. Most screen readers include a Braille output mode that interfaces to many different refreshable Braille displays via a USB port. These are only examples of product features; as is true for any computer application, rapid advances are common.

Many screen readers have applications for specific types of programs, procedures, or applications. Examples include SuperNova,† JAWS for Windows,‡ and Window Eyes.§ These applications, called **scripts**, are small computer programs that contain sequences of individual steps used to activate and control a wide variety of computer applications. Scripts are used to make screen readers and screen magnifiers work well with specific programs. The script runs when a user loads a document and provides a way for an application to be customized for a particular user. Each script or function contains commands that tell the screen reader how to navigate and what to read under different conditions. An example of a customization for a person with low vision might include the color combinations for the best contrast, font size, and overall spacing of elements. These features will be automatically loaded any time the application program is loaded. Scripts are used for software applications such as e-mail, Web browsing, word processing, and other applications. Screen readers generally allow modification of scripts and provide development tools for scripts used to make any application accessible with the screen reader. By analyzing what actions are taking place in a given application, the script can optimize the screen reader for the intended use. Scripts require access to a proprietary scripting language that varies by the screen reader/magnifier manufacturer. For computer users who are familiar with Braille, refreshable Braille displays can be more effective than screen readers. However, a combination of approaches may be most effective with Braille and speech combined.

* www.apple.com/accessibility/

† For example, Jaws for Windows from Freedom Scientific, St. Petersburg, Fla. (www.freedomsci.com); Zoom Text Magnifier/Reader from AI Squared, Manchester Center, Vt. (www.aisquared.com); Supernova ScreenReader from Dolphin Computer Access, San Mateo, Calif. (www.yourdolphin.com); Magnum and Magnum Deluxe from Artic Technologies, Troy, Mich.; Protalk32 for Windows; Window Eyes from GW Microsystems, Fort Wayne, Ind. (www.gwmicro.com)

‡ Freedom Scientific, St. Petersburg, Fla. (www.freedomsci.com)

§ Microsoft Corporation, Seattle, Wash. (www.microsoft.com/)

* Dolphin Computer Access, San Mateo, Calif. (www.yourdolphin.com/)

† Dolphin Computer Access, San Mateo, Calif. (www.yourdolphin.com/)

‡ For Example: JAWS, Freedom Scientific, St. Petersburg, Fla. (www.freedomsci.com)

§ GW Microsystems, Fort Wayne, Ind. (www.gwmicro.com)

The hardware and software designed for Braille can be used together with that developed for screen reading using speech synthesis.

Printed Braille output is produced by *embossers*. Embossers are available in both single sided and double sided formats.* The Viewplus Braille Embosser Series† are embossers that print in different paper weights at high speeds for use in production. The Mountbatten Brailler‡ is a Braille writer with a Braille keyboard, built-in memory, auto-correction features, and extensive formatting controls. The Mountbatten can be used as an embosser for a computer or as a Braille translation device. It can translate from print into Braille or Braille into print and is available in both AC and battery-operated models. All these embossers include internal software that accepts standard printer output from the host computer and converts it to either six- or eight-cell Braille embossed on heavy paper. American Thermoform Corporation§ makes a variety of Braille embossers. These cover applications from mass production to systems for individual users.

Braille translation programs are available from Duxbury Systems.|| These programs convert computer data (word processor text files, spreadsheets, or database files) to Grade 2 Braille in hard copy form for either Macintosh OS X or Windows operating systems. Duxbury Braille Translation provides translation and formatting capabilities to automate the process of conversion from regular print to Braille (and vice versa) and also provides word processing functions for working directly in Braille or print format. Braille characters can be displayed on the screen for proofreading before printing. This software is typically used both by individuals who do not know Braille and those who do. The Duxbury Braille Translator allows the user to create Braille for schoolbooks and teaching materials, office memos, bus schedules, personal letters, and signs. The software allows importing of files from popular word processors and other sources.

VISUAL ACCESS TO THE INTERNET

More multimedia representations involving complex graphics, animation, and audible sources of information are being included in Internet websites. This makes it difficult for people who are blind. Individuals who have learning disabilities and dyslexia also find it increasingly difficult to access complicated websites that may include flashing pictures, complicated charts, and large amounts of audio and video data. The challenges faced by these populations are discussed in Chapter 10. It is estimated that as many as 40 million persons in the United States have physical, cognitive, or sensory disabilities.[20] Thus it is important to make the Internet accessible for all.

Making the computer accessible using the input and output methods discussed in this chapter helps persons who have disabilities. Two useful sources of information regarding Internet access for people with disabilities are the World Wide Web Consortium Web Accessibility Initiative (W3C WAI; www.w3.org) and the Trace Center (www.trace.wisc.edu/world/web). The W3C consortium has provided guidelines for web content accessibility at www.w3.org/WAI/WCAG20/quickref/.

User Agents for Access to the Internet

A **user agent** is defined as software that is used to access Web content (www.w3.org/wai). This includes desktop graphical browsers, text and voice browsers, mobile phones, multimedia players, and software assistive technologies (e.g., screen readers, magnifiers, and keyboard emulators) that are used with browsers. Input devices that are used for Internet access include many of those described earlier in this chapter and in Chapter 7. Mouse and mouse-alternative pointing devices, head wands, keyboards and keyboard alternatives such as on-screen keyboards, Braille input keyboards, switches and switch arrays, and microphones can all serve as input devices for user agents. Output devices for Internet access are also those described in this chapter (e.g., screen readers, screen magnifiers, Braille displays, and speech synthesizers).

The W3C WAI project provides practical solutions for the development of accessible user agents based on existing and emerging technologies. The most useful commercial products maximize compatibility between graphical desktop browsers and dependent assistive technologies (e.g., screen readers, screen magnifiers, Braille displays, and voice input software). These developments will also benefit those who access the Internet through palmtop computers, telephones, and pad computers. Users may also have difficulty reading or comprehending text. Users who have low vision or blindness will require adaptations for computer access and user agents need to be accessible.

The W3C WAI user agent guidelines are based on several principles.* The first is to ensure that the user interface is accessible to a consumer using an adapted input system in the same way that it is accessible to a nondisabled person using standard keyboard, mouse, and video display. Second, the user must be able to control the style (e.g., colors, fonts, speech rate, and speech volume) and format of a document. Many of the screen magnifier approaches described earlier in this chapter (e.g., easy scrolling, and viewing windows that follow changes) help make access to content easier. When

* Enabling Technologies, Jenson Beach, Fla. (http://www.Brailler.com/index.htm); Pulse Data HumanWare, Concord, Calif. (http://www.pulsedata.com); GW Microsystems, Fort Wayne, Ind. (https://www.gwmicro.com/); View Plus, Corvallis, Ore. (http://www.viewplus.com)

† Pulse Data HumanWare, Concord, Calif. (http://www.pulsedata.com)

‡ Quantum Technology, Sydney, AU. (http://www.mountbattenbrailler.com/)

§ La Verne, Calif. (http://www.americanthermoform.com/index.html)

|| Westbury, Mass. (http://www.duxburysystems.com/)

* W3C WAI Web page (www.w3.org/wai)

using a screen reader or magnifier, a challenge for the user is to know where they are on a website or a linked website, if that is needed. We typically have this information visually, but when using speech or Braille or a magnified screen it is often hard to keep track of links on a Web site or to follow links to similar Web sites. Thus, a third principle for user agents is to help orient the user to where he is in the document or series of documents. This function can be accomplished by showing how many links the document contains and the number of the current link or other numerical position information that allows the user to jump to a specific link.

Web Browsers

Web browsers incorporate accessibility features to varying degrees. The W3C initiative describes standards for browsers at www.w3.org/standards/agents/browsers. There are many features of browsers that are independent of the operating system. Thus the accessibility of browsers varies. Cascading style sheets (CSS) allow a Web page to be viewed in any layout chosen by the user.[20] Style sheet layouts that are compatible with screen magnifiers, screen readers, and Braille are available. One example of an HTML accessibility standard is the alt = "text" HTML attribute. This function associates text with each graphic object. By pressing the ALT key on the keyboard, the text associated with the object is displayed. This can also be linked to a screen reader or Braille output device.

Microsoft Internet Explorer* contains a range of features for people with disabilities. These include keyboard navigation (among links, frames, and client-side image maps), optional display of text descriptions with images, multiple font sizes and styles, and an optional disabling of style sheets so that the user's font, color, and size settings (their personal style sheet) will be used. This allows turning sounds, videos, pictures, and backgrounds off or on. Tool bar button size and icon size, and text color, font, and size are all adjustable. Automatic fill-in of user names, passwords, web addresses, and routine forms is also included. Internet Explorer also uses the High Contrast function to increase legibility and incorporates Microsoft Active Accessibility to provide information about the document. Internet Explorer is compatible with most screen readers and magnifiers.

Safari† is a browser included with the Macintosh OS X operating system. It is also available for Windows and the mobile iPod Touch, iPhone, and iPad. Safari has features for accessible Web browsing. For example, the user can click on a box to prevent text from being displayed in a size smaller than the setting for the screen. There are also special features that aid in navigation of a webpage. Additional special accessibility features can be added using cascading style sheets (CSS) accessed through a pop-up menu. CCS-based adjustments to a Web page include color, font size, number of columns, and other ways of modifying the way Web pages are displayed.

Many individuals who have low vision or blindness are also seniors. They may not have had experience with computers and they may not be comfortable with the many features that are available on many screen readers/screen magnifiers. To meet the need for this population to have access to computer programs such as e-mail or Web browsing, Dolphin has developed the Dolphin Guide.* This program is based on a simple menu-driven user interface that makes it easier for a partially sighted person to access the computer. All commands and screen elements are available in both speech and enlarged text formats. Voice recognition (see Chapter 7) can also be used for input, creating a completely hands-free environment.

Evaluating Web Sites for Accessibility

There are a number of different approaches to the evaluation of a Web site to determine how accessible it is. The W3C initiative is a good source of information regarding how to determine if a Web site is accessible, where to find tools to aid in the determination of accessibility, an outline of a general procedure for evaluation, and tips for making accessible Web sites (http://www.w3.org/standards/webdesign/). Evaluation of accessibility varies for different disabilities and for different situations, such as development of a Web site versus on-going use. The W3C Web site also describes the pros and cons of using Web evaluation tools (www.w3.org/WAI/eval/). The main advantage of evaluation tools is the saving in time and effort. However, these tools do not replace human judgment, which may require manual testing of the Web site. Finally, the W3C Web site also lists considerations that are important to the selection of a Web evaluation tool.

MOBILITY AND ORIENTATION AIDS FOR PERSONS WITH VISUAL IMPAIRMENTS

For individuals who have low vision or blindness, mobility and orientation are major challenges. The blind traveler uses many methods to orient herself to the environment and move safely.[2] Attention to sensory inputs of smell, sound, air currents, and surface texture alert the blind person to the terrain and environment and helps her pick up cues regarding objects. Sound cues are derived from reflections, sound shadows, and echo location. Temperature changes are also important. For example, passing a window on a cold day or passing under a canopy on a warm day provides information that is used in orientation. Odors from restaurants and crowds and other strong smells also provide information. Input regarding the texture of a sidewalk or grass is provided by the kinesthetic sense. Travel

* Microsoft: Seattle, Wash.(www.microsoft.com/enable/)
† www.apple.com/safari

* www.yourdolphin.com/productdetail.asp?pg=1&id=30

aids are also used by some individuals. A variety of these aids are discussed in this section.

Mobility Aids Compared to Reading Aids

The requirements of devices that aid mobility for persons with low vision differ significantly from those for reading. There are several important differences between sensory input for reading and that for mobility.[23] Inaccuracies in reading results in loss of information, but errors in **orientation and mobility** can result in injury or embarrassment. **Reading aids** always sense information in a text or graphics form. Although there are differences in text fonts and reading needs, the differences across all reading materials are relatively small. Alternatively, the blind traveler needs to avoid obstacles as varied as a roller skate and a tree. The range of possible objects to be detected is large and dynamic. The environment changes frequently (e.g., a chair is moved to a new location or a parked car starts moving), and the blind person must be able to sense these differences. The obstacles of most concern to blind travelers are bicycles, streets, posts, toys, ladders, scaffolding, overhanging branches, and awnings.[2] **Mobility aids** for blind persons must accommodate for these large variations in the objects to be detected. *Orientation* refers to the "knowledge of one's location in relation to the environment."[30] There are five approaches used to aid blind travel: a sighted guide, guide dogs, the long cane, electronic aids for obstacle detection, and orientation and navigation systems. The last three are discussed in this section.

Long Canes

The most common mobility aid for persons with visual impairments is the long cane.[8] The standard cane consists of three parts: the grip, the shaft, and the tip. The entire cane is designed to maximize tactile and auditory input from the environment. The grip (which forms the handle) is made of leather, plastic, rubber, or other materials that easily transmit the tactile information to the user's hand. The shaft and tip work together to sense and then relay the tactile information to the grip. The tip (especially a metal tip being used on a hard surface such as concrete) is a major source of high-frequency auditory input used by pedestrians who are blind in order to detect obstacles and landmarks by echolocation (i.e., the reflection of sound from a near object is different in pitch than from a far object, likewise for a small [chair] or large [tree] object). A careful balance is obtained between sufficient rigidity to resist wind and bending and adequate flexibility to transmit the tactile and auditory sense of the surface texture. The advantages and limitations of the long cane are shown in Table 8-4. It takes between 6 and 12 weeks to develop proficiency in using a long cane.[26]

Many blind travelers use folding or telescoping canes, which offer the advantage of easy storage when not in use. Typically these are made of composite materials such as carbon fiber. When collapsed they can be placed in a pocket or purse.

TABLE 8-4 Pros and Cons of the Long Cane

Advantages	Limitations
Low cost	Only detects obstacles one step in front of the user.
Simplicity of use	Doesn't sense objects above waist level (e.g., the cane may pass between table legs, under the tabletop).
Well-developed training programs	Doesn't sense head-height obstacles such as tree branches.

Electronic Travel Aids for Obstacle Detection and Orientation

Roentgen et al (2008)[28] identified 12 devices designed specifically for obstacle detection and orientation. Often called **electronic travel aids (ETAs)**, these devices have been developed to overcome some of the limitations of the long cane. These aids supplement rather than replace the long cane and guide dog. Some of these aids add features to the long cane to increase the range or types of obstacles detected. Others are used with the long cane or guide dog to overcome limitations. ETAs also provide information not available from the cane such as the presence of more distant objects or the presence of overhangs. This information can assist with orientation for pedestrians who are blind.[30]

ETAs have the three components shown in Figure 8-1: an environmental interface, an information processor, and a user display. The **environmental interface** is typically both an invisible light source and a receiver (usually in the infrared range) or an ultrasonic transmitter and receiver. Both these technologies are similar to those used in television remote controls. The information processor may be a special-purpose electronic circuit or a microcomputer-based device. The user display may be either an auditory tone of varying frequency (e.g., higher as an object gets closer) or a haptic interface (pins that vibrate faster as an object is closer). Examples of the major types of ETAs are described in this section. A more complete listing of options can be found in Roentgen et al.[28]

Electronically Augmented Canes

Over the years several alternatives have been developed to extend the range of the standard cane and add the capability of detecting overhangs and/or sensing of drop-offs. Figure 8-12, *A*, illustrates the principle of operation of electronically augmented canes. From one to three narrow beams of laser light or high frequency sound (ultrasound) are projected from the cane. Commercial products have one, two, or three beams. One beam is directed upward, and it detects obstacles at head height. If an object is in the path of the beam, there is a reflection back to a receiver. This input generates either an auditory or tactile (through vibrating pins

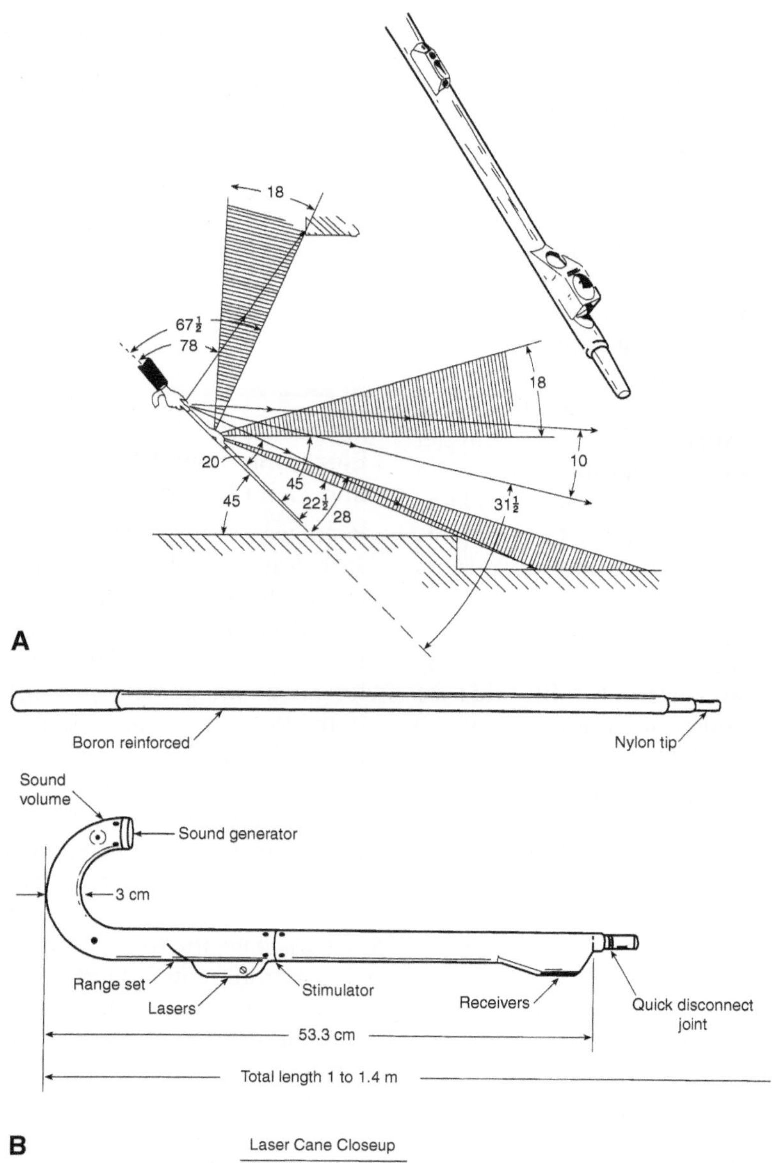

Figure 8-12 The laser cane. **A,** The triangulation method employed. **B,** The major components. (From Nye PW, Bliss JC: Sensory aids for the blind: a challenging problem with lessons for the future, *Proc IEEE* 58:1878–1879, 1970.)

in the handle) signal to the user. Another beam detects objects directly in front of the traveler. If an object is encountered in this beam, the reflected signal causes a different auditory or tactile signal to be sent to the user. The final beam is aimed downward, and it is intended to detect drop-offs (e.g., stairs or curbs) located in front of the cane tip. If the reflected beam is interrupted (because the drop-off does not reflect light back in the same way as a level surface), then a signal is sent to the user. For tactile response, the pins are located in the handle of the cane, where the fingers can comfortably rest on them (Figure 8-12, *B*). Auditory feedback is usually a tone that rises as objects get closer. In some cases different frequency tones will be used for different beams (e.g., a low tone from the drop-off sensor, a higher tone from the overhang sensor). The auditory and vibrating tactile inputs supplement the haptic input from the tapping of the cane on the ground transmitted up the shaft of the cane during normal use.

A current ETA based on the cane is the UltraCane,* which uses ultrasound. The UltraCane, shown in Figure 8-13, provides all the information normally obtained from the long cane and adds two ultrasound beams and sensors. One detects objects directly in front and one detects objects at head height. The ultrasound beam avoids the problems of transparent glass experienced by the laser cane since the ultrasound beam is reflected from glass or shiny surfaces without distortion. The user display (Figure 8-13, *B*) provides tactile feedback with three vibrating pins, located on each side and the middle, to indicate where the detected object is located. The intensity of the vibration indicates how close the object is. The UltraCane is collapsible and lightweight and is used in the same way as the standard long cane. The user sweeps the cane in an arc in front of her as she

* Sound Foresight LTD, Barnsley, UK (www.ultracane.com)

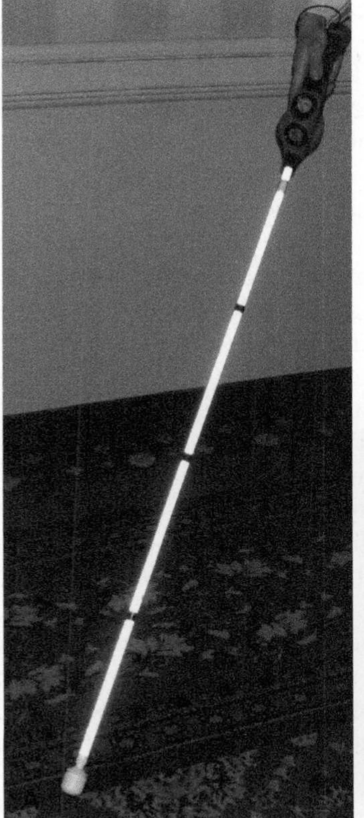

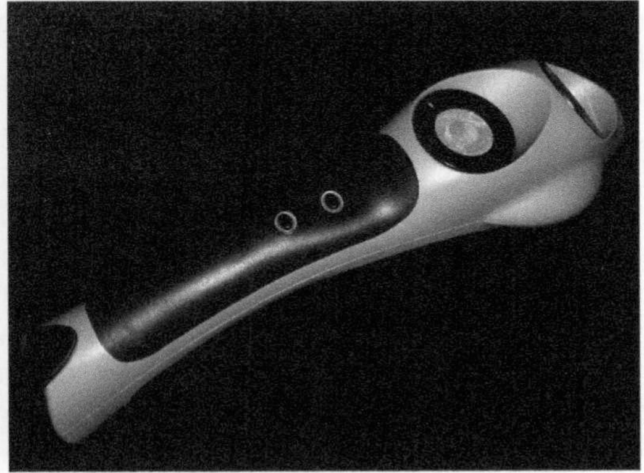

Figure 8-13 **A,** The UltraCane provides all the information normally obtained from the long cane. **B,** Two ultrasound beams and sensors are built into the handle.

walks. Although it is not quite as responsive as a standard long cane, primarily because of the added electronics in the handle, the laser cane can also provide conventional tactile and auditory information. One major advantage of the UltraCane is that it is fail-safe; if the batteries run down or an electronic failure occurs, the cane can be used like a standard long cane.

Augmented canes such as the laser cane or UltraCane can be used during mobility training, helping the trainee understand how to hold the cane correctly and move it in the correct arc.[24] After the training is completed, the trainee can choose either to use the standard cane or to continue with the electronically augmented cane.

The most significant disadvantage to augmented canes is the cost/benefit ratio. These devices are up to 8 times more expensive than the long cane, and each individual user must decide how important the additional information received from an augmented cane is to his work, lifestyle, or safety. There are a variety of specially designed augmented canes and devices that attach to the standard long cane.[28]

Hand-Held and Body-Mounted Obstacle Detection and Orientation Devices

Another approach to obstacle detection is the use of hand-held sensors that are used alone or with the cane. One example, the Miniguide,* is about the size of a rectangular flashlight and weighs less than 50 grams (about 2 ounces).[15] It has an ultrasound transmitter and receiver that emit and receive ultrasound pulses in an elliptical pattern. When an object is detected in the ultrasound beam, the device begins to vibrate gently in the hand. The vibrations become faster for objects that are closer. The typical use of the Miniguide is to scan the environment to locate specific familiar landmarks (e.g., a bus stop sign) or clear spaces such as doorways. It is small enough to be carried easily in a pocket or purse, and it is generally used to supplement other mobility and orientation devices. If two hands are used, it can detect overhangs with simultaneous use of the long cane. The Miniguide can be used when reaching and touching may be dangerous or undesirable, such as in a machine shop or hospital. It can also be placed on the floor and slowly rotated to find an object that has fallen. Finally, it can be placed on a desk used by a blind receptionist to indicate when someone is standing in front of the desk. The simplicity and relatively low cost of hand-held devices such as the Miniguide make them functional as supplements to other orientation and mobility devices.

Some devices are worn on the body and are used to supplement the long cane by detecting objects further away than the cane can reach or obstacles that are located above. An ultrasound transmitter and sensor are used for object detection. Feedback to the user is generally either vibrating pins or auditory signals as either speech (e.g., "stop" when an object is too close) or rising tone pitch as an object is getting closer. One example is the Ultra

* GDP Research, Adelaide, South Australia (http://www.gdp-research.com.au/index.html); available in North America from Sendros, Davis, Calif. (www.senderogroup.com/index.htm)

Body Guard.* This device can be held in the hand or mounted to the chest. A detected obstacle causes a vibration on the hand or the neck (depending on where the device is worn). This device also allows the user to store common routes and it then guides the individual along the known route.

Navigation Aids for the Blind

The electronic travel aids for obstacle avoidance do not address orientation that keeps an individual apprised of location and heading. In order to be effective a navigation system should: (1) keep track of the user's current location and heading as he moves through the environment, (2) find the way around and through a variety of environments, (3) successfully find and follow an optimally safe walking path to the destination, and (4) provide information about the salient features of the environment.[35] The major approach for descriptive information in navigation aids is synthetic or recorded speech cues and environmental descriptions. It is important that the presentation of auditory information not interfere with natural environmental cues (e.g., sounds of traffic, water, etc.).

User Preferences for GPS Systems

The satellite-based global positioning system (GPS) provides precise information regarding features, terrain, vehicles, or buildings that is ideally suited for use in navigation systems for persons who are blind. Golledge et al (2004)[13] conducted a survey of blind individuals to determine their preferences for the development of GPS-based navigation aids. The most common problems reported were dealing with street crossings, avoiding unknown obstacle hazards, learning new routes, and taking shortcuts. Difficulty in gaining access to navigational information was identified in several areas, including knowing and keeping track of the direction to walk to a destination, knowing which way the person was facing, knowing that they were at a street corner, where to turn, and location of specific landmarks such as stores and bus stops. The type of needed navigational information identified (in priority order) was information about: landmarks, streets, routes, destination buildings, and transit. All participants identified automatic speech recognition (see Chapter 7) as the most desirable form of input to the device. Other highly rated input choices were a QWERTY keyboard, Braille keyboard, and telephone keyboard. The most acceptable output device for providing navigational information to the user was a collar or shoulder-mounted speech or sound device. Based on the loss of ambient auditory information when using headphones, this mode was the least acceptable. The Wayfinding Group is collaborating on the development of GPS-based devices (www.senderogroup.com/wayfinding/).

GPS-Based Mobility Aids

There are three approaches used for GPS-based systems for the blind traveler: (1) stored digital maps or databases of locations, street names, and postal codes; (2) the use of databases only; and (3) systems that have no maps or databases and instead rely on the user generating their own route.[28] If using the first type of device, routes can be planned and information about the user's current location and points of interest in their environment are included. The second type uses only a database with checkpoints along a route to guide the blind traveler. For the third type of device the user must store a series of announcements (e.g., street names, waypoints, and individual points of interest with voice descriptions) that are used as landmarks during travel. All of the GPS-based systems are intended to be used in conjunction with other mobility aids such as a guide dog, cane, or ETA. Examples of each of these categories of navigation aids are described in this section.

One approach uses the PAC Mate Omni as a platform for the StreetTalk VIP software* combined with a GPS receiver resulting in a navigation aid with either Braille or speech output for the user. The database contains millions of points of interest such as restaurants, banks, and parks. Maps can be purchased for specific regions on flash cards that are inserted into the PAC Mate Omni. Routes that are repeated can be saved to aid in travel. The routes can be printed on embossed paper, uploaded and saved, or emailed to other users.

GPS LookAround† is a talking map that can be loaded on an iPhone. In operation, a shake of the iPhone will display the current heading, street, city, cross street, and nearest point of interest (POI). The POI information is based on the selection of a category from a database of points of interest that includes street names and other points of interest such as bus stops, favorite restaurants, frequently visited shops, friends' houses, public buildings, landmarks, and museums. At the press of a button a "Where am I?" feature is activated and the LookAround tells the user the current location. Another feature tells the user what points of interest are in the immediate vicinity.

The Trekker‡ is a palm-sized GPS device that includes digital maps and a points-of-interest database. Trekker provides information via speech and allows users to record both vocal and written notes. A wide variety of maps from Navteq are available that cover most Western countries. Maps can be downloaded from the Internet or obtained on CD or Compact Flash™ cards. Navteq§ creates and maintains a database containing all street names and ranges of addresses for urban areas, as well as over 1,500,000 points of interest both in North America and Europe. Trekker can be combined with the functions of

* RTB GmbH & Co. KG (http://www.rtb-bl.de/RTB/ultra-body-guard-2/?lang=en)

* www.freedomsci.com/

† Sendros, Davis, Calif. (www.senderogroup.com/index.htm)

‡ HumanWare, Concord, Calif. (http://www.humanware.ca/)

§ http://www.navteq.com/

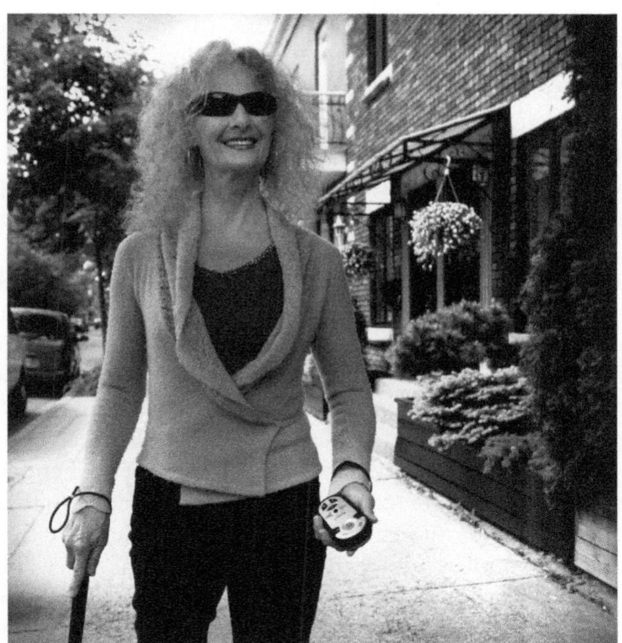

Figure 8-14 The Trekker Breeze is a handheld GPS system. (Courtesy of HumanWare.)

a PDA: agenda, text notes, voice notes, address book, DAISY reader (Victor Pocket Reader), media player, e-mail manager, Web browser, calculator, and clock and alarms in the Maestro system.

Trekker Breeze, Figure 8-14, is a simplified and less-expensive GPS navigation aid. Trekker Breeze can be controlled by one hand and it verbally announces names of streets, intersections, and landmarks during travel. When a single button is pressed, Breeze speaks the current location. When used in a vehicle, Trekker Breeze speaks the names of intersections. Breeze also provides locations and points of interest in the immediate vicinity of the user. It also records the path for a journey and allows it to be played back to repeat the path. Breeze can be used to record a path while guided by a sighted person and then play it back for independent travel at a later time.

The BrailleNote GPS* is a cell phone–size GPS receiver that is an accessory to portable Braille or voice note takers. It relays information from GPS satellites that can be used by the portable note taker to calculate where the user is and to plot a route to a destination of choice. The BrailleNote GPS includes Global Positioning System software with maps and hundreds of points of interest. The user can calculate the distance and direction to a street address or intersection, find out the relative location of points of interest, automatically create routes for either walking or riding in a vehicle, and provide detailed information about speed and the direction of travel.

The simplest devices for assisting with orientation are adapted compasses. The Braille compass has the major north, south, east, and west directions labeled in Braille and the intermediate points labeled with raised dots. The face opens, much like a Braille watch, so that the direction can be felt. The C2 Talking Compass* (Figure 8-15) uses spoken output to help orient the user. The user points the compass in one direction and presses a button. The compass then speaks the direction as north, east, south, west, or intermediate directions (e.g., northwest). The compass can be purchased with two languages installed, and 20 languages are currently available.

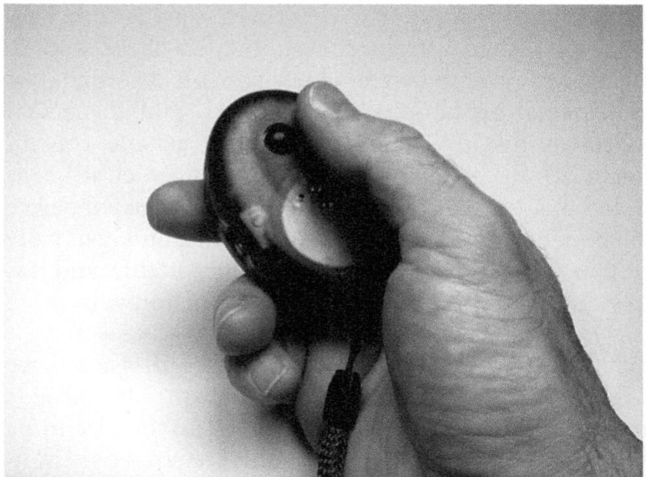

Figure 8-15 The C2 Talking Compass. (Courtesy of Radixon Group, Victoria, Australia.)

Navigation Aids Based on Environmental Adaptations

Another aid for travelers who are blind is Talking Signs.† Street signs and building signs provide a significant amount of our orientation as sighted travelers. Individuals who are blind or who have trouble reading require that same information in order to maintain their orientation as they travel. The Talking Signs voice message originates at the sign and is transmitted by infrared light to a handheld receiver at a distance. Because of the nature of infrared transmission, the transmission is directionally selective. When the user aims the receiver directly at the sign, the intensity and clarity of the message increases. This change allows the user to focus the Talking Signs system and orient herself to her actual location. In order to operate, Talking Signs transmitters must be installed as adjuncts to all signs. This is a large task, but many have already been installed. Talking Signs can also be used to label objects such as building entrances, drinking fountains, phone booths, or rest rooms.[30]

User Preferences for Sensory Aids for Mobility

There have been a number of studies that have evaluated the effectiveness of ETAs and the perception of their value by persons with visual impairments. Jutai et al (2009)[16]

* HumanWare, Concord, Calif. (http://www.humanware.ca/)

* Sensory Tools division of Robotron Group (www.sensorytools.com/c2.htm)

†Talking Signs, Inc., Baton Rouge, La. (www.talkingsigns.com)

and Roentgen et al (2008)[28] conducted systematic reviews of the published literature to summarize these studies. The studies reviewed were widely variable in number of participants, methodologies employed, and the actual devices evaluated. These factors make general conclusions difficult to obtain. However, Roentgen et al[28] concluded that in most of the studies, users evaluated device functionality as being beneficial. Participants generally felt that their travel was safer, more comfortable, and less stressful when ETAs were used in conjunction with more traditional mobility aids (e.g., guide dogs or canes).

Different types of technologies that aid vision have different levels of perceived effectiveness.[16] Optical aids are perceived as both effective and accessible. Electronic magnifiers (e.g., CCTV) are generally preferred over nonelectronic devices, but cost is a major factor in accessibility of these technologies. There is some evidence that visual aids for computer access are important for individuals who have low vision. Training of both the user and family and care givers in the use of aids can make a large difference in the eventual effectiveness of the sensory aid.

SPECIAL-PURPOSE VISUAL AIDS

In developing the HAAT model in Chapter 2, we defined three performance areas as part of the human component: self-care, work and school, and play and leisure. Persons with blindness or low vision may have needs in each of these areas, and there are special-purpose devices that can provide assistance. These devices are in addition to those serving needs for reading and orientation/mobility, which are used in all three performance areas. In this section we describe some of the special-purpose devices that serve these needs. The American Foundation for the Blind* (AFB), Sensory Access Foundation,† Smith-Kettlewell Eye Research Institute, Rehabilitation Engineering Center,‡ and New York Lighthouse, Inc.,§ are good sources of information regarding specific needs. Several companies sell large numbers of products for all three performance areas.‖

Devices for Self-Care

Auditory or tactile substitutes can be used for many household tasks. The American Foundation for the Blind¶ Web site lists almost 200 devices for use in household tasks, self-care, and independent living. For example, Braille tape (similar to the tape used for labeling, with raised letters) can be used to label canned foods and appliance controls. Another approach to identification of household objects is the use of bar codes and recorded speech.[6] Bar codes are typically used in supermarkets for checkout scanning. However, the codes used are stored in the grocery store computer, so they can't be read at home. Crabb[6] developed a device called the I.D. Mate* that allows a sighted individual to sweep a reader over the bar code and then record a short spoken message describing the contents (e.g., "Campbell's tomato soup"). This information is then played back to the user who is blind when he scans a similar can at the grocery store. Other household items can also be scanned. Approximately 90% of the items sold in the United States have bar codes on them, including playing cards, cassette tapes, CDs, and many other items.

There are two commercial products that read bar codes. Scan Talker™† is a bar code reading accessory for the PAC Mate™ portable note taker. It has a built-in database that matches the bar code with a wide variety of food and personal care products. The product information is provided to the user via speech. The ScanTalker also provides other information from product labels such as nutritional information and preparation instructions. There over 1.2 million codes stored on a flash card that inserts into the Pac Mate. There are more than 285,000 grocery and pharmaceutical items, more than 90,000 health and beauty aids, more than 530,000 general merchandise items, and more than 320,000 audio and video compact discs in the database. The user can also add items to the database.

The ID Mate Summit‡ is a self-contained device that has a unidirectional bar code reader and hand-held user display that provides product identification and extended information in speech form. Over 1 million items are contained in the ID Mate Summit database. The ID Mate can also be personalized by entering a bar code and recording a corresponding message. This method can be useful for labeling household objects, clothing, and similar personal items.

Voice output is also available on some mainstream appliances, such as microwave ovens, kitchen timers, thermometers, and alarm clocks, and it is available in both auditory and tactile forms. Talking wristwatches are used by individuals who are blind. Electrical appliances may have controls marked with tactile labels to allow a person who is blind to adjust the controls. Raised or enlarged-print telephone dials can also be obtained from local telephone companies. There are also devices that read paper money and speak the denomination of the bill. These are similar to change machines or those used for automatic purchase of public transportation tickets in many cities. A portable paper money reader is shown in Figure 8-16.§ When a paper monetary note of $1 to $100 value is inserted into the device, it automatically turns on and

* New York City (www.afb.org)
† Palo Alto, Calif. (http://www.visionaware.org/)
‡ San Francisco, Calif. (http://www.ski.org/)
§ New York (www.lighthouse.org)
‖ LS&S Group, Northbrook, Ill. (www.Lssgroup.com); Maxi Aids, Farmingdale, N.Y. (www.maxiaids.com); Independent Living Aids, Inc, Plainsview, N.Y. (www.independentliving.com), www.MaxiAids.com,
¶ www.afb.org/ProdBrowseCatResults.asp?CatID=3

* En-Vision America, Normal, Ill. (www.envisionamerica.com)
† Freedom Scientific, St. Petersburg, Fla. (www.freedomsci.com)
‡ Sendros, Davis, Calif. (www.senderogroup.com/index.htm)
§ Note Teller, Brytech, Ottawa, Ontario, Canada (www.brytech.com/)

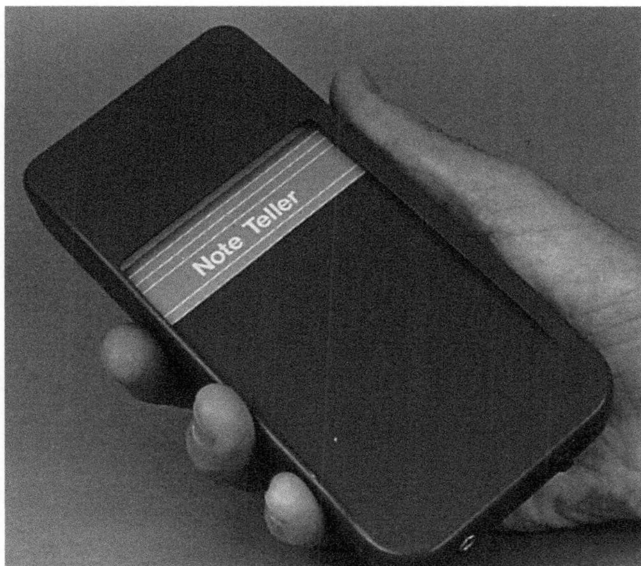

Figure 8-16 The Note Teller paper money reading device. (Courtesy Brytech, Nepean, Ont., Canada.)

speaks the denomination of the note. Both English and Spanish voice outputs are available, and a headphone may be used for privacy. When the note is removed, the unit automatically turns itself off. Versions are available specifically for U.S. and Canadian currencies in addition to a universal model.

The use of tactile labels (e.g., Braille) and speech output have made automatic teller machines (ATMs) useable by both sighted persons and persons with visual impairments. Banking over the Internet is also available for persons who are blind or have low vision. Regulations concerning ATMs are contained in the Americans with Disabilities Act Access Guidelines (ADAAG).* In Ontario, Canada, similar legislation is contained in the Accessibility for Ontarians with Disabilities Act.[1] These guidelines provide performance standards for people with vision impairments. To provide non-visual information from the ATM, Braille instructions and control labels are used. For user feedback during use, audible devices and handsets are recommended to provide access while maintaining privacy. Braille output is not required. Touch-screens with appropriate software and hardware can also be made accessible to persons who are blind. The major provisions of the standards are†: differentiation of each control or operating mechanism by sound or touch, provision of opportunity for input and output privacy, marking of function keys with tactile characters, provision of both visual and audible instructions for operation, dispensing of paper currency (if available) in descending order with the lowest denomination on top, and options to receive a receipt in printed or audible form, or both.

* http://www.access-board.gov/ada-aba/adaag/about/guide.htm#Automated
† Trace Center, University of Wisconsin (trace.wisc.edu)

A leading cause of blindness is diabetes. Insulin injection devices are available that provide independence for blind users, including adapted syringes and holders for bottles. The holder guides the syringe into the bottle, and the syringe can be set to allow only the amount necessary for one dose to be drawn out of the bottle. Other home health care devices include thermometers with speech output and sphygmomanometers (for blood pressure measurement) that use raised dots on the pressure meter face or synthesized speech output. There is also a prescription reader that reads information on "smart labels" with store prescription information provided by pharmacies.*

Devices for Work and School

The major needs within vocational and educational applications are for access to reading, mobility, and computers. The approaches and devices in the sections on reading and mobility in this chapter often meet these needs. In order to be operated as they were designed, many tools require the use of vision. It is possible to use either tactile or auditory adaptations to make these tools available to individuals who have visual impairments. A carpenter's level with a large steel ball and center tab has an adjustment screw on one end. The screw is calibrated with half a degree of tilt corresponding to one turn. To level the device, the carpenter adjusts the screw until the ball is at the center. She then knows how many degrees of tilt there are and can correct for the tilt. There is also a tactile tape measure with one raised dot at each quarter-inch mark, two at half-inch increments, and one large dot at each inch mark. Calipers, protractors, and micrometers use a similar labeling scheme. An audible device is used by machinists to determine depth of cut when using a lathe. There are also talking tape measures, calculators, scales, and thermometers. Many of these also have tactile versions.

Many electronic test instruments use digital (numeric) displays, and these displays are easily interfaced to speech synthesizers. The output of the meter (e.g., a voltage measurement by a technician) is heard instead of read. Oscilloscopes are also available in both auditory and tactile forms. Electronic calculators that have speech output provide an alternative to visual display-based devices. It is possible for a person with total visual impairment to perform virtually all the tasks required for electronic or mechanical design, fabrication, and testing using adapted tools and instruments. The Color Teller† is a handheld device that detects colors, tints and shades such as pink, pale blue-green, dark brown, and vivid yellow. The color is spoken in English, French, or Spanish with adjustable volume. It can also be used to determine whether the lights in a room are on or off.

* Envision America (www.envisionamerica.com/)
† Brytech, Ottawa, Ontario, Canada (www.brytech.com/)

Devices for Play and Leisure

Almost any common board game can be obtained in enlarged form. There are also enlarged and tactually labeled playing cards, and Braille or other versions exist for common board games and dice. Computer games that emphasize text rather than graphics can be used with computer screen–reading software.

More active games include "beeper ball," in which auditory signals replace visual cues. In this softball-like game, the ball contains an electronic oscillator that emits a beeping sound. The batter can aim for the sound. Bases are also labeled with sounds. Similar approaches are available for playing Frisbee, soccer, and football. In each case the object to be thrown or kicked emits a beep and goals are labeled with auditory markers. Individuals who are blind can snow ski with the assistance of both sighted guides and auditory signals from barriers such as slalom poles and fences.

CASE STUDY – CHANGING NEEDS FOR VISUAL AIDS

Ken has enrolled this fall semester as a student at the state college. He has retinitis pigmentosa. Retinitis pigmentosa is a midperipheral ring scotoma that gradually widens with time, so that central vision is frequently reduced by middle age. Night blindness occurs much earlier, and total blindness may eventually ensue. Ken has recently noticed that his vision seems to have deteriorated significantly. He would like to study to become a journalist. Ken lives alone in an apartment close to campus so he can walk to school or, when it is raining, take the bus. As Ken's retinitis pigmentosa advances, what types of assistive technology for sensory impairments might be useful to him in order to enable him to continue with his activities in the following areas: (1) school, (2) home/self-care, and (3) recreation/leisure?

SUMMARY

It is possible to improve performance by increasing size, contrast, and spacing of the material for persons who have low vision. Low-cost magnification aids and filters can help in this regard, but electronic aids provide much greater flexibility. Reading aids for persons who are blind rely on either tactile or auditory substitution. The most effective of these are language based (e.g., speech or Braille). Fully automated reading devices are capable of imaging print documents and converting them to speech using voice synthesis. Accessibility for people with low vision or blindness to mainstream technologies such as computers, smart phones, pad computers, and household appliances is available both as built-in adaptations and as separate products.

Electronic travel aids for persons who are blind serve a useful but limited purpose in aiding mobility and orientation for blind travelers. Just as reading aids use the alternative sensory pathways of auditory and tactile input, so do ETAs. The ETA converts the reflected light or ultrasound information to the audible or tactile display information presented to the user. Current technology provides only limited substitution or augmentation for the long cane. Future developments will most likely be in the extraction of useful features from the visual image for display to the blind traveler. By concentrating on achieving input that is more informative regarding obstacles and the orientation and location of objects in the environment, the utility and reliability of these devices will be greatly enhanced.

STUDY QUESTIONS

1. What are the two basic approaches to sensory aids in terms of the sensory pathway used?
2. List three output modes available for reading machines.
3. What is a GUI? What advantages does it provide for persons with disabilities?
4. What special problems does the GUI present for persons who are blind?
5. What are the three factors that must be considered when accommodating for low vision? How are they normally dealt with in access software?
6. What are optical and non-optical aids for low vision?
7. What are the primary assistive technology approaches to assisting individuals who have visual field problems?
8. Describe the relative advantages and disadvantages of software and hardware approaches to obtaining enlarged displays for persons with visual impairments.
9. What is the primary tactile method used for computer output?
10. What special adaptations are made to Braille specifically for computer output use?
11. What adaptations are made to provide hard copy for users with low vision?
12. What are the major challenges for people with low vision or blindness in using cell phones, including smart phones?
13. What adaptations are made to provide hard copy for users who are blind?
14. Describe the major benefits of computer use reported by individuals who are blind or have low vision.
15. What are the major barriers to computer use reported by individuals who are blind or have low vision?
16. What are the primary challenges in obtaining Web access for persons who have disabilities?
17. What is a Web browser? What features are necessary in a Web browser to ensure that people who have disabilities can use it?
18. List the major features of accessible Web sites. What tools are typically used to test accessibility of Web sites?
19. What are the major differences in the effects of errors in those low vision and blindness devices developed for reading and those developed for mobility?
20. What are the major limitations of the long cane for use as a mobility aid by persons who are blind?
21. What is an electronic travel aid?

22. Pick a tool or measurement instrument and figure out how to adapt it for both a person with low vision and one who is blind.
23. How are GPS systems used to aid people who are blind?
24. Pick one recreational activity and describe the ways that it can be adapted for people with low vision or blindness.

REFERENCES

1. *Accessibility for Ontarians with Disabilities Act, Bill 118, S.O, Chapter 11*, Toronto, ON, 2005, Legislative Assembly of Ontario.
2. American Foundation for the Blind: *How does a blind person get around?* New York, 1978, The Foundation.
3. Bailey RW: *Human performance engineering*, ed 2, Englewood Cliffs, NJ, 1989, Prentice Hall.
4. Blenkhorn P, Evans DG, Baude A: Full-screen magnification for Windows using DirectX Overlays, *IEEE Trans Neural Syst Rehabil Eng* 10(4):225–231, 2002.
5. Boyd LH, Boyd WL, Vanderheiden GC: The graphical user interface crisis: danger and opportunity, *J Vis Impair Blind* 84(10):496–502, 1990.
6. Crabb N: Mastering the code to independence, *Braille Forum* 24–27, 1998.
7. Doherty JE: *Protocols for choosing low vision devices*, Washington, DC, 1993, National Institute on Disability and Rehabilitation Research.
8. Farmer LW, Smith DL: Adaptive technology. In Blasch BB, Wiener RW, Welsh RL, editors: *Foundations of orientation and mobility*, New York, 1997, AFB Press, pp 231–259.
9. Fruchterman JR: In the palm of your hand: a vision of the future of technology for people with visual impairments, *J Vis Impair Blind* 97(10):585–591, 2003.
10. Galloway NR, Amoaku WMK, Galloway PH, et al: *Common eye diseases and their management*, ed 3, London, 2006, Springer-Verlag.
11. Gerber E: The benefits of and barriers to computer use for individuals who are visually impaired, *J Vis Impair Blind* 97(9):536–550, 2003.
12. Gerber E, Kirchner C: Who's surfing? Internet access and computer use by visually impaired youth and adults, J Vis Impair Blind 95(3):176–181, 2001.
13. Golledge RG, Marston JR, Loomis JM, et al: Stated preference for components of a personal guidance system for nonvisual navigation, *J Vis Impair Blind* 98(3):135–147, 2004.
14. Griffin HG, Williams SC, Davis ML, et al: Using technology to enhance cues for children with low vision, *Teaching Exceptional Children* 35(2):36–42, 2002.
15. Hill J, Black J: The Miniguide: a new electronic travel device, *J Vis Impair Blind* 97(10):655–658, 2003.
16. Jutai JW, Strong JG, Rusell-Minda E: Effectiveness of assistive technologies for low vision rehabilitation: a systematic review, *J Vis Impair Blind* 103(4):210–222, 2009.
17. Kane SK, Jayant C, Wobbrock JO, et al: Freedom to roam: A study of mobile device adoption and accessibility for people with visual and motor disabilities. In *ASSETS '09*, Pittsburgh, PA, USA, 2009, pp 115–122.
18. Kerscher G, Hansson K: DAISY Consortium—developing the next generation of digital talking books (DTB). In *Proc CSUN Conf*, 1998. http://www.csun.edu/cod/conf/1998/proceedings/csun98_065.htm.
19. Kirman JH: Tactile communication of speech: a review and analysis, *Psychol Bull* 80(1):54–74, 1973.
20. Lazzaro JJ: Helping the web help the disabled, *IEEE Spectrum* 36(3):54–59, 1999.
21. Lazzaro JJ: *Adaptive Technologies for Learning and Work Environments*, ed 2, Chicago, 2001, American Library Association.
22. Legge GE, Madison CM, Mansfield JS: Measuring Braille reading speed with the MNREAD test, *Vis Impair Res* 1(3):131–145, 1999.
23. Mann RW: Technology and human rehabilitation: prostheses for sensory rehabilitation and/or substitution. In Brown JHU, Dickson JF, editors: *Advances in biomedical engineering*, New York, 1974, Academic Press.
24. Mellor CM: *Aids for the '80s: what they are and what they do*, New York, 1981, American Foundation for the Blind.
25. Ministry of Industry: *Participation and Activity Limitation Survey 2006: Analytical Report*, Ottawa, ON, 2007, Canadian Ministry of Industry.
26. Ramsey VK, Blasch BB, Kita A, et al: A biomechanical evaluation of visually impaired persons' gait and long-cane mechanics, *J Rehabil Res Dev* 36(4):323–332, 1999.
27. Ratanasit D, Moore MM: Representing graphical user interfaces with sound: a review of approaches, *J Vis Impair Blind* 99(2):69–93, 2005.
28. Roentgen UR, Gelderblom GJ, Soede M, et al: Inventory of electronic mobility aids for persons with visual impairments: a literature review, *J Vis Impair Blind* 102(11):702–724, 2008.
29. Sardegna J, Shelly S, Rutzen AR, et al: *The encyclopedia of blindness and vision impairment*, 2002 Facts on File.
30. Scadden LA: Technology and people with visual impairments: a 1997 update, *Technol Disabil* 6(3):137–145, 1997.
31. Servais SP: Visual aids. In Webster JG, et al, editors: *Electronic devices for rehabilitation*, New York, 1985, Wiley and Sons.
32. Smedema SM, McKenzie AR: The relationship among frequency and type of Internet use, perceived social support, and sense of well-being in individuals with visual impairments, *Disabil Rehabil* 32(4):317–325, 2010.
33. Stelmack JA, Rosenbloom AA, Brenneman CS, et al: Patients' perceptions of the need for low vision devices, *J Vis Impair Blind* 97(9):521–535, 2003.
34. Tobias J: Information technology and universal design: an agenda for accessible technology, *J Vis Impair Blind* 97(10):592–601, 2003.
35. Walker BN, Jeffery J: Using virtual environments to prototype auditory navigation displays, *Assist Technol* 17(1):72–81, 2005.
36. Wolffe KE: Wired to work: an analysis of access technology training for people with visual impairments, *J Vis Impair Blind* 97(10):633–645, 2003.
37. Wolffe KE, Candela T, Johnson G: Wired to work: a qualitative analysis of assistive technology training for people with visual impairments, *J Vis Impair Blind* 97(11):677–694, 2003.
38. World Health Organization: *Cumulative Official Updates to ICD-10*, 2010. http://www.who.int/classifications/icd/Official_WHO_updates_combined_1996_2009VOL1.pdf.

CHAPTER 9

Sensory Aids for Persons with Auditory Impairments

LEARNING OBJECTIVES

Upon completing this chapter, you will be able to do the following:

1. Describe the major types of hearing loss and their cause
2. Describe the types of hearing aids and their features
3. Describe how common devices can be adapted for use by a person who is hard of hearing or deaf
4. List ways that people who are hard of hearing or deaf can use telephones
5. Describe how computer outputs are adapted for individuals with auditory limitations
6. Discuss the major approaches used to support communication for individuals who are deaf and blind

KEY TERMS

Alerting Devices
Alternate Sensory Pathways
Assistive Listening Devices
Closed Captioning
Cochlear Implants
Hearing Aids
Hearing Carry Over (HCO)
Short Message Service (SMS)
Visual Substitution
Voice Carry Over (VCO)

CHAPTER OUTLINE

When an individual has a sensory impairment, access to information via vision or hearing is restricted. Assistive technologies can provide assistance in the input of information via sensory systems. In this chapter we focus on assistive technologies designed to meet the needs of persons with auditory limitations. This includes sensory aids that are intended for *general use* as well as assistive technologies that are used specifically for providing auditory access to computers.

AUDITORY FUNCTION

Auditory function can be measured in several ways. *Auditory thresholds* include both the *amplitude* and *frequency* of audible sounds. The amplitude of sound is measured in decibels (dB). The minimal threshold for hearing is 20 dB and is equivalent to the ticking of a watch under quiet conditions at 20 feet away. Figure 9-1 shows sound pressure levels for a variety of typical sounds.[1] The typical range of frequencies that can be heard by the human ear is 20 to 20,000 hertz (Hz), but the ear does not respond equally to all frequencies in this range.[13] There are several types of tests that audiologists use in assessing hearing. Pure tone audiometry presents pure (one-frequency) tones to each ear and determines the threshold of hearing for that person. The intensity of the tone is raised in 5-dB increments until it is heard; then it is lowered in 5-dB increments until it is no longer heard. The threshold is

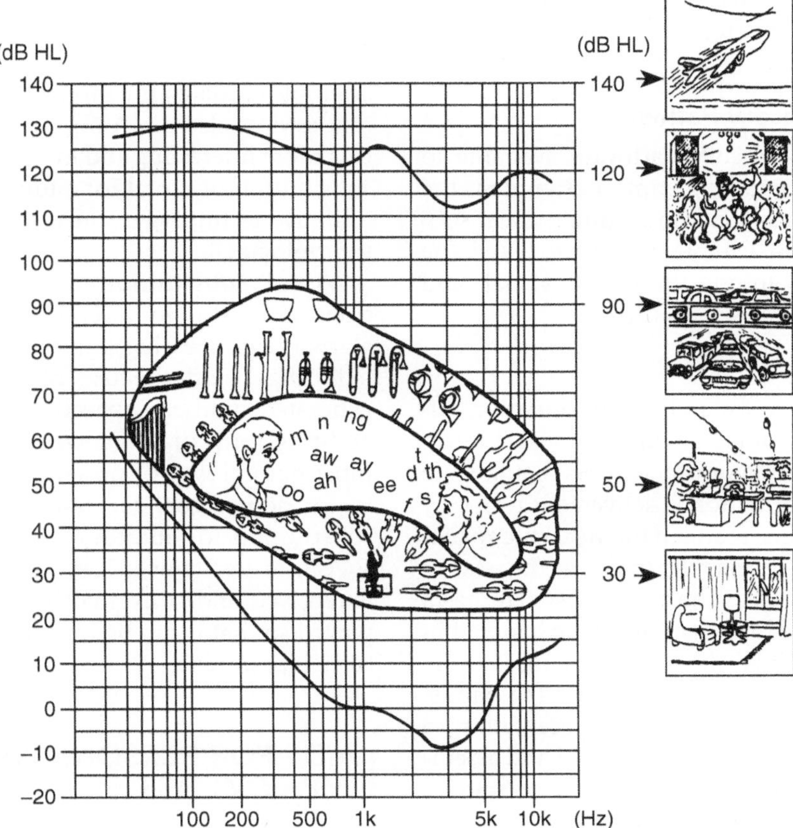

Figure 9-1 The sensitivity of the human ear to frequency is shown on the plot. This curve is normalized to zero dB at 1000 Hz. The reference pressure is 0.0002 dynes/cm^2. Along each side and in the center of the plot are shown frequencies and intensities of common sounds and speech. (From Ballantyne D: *Handbook of audiological techniques*, London, 1990, Butterworth-Heinemann.)

the intensity at which the person indicates that he or she hears the tone 50% of the time. Although the frequencies presented in the pure tone test are in the range of speech (125 to 8000 Hz), this test alone does not indicate the person's ability to understand speech. To evaluate this function, the audiologist uses a speech recognition threshold test. In this evaluation, speech is presented, either live or recorded, at varying intensity levels, and the person's ability to understand it is determined. The person is asked to repeat either words or sentences presented at these varying intensities.

HEARING LOSS

On the basis of these and other tests, the audiologist determines both the degree of hearing loss and the type of loss. Four types of hearing loss are typically defined.[13] These are (1) conductive loss associated with pathological defects of the middle ear, (2) sensorineural loss associated with defects in the cochlea or auditory nerve, (3) centrally induced damage to the auditory cortex of the brain, and (4) functional deafness resulting from perceptual deficits rather than physiological conditions. Auditory impairment is considered slight if the loss is between 20 and 30 dB, mild if from 30 to 45 dB, moderate if from 60 to 75 dB, profound if from 75 to 90 db, and extreme if from 90 to 110 dB.[13] Causes of hearing loss include congenital loss, physical damage, disease, aging, and effects of medications.[13] These conditions can affect the outer, middle, or inner ear.

FUNDAMENTAL APPROACHES TO AUDITORY SENSORY AIDS

In Chapter 8 we describe the fundamental approaches to sensory aids. Figure 8-1 applies to auditory as well as visual sensory aids. Augmentation of an existing pathway and use of an alternative pathway are the two basic approaches to sensory assistive technologies. When applied to the auditory system, the alternative pathways are tactile and visual. We discuss each of these approaches in this chapter.

Augmentation of Existing Pathway

When someone is hard of hearing, the primary pathway (i.e., the one normally used for input) is still available, but it is limited. Insufficient intensity means that the signals are too weak to be heard, and an amplifier is required. Certain frequencies may be more limited than others for people who are hard of hearing, and the hearing aid must be designed or specified to take this into account. For example, in aging there is usually a greater hearing loss in high than in low frequencies. Augmentation of the auditory pathway is via hearing aids, cochlear implants, or assistive listening devices.

Use of Alternative Sensory Pathway

There are two **alternate sensory pathways** available to someone who is deaf. The most common example is the use of manual sign language and lip reading (visual substitution for auditory). In Chapter 8 we discussed the fundamental differences among the tactile, visual, and auditory systems.

Tactile Substitution

Substitution of tactile input for auditory information differs from the substitution of tactile input for visual information (i.e., Braille). One major difference is that the rate at which the auditory information is delivered is relatively high compared with the time required for the tactile system to input information. Engineers refer to this as the relative *bandwidths* of the two systems. The auditory system has a broader bandwidth (more information can be handled in a given amount of time) than the tactile system. Because auditory information is a sequence of sounds, these must be translated into tactile information for presentation to the user. These tactile signals are then detected and assembled into meaningful units by the central nervous system. Because the tactile system requires spatial and temporal information, its rate of input is slower than for the auditory system. Another major limitation of the tactile system for auditory input is that it lacks a means of converting sound (mechanical vibrations) into neural signals. This is the function normally carried out by the cochlea.

The only tactile method for input of auditory information that has been successful is the *Tadoma method* employed by individuals who are both deaf and blind. In this method, used by Helen Keller, the person receives information by placing his hands on the speaker's face, with the thumbs on the lips, index fingers on the sides of the nose, little fingers on the throat, and other fingers on the cheeks. During speech, the fingers detect movements of the lips, nose, and cheeks and feel the vibration of the larynx in the throat. Through practice, kinesthetic input obtained from these sources is interpreted as speech patterns. One reason for the success of this method is that there is a fundamental relationship between the articulators (reflected in the movements of the lips, nose, and cheeks) and the perceived speech signal, and this relationship is at least as important as the acoustic information (pitch and loudness) in the speech signal for individuals using the Tadoma method.[10]

Visual Substitution

Visual displays of auditory information can take several forms. One example, sometimes used in speech therapy or as an aid to deaf individuals who are learning to speak, is to display a picture of the speech signal on an oscilloscope-like screen. Often a model pattern portraying the ideal speech signal is placed on the top half of the screen, and the pattern from the person learning to speak is placed on the bottom half of the screen. The learner attempts to match the model through practice. Some current devices also use computer graphics to make the process more interesting and motivating. This type of sensory substitution of visual for auditory information is a rehabilitative technology, and it is not practical for assistive technologies.

Visual substitution for auditory information has been successful in several areas. These include visual alarms (e.g., flashing lights when a telephone or doorbell rings) and the use of text labels for computer-generated synthetic speech. Speech is the most natural auditory form of language. Likewise, written text is the most natural way of presenting visual language. Thus a major design goal for assistive devices that use visual substitution for auditory communication is to provide speech-to-text conversion. In this type of device, speech is received and converted by computer to text and displayed so that it can be read by the person with an auditory impairment.

AIDS FOR PERSONS WITH AUDITORY IMPAIRMENTS

Helen Keller, who was both deaf and blind, is reported to have been asked whether she would prefer to have her vision or her hearing if she could have one or the other. She responded that she would prefer to have her hearing, since she felt that people who are blind are cut off from things, whereas those who are deaf are cut off from people. It is important to keep this concept in mind as we discuss aids for persons who are deaf or hard of hearing. Auditory impairment is often not as obvious as visual impairment, and society does not view it as having the same degree of significance as visual impairment. It is natural for a person to wear glasses as a part of the inherent process of aging. However, many people are embarrassed to admit hearing loss sufficient to require a hearing aid. Despite these considerations, hearing loss is significant, and it can be socially isolating. Assistive technologies can provide great improvement in the lives of persons who have either partial or total auditory impairments.

Hearing Aids

Hearing aids are often conceived of as simple devices that amplify sound, primarily speech. Although hearing aids do contain amplifiers, hearing loss is rarely consistent across the entire speech frequency range. Hearing loss is generally greater at some frequencies than others. This presents a problem in the design of hearing aids. If we amplify all frequencies the same amount, the sound will be unnatural to the user. An additional difficulty encountered in providing hearing aids of high fidelity is that the components are small, and this miniaturization can limit the frequency response of the microphone and speaker, further reducing the quality of the aided speech.

Approximately 60% of the *acoustic energy* of the speech signal is contained in frequencies below 500 Hz.[3] However, the speech signal contains not only specific frequencies of sound, but also the organization of these sounds into meaningful units of auditory language (e.g., phonemes), and over 95% of the *intelligibility* of the speech signal is associated with frequencies above 500 Hz. For this reason, speech intelligibility rather than sound level is often used as the criterion for successful application of hearing aids.

Types of Hearing Aids

Conventional hearing aids can be divided into two types: air conduction and bone conduction. All air conduction hearing aids deliver the hearing aid output into the listener's ear canal. However, some people are unable to use air conduction hearing aids due to chronic ear infections or malformed ear canals. For these individuals, a bone conduction hearing aid is most appropriate. The most common type of bone conduction hearing aid is a BAHA (Bone Anchored Hearing Aid); see Figure 9-2. Inputs to this type of hearing aid are converted to mechanical vibrations that shake the skull and stimulate the receptors in the cochlea. BAHAs take advantage of the fact that, at a sensory level, it does not matter whether sounds come from an air conducted hearing aid or a bone conducted hearing aid.[18]

Air conduction hearing aids are available in several different configurations.[19] Figure 9-3 illustrates several commonly used types of aids. The major types of ear-level aids are behind-the-ear (BTE), in-the-ear (ITE), in-the-canal (ITC), and completely in-the-canal (CIC). Body-level aids are used in cases of profound hearing loss. The processor is larger to accommodate more signal processing options and greater amplification and is mounted at belt level. The body-level aid is usually used only when other types of aids cannot be used.

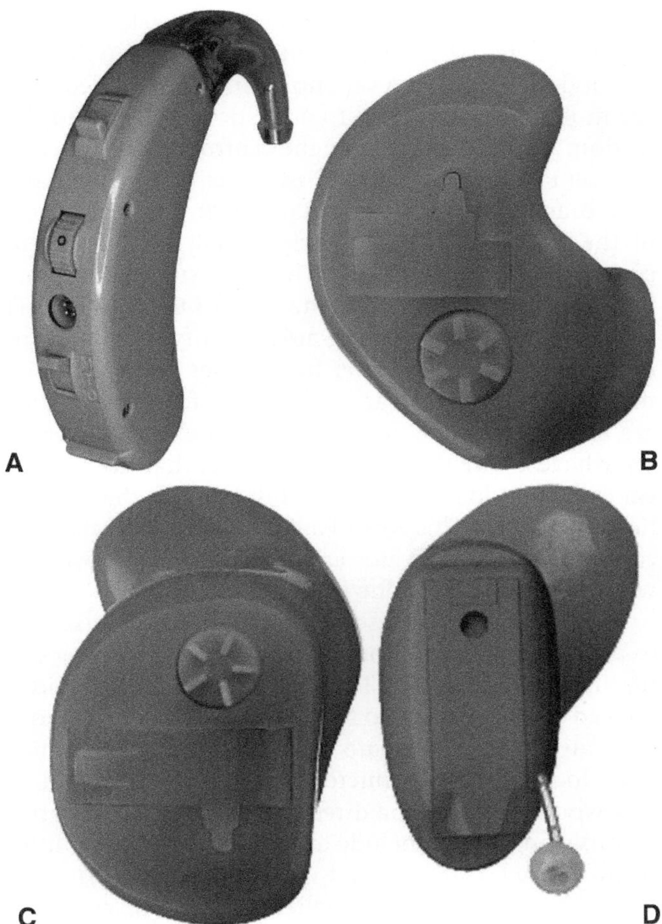

Figure 9-3 Types of hearing aids. **A,** Behind the ear (BTE). **B,** In-the-ear (ITE). **C,** In-the-canal (ITC). **D,** Completely in-the-canal (CIC). (Courtesy Siemans Hearing Instruments, Inc.)

BTE hearing aids fit behind the ear and contain all the components shown in Figure 9-4. The amplified acoustic signal is fed into the ear canal through a small ear hook that extends over the top of the auricle and holds the hearing aid in place. A small tube directs the sound into the ear through an ear mold that serves as an acoustic coupler. This ear mold is made from an impression of the individual's ear to ensure comfort to the user, maximize the amount of acoustical energy coupled into the ear, and

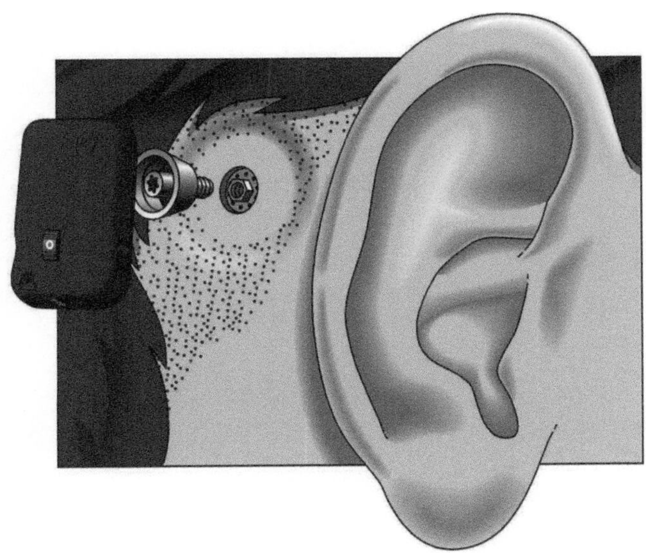

Figure 9-2 Bone-anchored hearing aid. (Courtesy Entific Scientific.)

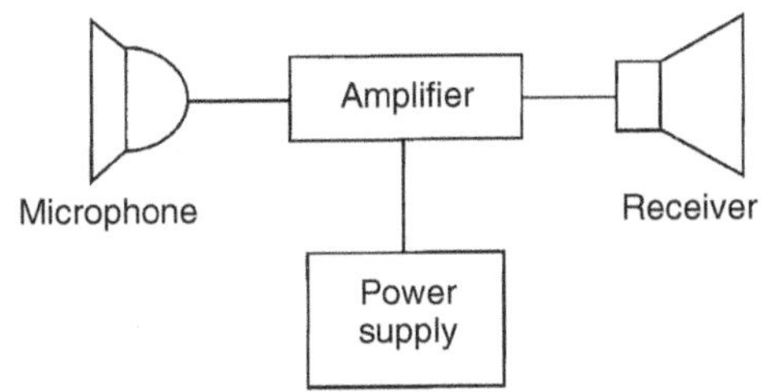

Figure 9-4 The major components of a hearing aid.

prevent squealing caused by acoustic feedback. When the mold is made, a 2-ml space is included between the coupler and the eardrum. A vent hole can also be added to an ear mold, which can add to acoustic feedback and distortion, as well as preventing the ear from being blocked. The vent hole allows sound to travel to the tympanic membrane directly. An external switch allows selection of the microphone (M), a telecoil (T) for direct telephone reception, or off (O). The MTO switch and a volume control are located on the back of the case for BTE aids. Some types of hearing aids amplify only high frequencies because the lower frequencies are within normal hearing limits. Hearing aids used for this situation are called *open fit* because they do not use an ear mold. They have a wire that runs to a speaker that fits into the ear canal but does not block out the sounds that are still heard normally. This type of aid is called a receiver in the canal (RIC). Open fit aids are often used for individuals whose hearing loss is due to aging.

The ITE aid makes use of electronic miniaturization to place the amplifier and speaker in a small casing that fits into the ear canal. The faceplate of the ITE aid is located in the opening to the ear canal. The microphone is located in the faceplate. This provides a more "natural" location for the microphone as it receives sound that would normally be directed into the ear.[19] External controls on the ITE include an MTO switch and volume control. The ITC is a smaller version of the ITE. The CIC type of hearing aid is the smallest, and it is inserted 1 to 2 mm into the canal with the speaker close to the tympanic membrane. Because this type does not protrude outside the ear canal, it is barely visible. Any controls for the aid are fit onto the faceplate of the ITE, ITC, and CIC types of aids. The basic components of analog and digital hearing aids are described by Cook and Polgar in *Cook and Hussey's Assistive Technologies: Principles and Practice.*[5]

Hearing Aid Accessories

Modern digital hearing aids have many capabilities. For example, there are programs that amplify speech selectively in a noisy environment. Directional microphones can be adjusted to pick up sound from the side, front, or back. Volume levels can be adjusted for each ear independently. These and other features are often controlled through a handheld remote control. Many hearing aids phones also have a Bluetooth link that can be used with a mobile phone or entertainment appliance (i.e., TV, DVD, or music player). The Bluetooth linkage makes it possible for the person using the hearing aid to selectively adjust volume and perform other features (e.g., answering a mobile phone) without disturbing others.

Cochlear Implants

If there is damage to the cochlea of the inner ear, an auditory prosthesis can provide some sound perception. These devices, termed **cochlear implants,** have the components shown in Figure 9-5.[6,15] As long as the eighth cranial nerve is intact, it is possible to provide stimulation via implanted electrodes. Cochlear implants have been shown to be of benefit to adults and young persons who have adventitious hearing loss (i.e., hearing loss after acquiring speech and language).[19] Significant benefits have also been reported for cochlear implants in young pre-lingual children.[2,20] The main distinguishing characteristics, shown in Box 9-1, are discussed in depth by Loizou (1998)[11] and summarized in this section.

There are two major parts of most cochlear implants.[16] External to the body are a microphone (environmental interface), electronic processing circuits that extract key parameters from the speech signal, and a transmitter that couples the information to the skull. The implanted portion consists of an electrode array (1 to 22 electrodes), a receiver that couples the external data and power to the skull, and electronic circuits that provide proper

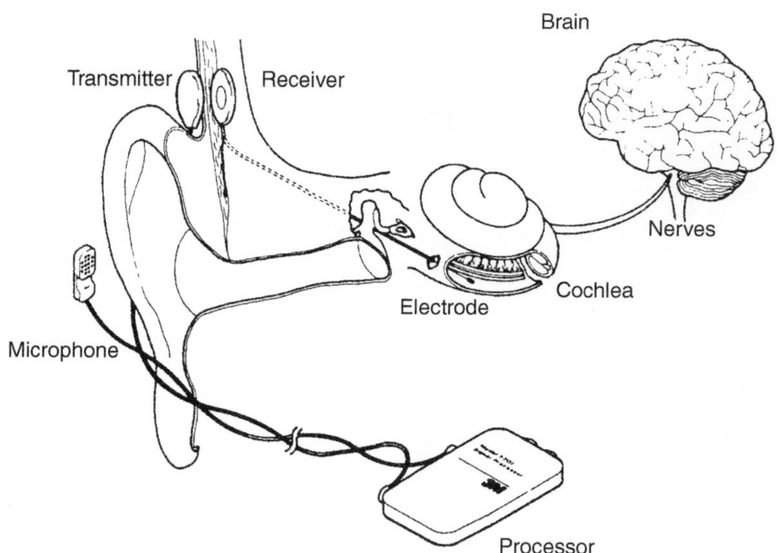

Figure 9-5 The components of a cochlear implant. (From Radcliffe D: How cochlear implants work, *Hearing J*, p 53, November 1984).

BOX 9-1 Varying Characteristics of Cochlear Implant Systems

Electrode design: number of electrodes, electrode configuration
Type of stimulation: analog or pulsatile
Transmission link: transcutaneous or percutaneous
Signal processing: waveform representation or feature extraction

From Loizou P: Mimicking the human ear, *IEEE Signal Process Mag*, 15:101–130, 1998.

synchronization and stimulation parameters for the electrode array.

Surgical procedures consist of insertion of the electrode array into the cochlea and implantation of the internal components and linking antenna for transcranial transmission of data and power. After the implant is inserted, a period of one month or so is allowed for healing and a process of "switch-on and tuning" is carried out (Ramsden, 2002).[16] Two thresholds are measured: minimal perception of sound and the level at which the sound just ceases to be comfortable. Then the electrode array is tested and signal processing is applied. Current commercial approaches to cochlear implants differ in several important respects. User evaluation research is summarized in Box 9-2.

BOX 9-2 What the Research Says: Cochlear Implant User Evaluation Results

- Almost all postlingually deaf individuals can obtain some degree of speech perception without lip reading using cochlear implants (Ramsden, 2002).[16]
- Some users can also communicate over the telephone.
- Effective auditory perception is critical for pre-lingual children to develop spoken language.
- For deaf children, the cochlear implant has been shown to facilitate development of language at a rate comparable to typical hearing children.[2]
- Results are dependent on a number of factors including age at implantation, length of deafness, and length of use (habituation to the cochlear implant).[20]
- The minimum age is 12 months; implantation before 5 years results in better performance on speech perception tests than implantation for children who are older; and children who receive an implant before the age of two perform equally well with children who receive their implant between 2 and 5.
- Children who use the cochlear implant full-time perform significantly better than those who do not.[2]
- Performance improves as the duration of use increases.[2,20]
- Word recognition scores increased from < 1% prior to implantation to 8.9% (1 year), and 30% (3 years) to a maximum of 65%; sentence recognition scores increased from 18% (1 year) to 42% (3 years) to a maximum of 80%.[20]

Telephone Access for Persons Who Are Deaf

The isolation imposed on deaf persons by the telephone is ironic given that Alexander Graham Bell was working on an aid for the deaf when he invented it. For some individuals, additional amplification is sufficient to make the telephone accessible. This is most often built into the person's telephone. For many individuals with severe hearing loss even increased amplification does not make the telephone signal audible, and a device that can visually send and receive telephone information is used. These individuals also often make use of devices that either amplify the ringing of the telephone or connect the ringer to a table lamp that flashes when the telephone rings.

Telephone Devices

Electronic visual telephones are referred to as TTYs.* They use a keypad, a visual display, and a means of connecting to a phone line or cellphone. Connection to the telephone service is by one of three methods: (1) an acoustic coupler that couples the pulses directly to the telephone handset, (2) direct connection to the telephone line via a cable, (3) cable connection to a cell phone. Some TTYs also function as telephones with additional amplification for users who are hard of hearing. Several models of current TTYs are lightweight, battery-powered devices for portable use†. Additional features include built-in printers or connections for external printers, automatic answering messages, storage of phone numbers, answering machine capability, storage of conversations, and identification to the person you are calling that you are using a TTY. An example of a TTY is shown in Figure 9-6. Other TTY features include use with an answering machine, remote retrieval of messages, message notification via paging, and a printer. The printer function gives both a permanent record of the conversation and a chance to review messages before responding to them. Some TTYs also include the "StickyKeys" feature (see Chapter 7, Table 7-1) that supports one-handed typing for modifier keys such as SHIFT and CTRL. Many TTYs plug directly into cellular and cordless telephones to allow mobile use. Some are designed for battery-powered portable use.

---

* Years ago, deaf individuals used teletype (TTY) devices designed for sending weather and news information over telephone lines to provide a "visual telephone." The original TTY, now obsolete, consisted of a typewriter and electronic circuitry for converting the typed letters to pulses that could be sent over the telephone line to another TTY. The second TTY converted the pulses back into text that was typed on paper on the remote TTY. Because of their low cost, especially for surplus units, TTYs were very popular with deaf individuals, and some are still in use. These devices used a special code for transmission called Baudot. To maintain compatibility any current devices still use that code or have it as an option. A good source of information is the Gallaudet University Technology Assessment Program (http://tap.gallaudet.edu).

† For example the Clarity (http://shop.clarityproducts.com/products/ameriphone/); Krown Manufacturing (http://www.krownmfg.com/us/products/tty.html); Ultratec (http://www.ultratec.com/products.php)

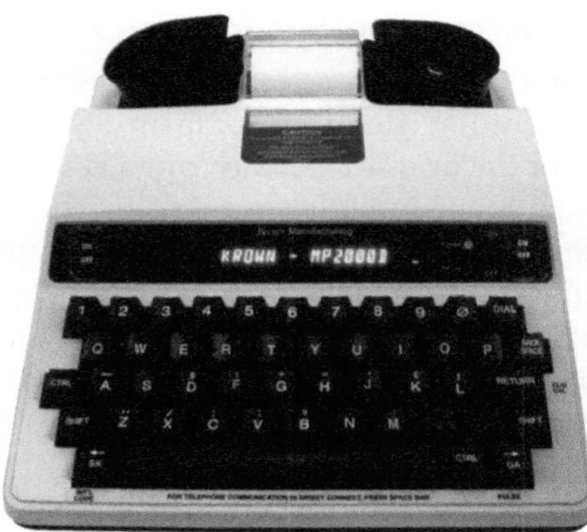

Figure 9-6 A typical TTY has an electronic display and a keyboard for typing messages. (Courtesy of Krown Manufacturing, krownmfg.com.)

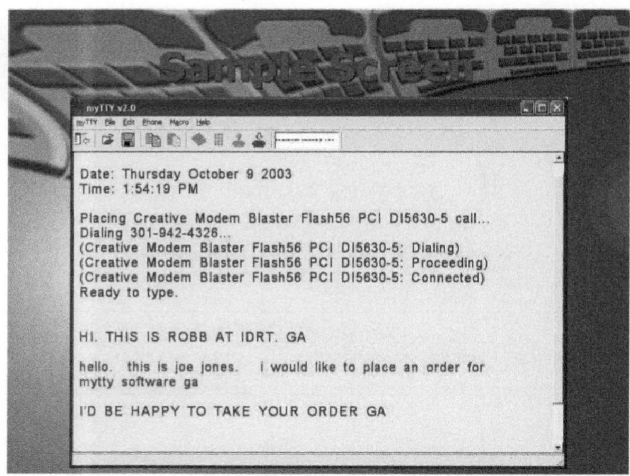

Figure 9-7 A screen shot of a software-based TTY system. (Courtesy of SoftTTY, Inc.)

There are two primary ways to use the TTY with the telephone. If both parties have a TTY, then each simply types her message, sends a "go ahead" command (the letters *GA*) to indicate that she is finished, and then waits for an answer. Some TTYs include a button that sends GA with one key press. If the deaf person needs to talk to someone who does not have a TTY, then a relay operator is provided by the telephone company. The operator has a TTY, and he reads the message sent by the deaf person to the hearing person. The response is then spoken to the operator, who types the message to the deaf person's TTY. For people who can speak but not hear, **Voice Carry Over (VCO)** phones allow communication by both voice and text. These individuals can use the relay service by speaking naturally and reading the responses on the screen. For those who can hear but not speak, **Hearing Carry Over (HCO)** allows individuals to type their message and listen to the response. The HCO user types a message for the Relay Operator to read aloud to the other party. TTYs also support **Short Message Service (SMS),** the text communication protocol that enables text messaging using cell phones.

There are a large number of deaf persons who have and use TTYs (Baudot protocol), and there are also many individuals who have personal computers with modems that use the ASCII protocol. Therefore, current TTYs often include both ASCII and Baudot, and computer programs that convert from one code to another are available. To use a computer for TTY communication, the user must have both TTY software and a modem that can emulate a TTY (Baudot at 300 baud)*. The TTY software generates the Baudot codes and sends information to the TTY modem (hardware plugged into the computer). The modem then communicates with a stand-alone TTY at 300 baud. The modem must meet all the transmission protocols (e.g., frequency, 5-bit code, half-duplex communication) of the Baudot TTY in order for the communication to be successful. These protocols are not available on standard computer modems, and that is the reason that a special TTY modem (with a setting of 300 baud to communicate in Baudot code with other TTYs) is required for successful communication with a TTY. A typical screen shot of a software-based TTY program in use is shown in Figure 9-7. Several windows are used including incoming and outgoing messages, a phone book, and a log of past messages.

CASE STUDY – SELECTING A TTY PROGRAM

The educational audiologist at a local school has approached you for advice regarding a young child who is profoundly deaf. The family does not have a stand-alone TTY, but they do have a computer. They are interested in using it as a TTY. The computer has the advantage of being a full-screen, full-keyboard computer that may be easier for the child to use and to read than one-line, cramped-keyboard traditional models. However, the computer is not as portable. Also if the phone rings with a TTY call while the computer is off, the call will be missed. The price of each approach is about the same. What approach would you take to help the family make this choice? Pay special attention to helping them (1) decide if their computer and modem will work with TTY software and (2) determine the trade-offs between the stand-alone TTY and a computer-based TTY with TTY software.

Visual Telephones

Because it requires typing of each utterance, TTY telephone transmission is slow, typically one third to one fourth the rate of human speech.[7] Visual sign language, on the other hand, results in communication rates comparable to human speech, and it is the primary form of communication used by individuals who are deaf. It does, of course, require that both the speaker and the listener understand sign language or that an interpreter be

*For example: Next Talk NXi Communications, Inc. (http://www.nextalk.net/nextalk62/nextalk.pl?rm=homepage); Phone-TTY, Inc. (www.phone-tty.com); Ultratec, Inc. (www.ultratec.com)

available. There are many situations in which this option is unavailable or impractical. For example, in a work setting it is not always practical to have an interpreter available for casual or unscheduled conversations. If standard telephone lines could be used to send visual images of manual signs, it would significantly increase communication rates over those obtained using TTYs.

The use of PCs and local area networks (LANs) can provide many of the same benefits as the visual telephone in a work environment. LANs are typically used to transfer data and messages (e.g., e-mail) from one PC to another within an office or over a wider network. When PCs and LANs are used in conjunction with a simple video camera and software, visual images can be sent from one computer to another.[8] This allows two individuals with hearing impairments to communicate via sign language. Another, far more reaching application is to use a LAN to provide interpretive services to a deaf employee or customer. The interpreter can be connected via video on the network to the employee. A speakerphone provides audio connection from the meeting to the interpreter and from the hearing impaired person (via the interpreter) to others at the meeting. The network video provides signed interpretation to the individual with a hearing impairment from the interpreter and from the hearing-impaired individual to the interpreter for voice relay to the meeting.

The use of PCs with software can replace the TTY function. This can be extended to provide telephone service for the deaf by expanding to the Internet to create *text over IP* (i.e., sending text messages using the Internet instead of phone lines). This approach has fewer restrictions than traditional TTYs because it uses standard computers and the Internet. It does require some means of alerting the deaf person that a call is coming in, but that can be included in either hardware or software. Applications that support relay calling are also available for mobile phones.*

Another approach is to take advantage of the Internet and use an interpreter located at a remote location who hears the conversation and then signs it over video for the individual who is deaf.† This approach is enabled by a broadband videophone specifically designed for deaf and hard-of-hearing individuals.‡ The Sorenson videophone also includes the recording of messages in sign language (called SignMail) by Sorenson interpreters and integration with the video relay service.

Sorenson Video Relay Service (VRS) is a free service to conduct video relay calls with family, friends, and business associates through a certified sign language interpreter, using the Sorenson videophone, a TV, and a high-speed Internet connection. The deaf user sees an interpreter on their TV and signs to the interpreter, who then contacts the hearing user via a standard phone line and relays the conversation between the two parties.

The use of an intermediary relay operator has been extended by one company (CapTel) to include a person who listens to the call as it comes in and captions the auditory information onto a small display built into the telephone.* Figure 9-8 shows how the system works. With this system, the user dials a call as they would on any other telephone. As the call is dialed it is also connected to a captioning service. When the call is completed the other party speaks to the caller in the normal way, and the captioning service transcribes everything the other party says into written text, using voice-recognition technology. The written text appears almost simultaneously with the spoken word on a visual display on the captioning phone. The cost of the captioning service is covered by Telecommunications Relay Service (TRS) funds as part of Title IV of the Americans with Disabilities Act (ADA). This approach requires both a special phone and the availability of the CapTel captioning service as part of the relay service. This system also works with external voice answering machine messages.

Access to Mobile Phones

Mobile phones are used by people who are deaf to meet needs in six broad categories: social, safety, communication, transportation, consumption, and entertainment.[4] These are inter-related, with social linkages being the most important. There are mobile phone features that would be useful in order to meet these needs. Many people who are deaf rely on short message service (SMS—generally referred to as "texting") for their mobile phone communication.[14] Deaf users of mobile phones indicated that touch screen keyboards, handwriting recognition, and QWERTY keyboard layouts support SMS capability.[4] As we have described, visual telephones are used to support sign language conversations. Deaf users would like this capability to be included in mobile phones.[4] Specific features that would support signing are cameras located on the same side as the display and large screens. A number of needs are met through smart phone access to the Internet. For those functions people who are deaf desire WiFi and wireless network linkages. Other desirable features are text-to-speech for monitoring of speech input to the device and improving communication with others, and speech-to-text for presenting received auditory content in readable form.[4]

Some people who are deaf want to use their mobile phone as a TTY. This usually requires an adapter of some sort (often just a cable) and an application that provides TTY functionality. A number of mobile phones provide this capability.†

* For example, the iPhone (http://www.purple.us/)

† Sorensen Communications, Inc., Salt Lake City, Utah (http://www.sorenson.com/)

‡ Sorenson VP-200™, Sorensen Communications, Inc., Salt Lake City, Utah (http://www.sorenson.com/)

* CapTel, Ultratec (www.captel.com/)

† http://reviews.cnet.com/4566-6454_7-0-3.html?filter=1101535_7060785_&tag=mncol;page

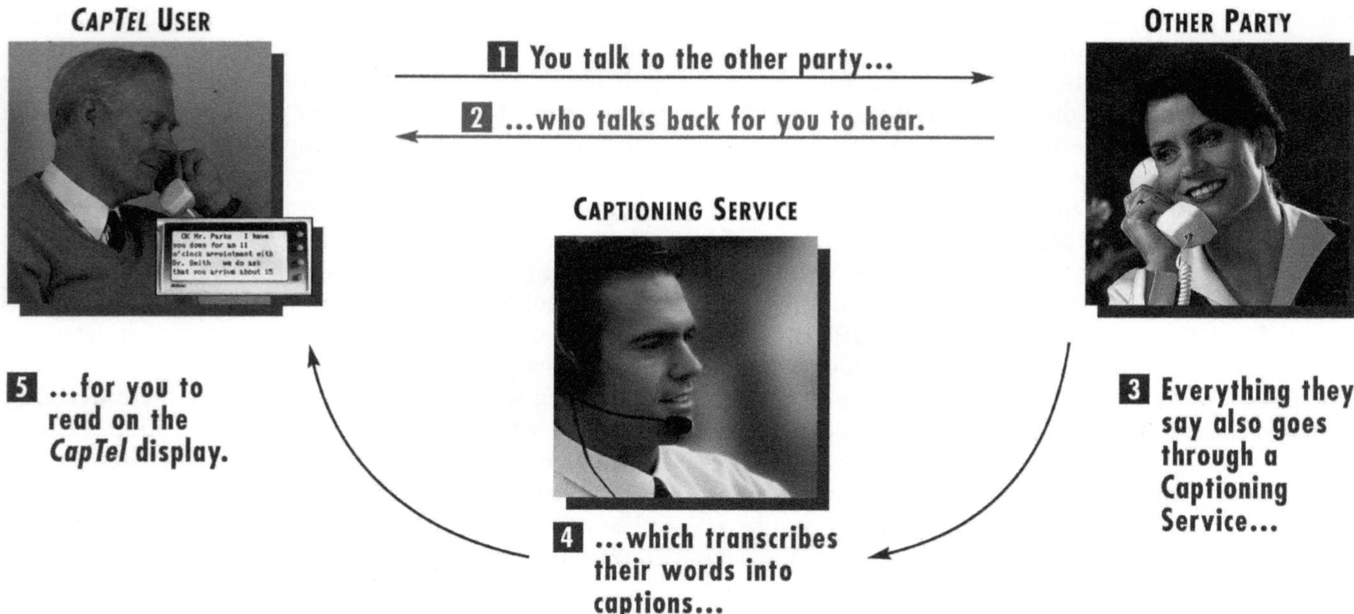

Figure 9-8 The CapTel private phone captioning system is built on the same concept as a telephone relay operator. (Courtesy of CapTel.)

Technology for Face-to-Face Communication Between Hearing and Deaf Individuals

The Sorenson method can be effective for face-to-face conversations, but it requires time for setup and must be planned in advance for work meetings or casual conversations. For these purposes, assistive technologies that allow communication without speech or sign language interpretation can be very effective. One product, the Interpretype* is designed specifically for this application. This system consists of a preprogrammed laptop-style computer that is able to send typed messages to other TTY units or another computer.[9] A built-in display shows the text that is received from the communication partner and displays messages typed into its keyboard. The major advantage of this approach is its simplicity; however, these stand-alone devices are expensive relative to TTYs. For this reason some individuals have developed simple modifications to TTYs to allow them to be used as face-to-face communication devices.† In this case, the TTYs are interconnected rather than being connected to a telephone line. Once connected they function like the TTY: one person types and his text shows up on the other person's screen. The primary advantage of using simple technology for face-to-face communication is that it is simple to set up, lightweight to carry, and intuitive to use. Since many deaf individuals have portable TTYs, the modification for face-to-face use is more cost effective. They still need to buy a second unit, but the total cost for both units can be under $600 and the total weight can be less than 3 lbs (1.5 kg).‡

* ITY, Interpretype (http://www.interpretype.com/index.php)
† Modern Deaf Communication, Inc., Danbury, Conn. (www.danbury.org/moderndeafcommunication/about_comm_equip.htm)
‡ Modern Deaf Communication, Inc. (www.danbury.org/moderndeafcommunication/about_comm_equip.htm)

Alerting Devices for Persons with Auditory Impairments

There are many environmental sounds other than speech about which a person who is deaf needs to know. Examples are telephones, doorbells, smoke alarms, and a child's cry. There are **alerting devices** available that detect these sounds and then cause a vibration, a flashing light signal, or both to call attention to the sound. Some devices are very specific. For example, one device is tuned to the frequency of a smoke alarm and it responds only to that sound. When the smoke alarm auditory signal is detected, the visible smoke detector transmits a flasher, which can be connected to a standard lamp. The lamp flashes as long as the smoke detector is active.

Telephone alerting devices include amplified ringers that plug into a standard telephone jack and provide up to 95 dB of ringing sound.[12] Another approach is to use a flashing light that is connected to the telephone line. This can alert the person who is deaf that there is an incoming TTY call. Some systems have a strobe light connected to them; others use a table lamp plugged into the alerting device. The only modification required for these adaptations is a two-plug telephone adapter to allow plugging in of both the adapted alerting device and the telephone.

Doorbells can be either directly wired into a flashing light or detected by a microphone and then converted into a visible (typically a flashing light) or tactile (vibration) signal. For more general sound detection there are silent alarms that can detect any signal and then transmit to a wrist-worn receiver. This both vibrates and flashes a light to indicate that the sound has occurred. Some devices can accommodate 16 or more channels and different lights flash for each sound.

A microphone and transmitter can be placed in each of the locations where an important sound may occur. For example, one can be near the front door, another near the telephone, another in the baby's room, and a final one near the back door. When a sound is detected at any of these locations, the wrist unit vibrates and one light is illuminated to indicate which sound has been detected.

Alarm clocks for persons who are deaf generally are either visible (flashing light on a bedside table) or tactile (vibration under the pillow). They may either be built into an alarm clock (e.g., the entire face of the clock flashes) or they may detect the clock's alarm and then cause the vibration or flashing light (or both).

CASE STUDY – LIVING WITH HEARING LOSS

Sandra Robinson lives alone in the home that she and her deceased husband Russell bought 40 years ago. She is very attached to the house and wants to continue to stay there. Unfortunately, her hearing loss has been steadily increasing and she is unable to hear the telephone, doorbell, kitchen timer, microwave beeper, and alarms (i.e., smoke and home security system). Her daughter, Ann, is concerned about her mother's increasing isolation. You have been asked to recommend things that might help her become more connected to her family (some of whom live several hundred miles away) and to feel safer in her home surroundings. What would you recommend?

Assistive Listening Devices (ALDs)

All the devices we have discussed in this chapter have been designed for use by hearing-impaired individuals. There is also a class of assistive devices that are intended to be used in group settings, such as lecture halls, churches, business meetings, courtrooms, and broadcast television. These are called **assistive listening devices**.

For many individuals who have auditory impairments, hearing aids are only effective for one-on-one conversations at close range (and possibly for telephone use). These individuals may also have difficulty if the environment has reverberations, such as a "live" room with echoes. Because of the abnormalities in the auditory system, the speech signal becomes buried in the background noise. A hearing aid amplifies both the desired signal (e.g., speech) and the background noise to the same degree. The person with a hearing loss will have increased difficulty hearing when there is background noise present. In order for the person using a hearing aid to be able to distinguish speech from background noise, the speech must be 5 to 10 times louder than the noise. Wireless technology can preserve speech in the presence of background noise. Sometimes these systems are referred to as *small-group* or *personal listening devices*.

FM systems consist of a microphone and a battery-powered radio transmitter that are worn by the speaker and a receiver that is carried by the person with an auditory impairment. The output of the receiver can either be fed into earphones (personal FM system) or coupled directly to the hearing aid. If the person does not normally use a hearing aid or the hearing aids used do not accommodate direct coupling of the signal, earphones are used. The speaker uses a microphone and whatever she says is then transmitted to the listener with a high signal-to-noise ratio. For small-group meetings with several participants, the microphone can be placed in the middle of the conference table to pick up all the voices. Small-group devices can have multiple receivers for one transmitter if there is more than one person requiring amplification.

Several manufacturers produce devices that combine a conventional BTE hearing aid with an FM system.* Some manufacturers use a "boot" that fits over the bottom of the BTE device and directly couples the amplified sound to the hearing aid. Other manufacturers have built the FM receiver directly into the case of the BTE. In either case, a transmitter sends the radio signal from the person who is speaking to the wireless receiver attached to or built into the BTE device. The hearing aid user can switch between the hearing aid–only, hearing aid plus FM, and FM-only modes. In the FM-only mode, the user would hear only the speech of the person wearing the transmitter. However, if the user wanted to monitor his/her own voice or hear another child's answer to a question in class, the HA plus FM mode might be more appropriate.

Digital FM systems pair the transmitter and receiver so that multiple users can each receive private messages from different speakers.† Digital transmission is also more reliable than analog systems. The specificity of digital transmission makes it possible to have an increased level of security over previous analog systems. Each transmitter and receiver is paired by the transmitter sending a coded key to the receiver.

One approach to achieving uniform sound throughout the room and avoiding the problems of distance from the speaker is the use of *sound field systems*.[‡,17] As shown in Figure 9-9, the speaker's voice is transmitted to speakers located around the room using FM or infrared radio transmission. The presenter's (e.g., teacher, preacher, or meeting speaker) voice is amplified so it is just louder than the background nose and their voice is presented uniformly throughout the room. A presenter's voice (e.g., a classroom teacher) is at a level only about

* For example, the Extend Ear, AVR Communication Limited, Eden Prairie, Minn. (http://www.avrsono.com); Microlink, Phonak Staeta, Switzerland (http://www.phonak.com)

† For example, the Comfort Contego (http://www.comfortaudio.com/for-users/finding-the-right-hearing-product/product-overview/comfort-contego/product-information/)

‡ For example, Pnonic Ear Front Row Systems (http://www.phonicear.com/SF.aspx)

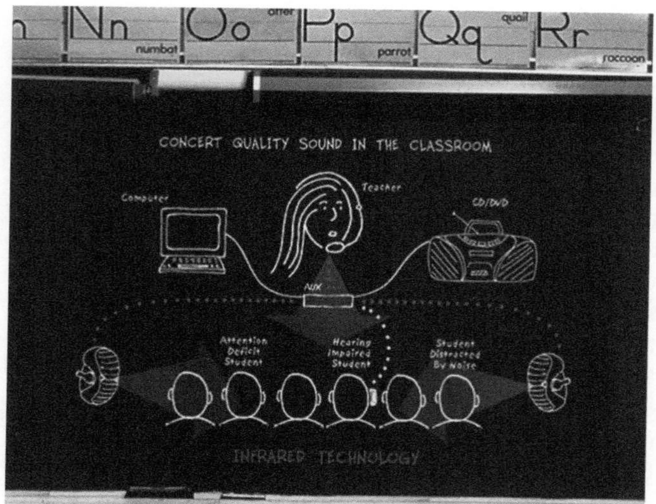

Figure 9-9 A typical sound field system set-up. (Courtesy of Telex.)

6 dB above background noise. A sound field system can boost this to 8 to 10 dB, which is a much more suitable signal-to-noise ratio (SNR).[17] Individuals with mild hearing loss and those with attention deficit and learning disabilities gain the maximum benefit of sound field systems. For those with more profound hearing loss, sound field systems also allow direct transmission to an individual student through earphones by coupling to a personal FM system.

Hearing in the presence of background noise can also be difficult for individuals with hearing loss in large meeting rooms such as concert halls, lecture auditoriums, and churches. Under the provisions of the ADA, these areas must be equipped with assistive listening devices. There are several approaches possible, all of which are directly coupled to the public address system of the facility being equipped. These are (1) hard-wired jacks for plugging in earphones, (2) FM or infrared transmitter-receiver setups similar to small-group devices, and (3) audio induction loops for transmission to hearing aids equipped with telecoils (http://www.asha.org/public/hearing/treatment/assist_tech.htm). Other assistive listening devices (ALDs) have been developed for television viewing and for use as personal amplifiers.[19] Personal amplifiers are hard-wired microphones connected to an amplifier and to earphones worn by the person who is hard of hearing. They are used in hospitals and similar situations for temporary amplification when hearing aids are not available or not worn. Television listeners are ALDs that connect directly to the audio of the television set and transmit the signal to a receiver via FM or ultrasound. The user has earphones connected to the receiver.

Captioning as an Auditory Substitute

Captioning is a process whereby the audio portion of a television program is converted to written words, which appear in a window on the screen. Captioning substitutes visual (text) information for auditory information (i.e., dialogue, narration, and sound effects). Originally focused on broadcast television and films, captioning has been expanded to include cable television, Webcasting, home video and DVDs, and government and corporate video programming. Captioning is also used as an alternative to sign language interpreters in classrooms and meetings and for face-to-face conversations.

The National Captioning Institute* (NCI) in the United States is a leading provider of closed captioning and other media access services. NCI provides subtitling and language translation services in over 50 languages and dialects. The NCI can also caption live programs such as news broadcasts, presidential speeches, and coverage of the Olympics. Captions can aid those learning English as a second language and provide assistance in efforts to eradicate illiteracy. The European Captioning Institute† (ECI) provides similar services throughout Europe. Similar organizations exist in most countries.

Closed-Captioned Television and Movies

When captioning is used in public media (i.e., television or movie theatres) it is **closed captioning.** It is called "closed" because the words are not visible unless the viewer has a closed-caption decoder. In the United States, the Telecommunications Act of 1996 resulted in FCC regulations requiring television broadcasters to provide closed captioning for all new programming released after January 1, 1998, so that the programs are "fully accessible." *Fully accessible* means that 95% of the nonexempt programming must be closed captioned. Most other countries have passed similar legislation. All television sets currently being produced have a built-in closed caption converter. It takes between 20 and 30 manhours to close caption a 1-hour television program. The individual broadcasters make decisions regarding which programs are captioned consistent with the local regulations. Some programs, such as live newscasts, are captioned on the fly, whereas others are captioned in postproduction. Many DVDs and much network, cable, and independent programming are now available in closed-caption form. Closed captioning includes movies, network news, comedies, sporting events, and dramas as well as educational, religious, and children's programming. In excess of 550 national advertisers have closed captioned more than 13,000 commercials.

Real-Time Captioning for Education and Business Applications

Computer Assisted Realtime (or Remote) Transcription (CART) has been applied in several different ways (Figure 9-10). For lectures or meetings where there is one deaf participant, CART can be provided one-on-one, where a stenographer translates speech into text in real

* http://www.ncicap.org
† http://www.ecisubtitling.com/

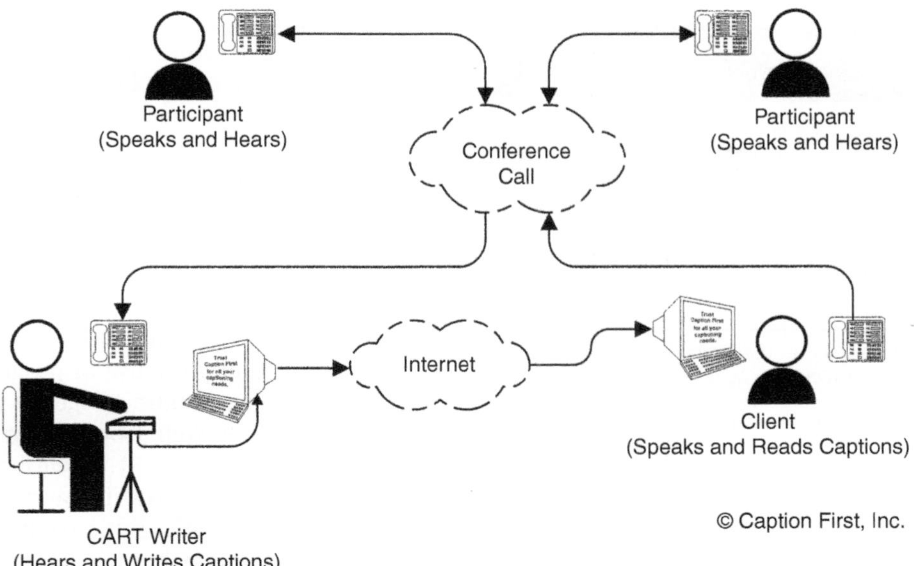

Figure 9-10 Schematic representation of a Computer Assisted Realtime (or Remote) Transcription (CART). (Courtesy of Caption First, http://www.captionfirst.com/.)

time. It is displayed on a monitor for the individual who is deaf. For meetings in which there is more than one deaf participant, the text output is projected on a screen, generally from a computer. The Internet can also be used to assist deaf individuals with spoken language interpretation. The stenographer has voice connection via the Internet to the meeting or classroom and enters text with a stenotype machine. The text is translated through computer software to text, transmitted over the Internet back to the classroom or meeting, and then read by the deaf individual. Several vendors provide CART services.*

Another example is computer assisted note taking (CAN).[21] A fast typist enters text using a standard computer keyboard using abbreviations (see Chapter 11) to maximize speed of data entry. As in the CART method, text is displayed on a screen. The rate of entry is too slow for the speech to be converted directly to text so a summary is used. The accuracy of the summary is estimated to be in the 90% to 95% range. In an evaluation study Youdelman and Messerly (1996)[21] identified that note takers found this approach to be superior to pencil and paper methods since speed could be increased without sacrificing legibility; text could be easily edited; printed copies could be made available to students immediately; and emphasis of important points could be enhanced by bold, italic, or underline formats. When evaluating the approach, the teachers felt that CAN helped students obtain more information than they had with previous methods and that the printed method improved spelling skills. Since the CAN was applied to uncaptioned videotapes and other media it had an additional benefit. The teachers also noted a positive impact on the entire class, not just the hearing-impaired students, because it helped the entire class focus on the material covered and helped them develop good note-taking skills. The hearing impaired students stated that CAN helped them understand the material and keep up with the teacher. The children without hearing impairments observed that it was helpful to glance at the display as the teacher was talking to gain information missed orally. They also benefited from the printed notes.

* For example, Hear Ink (www.hearink.com/); Caption First (www.captionfirst.com/)

Computer Adaptations for Auditory Impairments

The basic characteristics of the Graphical User Interface (GUI) are described in Chapter 8. Increasingly, there is auditory information that is included with programs or Web pages. For persons who are deaf this information may be inaccessible. If an individual is hard of hearing, the system volume can generally be increased. It is also possible to use headphones and link more directly to the user's auditory system. Computer interaction is bidirectional, and the ATP must understand how computer outputs can be adapted for persons with sensory impairments. Persons who are deaf or hard of hearing also may experience difficulties in recognizing auditory computer outputs such as sounds or speech.

Built-in Options to Increase Usability by Persons Who Are Deaf

Adaptations that facilitate some of these functions and that are included in the Accessibility Options in Windows and Macintosh are shown in Table 9-1. ToggleKeys (Windows XP™) generates a sound when the CAPS LOCK, NUM LOCK, or SCROLL LOCK key is pressed. *Spoken dialog* displays captions for speech and sounds to indicate that activity has occurred such as a document started or finished printing. Visual notification is an alternative feature of some operating systems that allows deaf or

TABLE 9-1 Simple Adaptations for Auditory Impairment*

Need Addressed	Software Approach
User cannot hear speech and sounds produced by programs or Web pages	ShowSounds[†] Flash Screen[‡] Visual Notifications[§]
User cannot hear sounds used to signal change of operations or errors during program operation.	SoundSentry

* Software modifications developed at the Trace Center, University of Wisconsin, Madison. These are included as before-market modifications in most personal computers.
†Windows XP™, Microsoft, Seattle, Wash. (www.microsoft.com/enable/)
‡Macintosh, Apple Computer, Cupertino, Calif. (www.apple.com/education/accessibility/technology/)
§Windows Vista™, Microsoft, Seattle, Wash.

hard-of-hearing users to receive a visual alert of a warning or error message that might otherwise be issued by sound. In the Apple Macintosh operating system, visual notification is called *screen flash.** This notification can be a simple beeping sound or the entire screen can light up like a camera flash.

In addition to the benefit to hearing-impaired students, non–hearing-impaired students may also appreciate the option of having visual rather than auditory alerts. A variety of screen flash options are available in Microsoft operating systems.[†] Visual notifications are used to replace system sounds with visual cues, such as a flash on the screen, so that system alerts are announced with visual notifications instead of sounds. The way in which the warnings from Sound Notifications are presented is also variable.

Access to the Internet when Auditory Information Is Difficult for the User

Hard of hearing refers to individuals who have a mild to moderate hearing limitation. These individuals may require amplification of sound levels, transcripts, or captions for audio content to use the Web.[‡] Adaptations that may be useful for this group of people are media players that display captions provided for audio content, options to turn off any background audio, and options to adjust the volume of the foreground audio.

People who are deaf need access to the same multimedia Web information as hearing individuals.[§] They rely on transcripts or captions for audio content and the display of captions provided for audio information on media players. Additional assistance may be provided for some people by simplifying language or clarifying it by combining pictures, graphs, and other images to highlight content. Other Internet users who are deaf may prefer to make use of sign language provided through the picture-in-picture format. However, not all people who are deaf know sign language.

Since Web pages are a mixture of text, graphics, and sound, they can present challenges to individuals who are deaf or hard of hearing. As the amount of auditory Web content increases, people who are deaf are also prevented from accessing that information. We described general issues of access and how Web pages are developed in Chapter 8, including the use of programming languages such as Hypertext Markup Language (HTML). The W3C WAI (World Wide Web Consortium Web Accessibility Initiative—see Chapter 8) recommendations include accessibility for hard-of-hearing and deaf users.

The W3C accessibility initiative has identified a number of barriers faced by hard-of-hearing and deaf individuals. These include*:

- Lack of captioning or transcripts for material containing audio (e.g., voices or sounds in videos).
- Web applications that do not contain captioning or transcripts for auditory information or depend on voice for input.
- Lack of sign language, images, or other highlights to support long passages of text.

AIDS FOR PERSONS WITH BOTH VISUAL AND AUDITORY IMPAIRMENTS

Individuals who are both deaf and blind must use tactile input to obtain information about the environment and to communicate. Two basic methods are used by this group of people. The Tadoma method (described earlier in this chapter) is used to understand speech. Finger spelling, with the deaf-blind individual sensing the signs in his hand, is used when both persons in the conversation know signing or when one person acts as an interpreter.

Devices for Face-to-Face Communication with Individuals Who Are Deaf and Blind

A common approach to communication between a non-disabled person and an individual who is both deaf and blind is to use a standard keyboard and visual display for the non-disabled person and a Braille keyboard and display for the person who is deaf and blind.[†] This configuration enables direct face-to-face communication with individuals who have no knowledge of sign language or

* http://www.apple.com/accessibility/
† http://www.microsoft.com/enable/
‡ http://www.w3.org/WAI/EO/Drafts/PWD-Use-Web/2009/disabilities#hardofhearing
§ http://www.w3.org/WAI/EO/Drafts/PWD-Use-Web/2009/disabilities#hardofhearing

* http://www.w3.org/WAI/EO/Drafts/PWD-Use-Web/2009/disabilities#hardofhearing
† For example: ITY, Intertype, Rochester, N.Y. (www.interpretype.com/index.php); FSTTY and FSCommunicator, Freedom Scientific, St. Petersburg, Fla. (www.freedomscientific.com/fs_products/FlyerPDFs/FSTTYFlyer.pdf); Braille-TTY telephone, Krown, Ft. Worth, Tex. (http://www.krownmfg.com/us/products/vtouch.htm); Braillephone (http://www.av-mart.com/Braillephone.htm)

Braille to communicate with a person who is both deaf and blind. It does require knowledge of Braille by the person with the disabilities.

The FaceToFace* uses a portable note-taking device (PACMate) with a built-in Braille keyboard and refreshable display (see Chapter 8) together with a software application on a PDA or portable computer. The two devices communicate via Bluetooth. The person who is deaf and blind types a message on the Braille keyboard, and it is displayed as text on the PDA or computer screen. The communication partner types on the PDA or computer and it is shown on the Braille display. A similar approach is available in the Deafblind Communicator† from Humanware.

The Braillephone‡ and Krown VTouch TTY§ extend the FaceToFace concept to include a Braille display, TTY, QWERTY keyboard, and visible display all built into the same case. These devices allow communication between a person who is deaf and blind and another person using deaf relay services, and face-to-face communication between a disabled person and one who is deaf and blind, or between two people who are deaf and blind. A vibrating cell provides notification of incoming data including phone calls. Software options allow the Braillephone to be used to access Microsoft Windows applications. Connection to the phone line is through an acoustically coupled modem or a direct connection.

The TTY function provides the capability for the person who is deaf and blind to talk to other people who have a TTY or, through a relay operator, or to anyone with a telephone. The keyboards (Braille and QWERTY) and displays (Braille and visual) allow face-to face communication. Finally, another approach uses two separate devices connected by cable or wireless transmission.‖ Both the hearing and the deaf and blind user have a keyboard and display, which may be a QWERTY or Braille keyboard and a visual or Braille display. The advantage of this approach is that the two people communicating can have a more comfortable physical spacing as they communicate because they each have their own device. The device can either be a stand-alone system designed for this purpose or a computer running special software.

SUMMARY

Hearing aids provide assistance for persons whose hearing is inadequate for conversation. Recent trends in hearing aid design have focused on improved fidelity and digital speech processing. When an individual has damage to the cochlea, he may benefit from the use of cochlear implants. Aids for persons who are deaf use either visual or tactile systems as alternatives. Speech-to-text (sound-to-visual display) devices are not as well developed as text-to-speech aids, and visual information is most commonly used for alarms rather than for communication. Exceptions to this are telephone communication using telephone devices for the deaf (TTYs).

Aids for persons who are both deaf and blind must use tactile substitution. The major approach is Braille output with a text-based keyboard for communication between a sighted and a deaf-blind individual. A mechanical device that emulates finger spelling (commonly used by deaf-blind persons) and is driven by a computer with keyboard entry provides communication between a sighted person who does not know finger spelling and a deaf-blind person who does.

* Freedom Scientific, St. Petersburg, Fla. (www.freedomscientific.com/)

† www.humanware.com

‡ Braillephone (http://www.av-mart.com/Braillephone.htm)

§ Braille-TTY telephone, Krown. Ft Worth, TX (http://krownmfg.com/us/products/vtouch.htm)

‖ ITY, Intertype, Rochester, N.Y. (http://www.interpretype.com/index.php)

STUDY QUESTIONS

1. What are the major types of hearing loss?
2. List the major cause of hearing loss.
3. How is the visual system used to substitute for auditory input for people who are deaf?
4. How is the tactile system used to substitute for auditory input for people who are deaf?
5. Discuss the major differences between blindness and deafness in terms of the effect on the individual's social, work, or school and private lives.
6. What are the types of hearing aids?
7. How does a BAHA function and when is it used?
8. List the major functions that a cochlear implant must accomplish.
9. What is a TTY?
10. What is CapTel and how does it work?
11. What is required to make a computer communicate with a TTY?
12. List the major ways that mobile phones are used by individuals who are deaf.
13. What is required to make a mobile phone communicate with a TTY?
14. What is CART and how does it apply to education, business, and personal use?
15. What are "alerting devices"? For what purposes are they normally used?
16. What is a group listening device?
17. Describe how a group listening device could be used by a church or other public organization?
18. How could you use an FM assistive listening system in a group home or skilled nursing facility?
19. How is assistive technology used to support communication for deaf-blind individuals?

REFERENCES

1. Bailey RW: *Human performance engineering*, ed 2, Englewood Cliffs, NJ, 1989, Prentice Hall.
2. Balkany TJ, Hodges AV, Eshraghi AA, et al: Cochlear implants in children–a review, *Acta Otolaryngol* 122(4):356–362, 2002.

3. Berger KW, Hagberg EN, Rane RL: *Prescription of hearing aids: rationale, procedures and results*, Kent, Ohio, 1977, Herald.
4. Chiu H-P, Liu C-H, Hsieh C-L, et al: Essential needs and requirements of mobile phones for the deaf, *Assist Technol* 22(3):172–185, 2010.
5. Cook AM, Polgar JM: *Cook and Hussey's Assistive Technologies: Principles and Practice*, St Louis, 2008, Mosby.
6. Feigenbaum E: Cochlear implant devices for the profoundly hearing impaired, *IEEE Eng Med Biol Mag* 6(2): 10–21, 1987.
7. Galuska S, Foulds R: A real-time visual telephone for the deaf. In *Proc 13th Ann RESNA Conf*, 1990, pp 267–268.
8. Galuska S, Grove T, Gray J: A visual "talk" utility: using sign language over a local area computer network. In *Proc 15th Ann RESNA Conf*, June 1992, pp 134–135.
9. Gan K: Interpretype–assistive technology for face-to-face communication. In *Proc. CSUN Conference*, 2005. retrieved from http://www.csun.edu/cod/conf/2005/proceedings/2168.htm.
10. Lieberman P: *Intonation, perception, and language*, Cambridge, Mass, 1967, MIT Press.
11. Loizou PC: Mimicking the human ear, *IEEE Signal Processing Mag* 15(5):101–130, 1998.
12. McFadden GM: Aids for hearing impairments and deafness. In Galvin JC, Scherer MJ, editors: *Evaluating, selecting, and using appropriate assistive technology*, Rockville, Md., 1996, Aspen Publishers.
13. Martin FN, Clark JG: *Introduction to Audiology*, ed 11, Upper Saddle River, NJ, 2012, Allyn & Bacon.
14. Power D, Power MR, Rehling B: German deaf people using text communication: short message service, TTY, relay services, fax, and e-mail, *Am Ann Deaf* 152(3):291–301, 2007.
15. Radcliffe D: How cochlear implants work, *Hear J* 53, November 1984.
16. Ramsden RT: Cochlear implants and brain stem implants, *Br Med Bull* 63(1):183–193, 2002.
17. Ross M, Levitt H: Classroom Sound-Field Systems, *Volta Voices* 9(2):7–8, 2002 Mar/Apr. 2002.
18. Snik AF, Mylanus EA, Cremers CW, et al: Consensus statements on the BAHA system: where do we stand at present? *Ann Otol Rhinol Laryngol Suppl* 195:2–12, 2005.
19. Stach BA: *Clinical audiology: an introduction*, San Diego, 1998, Singular Publishing Group.
20. Waltzman SB, Cohen NL, Green J, et al: Long-term effects of cochlear implants in children, *Otolaryngol Head Neck Surg* 126(5):505–511, 2002.
21. Youdelman K, Messerly C: Computer-assisted note taking for mainstreamed hearing-impaired students, *Volta Review* 98(4):191–200, 1996.

CHAPTER 10

Assistive Technologies to Aid Cognitive Function

CHAPTER OUTLINE

LEARNING OBJECTIVES

Upon completing this chapter, you will be able to do the following:

1. Apply the HAAT model to help identify appropriate assistive technologies for individuals with cognitive disabilities
2. Identify cognitive skills that underlie functional performance for persons with cognitive disabilities
3. Understand what cognitive faculties are commonly compromised in specific disorders
4. Understand the role of assistive technologies in aiding cognitive function
5. Identify and describe some of the assistive technologies that are currently available to assist individuals with cognitive impairments

KEY TERMS

Alternative Input
Alternative Output
Attention
Attention Deficit Hyperactivity Disorder (ADHD)
Autism Spectrum Disorder (ASD)
Cerebral Vascular Accidents (CVAs)
Cognition
Cognitive
Cognitive Prosthesis
Dementia
Generalization
Information Processing
Intellectual or Developmental Disabilities
Knowledge Representations
Learning Disabilities (LD)
Media Presentation
Memory
Mild Cognitive Disabilities
Problem Solving
Prompting
Stimuli Control
Smart House
Tracking and Identification
Traumatic Brain Injury (TBI)
Vigilance

"**Cognition** is the mental process of knowing, including aspects such as awareness, perception, reasoning, and judgment."* **Cognitive** is the adjective referring to cognition. Cognitive disabilities may be present at birth or result from injury or disease.

---

*The Free Dictionary (http://www.thefreedictionary.com/cognition)

Of those present at birth, some are genetically transmitted, others result from prenatal or perinatal conditions, and there is no identifiable cause for many other cases. Acquired cognitive disabilities are the result of injury or disease. Needs that result from cognitive disabilities include memory loss, dementia, language disorders, the inability to make decisions, and the incapacity to function independently. For any individual with a particular cognitive disability, existing skills and possible limitations can be identified.

There are over 20 million individuals with a cognitive disability in the United States.[7] This number can be broken down into categories: mental illness: 27%; Alzheimer's disease: 20%; brain injury: 27%; mental retardation/developmental disabilities: 22%; and stroke: 4%.

The HAAT model (see Chapter 2) consists of four elements: Human, Activity, Context, and Assistive Technology (Figure 2-1). In this chapter we focus on human cognitive skills and activities that require those skills. For example, the *activity* might be carrying out a sequence of steps, such as for making a bed in the *context* of the home. Alternatively, as shown in Figure 10-1, the context might be the broader community, where devices that provide assistance for independent navigation are important. When we know the activity and the context we can determine the required set of skills to accomplish the activity. If there is a gap between the abilities required to complete the task and the individual's skills, we can look for assistive technologies that can aid or replace the required skill. The expected skills and limitations presented in this chapter are general and every individual is unique. The case study "Intellectual Disability and the Tasks of Daily Living" illustrates how assistive technologies can be identified and applied to meet cognitive needs.

CASE STUDY – INTELLECTUAL DISABILITY AND THE TASKS OF DAILY LIVING

William is a 38-year-old man with an intellectual disability. He lives in a group home with five other men. He is expected to carry out duties to contribute to the program at the home. His task is to set the table for dinner. Currently he is only successful in completing this task if he has continuous prompting from a member of the staff. This is limiting both for William—because he is not independent—and for the home, because the staff is occupied making dinner during the time William is to carry out this task. Fortunately there are assistive technologies available to assist William in this task. List the characteristics you think such a technology should have and then look later in this chapter at the descriptions of approaches that have been taken. Did you come up with better ideas than what is currently available?

COGNITIVE SKILLS

Understanding the cognitive demands of various tasks can help us understand why an individual may find a seemingly simple task to be very difficult, while a seemingly difficult task may be carried out virtually effortlessly. Some cognitive skills such as **memory, attention, information processing**, and **problem solving** are better understood than others.[43] The definitions of some of the cognitive skills for which assistive technologies have been developed are listed in Box 10-1. Each skill listed will be described briefly in this section; for more detailed descriptions, refer to a cognitive psychology textbook.[43]

Perception

Perception is the interpretation of sensory information received through our eyes, ears, and skin, i.e., what we see, hear, and feel.[2] Perception is a very basic cognitive skill that is integrated with higher-order cognition to achieve various skills, such as sequencing the steps required to make a bed. Impairments that affect perception limit an individual's ability to use information from the environment to assist her daily activities. For example, someone with reduced visual acuity may have difficulty perceiving text that is presented on a computer screen. In this case, enlarged letters and auditory feedback may aid her when using a computer for word processing.

Attention

Attention is the ability to focus on a particular task.[50] For example, selective attention refers to the ability to shift attention between competing tasks, which requires selectively attending to one stimulus while ignoring another.[21] The characterization of different types of attention provides insight into different areas in which people may have strengths and weaknesses and for which assistive technologies may be able to help.

Attention has been characterized by different levels. Any task can involve more than one type of attention. The first of these is the detection or observation of a particular stimulus or signal (e.g., an object or event occurring in the environment). We can detect a signal in two ways. **Vigilance** refers to paying close and continuous attention over a prolonged period in order to detect a signal. Sustained attention is similar to vigilance, but there isn't necessarily a competing stimulus present in sustained attention. *Search* is the active scanning of the environment to find a particular stimulus or particular features. Vigilance and sustained attention require the person to wait for the signal to appear, and search requires the person to actively seek out a target.

Using *selective attention*, we filter out distractions and focus on the event we have chosen.[3] Variability in our selective attention skills is common, especially when there are distractions. For some individuals, the influence

		Attention				Perception	Memory					Information Processing/ Orientation				Knowledge Representation and Organization					Problem Solving								Language	Learning			
		Signal Detection		Selective	Divided		Storage		Encoding	Retrieval		Quantitative	Visuospatial	Temporal	Personal	Categorization	Sorting	Sequencing	Mental Representations		Identify Problem	Judgment	Decision Making	Reasoning		Planning	Evaluation and Iteration	Generalization		General	Mathematics	Reading	Writing
		Vigilance	Search				Short Term	Long Term		Recognition	Recall								Declarative / know what	Procedural / know how				Deductive	Inductive								
Memory Aids	Recorders	X				X	R	R			R			A					R	X									X	X			
	Word completion/prediction	X	X		X	X		X		X	A								A	X			X				X		X	A		X	A
	Information retrieval		X		X	X		X		X	A					X		X	A	X			X				X		A	A			A
Time Management			X	X		X	R	R		X	R			R						X			X						X	X			
Prompting / Cueing		A			X	X	R	R		R	R	A		R					R	R	A	R	R	R	R	R	R	A	X	R	R	R	R
Stimuli Control	Auditory (noise reduction)	A	A	A		A																								A			
	Visual field		A	A		R							A																	A		A	
	Media presentation	A	A	A	A	A																							X	A		A	
Concept organization		A	X	A	A	X	A	A	A	A	X		A			A	A	A	X	X			A	X	X	A	X	A	X	A		X	X
Language Tools		X	X		X	X		X		X	R					X		X	A	X			X				X		A	A		A	A
Alternative Input			X			X														X							X		A	X			
Alternative Output		X		X		R																							A	A	A	A	A
Tracking							R				R	A	R						R		R						R						
ID							R	R		R	R		A		R				R	X													

Figure 10-1 Skills versus assistive technology matrix. An "X" means that the cognitive skill is required to use that type of assistive technology. An "A" means that type of assistive technology might aid the cognitive skill in an activity. An "R" means that the type of assistive technology might replace the requirement for that cognitive skill in an activity. Note that these entries are with respect to the assistive technology.

BOX 10-1 Definitions of Cognitive Skills

PERCEPTION

Interpretation of the sensations received from environmental stimuli (through the sense organs)

ATTENTION

Link between the limited amount of information that is actually manipulated mentally and the enormous amount of information available through the senses, stored memories, and other cognitive processes

Signal detection: Detecting the appearance of a particular stimulus

Vigilance: Paying close and continuous attention

Search: Active scanning of the environment for particular stimuli or features

Selective: Tracking one stimulus or one type of stimulus and ignoring another

Divided: Allocating available resources to coordinate performance of more than one task at a time

MEMORY

Drawing on past knowledge to use it in the present.

Encoding: Physical and sensory input is transformed into a representation that can be stored in memory

Storage: The movement of encoded information into memory and the maintenance of information in storage

Sensory: The smallest capacity for storing information (i.e., for only a fleeting sensory image) and the shortest duration for memory storage (i.e., for only fractions of a second)

Short-term: A modest capacity (i.e., for about seven items) and a duration of a number of seconds unless strategies (e.g., rehearsal) are used for keeping the information in the short-term store for longer periods of time

Long-term: A greater capacity than both the sensory store and the short-term store, and it can store information for very long periods of time, even indefinitely

Retrieval: Recovery of stored information from memory, by moving the information into consciousness for use in active cognitive processing

Implicit: Enhanced performance on a task, as a result of prior experience, despite having no conscious awareness of recollecting the prior experience

Explicit: Consciously recalling or recognizing particular information

Recall: Retrieving memories with no hints

Recognition: Retrieving memories with hints

ORIENTATION

Knowing and ascertaining one's relation to self, to others, to time, and to one's surroundings

Person: Awareness of one's own identity and of individuals in the immediate environment

Place: Awareness of one's location, such as one's immediate surroundings, one's town or country

Time: Awareness of day, date, month, and year. Also, time management: ordering events in chronological sequence, allocating amounts of time to events and activities

Quantity: Activity involving numbers (counting) and other incremental problems

KNOWLEDGE REPRESENTATION

The mental representation of facts, objects, and skills

Mental Representation

Declarative: Recognition and understanding of factual information about objects, ideas, and events in the environment ("knowing that")

Procedural: Understanding and awareness of how to perform particular tasks or procedures ("knowing how")

Grouping

Categorization: The characterization of the relationship among objects, concepts, or thoughts

Sorting: Organizing objects, concepts, and thoughts into defined categories

Sequencing: Ordering objects or activities according to a set of rules

PROBLEM SOLVING

A process for which the goal is to overcome obstacles obstructing a path to a solution

Problem identification: Awareness of and definition of the problem

Judgment: Ability to make sound decisions, recognizing the consequences of decisions taken or actions performed

Decision making: Selecting a course of action from defined alternatives

Reasoning

Deductive: To draw a specific conclusion from a set of general propositions

Inductive: To reach a probable general conclusion on the basis of specific facts or observations

Planning: Anticipating events so as to formulate a course of action to achieve a desired outcome

Evaluation and iteration: Monitoring the status of the problem, evaluating if the goal has been achieved, and, if not, making another iteration of the problem-solving cycle

Transfer: The carryover of knowledge or skills from one context to another

LANGUAGE

A system of communicating objects, concepts, emotions, and thoughts through the systematic use of sounds, graphics, gestures, or other symbols

Data from Sternberg RJ: *Cognitive psychology*, ed 3, Belmont, Calif., 2003, Wadsworth.

of distractions is such that they are unable to focus on a task when another stimulus (e.g., a conversation) is occurring in the background. For example, individuals with attention deficit disorder have difficulty focusing on the teacher in class. There are other situations in which we are required to devote attention to two or more tasks at the same time using *divided attention.* One example is listening to a lecture and taking notes. Students need auditory attention and processing skills to understand what the teacher is saying, and additionally require visual and tactile skills to take notes. While the activities of listening to a lecture and taking notes appear to be concurrent, in fact attention is moving quickly between the two tasks.

Memory

Memory draws on past knowledge to use it in the present. *Short-term memory* refers to storage of information for up to about 20 seconds. Various strategies, such as rehearing the information to be remembered, can be used to maintain information in the short-term memory. For something to be remembered for a longer period of time, it is necessary for it to be transferred to *long-term memory.* In order for memory to be useful, the input must be perceived, recognized as something that is important to retain, encoded, stored, and then retrieved. Memory impairment can occur at any one of these parts of the process.

Two common ways of retrieving information from memory are *recall* and *recognition.* Free recall tasks provide virtually no hints at all, while cued recall tasks add in a small amount of information about the material the participant is supposed to recall.[50] *Recognition* tasks provide the target (material to be remembered) along with other material meant to distract the person; for example, recognition is often involved in multiple choice questions.

Orientation

A simple walk down the street during lunch hour provides an abundance of information about a noisy construction site, the smell of flowers, or the number of cars waiting at a stoplight. These things, as well as all the other information that we attend to on a constant basis, help us to orient ourselves. Orientation can be interpreted in different ways, depending on the perspective. To someone who works with an individual with a visual impairment, orientation means moving about the environment. For an individual with a cognitive impairment, the link to movement is not required, but it is often an important part of orientation. There are three types of orientation that are important: person, place and situation, and time.

Our awareness of our own identity and that of others in our environment is called *orientation to person.*[49] Orientation to person is commonly affected in disorders such as dementia and traumatic brain injury (TBI), where people forget not only who others are, but also who they are. A simple assistive technology that can aid orientation for a person is a card that lists the person's address and phone number, which can be presented to a passerby if they become lost.

We are constantly made aware of where we are and where we are going by paying attention to clues such as streets and landmarks, or by knowing that home lies east of where we are. More importantly, the ability to guide ourselves from point A to point B using these clues is called *orientation to place.*[49] Assistive technology way-finding devices can aid people who have orientation-to-place limitations.

Orientation to time is what permits us to know it is lunch time and that we can go on our daily walk.[49] For individuals who have difficulty reading standard clocks, there are assistive technologies that provide a sense of when events are to occur and the amount of time that must elapse before the event occurs. Orientation to time is broader than simply the time of day; often the question for an individual is "What day is it?" It also involves orientation to things such as time of year (e.g., certain holidays, which are cues for behaviors and activities).

Knowledge Representation

Knowledge representations help us relate to things, ideas, and events. The mental representation of facts (e.g., "gravity makes things fall"), objects (e.g., our house or car), and skills (e.g., how to wash our hands) is also related to memory. *Declarative memory* is what allows us to know what an object is (e.g., a ball). *Procedural memory* allows us to correctly remember a sequence of operations necessary for performance of a task or procedure (e.g., tying a shoe). Both of these can be important in the application of assistive devices to aid cognitive function.

Grouping like items together is important in representing knowledge. *Categorization* is the basis for ordering and organizing objects based on their characteristics and how they relate to each other. Categorizing of clothes could identify the type of clothing (e.g., socks, pants, or skirts) or the color or the style or many other features. Once we have decided on a set of categories, the objects, concepts, or thoughts can be organized into defined categories by *sorting,* the second step of organizing. If the objects, concepts, or thoughts to be organized have a numerical relationship, then the sorting task is called *sequencing* (i.e., placing the items in the correct numerical order). Sequencing could refer to the steps required to set the table, make a bed, or take a bus to work. Assistive technologies exist that can help individuals who have difficulty sequencing.

Problem Solving

Problem solving is the process of working through details of a problem to reach a solution. In the hierarchy of Box 10-1, the first step in problem solving is *identification of the problem.* If a person has difficulty identifying problems, various devices such as ones that prompt or cue may help.* *Judgment* is the ability to make sound decisions and recognize the consequences of decisions taken or actions performed. *Decision making* is the cognitive process of selecting a course of action from defined alternatives. Two types of *reasoning* are deductive reasoning and inductive reasoning. *Deductive* reasoning is a process by which an individual tries to draw a logically certain and specific conclusion from a set of general propositions. For example, when using an assistive device that requires touching a screen location (a button) to create an action, the statements "All buttons make something happen when you push them" and "This is a button" lead to the conclusion, "Something will happen if this button is pushed." *Inductive* reasoning is a process by which an individual tries to reach a probable general conclusion based on a set of specific facts or observations. This conclusion is likely to be true, based on past experience, but there is no guarantee that it will absolutely be true.[26] In assistive technology design the existence of various types of reasoning implies that the steps required for operation of a device must be logical and intuitive from the user's point of view, not just from the designer's point of view. For example, a navigational aid designed for someone with intellectual disabilities needs to present information via voice in simple direct commands (e.g., "go to the white building") rather than in more abstract general terms (e.g., "turn right 45 degrees and walk 20 meters, then turn right 30 degrees").

Planning is the process of anticipating future events so as to formulate a course of action to achieve a desired outcome. A person's ability to perform these tasks may be impacted by congenital conditions affecting brain development or by injury or disease. For these individuals, the best approach is often to reduce the number of alternative solutions, make the options clear, and reduce the reliance on anticipation of future consequences of decisions.

Once a problem solution has been derived, the next step in problem solving involves *confirming the successful conclusion of the task*. The problem solver must *evaluate* the outcome of his or her actions and determine whether the task has ended successfully, or whether it requires continuation or repetition (called *iteration*). **Generalization** is the carry-over of knowledge or skills from one kind of task or one particular context to another kind of task or another context. Knowledge is most likely to be generalized when the conditions under which the knowledge is to be used are very similar to those under which the knowledge was acquired.[26]

Language and Learning

Language is fundamental to cognitive task representation. Through language and the process of exchanging information, we can express our thoughts, needs, and ideas. *Language* is a method of communication and is composed of rules (grammar) and symbols, expressed by gestures, sounds, or writing. When teaching a skill or task, language is used to portray the desired outcome. *Learning* is the process by which knowledge, skills or attitudes are acquired and it can be attained through study, experience or teaching. In Figure 10-1 we have placed learning at the end of the hierarchy because we believe it builds upon the previously mentioned skills, like building blocks. *General learning* refers to the basic ability to acquire the knowledge, skills, or attitudes that are necessary for the more specific types of learning: *mathematics, reading,* and *writing*. The ability of someone to learn and comprehend in each of these categories helps define both the features the assistive technology must have as well as the skills the person needs in order to use it. Examples of AT for learning are discussed in Chapter 11.

*For example, the Independent Living Suite, Ablelink Technologies, Colorado Springs, Colo. (www.ablelinktech.com)

DISORDERS THAT MAY BENEFIT FROM COGNITIVE ASSISTIVE TECHNOLOGIES

Cognitive skills may be compromised as a consequence of a number of disorders. Congenital disorders (those present at birth) include intellectual or developmental disabilities (DD), learning disabilities (LD), attention deficit hyperactivity disorder (ADHD), and autism spectrum disorder (ASD). Acquired disorders that can lead to cognitive limitations include dementia, traumatic brain injury (TBI), and cerebral vascular accidents (CVAs). The characteristics of these disorders are summarized in Table 10-1.

There are other conditions that are typically thought of in terms of their motor limitations that may also have some cognitive involvement. Cerebral palsy (CP) is a primarily motor congenital disorder that may have a concurrent intellectual disability. In addition to the progressive motor limitations, multiple sclerosis (MS) may result in cognitive involvement and include behavior changes as the disease progresses. Aging is a physical process that limits motor function and also affects cognitive skills such as memory.

Congenital Disabilities

Intellectual Disabilities

Intellectual disability is typically defined as a disability where one has a below-average score on an intelligence or mental ability test as well as a limitation in functional skills.[47] These functional skills include (but are not limited to) communication, self-care, and social interaction. The terms *developmental disability, cognitive disability,* and *mental retardation* are often used to describe individuals with intellectual disabilities. Intellectual disability can range in severity from mild to severe.

Learning Disabilities

Learning disabilities (LD) are disorders in which one has near-normal mental abilities in general, but a deficit in the comprehension or use of spoken or written language. These disabilities may be manifested as a significant

TABLE 10-1 Disorders That May Benefit From Cognitive Assistive Technologies

Disorder	Incidence	Characteristics
Intellectual disability	8 individuals per 1000 (http://www.cdc.gov/mmwr/preview/mmwrhtml/00040023.htm)	Limitations in functional skills; impairments in memory, language use, communication, abstract conceptualization, generalization, and problem identification/problem solving[47]
Learning disability	2% of children	Significant difficulties in understanding or in using either spoken or written language; evident in problems with reading, writing, mathematical manipulation, listening, spelling, or speaking[19]
ADHD	4%[12] and 5% to 7% (www.adhd.com)	Typical capacity to learn and to use their skills confounded by factors that make it difficult to fully realize that potential; easily frustrated, have trouble paying attention, prone to daydreaming and moodiness; fidgety, disorganized, impulsive, disruptive, or aggressive[41] (www.adhdcanada.com)
ASD	1 child per 165, 25% exhibit intellectual disability, 4 times more prevalent in boys than girls[6]	Varying degrees of impairment in communication and social interaction skills or presence of restricted, repetitive, and stereotyped patterns of behavior
Dementia	0.5% to 1% (<65 years), 7% to 10% (65 to 75 years), 18% to 20% (75 to 85 years), 35% to 40% (>85 years)	(1) Decline of cognitive capacity with some effect on day-to-day functioning, (2) impairment in multiple areas of cognition (global), and (3) normal level of consciousness[39]
TBI	Mild: 131 per 100,000 Moderate: 15 per 100,000 Severe: 14 per 100,000 people (21 per 100,000 if prehospital deaths included)[17]	See Table 10-6
CVA	160 per 100,000 (overall), 1000 per 100,000 (age 50 to 65 years), 3000 per 100,000 (>80 years)[18]	Visual neglect, apraxia, aphasia, dysphagia, perceptual deficits, impaired alertness, attention disorders, memory disorders, impaired executive function, impaired judgment, impaired activities of daily living[38]

difficulty with reading, writing, reasoning, and/or mathematical ability. Because students with learning disabilities tend to perform poorly on standardized tests, it was long thought that learning disabilities were a mild form of intellectual disability. This assumption is untrue; learning disabilities can be thought of as a deficit in the processing and integration of information in an area (e.g., reading) as opposed to limitations in the basic ability in that specific area of learning. People with LD have typical age-related capacity in all areas. Table 10-2 lists abilities associated with learning disabilities. However, processing deficits lead to the problems in learning identified above.[27]

TABLE 10-2 Categorization of Abilities Associated with Learning Disabilities

Explicit Abilities	Implicit Abilities
Reading skills (dyslexia)	Visual or auditory discrimination
Mathematical skills (dyscalculia)	Visual or auditory closure
Writing skills (dyslexia, dysgraphia)	Visual or auditory figure-ground discrimination
Language skills (dysphasia)	Visual or auditory memory
Motor-learning skills (dyspraxia)	Visual or auditory sequencing
Social skills	Auditory association and comprehension
	Spatial perception
	Temporal perception

Attention Deficit Hyperactivity Disorder (ADHD)

Attention Deficit Hyperactivity Disorder (ADHD) is defined as a pattern of inattention, hyperactivity, and/or impulsivity that is more frequent or severe than for typical people of a given age (http://www.nimh.nih.gov/health/publications/attention-deficit-hyperactivity-disorder/complete-index.shtml). The delay aversion hypothesis of ADHD posits that the ADHD child distracts himself from the passing of time when he is not in control, which explains daydreaming, inattention, and fidgeting.[41]

Children (and adults) with ADHD have a normal capacity to learn and to utilize their skills, but suffer from confounding factors that make it difficult to fully realize that potential.[41] Particularly, those with ADHD can be easily frustrated; have trouble paying attention; are prone to daydreaming and moodiness; and are fidgety, disorganized, impulsive, disruptive, and/or aggressive (www.adhdcanada.com).

Autism Spectrum Disorder (ASD)

Autism Spectrum Disorder (ASD) is a developmental disorder that is characterized by varying degrees of impairment in communication and social interaction skills, or the presence of restricted, repetitive, and stereotyped patterns of behavior. A commonly used definition for autism is that of the Diagnostic and Statistical Manual of Mental Disorders – Fourth Edition (DSM-IV),[1] which classifies autism as a *pervasive developmental disorder (PDD)*. As the term implies, this disorder covers a wide spectrum of conditions, with individual differences in the number and kinds of symptoms, levels of severity, age of onset, and limitations with social interaction. Major subtypes of ASD include *Autistic Disorder, Asperger Syndrome, Rett Syndrome, Childhood Disintegrative Disorders,* and *Pervasive Developmental Disorder Not Otherwise Specified (PDD-NOS)*.

Individuals with ASD typically demonstrate deficits in communication skills, including delay in, or total lack of, spoken language and *spontaneous speech*; unusual speaking patterns (e.g., *echolalia* or idiosyncratic language); and underdeveloped social interaction skills (including problems interpreting facial expressions, gestures, and intonation while interacting with other people). They might also seem evasive, avoid eye contact, and appear to lack initiation and the desire to share joy or interest. Children with ASD also have inflexible adherence to specific routines and demonstrate unusual persistence and intense focus on a specific subject or activity. Many children with ASD have unusual (hypersensitive or hyposensitive) responses to sensory information, which could lead to the lack of response or an aversive response to sensory input.

Individuals with ASD also have strengths and unique abilities. For example, some individuals with ASD have unusually good spatial perception and visual recall, have an accurate and detailed memory for information and facts, are able to concentrate for long periods of time on particular task or subjects, and are more attentive to details than most other people. These abilities may allow them to excel in music, science, math, physics, and other specialized areas.

Acquired Disabilities

Dementia

The word *dementia* comes from the Latin *de mens* which means "from the mind." **Dementia** is best defined as a syndrome, or a pattern of clinical symptoms and signs, which can be defined by the following three points: (1) a decline of cognitive capacity with some effect on day-to-day functioning; (2) impairment in multiple areas of cognition (global); and (3) a normal level of consciousness.[39] Dementia is distinguished from congenital cognitive disorders (such as intellectual disability, learning disabilities, etc.) by its age of onset and its degenerative component. It is also important to note that although it affects multiple areas of cognition, not all areas are affected.

Rabins, Lyketsos, and Steele (2006)[39] define the "Three pillars of dementia care." The first is to treat the disease, which helps identify current needs as well as future necessities as the disorder progresses. The second is treatment of the symptoms. By treating the symptoms, the patient's quality of life will improve in the cognitive, functional, and behavioral domains. Medications and technology are the two main ways to accomplish this task. Third, patient support is important and leads to ensuring that the patient's needs are met and the quality of life is improved as much as possible.

Traumatic Brain Injury (TBI)

People who experience a **traumatic brain injury (TBI)** often lose significant cognitive function. A TBI may occur when the head or brain is struck by an external force, such as from a fall, a gunshot wound, or a motor vehicle accident (Table 10-3). The extent of the trauma to the brain, and not the injury itself, is the determining factor in diagnosing TBI. For instance, it is possible to incur TBI as the result of both open-head injuries (the brain is exposed to air) and closed-head injuries (no brain exposure). The effect of a TBI on an individual's cognitive ability varies from case to case, in terms of both severity and the set of skills affected.

Not all head injuries give rise to TBI, and there is an accepted scale for diagnosing such an injury. One tool available to assist with diagnosis is the Glasgow Coma Scale (GCS), a rating system used for describing the severity of a coma.[17] The Glasgow Coma Scale ranks comas on a scale of from 3 (most severe) to 15 (mildest) in the eye response, verbal response, and motor response categories. A score on the GCS of 12 or higher is a mild brain injury, and below 8 is considered a severe injury.[17]

If the GCS does not indicate TBI, one of the following two criteria must be satisfied for a TBI diagnosis: either the patient has amnesia from the traumatic event, or the patient has a documented loss of consciousness. It is common to have a *recovery period* following the injury. This recovery usually plateaus within 12 months post-injury, and the extent of recovery is both variable and unpredictable.[9]

TABLE 10-3 Data on Causes of Traumatic Brain Injury (Injury Control Research Center)

Cause	Percentage of Total
Motor vehicle crashes	64%
Gunshot wounds	13%
Falls	11%
Assault	8%
Pedestrian	3%
Sports	1%

Data from TBI Inform, June, 2000. Published by the UAB-TBIMS, Birmingham, AL. © 2000 Board of Trustees, University of Alabama, http://main.uab.edu/tbi/show.asp?durki=27492&site=2988&return=57898#cause.

TABLE 10-4 Return to Prior Activities

	Student	Employed	Home	Retired	Unemployed
Onset	11%	57%	1%	11%	21%
6 months	7%	17%	None	10%	67%
12 months	7%	26%	None	8%	57%

Data from IRCR Study, 1999, http://www.neuroskills.com/whattoexpect.shtml.

A good measure of the extent of a TBI patient's recovery is his or her return to the preinjury activities of daily living. Two main recovery indicators are the return to work and the return to driving, both important tasks for independent living. Data on returning to work are summarized in Table 10-4, and similar data for returning to driving are shown in Table 10-5.[37] In both cases, very little improvement was observed beyond 12 months post-injury.

Typical cognitive and behavioral difficulties that a person with TBI may encounter are listed in Table 10-6.[37,40] Two areas of importance are memory and language skills, as these may benefit from intervention with assistive technology.

TABLE 10-5 Return to Driving

	PERCENT RETURN TO DRIVING		
	No	Partially	Yes
6 months	69%	13%	19%
12 months	60%	10%	30%

Data from ICRC study, 1999, http://www.neuroskills.com/whattoexpect.shtml.

TABLE 10-6 List of Typical Cognitive and Behavioral Difficulties after TBI

Type of Difficulty	Examples
Cognitive	Processing of visual or auditory information Disrupted attention and concentration Language problems (i.e., aphasia) Difficulty storing and retrieving new memories Poor reasoning, judgment, and problem solving skills Difficulty learning new information
Behavioral	Restlessness and agitation Emotional lability and irritability Confabulation Diminished insight Socially inappropriate behavior Poor initiation Lack of emotional response Projecting blame on others Depression Anxiety

Stroke

A *stroke,* or **cerebral vascular accident (CVA)**, is an incidence of irregular blood flow within the brain causing an interruption in brain function. A stroke may arise from a lack of blood flow to the brain (known as an *ischemic stroke*) or from ruptured blood vessels in the brain (a *hemorrhagic stroke*).[25] The neurological damage incurred as the result of a stroke produces symptoms that directly correspond to the injured area within the brain.[38] A CVA causes acute damage to the brain; there are no degenerative effects after the onset of injury. As with TBI, persons who have sustained a stroke often have a recovery period where portions of the brain learn to compensate for damaged areas. Typical cognitive and behavioral difficulties associated with stroke are shown in Table 10-7. Most recovery (as observed by the return to activities of daily living) occurs within 6 months after onset.[8] The majority of persons with CVA are able to return home following their initial hospitalization period. A summary of discharge locations following hospitalization for stroke is shown in Table 10-8. These data suggest that the number of people returning home following a CVA is increasing, which might be attributed to improvements to hospital

TABLE 10-7 List of Typical Cognitive and Behavioral Difficulties after Stroke

Type of Difficulty	Examples
Cognitive	Visual neglect, hemianopsia Apraxia Language problems (i.e., aphasia, dysarthria) Perceptual deficits (i.e., figure-ground impairment, disorientation) Impaired alertness, attention disorders Memory problems, both short-term and long-term Perseveration Decreased executive function
Behavioral	Impaired judgment Impulsiveness Emotional lability Confabulation Poor initiation Mood alterations Depression

TABLE 10-8 Discharge Data for Stroke from the Canadian Heart and Stroke Foundation

Discharge Destination	1993	1999
Home	33%	56%
Inpatient rehabilitation	41%	32%
Nursing home or long-term care	26%	11%

Data from Heart and Stroke Foundation of Canada. Stroke statistics: http://ww2.heartandstroke.ca/Page.asp?PageID=33&ArticleID=428&Src=stroke&From=SubCategory/. Accessed April 16, 2005.

care at the onset of stroke. Children may have a more pronounced recovery than adults, as their brains have a greater degree of plasticity. Also, women may display greater recovery of lost language skill than men, as the language centers of the brain are larger in women than in men.[8]

COGNITIVE SKILLS RELATED TO SPECIFIC DISORDERS

Figure 10-2 relates the disorders described in Table 10-1 to the cognitive skills described in Box 10-1. Items marked with an *X* are the skills that may be limited or absent in the corresponding disorder. The cognitive skills are roughly arranged such that, moving from left to right in Figure 10-2, the skills build on each other. This figure illustrates *possible* skills that may be affected for a person with a specific disorder, but each case must be considered to determine specific impacts for a given individual. Most of the disorders and disabilities that have cognitive implications are quite variable from individual to individual, and not all of the possible limitations included in Figure 10-2 will necessarily exist for any specific person. The listed cognitive skills are judged to be those that may be aided or replaced through the use of assistive technologies. Figure 10-2 can serve as a checklist to ensure that all of the skills that might be affected and aided by assistive technologies are identified.

ADDRESSING COGNITIVE NEEDS THROUGH ASSISTIVE TECHNOLOGIES

Assistive technologies are being applied to meet the needs of individuals with a wide range of cognitive problems. These applications vary by the type and severity of the cognitive limitations faced by the individual. In this section we first discuss aspects of AT application specific to three broad categories of cognitive need: congenital disabilities categorized as mild; congenital disabilities categorized as moderate to severe; and acquired cognitive disabilities. Both the general characteristics of cognitive assistive technologies and technologies designed to meet specific needs are described.

			ID	LD	ADHD	ASD	DEMENTA	TBI	CVA
Perception				X		X		X	X
Attention	Signal Detection	Vigilance			X			X	X
		Search			X	X		X	X
	Selective				X		X	X	X
	Divided				X	X	X	X	X
Memory	Encoding						X	X	X
	Storage	Short Term		X	X		X	X	X
		Long Term					X	X	X
	Retrieval	Recognition					X	X	X
		Recall					X	X	X
Orientation	Place			X		X		X	X
	Time			X		X	X	X	X
	Person			X			X	X	X
	Quantitative			X		X		X	X
Knowledge Representation and Organization	Mental Representations	Declarative/know what				X	X	X	X
		Procedural/know how				X	X	X	X
	Grouping	Categorization				X		X	X
		Sorting				X		X	X
		Sequencing				X		X	X
Problem Solving	Identify Problem					X		X	X
	Judgment			X	X	X	X	X	X
	Decision Making			X	X	X		X	X
	Reasoning	Deductive				X	X	X	X
		Inductive				X	X	X	X
	Planning					X		X	X
	Evaluation and Iteration					X	X	X	X
	Transfer/Generalization					X		X	X
Language						X		X	X
Learning	General			X		X		X	X
	Mathematics			X		X		X	X
	Reading			X		X		X	X
	Writing			X		X		X	X

Figure 10-2 Skills versus disorder matrix. *ID,* intellectual disability; *LD,* learning disability; *ADHD,* attention deficit hyperactivity disorder; *ASD,* autism spectrum disorder; *TBI,* traumatic brain injury; *CVA,* cardiovascular accident (stroke).

Considerations for Individuals with Mild Cognitive Disabilities

Individuals with **mild cognitive disabilities** have needs that are more subtle and harder to define than in the case of physical disabilities or more severe cognitive disabilities. For example, learning disabilities typically involve significant challenges in understanding and/or using either spoken or written language or both, which may be evident in problems with reading, writing, mathematical manipulation, listening, spelling, or speaking.[19] While there are assistive technologies that are specifically designed to address these areas (discussed later in this chapter), many of the technological tools are useful for all students and are part of existing instructional technology.[4] Even the identified assistive technologies (e.g., multimedia, synthetic speech output, and voice recognition input) have features that are useful to all learners.

In Chapter 1, we distinguish between educational technologies (or instructional technologies) and assistive technologies. This distinction works well for sensory and motor assistive technologies. The distinction is much more blurred for cognitive assistive technologies.[4,19] For example, some spell checkers, word prediction programs, and talking word processors have been specifically designed for individuals with learning disabilities.* We discuss these programs later in this chapter. As Ashton points out, each of these technologies is potentially useful to all students, not just those with learning disabilities.[4] In that sense they are educational or instructional technologies. The issues surrounding assistive technologies and competency are described in Box 10-2.

BOX 10-2 Compensation vs. Remediation

What constitutes independence?

Do we care how the function is accomplished as long as the activity can be satisfactorily completed?

Sensory or motor disabilities: Questions such as how much energy it takes to walk vs. use a powered wheelchair for someone with severe cerebral palsy are matters of personal choice.

Cognitive disabilities: Should a child in our example be required to learn the presidents' names (remediation) or be allowed to use an assistive technology (e.g., Ask Jeeves) as a compensatory tool, and why is its use considered "cheating" by some educators and parents?[19]

The role of time:

- In community settings time is not as critical (e.g., allowing additional time for an individual who is blind to cross the street using a long cane is an accepted part of human performance).
- In vocational settings, completion time for a task also varies from individual to individual and is acceptable within wide limits.
- Why, then, in educational contexts is time fixed (e.g., for an exam) and accomplishment variable?[19]
- Restricting time, learning activities, instructional approaches, and other classroom variables to a "one-size-fits-all" constraint in educational settings means that high standards of performance cannot be achieved. (Edyburn, 2005)[19]
- While many students with special needs are given extra time to complete an exam, the level of competence they achieve is still variable and time (even expanded time) is fixed.
- If achievement were to be fixed, then each student would be allowed as much time as necessary to complete the task.
- If uniformly high performance and preparation for later vocational success are the goals, then compensation, using both hard and soft assistive technologies, must be as much an alternative for individuals with mild cognitive disabilities as it is for their counterparts with motor, sensory, or communication disabilities.
- Time considerations can also apply in other rehabilitation settings. For example, if caregivers/teachers/CNAs intervene to speed up a task (such as dressing or feeding) due to time limitations, it can decrease the individual's independence, confidence, and self-esteem and increase the learned helplessness cycle.

Considerations for Individuals with Moderate to Severe Cognitive Disabilities

One method of characterizing assistive technology applications for individuals who have intellectual disabilities is based on the specific type of cognitive impairment exhibited. Some examples of specific impairments are: memory, language use and communication, abstract conceptualization, generalization, and problem identification/problem solving.[47] General assistive technology characteristics that address these impairments include simplicity of operation; capacity of the technology to support repetition; consistency in presentation and use; and inclusion of multiple modalities (e.g., speech, sounds, and graphical representations). Wehmeyer, Smith, and Davies (2005)[47] discuss assistive technology characteristics and approaches for each of these impairments. Research studies related to the use of assistive technologies with individuals who have intellectual disabilities are shown in Box 10-3.

Granlund, Bond, Linstrom, and Wennberg (1995)[23] take a different approach and define five content areas for technological assistance to individuals who have moderate to severe intellectual disabilities. The five content areas, based on cognitive structures, are:

1. Quality (What is this?)
2. Causal patterns (Why? And if so?)
3. Space (Where?)
4. Quantity (How much? How big?)
5. Time (When? Duration?)

Within these content areas individuals with intellectual disabilities typically have difficulties in organization and reorganization, performing operations with cognitive structures, and symbolic representation. Within these content areas adults with cognitive disabilities may encounter problems in activities such as: choosing a leisure activity, using public transportation, being on time for work, and

*Co:Writer and Write:OutLoud, Don Johnston, Inc., Volo, Ill. (www.donjohnston.com)

BOX 10-3 What the Research Says: AT for Intellectual Disabilities

PDA PROMPTING AND DECISION MAKING SUPPORT[15]

A pilot study* with a PDA-based device* using graphic and audio prompts to guide the user through a decision-making process.

Decision points are identified with picture and audio labels.

User can move through the sequence of instructions using a touch screen on the beginning with START and then NEXT after each step is completed.

Forty participants who had intellectual disabilities participated in an activity to package different pieces of software using a sequence of prompted steps.

Participants using the device made fewer errors performing the task, fewer errors in decision points, and less assistance was required using the PDA than when they had only a job coach.

Conclusion: that technology can significantly assist persons with intellectual disabilities in accomplishing relatively complicated work-related tasks independently.

PDA-BASED TIME MANAGEMENT AND SCHEDULING SYSTEM[15;†]

Designed for individuals who have intellectual disabilities.

Schedule of daily events entered into the Schedule Assistant by care provider.

12 participants with intellectual disabilities completed an 8-item schedule using the Schedule Assistant and a traditional written schedule.

Device provided visual and auditory prompts corresponding to the appropriate time for entered events.

Results showed that participants required significantly less assistance when using the Schedule Assistant than with the written instructions.

The study concluded that electronic scheduling and prompting systems have value for individuals who have intellectual disabilities.

WEB BROWSING[13]

Twelve participants evaluated a specially designed Web browser (Web Trek)‡ compared with a standard browser.§

Three tasks: searching for Web sites, saving Web sites to a favorites list, and retrieving sites from the favorites list.

Three measures of performance: independence (fewer prompts), accuracy (errors made), and task completion (completed with 3 or fewer prompts).

All three measures showed statistically significant differences favoring the Web Trek browser, indicating that Internet access for persons with intellectual disabilities is feasible.

*Pocket Compass, AbleLink technologies, Colorado Springs, Colo. (http://www.ablelinktech.com/_handhelds/pocketcompass.asp)
†Schedule Assistant, AbleLink Technologies (www.ablelinktech.com/_handhelds/scheduleassistant.asp)
‡Web Trek, AbleLink technologies, Colorado Springs, Colo. (www.ablelinktech.com/_desktop/webtrek.asp)
§Internet Explorer, Microsoft, Inc., Redmond, Wash. (www.microsoft.com)

preparing meals. Typical evaluation questions and assistive technology examples for each content area are listed in Table 10-9.

Wehmeyer, Smith, Palmer, Davies, and Stock (2004)[48] described eight primary factors of cognitive ability: (1) language, (2) reasoning, (3) memory and learning, (4) visual perception, (5) auditory perception, (6) idea production, (7) cognitive speed, and (8) knowledge and achievement. They argue that the promise of technology for aiding individuals with intellectual disabilities lies in enhancing human capacity in these areas rather than in compensating for deficits. An important element in this approach is the application of the principles of universal design (see Chapter 1) to ensure that mainstream technologies are designed in such a way that individuals with a range of intellectual abilities can access them. The design of the human-technology interface (see Chapter 2) in the HAAT model is an example of the difference between a

TABLE 10-9 Assessment Questions and Assistive Technology Examples

Content Area	Typical Assessment Questions	Examples of Applicable Assistive Technology
Quality	How does person classify objects? Are one, two, or more dimensions used?	Sorting jigs, graphic symbol labels for categories
Causal patterns	How many steps in a process or chain can be understood? Can outcomes of accomplishing a task in different ways be compared?	Sequencing jigs, PDA-based prompting and cueing
Space	Can the person find his or her way with a map? Does he or she use shortcuts? Can he or she ask directions?	Paper maps, dynamic display on GPS, or PDA with speech output
Quantity	How is money handled? Is conservation of volume present?	Money-sorting jigs, matching task rather than counting, parts-counting jigs
Time	Can a watch be used? Is the duration of an activity or waiting period understood?	Quarter hour watch, electronic pocket calendars with reminders, PDA with reminder and voice output

From Granlund M et al: Assistive technology for cognitive disability, *Technol Disabil* 4:205–214, 1995.

compensation approach and the concept of enhancement of the technology characteristics to make it more accessible. If an individual with an intellectual disability has difficulty accessing a screen because of language problems (e.g., reading), a compensatory approach is to provide auditory output instead of text, avoiding the necessity for reading. If the problem is too much clutter on the display, then the best approach may be to simplify the display (i.e., enhance it) so that the information is more accessible. For individuals with intellectual disabilities, Wehmeyer et al. presented a thorough literature review of approaches that have been taken to enhance performance in each of the eight cognitive factors.[48]

Considerations for Individuals with Acquired Disabilities

Individuals with acquired cognitive disabilities due to injury (e.g., traumatic brain injury) or disease (e.g., stroke [CVA] or dementia) retain a wide variety of cognitive skills. The majority of assistive technologies and strategies that have been used to aid persons with acquired cognitive disabilities are designed to compensate for deficits by building on remaining strengths.[32] Collective technologies and strategies that help a person with cognitive deficits function more independently in certain tasks have been called *assistive technology for cognition* (ATC) or **cognitive prosthesis.**[11,32] An ATC or cognitive prosthesis is an entire system of hardware, software, and personal assistance that is individualized to meet specific needs. As the HAAT model (see Chapter 2) implies, a cognitive prosthesis includes a custom-designed computer-based compensatory strategy that directly assists in performing daily activities.* It may also include additional technologies such as a cell phone, pager, or digital camera or low tech approaches.

Characteristics of Cognitive Assistive Technologies†

In order to be useful to people who have cognitive disabilities, technologies must be accessible. Accessibility in this case means that complexity is reduced, multiple modes of presentation of choices are available, and operation is consistent with the cognitive skills of the potential user. To achieve this level of accessibility, commercial developers of technology must incorporate cognitive accessibility into their products by utilizing universal design principles (see Chapter 1). Support tools and services must also be developed to ensure they can be used by as wide a range of users with cognitive disabilities as possible. Currently, this level of cognitive accessibility is rarely achieved for mainstream technologies; instead, individuals who have cognitive disabilities must rely on specially designed assistive technologies to meet their needs.

Categories of assistive technologies for cognitive assistance are listed in Table 10-10. This categorization

*Institute for Cognitive Prosthetics (http://www.brain-rehab.com/definecp.htm)

†Dan Davies of AbleLink Technologies, Inc., provided significant insight to this section.

TABLE 10-10 Categories of Assistive Technologies to Aid Cognitive Function

AT Category	Needs Served	Examples:
Memory aids	Augment or replace the primary memory functions.	Recording/playback, word completion/prediction, information retrieval.
Time management	Planning, prioritizing, and execution of daily and time-dependent tasks.	Alternative formats, reminders, schedulers. Some prompt visually or auditorily as well as alarm for reminder.
Prompting/cueing	Guidance for procedural or navigational sequencing of tasks.	Auditory (verbal and sounds), visual (pictures or drawings), or word-based. Can be customized for individual tasks. May use other data such as GPS location.
Stimuli control	Address attention or perception problems by limiting or manipulating the information presented to the user.	Noise reduction techniques, visual field manipulation, and media presentation techniques.
Language tools	Assist with writing.	Word completion/prediction, spell checking, concept mapping.
Alternative input	Assist with reading.	Voice recognition software, simplified user interface, and desktop.
Alternative output	Assist with reading and writing.	Synthesized or digitized speech output; graphic alternatives to text; e-books; variation in font size, background/foreground color combinations, contrast, and spacing between words, letters, and paragraphs.
Tracking and identification	Safety for users that might not have the cognitive skills required to work their way out of problematic situations.	Wearable electronic monitoring devices, home monitoring systems.

is similar to that used by others.[7,11,19,23,32,33,37,38] Specific needs served by the type of assistive technology and examples of specific devices are also shown in Table 10-10 for each category. Some devices fit in more than one category. For example, time management requires memory, and prompting can have a temporal element if sequencing of tasks is required.

Many of the functions included in mainstream technologies such as mobile phones and computers are as useful to individuals with cognitive disabilities as to those without cognitive disabilities. Specific functions of mainstream technologies that are important to all users, including those who have cognitive disabilities, support activities of productivity, leisure, and self-care (i.e., communicate, remember schedules, learn new information, listen to music, access online information and services, etc.). For someone who has a cognitive disability, these features may be even more important because the individual depends on them to carry out independent daily activities.

Mainstream technologies can be complex to use. Specially designed cognitive support technologies have been developed to compensate for cognitive limitations when the mainstream options that are available are too complex to operate. Different applications for the same person could use the same technology device, and there could be further confusion for the person with a cognitive disability. For example, PDAs, mobile phones, pad computers, and other mainstream devices have been programmed to function as augmentative communication devices (see Chapter 11) and as cognitive assists. Many applications utilize as their input method either a touch screen or small keyboard, and they both have an output of either speech or visual characters and text. As these two diverse applications illustrate, these are superficial features that may be operated in many different ways. The surface features of the two applications may appear to be identical, and indeed the same device could be used for both applications with a change in software. However, the function will be very different because of the characteristics of the software loaded into the device. If the user attends only to the existence of the input and output features and the size, color, and shape of the device, then some of the operational parameters of the device may not be understood.

For individuals who have cognitive disability to effectively use the technology (either mainstream technology or specialized AT), the technology must have been made cognitively accessible. However, the availability of accessible technology alone is only the starting place for success. Success is dependent on the availability of soft technologies (see Chapter 1), including the effective selection, training, implementation, and recalibration of technology solutions provided by support individuals. Support can come from a wide variety of individuals (and usually multiple individuals) that are part of the life of individuals with cognitive disabilities, including OTAs, PTAs, speech assistants, parents, teachers, living skills counselors, home health care providers, friends, and other family members. These individuals typically represent a wide range of knowledge and experience in using technology with individuals with disabilities. However, unlike some categories of rehabilitation technology that have been around for several decades (AAC, vision products, etc.), most of the technology that is considered "cognitively" accessible is less than a decade old. Therefore there is often a lot of new learning necessary on the part of all individuals, regardless of their knowledge of other areas of assistive technology. Tips for supporting people who use cognitive assistive technologies are listed in Box 10-4.

BOX 10-4 Tips for Supporting Individuals Who Have Cognitive Needs

Dan Davies, President of AbleLink Technologies, a developer of cognitive technologies, provided these tips that address some of the issues that are particularly important for individuals, such as caregivers, siblings, parents, or spouses, who are responsible for supporting assistive technology application:

- Start small. Individuals with cognitive disabilities, as well as caregivers, can easily become overwhelmed by technology. It is best to identify the most important needs an individual has for the technology, and begin with meeting one of those needs. When the individual becomes comfortable with the use of the technology and experiences success with using it, then addressing another need with the technology can be added.
- Understand the different user settings that can be changed to simplify the program to meet a particular individual's needs. Then start the individual with the interface that best meets his or her current need for support. Well-designed cognitive support technology will provide the ability to modify the user interface for different individuals to ensure that the interface is not cluttered with buttons and other program options that the individual will not be using.
- Talk with others that have used cognitive support technology. The nature of cognitive technology is that it can be often be used in many different ways to help people with cognitive disabilities, even ways not envisioned by the developer of the technology. It is good to learn from others, such as through online communities, and contribute as well so others can learn from your experiences.
- Cognitive technologies are usually not designed as "out of the box" solutions that are "one size fits all." Good cognitive technologies are usually best applied by adding content that is appropriate for the individual. For example, the best task prompting systems come with

(Continued)

BOX 10-4 Tips for Supporting Individuals Who Have Cognitive Needs—cont'd

authoring tools to allow the caregiver to create a task that meets the specific needs of the individual they are serving, such as specific instructions for how to do his or her laundry. Generic instructions for performing activities of daily living are rarely useful for individuals with cognitive disabilities, other than for a general orientation to the task. Actually performing the task independently will often require customized steps with pictures of the individual's own washer and dryer (for example), and audio instructions designed for the cognitive level of the individual. Sometimes task libraries may be available (e.g., www.aimsxml.com) where previously created tasks can be downloaded and then customized with new pictures and audio files to make the downloaded task meet the needs of the particular individual. To get the most benefit out of cognitive technologies, it is very important to make full use of the ability to customize the relevant content to meet the unique needs of the individual with the cognitive disability. The time spent in creating custom content is well worth it given that the individual will then be able to do many things that they have been dependent on others for in the past.

- Use cognitive technology to help learn how to use cognitive technology. One of the unique benefits of cognitive support technology is that it can be used to provide very easy-to-follow instructions for using the technology itself.*

(Courtesy of Dan Davies, AbleLink Technologies)

*For example the Learning Library (http://trainer.aimsxml.com/) from AbleLink Technologies is a cognitively accessible Web-based training system using step-by-step prompting technology to provide picture, audio, and video-based instructions for how to use cognitive support technologies. See text for more information.

Assistive Technologies to Aid Cognitive Function

Memory Aids

Memory aids are those devices or software packages that augment or replace the primary memory functions. These devices can be subdivided into three categories based on their primary function: recording, word completion/prediction, and information retrieval. Recorders are devices that address storage of information to aid either short- or long-term memory loss. Stored information can be retrieved at a later time to aid in the recall of facts or appointments. Devices that record voice information as short memos are the most common in this category. Voice memo recording is often built into Personal Digital Assistants (PDAs), cell phones, and small digital recorders.

Reminding people to take their medication is one of the main uses of memory assistance technologies. Low tech medication reminders (i.e., boxes with seven or more compartments labeled by the day and/or type of medication), have been in widespread use for many years. However, these devices do not alert the person that it is time for the medication. If an alert is needed, then electronic medication reminders are required.[34] A watch-based medication reminder such as the Cadex Medication Reminder Watch* provides up to 12 daily reminders that have an audible alarm and a display of the required medication. While this format is convenient due to its small size, it has a small display and limited memory. Pagers and cell phones are also used as medication reminders with dosage, type of medication, and instructions provided via text messaging from a central service. Software for PDAs† provides medication alerts with detailed information regarding pill type and dosage, a medication log, refill reminders, and emergency information .[34]

*Cadex Medication Reminder Watch (http://www.cadexwatch.com/)
†For Example: On-Time-Rx for Palm OS (www.ontimerx.com)

Word completion and prediction solutions are software packages that rely on recognition memory to aid word finding during written communication. When a letter or series of letters are entered, a list of words is presented that begins with that set of letters. The user then chooses from the list using recognition memory skills. Word completion and prediction is also used to speed up time to input text, or to reduce the number of required keystrokes for individuals with motor limitations (see Chapter 5).

AT for Time Management

Time management technologies are those devices that aid in the planning, prioritizing, and execution of daily and time-dependent tasks. One class of devices uses an alternative format for representing time to make it more accessible to individuals with intellectual disability. One example is the Quarter Hour Watch* (Figure 10-3), which offers an alternative and potentially more intuitive representation of the passage of time.[23] The Quarter Hour

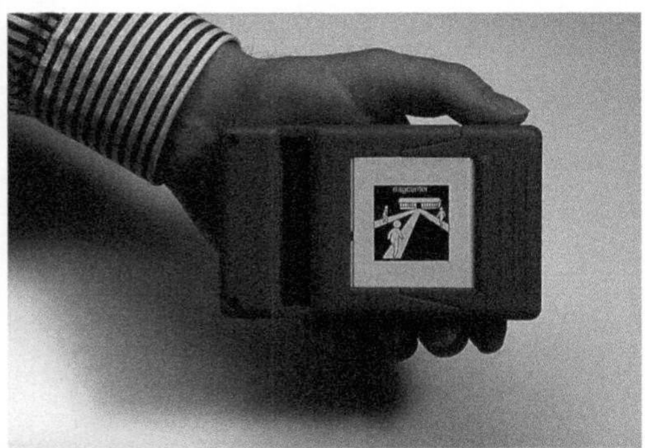

Figure 10-3 The Quarter Hour Watch. (Courtesy Zygo Industries© GEWA, AB, Portland, Ore., www.zygo-usa.com.)

*Made by Handitek AB, Sweden. Available from Zygo Industries, Fremont, California, (www.zygo-usa.com)

Watch uses an entirely different concept of time by presenting a two-hour time frame in 8 one-quarter-hour steps. Rather than clock hands or numbers, the watch display has 8 dots, one for each quarter hour up to two hours. The user of the watch must understand elapsed time rather than absolute time based on standard clocks. Events are represented by pictures on plastic chips (about 2 inches square) that are placed into the Quarter Hour Watch. A care provider sets the time of the event on the back of the plastic chip that is read by the watch. The front of the chip has a picture or symbol representing the upcoming event. When the chip is inserted into the watch, the display indicates how much time remains until the event should occur. If the time to the event is greater than two hours, then all 8 dots are dark. After each quarter hour, one dot turns from dark to light until they are all light. At that time a signal sounds and the dots flash. The individual using the watch chooses the chip (e.g., time for favorite TV program, or time to go to work) and then is able to tell when that time has arrived.

The 24-hour Electronic Time Panel,* (Figure 10-4) is a planning board or day planner that uses a lighted display on the one side with increments of 15 minutes from 7:00 AM to 11:00 PM. Like the Quarter Hour Watch, this device facilitates the sequencing and organization of an individual's tasks and events for a given period of time, and it helps teach concepts such as understanding units of time (e.g., "How long is an hour?") and elapsed time (e.g., "Why can't I have lunch now?"). It can also help individuals to independently answer daily life questions (e.g., "Do I have time to eat before the bus comes?" or "How long until we go swimming?"). A similar column of lights on the other side of the panel shows the times from 11:00 PM until 7:00 AM. The time slot adjacent to each light can be labeled with an activity using text, pictures, or other symbols. The current time is represented either by a column of lights starting with the current time and proceeding in 15 minute intervals, or by a single dot of light. The time until a desired activity is indicated by the length of the column of lights from the present time to the start time of the event. Alarms can be set for each 15-minute increment. The Electronic Time Panel can be used in an individual living arrangement, a group living setting, or a classroom.

*Saltillo (https://www.saltillo.com/shop/catalog/product_info.php?cPath=22&products_id=74)

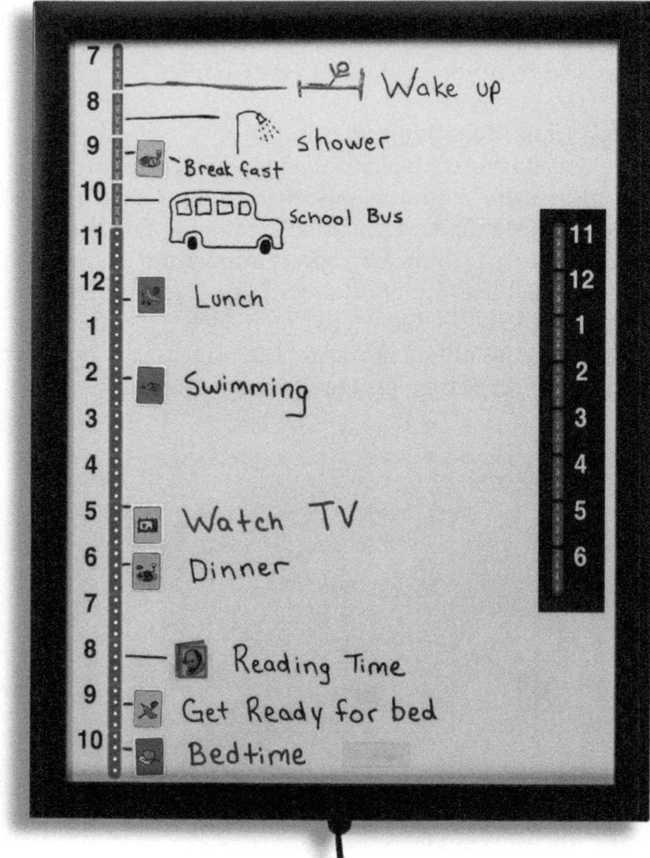

Figure 10-4 The 24-hour Electronic Time Panel. (Courtesy Saltillo, www.saltillo.com.)

The MEMOdayplan* (Figure 10-5) is a device that reminds a user when a given, preprogrammed task or event is scheduled to occur. This device was designed for people with ADD, ADHD, LD, chronic diseases, stroke, or brain injury. A silent, vibrating reminder system or beeping alert with 30 programmable alarms is included with both a training and a reminder mode. The reminder mode is for remembering specific tasks such as taking medication and doing homework or chores. The training mode is for behavior change and self-monitoring. Box 10-5 shows preset messages for the WatchMinder2. This device can also be programmed with three personalized messages. The WatchMinder2 has two possible schedule modes: *fixed* (every 2, 3, 5, 10, 15, 20, 30, 45, or 60 minutes) or random (the CPU randomly chooses from 2, 3, 5, 10, 15, 30, and 60 minutes). The person programming the device chooses one of these modes and the daily start (S) time and end (E) time.

*Abilia Products, Sweden, (http://www.abilia.org.uk/produkter/index.aspx?intshopcmd=&group=1306&prod=1517)

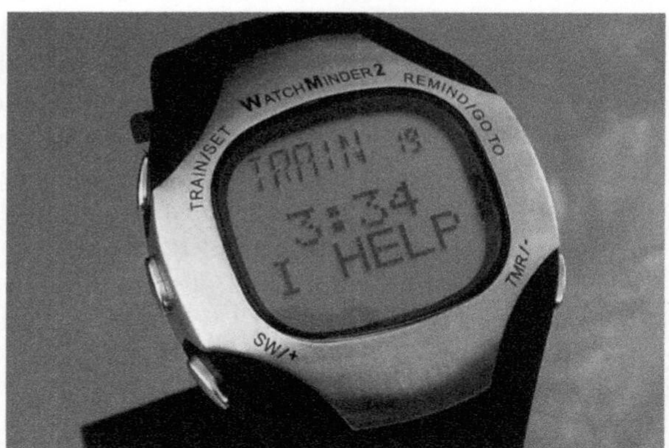

Figure 10-5 Watchminder. (Courtesy WatchMinder, Irvine, Calif., http://watchminder.com/.)

BOX 10-5 Examples of WatchMinder2 Preset Messages:*

BATHRM (bathroom)
BE POS (be positive)
BREATH (breathe)
COUGH
FOLDIR (follow directions)
FOLRUL (follow rules)
GIVPOS (give positive reinforcement)
GOODJB (good job)
HANDUP (raise hand)
IGNORE
POSIMG (positive image)
POSTUR (posture)
PRAY
PYATTN (pay attention)
RELAX
REST
SIT
STOP
STRTCH (stretch)

*Irvine, Calif. (www.watchminder.com)

Memory Message* (Figure 10-6) is designed to assist individuals by reminding them of activities and tasks throughout the day. The small size (6.3 inches × 4 inches × 1.1 inches, 12.5 oz) makes the device easy to carry. A standard clock face built into the front of the device shows the current day and time, and a button is available to provide audible time information. Up to 280 alarms can be set with 40 separate recorded instruction messages. When an alarm occurs, the user can either acknowledge the alarm (by pressing "OK") or have it repeated (by pressing "?"). A caregiver programs alarms and messages through a keyboard. Alarms can be set for a single event or for a recurring activity.

*Saltillo (www.saltillo.com/)

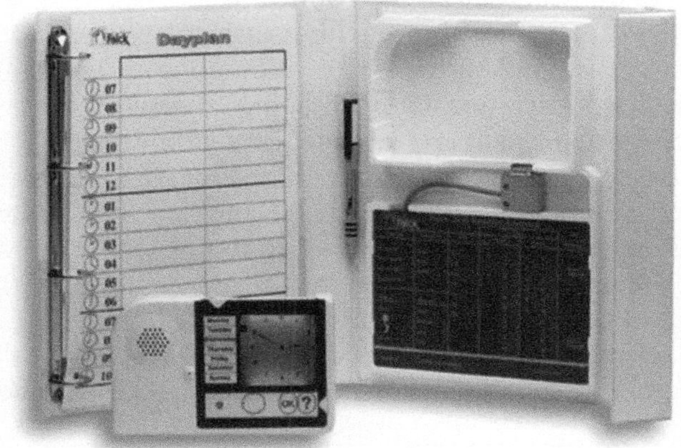

Figure 10-6 The Memory Message system provides reminders of activities throughout the day. (Courtesy Saltillo, www.saltillo.com.)

Figure 10-7 shows a PDA-based system in use.* Systems like this include daily schedulers and reminder alarm devices that are of benefit to people with TBI [29,46] and CVA, and with aging and intellectual disabilities.[29,45-47] Software packages for these devices have also been designed to include prompting cues to aid memory.[5] These specially designed systems can be customized to meet the needs of a specific user, they have user-friendly interfaces, and they are easy to carry.[22] The PDA-based information retrieval aids require the user to display some degree of sensory perception, language use, memory, and/or learning skill to be of practical benefit. The case study "Memory Challenges Following TBI" illustrates the application of a PDA as a memory and organization aid.

CASE STUDY – MEMORY CHALLENGES FOLLOWING TBI

Darrell is a 30-year-old man who suffered a traumatic brain injury three years ago. His ability to read and write was severely affected, but he is able to communicate well through speech. Darrell also has trouble with time management and often forgets to complete daily tasks. He acknowledges his weaknesses and has been actively seeking out technologies that could help him to live more independently. One of Darrell's main concerns is addressing his forgetfulness. Ever since returning to work, he has had to rely on constant reminders from his supervisor in order to complete tasks. He has found that his inability to read or write was not affecting his job performance, but it was limiting his ability to use written reminders to help with his memory difficulties. In addition to seeking help completing his work duties more independently, Darrell was also hoping to find something that would help him remember to take his medication at the right times throughout the day.

Essentially, what Darrell requires is both a "Things-to-do" checklist and an alarm capable of signaling reminders at preset times throughout the day. One major[5] restriction is that he must be able to interact with the device in some way that does not require reading or writing. Aside from that, Darrell has said he would prefer that the device be portable and that it should have at least enough battery life to last an entire 8-hour work shift.

A PDA device with voice recognition software was recommended for Darrell. After a brief training period, he was able to dictate a list of things he needed to do, store them in the PDA's memory, and then play them back for future reference via the device's text-to-voice synthesizer. In this manner, Darrell was able to set up a schedule in the morning and complete his work duties

(Continued)

*For example, Community Integration Suite, AbleLink Technologies (www.ablelinktech.com /)

CASE STUDY – MEMORY CHALLENGES FOLLOWING TBI—cont'd

without constant reminders from his supervisor. He was also able to program a spoken reminder that indicated when it was time to take his medication. Darrell enjoyed the flexibility of this system and, with some additional training with the device, he was able to program new checklists and alarms as needed. Overall, he was very satisfied with the independence he gained from using the device.

What other alternatives to voice input/output would be appropriate for Darrell's needs? If Darrell was able to read and write, would this affect the choice of technology? Could the same functionality be obtained with a less-costly device or combination of devices? Is there a "low tech" solution that might work equally well?

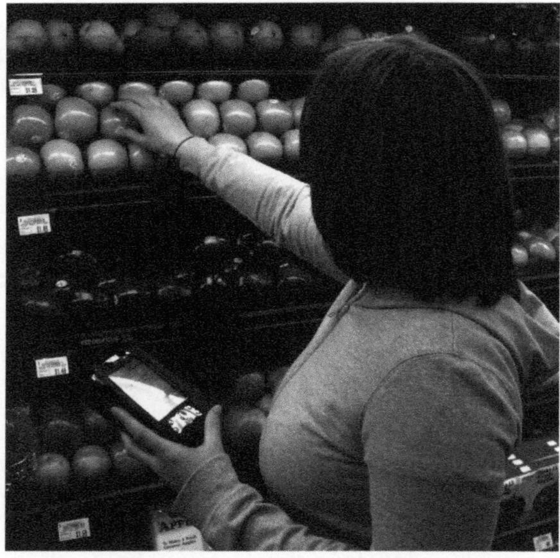

Figure 10-7 A specially programmed PDA can help an individual with a cognitive disability to achieve a greater level of independence. (Courtesy AbleLink Technologies, http://www.ablelinktech.com/.)

Another application that helps create access to portable electronic systems for people who have intellectual disabilities, autism, Down syndrome, traumatic brain injury, or Alzheimer's disease is the Pocket Ace.* This software application creates a simplified interface for cell phone use. Pocket Ace uses audio messages and images to navigate the phone structure to make and receive phone calls. A central element is a picture-based address book that allows a user to merely tap on the picture of the person he or she wants to talk to in order to place the call. Likewise, pictures of incoming callers who are in the address book are displayed and the user can recognize the caller and answer by tapping the picture. The Pocket Ace software runs on the Pocket Ace phone and allows individuals to make personal, business, and emergency phone calls without assistance.

*http://www.ablelinktech.com/

The Schedule Assistant* is a PDA and smart phone application intended for use by individuals who are unable to use mainstream text-based scheduling because of literacy limitations. It uses a multimedia approach that presents information in visual (picture or symbol) or auditory form. Appointments or events are entered into the system by recording an audio message and selecting a relevant digital picture or icon to be displayed when the message is activated. The day(s) and time(s) for the message to activate are also selected. The Schedule Assistant can be used for meeting bus schedules, medication reminders, taking work breaks, and maintaining classroom schedules or morning routines. Schedule Assistant is available as part of the Community Integration Suite or Pocket Endeavor Suite of products from AbleLink Technologies.†

Devices that Provide Prompting/Cueing/Coaching

Prompting systems are devices or computer programs that inform a user that an action should be taken. They also provide visual, verbal, and/or auditory cues as to how to accomplish a task. In most cases the systems allow a care provider to enter the relevant information regarding events, times, and frequency of repetition of the task. Some devices also allow collection of data regarding ease of use, and others feature communication with a central station for data logging, emergency assistance requests, and/or tracking of an individual's actions and location.

Prompting devices require a number of cognitive skills in order to be effective. One of these skills is *attention to task:* the ability to focus on a particular task.[50] *Vigilance, sustained attention,* and *selective attention* are also important. Prompting devices also require recognition memory and categorization in order to use the devices for procedural sequencing such as the steps required to set the table, make a bed, or take a bus to work.

For individuals who have difficulty understanding text and who need assistance with sequential activities, the Visual Assistant‡ provides task prompting using digital pictures and custom-recorded audio or video messages. Step-by-step instructional supports are provided by allowing caregivers to set up the instructional tasks. To provide multi-modal cues for task completion, each step has recorded instructions and corresponding pictures. The most useful pictures are of the user performing the step in the actual environment. The Visual Assistant can be used for more complex or detailed tasks where the addition of a picture or video clip can increase accuracy.

*http://www.ablelinktech.com/
†www.ablelinktech.com/_solutions/
‡http://www.ablelinktech.com/

Instructions can branch to different alternative sequences based on the choices made by the end user. Any step can be time based to advance automatically or provide periodic reminders to complete the current step.

The ISAAC™ Cognitive Prosthesis* System is a wearable and highly customizable device that provides procedural information and personal information storage.[10] This system is a fully individualized cognitive prosthetic system that assists the user to live and work more independently through the organization and delivery of individualized prompts and procedural and personal information. A care provider enters the content using an authoring system. The content is then delivered to the individual with a cognitive disability in English or Spanish as synthesized speech audio, text, checklists, or graphics. Prompts can be delivered on the basis of specified conditions, such as the time of day, to prompt for an action by the user. User input is through a pressure sensitive touch screen.

Mihailidis, Fernie and Barbenel (2001)[36] developed a prompting system for hand washing to assist individuals who have dementia. The system, called COACH, uses a video camera, personal computer, and artificial intelligence software. The system monitors the person's progress and provides auditory prompts when steps are skipped or mistakes are made. The system also learns the patterns of the individual users and adapts its settings and cues to match them. In a single subject design study with 10 elder participants, the COACH system led to significant improvement in completion of hand-washing tasks without caregiver assistance.[35]

A navigational device based on a GPS cell phone, called Opportunity Knocks, was designed specifically for people with cognitive limitations.[28] This device learns the patterns of the user, and uses those patterns to help the user find the most familiar (not necessarily the shortest) route, recover from mistakes, and receive prompts when needed. If an error occurs (e.g., a user misses a bus stop that is routinely taken), the device verbally prompts the user with prompts such as "I think you made a mistake" or "May I guide you to [location]." The user can indicate which location by touching a picture of it on the display of the cell phone. Then a mode of transportation (e.g., walk or bus) is chosen in the same way. Using the stored patterns, the system then directs the user to that location. Using stored information, the system can also determine if the user is on the wrong bus, and direct him to get off at the next stop. Instruction can then be provided to get the person back on track to their destination. These concepts have been realized in a number of smart phone and iPhone applications.† Voice output for navigations helps individuals who cannot read.

*www.cosys.us/

†For example, Google Maps Navigation (http://www.google.com/mobile/navigation/); and iNav (http://www.inavcorp.com/?gclid=CKSmhcPQ2qMCFVjW5wodkVDR9g)

WayFinder* is a smart phone-based application that is designed to enable people with intellectual and other cognitive disabilities to travel more independently via bus or light rail using generated audio and visual cues based on their GPS location. WayFinder includes an optional tracking feature that allows a family member or caregiver to track the location of the user using instant messaging and Google Maps.

The Planning and Execution Assistant and Trainer (PEAT)† is a PDA-based personal planning assistant designed to assist individuals with cognitive disorders due to brain injury, stroke, Alzheimer's disease, and similar conditions.[31] PEAT employs artificial intelligence to automatically generate plans and also to revise those plans when unexpected events occur. PEAT uses a combination of manually entered schedules and a library of stored scripts describing activities of daily living (e.g., morning routine or shopping). Scripts can be used for both planning and for execution. Planning involves a simulation of the activity with key decision points presented and necessary prompts (auditory and visual) supplied to aid the individual through the planning process. The plan to be executed can be either the stored script or a modified script based on the simulation. The PEAT artificial intelligence software generates the best strategy to execute the required steps in the plan.[32] PEAT also automatically monitors performance and corrects schedule problems when necessary.

Low tech devices can also aid a user in performing a task by providing concrete feedback as to the proper course of action to undertake. One approach is to design a *button shield* for a specific task to be placed over the buttons on a microwave oven. For example, if a meal is to be heated, only the buttons required for that task would be exposed. The shield is labeled with a picture of the meal or a general picture of re-heating. The places where buttons are to be pressed are labeled and times are labeled so the user can merely copy the numbers. For defrosting a frozen meal, a different shield is used. If the individual can distinguish the tasks, then the shields helps them use the microwave appropriately and independently.

Task specific *jigs* enable people to perform tasks that they may not otherwise be able to perform. For example, weighing and counting tasks in manufacturing and assembly can be difficult for workers who have cognitive disabilities. One approach to modifying weighing and counting is to use a talking scale connected to a controller that provides prompting and feedback as necessary.[20] For counting tasks, a set of bins, each holding one nail, is weighed. If the bins are properly filled the weight is correct and the user is prompted to proceed with the next step. If the weight is too low, the user is told to check all the bins,

*AbleLink Technologies (http://www.ablelinktech.com/)

†Attention Control Systems, Mountain View, Calif. (www.brainaid.com/)

and if it is too high the user is prompted to be sure only one element is in each bin. For weighing, objects placed on the scale are compared with stored weight limit values, and the user is prompted if the weight is above or below the weight range. Erlandson and Stant (1998)[20] describe the successful use of this system in a nail counting task for a construction supply company by a woman with mild intellectual disability. These jigs require the worker to fill the available spaces and then transfer the total number of items to a bag or other container. Thus, the worker does not need to be able to count: he just needs to have procedural memory skills sufficient to fill up the jig and then go to the next step.

Stimuli Control

For some individuals the influence of distractions is such that they are unable to focus on a task when another stimulus (e.g., a conversation) is occurring in the background. For example, individuals with attention deficit disorder have difficulty focusing on the teacher in class. There are other situations in which we are required to devote attention to two or more tasks at the same time using *divided attention*. One example is listening to a lecture and taking notes. Students need auditory attention and processing skills to understand what the professor is saying, and additionally they require visual and tactile skills to either write or keyboard as they take notes. While the activities of listening to a lecture and taking notes appear to be concurrent, in fact attention is moving quickly between the two tasks. Sustained attention is similar to vigilance, but differs in that there isn't necessarily a competing stimulus present.

Stimuli control devices include technologies that can be subdivided into three categories based on their intended application: noise reduction techniques, visual field manipulation, and media presentation techniques. Auditory (noise reduction) are those devices that filter out extraneous noise so the user may focus on one specific source. An example of such a system is a transmitter/headphone receiver link between a student and teacher in a classroom setting similar to those used for students who are hard of hearing (see FM systems in Chapter 9). Visual stimuli can be altered in a similar fashion, through the use of prism glasses or special lenses that correct for double vision or visual neglect (e.g., in TBI or CVA) (see prism glasses in Chapter 8).

Media presentation is an important design consideration for many visual display applications. Websites, computer monitors, and other visual displays need to be carefully designed to avoid extraneous information that might be distracting to a person with an attention disorder. By reducing clutter, increasing clarity, and simplifying visual displays, information can be presented in a way that is best perceived and understood by a broad target audience. Key concepts in Web page design for individuals with cognitive disabilities are shown in Table 10-11.

TABLE 10-11 Key Concepts in Web Design for Individuals with Cognitive Disabilities

Challenges	Solutions
Users may become confused at complex layouts or inconsistent navigational schemes.	Simplify the layout as much as possible. Keep the navigational schemes as consistent as possible.
Users may have difficulty focusing on or comprehending lengthy sections of text.	Where appropriate, group textual information under logical headings. Organize information in manageable "chunks."
One method of input may not be sufficient.	Where appropriate, supplement text with illustrations or other media, and vice versa.

Data from WebAIM, http://www.webaim.org/techniques/cognitive/.

The WebAim project* has many useful resources for making Web sites accessible to individuals who have cognitive disabilities. These include evaluation packages to check Web sites for accessibility, guidelines for developing accessible Web sites, and tools for making Web sites more accessible to this population.

Internet access for individuals with intellectual disabilities can provide benefits in self-esteem and self-confidence, independence in vocational and living contexts, opportunities for training, self-directed activities, and use of their time for pursuits that are stimulating and informative.[13] Unfortunately, access to the Internet for this population is often limited by standard Web browsers that require high level cognitive skills, particularly in reading and writing. A pilot project was designed to compare a specially designed Web browser (Web Trek)† with a standard browser‡ (see Box 10-3, "What the Research Says").[13] Web Trek uses graphics, reduced screen clutter, audio prompts, and personalization and customization to maximize accessibility to individuals with intellectual disabilities. Web Trek is also a part of the AbleLink technologies Endeavor Desktop Environment discussed in a later section.

Language Tools

Many forms of assistive technology are *language tools* that assist with reading or writing. Many devices focus on the memory requirements of language. For example, word completion programs (see Chapter 5) are useful

*Center for Persons with Disabilities, Utah State University (www.webaim.org)

†Web Trek, AbleLink Technologies, Colorado Springs, Colo. (www.ablelinktech.com/_desktop/webtrek.asp)

‡Internet Explorer, Microsoft, Inc., Redmond, Wash. (www.microsoft.com)

for people who are poor at spelling. They predict whole words based on the first few letters typed by the user. A list of possible word choices is presented, and the user need only recognize the intended word from that list. Dictionaries and thesauruses are low tech alternatives to word completion programs, as they also operate on the basis of using word recognition to rectify deficiencies in word retrieval. For individuals with TBI, word prediction software programs have all shown to be useful in clinical trials.[46]

Word prediction has been shown to be a promising strategy for improving the text entry speed of students with learning disabilities as they move from handwriting to computer writing using a word processor.[30] Word prediction programs written specifically for students with learning disabilities* include features that make them more effective. In addition to simple word prediction, these programs often include dictionaries to suggest alternatives that increase the richness and interest of the writing based on the topic being discussed, and they can be personalized for an individual student. Another program is WordQ,† which takes into account phonetic spelling mistakes.

Studies of the impact of word prediction on writing abilities of students with learning disabilities have led to mixed results.[42] In small sample studies, word prediction programs have been shown to improve writing by addressing word finding problems. When coupled with speech synthesis, the results are improved further. Results vary for word completion vs. word prediction (see Chapter 5), with word prediction being more effective since it includes the context of the sentence as well as that of the word.

Spell checking programs are helpful to students with learning disabilities as editing tools.[30] Spell checking programs are designed to primarily detect typographical errors, not misspellings due to phonetic errors.[4] Thus, the target word for a student with a learning disability, who is spelling phonetically, is often not the first word listed by the spell checking program. Despite this limitation, students with learning disabilities were able to detect their target word 95% of the time, even if it was not the first word listed.[4] When evaluated based on the types of spelling errors made by students with learning disabilities, spell checkers vary widely in effectiveness.[42] Spell checking programs are most effective when they are integrated into a word processing program. Grammar checkers are not helpful to students who have learning disabilities because they often rely on correct spelling in the text.[30]

Concept mapping is a process of conceptualizing information using graphics and text. The Inspiration® concept mapping software* is designed to help students in the 6th to 12th grades plan, organize, and write research papers. As shown in Figure 10-8, its alternative format for representing ideas with both text and graphics, its ability to import concepts from the Internet and other sources, and the provision of a large number of templates make Inspiration useful to students who have learning disabilities.[4,32] Inspiration also allows the student to toggle between the text and the concept map as they develop their report. Using Inspiration, 8th grade students who had learning disabilities produced essays that were significantly above their pretest levels in number of words, concepts included, and holistic writing scores.[44]

*For Example, the Co:Writer, Don Johnston, Inc., Volo, Ill. (www.donjohnston.com)

†http://www.synapseadaptive.com/quillsoft/WQ/wordq_description.htm

Alternative Input

Alternative input technologies offer the user different modalities for providing input commands and/or information to a device. Voice recognition software (see Chapter 6) can be useful for text input by individuals with cognitive disabilities that limit their ability to write.[32] Users are able to enter information or commands to a computer through voice dictation instead of mouse and keyboard. For TBI, speech recognition programs have all shown to be useful in clinical trials.[29,46] Voice recognition can also be effective in improving writing for students with learning disabilities who have difficulty visually processing words.[42]

An advantage of PDAs is that software can be customized and the complexity of operating functions can be adjusted to fit the skills of a wide variety of users. One example of customization of the user interface is AbleLink's Pocket Discovery Desktop.† This software tool is helpful for people who have difficulty using PDAs because of their complexity. The Pocket Desktop software interfaces to the traditional Windows Pocket PC desktop and provides a simplified interface for accessing programs. Picture or audio-based messages can be programmed into on-screen buttons for any application on the PDA. The pictures and audio labels help users identify different programs. Pocket Discovery Desktop can avoid accidental activation of the physical buttons by deactivating or causing them to have specific functions on the PDA. The Pocket Discovery Desktop is available as part of the Community Integration Suite from AbleLink Technologies. The AbleData PDA-based technologies are being replicated for the Android smart phone operating system.[16]

Endeavor Desktop Environment (EDE)‡ is designed for people who need a simplified Windows desktop. The program provides a picture-based log-in screen and allows the creation of custom, single-click picture buttons for everyday technologies, such as social networking, online access and communication, and productivity. EDE incorporates the Web Trek accessible browser to enable Web browsing, Endeavor Email

*Inspiration Software, Inc., Beaverton Ore. (http://www.inspiration.com/)

†http://www.ablelinktech.com/_handhelds/pocketdiscovery.asp

‡http://www.ablelinktech.com/

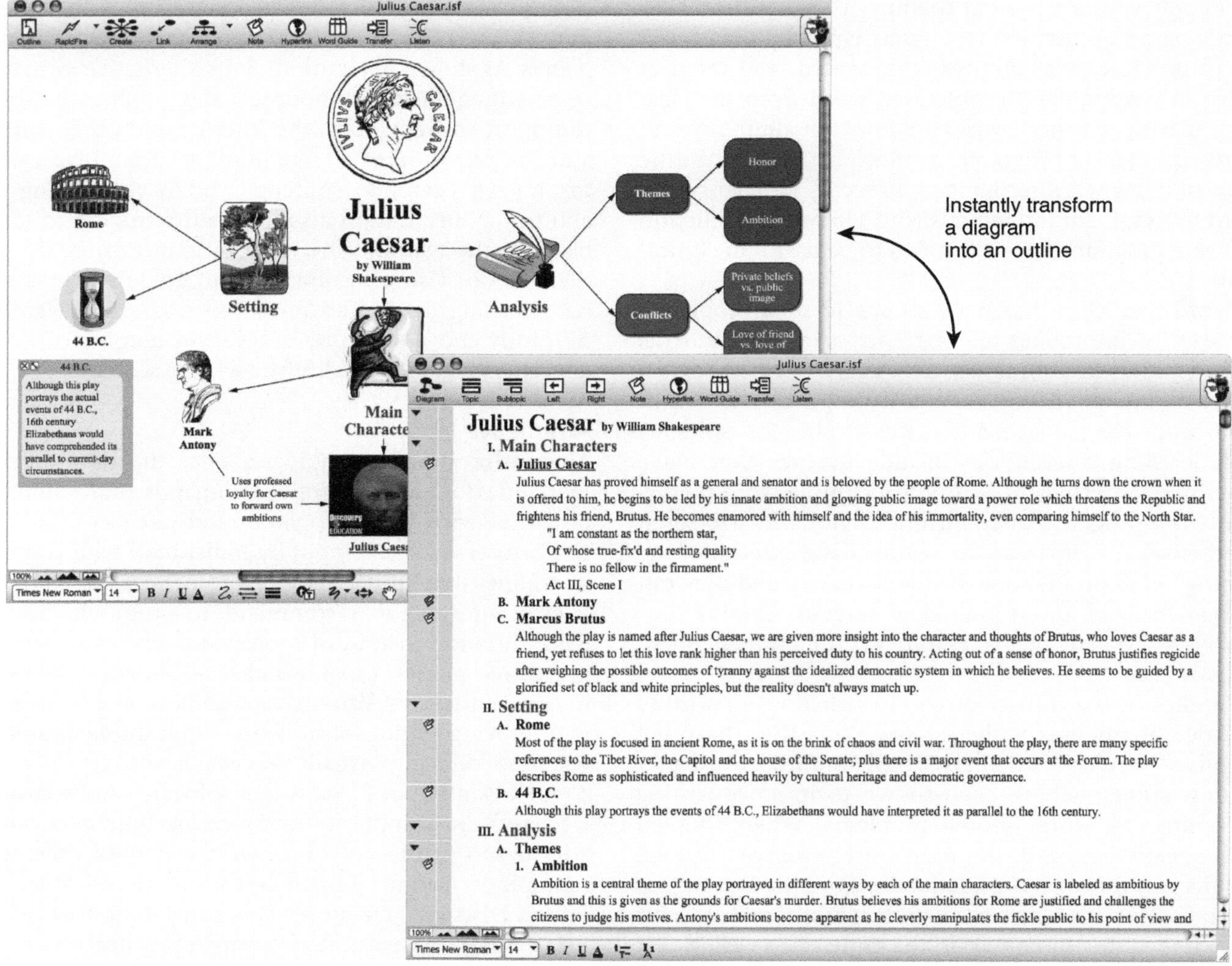

Figure 10-8 Inspiration software allows the development of ideas in a graphical format and automatic conversion to text. (Courtesy Inspiration Software, Inc, Beaverton, Ore., http://www.inspiration.com.)

(a picture-based address book), a visual media player, and access to news via an accessible RSS reader. Within each user's custom desktop, personalized content is available using dynamic buttons configured with descriptive images and audio to facilitate access. Because multiple users can each have their own unique desktop on a single computer, Endeavor Desktop Environment is useful in classrooms or group living settings. The desktop also identifies the user so that any programs customized for that user will be loaded, if available. EDE is available as part of the Computer & Web Access Suite or as part of the Smart Living Suite from Able Link Technologies.

Alternative Output

Alternative output technologies offer users a nontraditional means of acquiring feedback or information from a device. Some individuals are more visually oriented and print or screen displays work well for them. For others information is easiest to access in auditory form. Synthesized or digitized speech output is often used for auditory information. We discuss the principles of electronically generated speech and its application in augmentative communication systems in Chapter 7. Many devices that were originally developed for individuals who have limited vision make use of synthesized speech to enhance or replace a typically visual output. Examples of these devices include text-to-speech screen readers for computer applications, talking calculators, a tape measure with speech output, and barcode scanners (see Chapter 8).

Synthesized speech and digitized speech (see Chapter 7) are both used to provide auditory information to children and adults with intellectual disabilities (see the prompting and cueing section in this chapter). Synthesized speech associated with a word processor* for individuals who have learning disabilities can provide an additional modality that is helpful in writing and editing. The greatest benefit may be in reducing the most common misspellings (i.e., those that are "non-real" words) (e.g., "thar" for "there") as opposed to word substitutions (e.g., "to" for "two").[30] Synthetic speech output was also

*For Example, Write:OutLoud, Don Johnston, Inc., Volo, Ill. (www.donjohnston.com)

useful when the spell checker could not suggest any words due to gross misspelling. This technology can also benefit adults who have sustained a TBI or who have expressive language difficulties such as aphasia (see Chapter 11 for more information).

The impact of speech output is more significant for younger learners than for secondary students. In some cases, the impact of speech synthesizers in providing writing assistance to students with learning disabilities is less significant than the effective use of spell checkers and word prediction.[30] However, as illustrated by the case study "Learning Disability and Alternative Input for Reading," auditory output via speech synthesis is an effective tool for students with reading or writing difficulties associated with learning disabilities.[42] Students can often detect errors in their writing easier if they hear the words as opposed to reading them in written form. Adding speech synthesis to the presentation of screen-based text provides a multi-modal output that also assists in reading and writing.

CASE STUDY – LEARNING DISABILITY AND ALTERNATIVE INPUT FOR READING*

Daniel is a student in a regular educational program. He has a learning disability that makes it difficult for him to read printed material. The system provided for Daniel allows him to have an alternative input modality for his reading. He completes the printed lesson that requires him to fill in blanks on a worksheet by using a scanner that digitizes his lesson and puts it into a word processor. He listens to the text using earphones so as not to disturb the other students. With this system he is able to mark and copy the text using a reading program like the ones described in this section. He also makes use of word prediction, spell checking, and grammar checking applications in completing his assignments.

*Based on a case study listed by SEN-IST-NET

Because many individuals with learning disabilities have greater comprehension of auditory than written information, synthesized speech output in "talking books" or "e-books" has been shown to be effective in improving reading abilities.[4] E-books have a number of features that are useful for students who have learning disabilities. For example, words can be highlighted in the text as they are spoken or the document can be presented in an enlarged font. For students who need spelling practice, a spelling activity can be selected that uses the words from the story. Using software and on-line tools, teachers can create their own e-books.[4]

The Readingpen®,* an assistive reading device (Figure 10-9), is a handheld scanner that is designed specifically for school-age reading levels. This can also

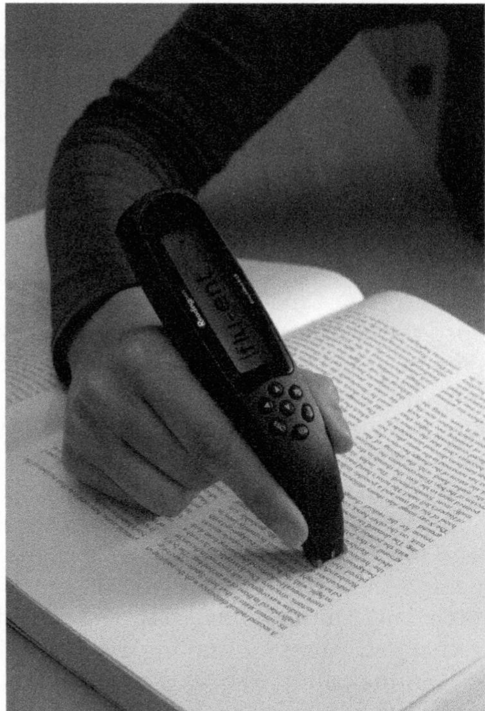

Figure 10-9 The Readingpen text-to-speech reading aid. Text is scanned into the pen's memory. (Courtesy WizCom Technologies, Marlborough, Mass., www.wizcomtech.com/.)

be useful for adults who have intellectual disabilities and need assistance with reading. As the pen is moved across a word or full line of text, the text is spoken aloud. Using a children's dictionary and thesaurus, the device also provides information to the student about word meaning and alternative words through a three-line built-in display. The pen provides a portable way for people with reading difficulties, learning disabilities, or dyslexia to get immediate word support when they are reading. The scanned text may be spoken word by word or line by line. An earphone connection is available for privacy.

Altering the visual appearance of the computer screen can also aid individuals with disorders such as dyslexia.[32] Changing features such as font size, background/foreground color combinations, contrast, and spacing between words, letters, and paragraphs and using graphics can all improve access to screen-based information.

Tracking and Identification

Individuals with Alzheimer's disease often experience periods of forgetfulness and disorientation. The disorientation can lead to wandering behavior that is unsafe to the person and very worrisome to the caregivers and family. Devices for **tracking and identification** of people or items often provide an extra degree of safety for users who might get lost or disoriented due to limitations in cognitive abilities required to work their way out of problematic situations. Global positioning

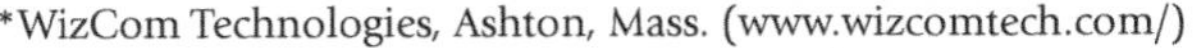

*WizCom Technologies, Ashton, Mass. (www.wizcomtech.com/)

systems (GPS) have been used to assist these individuals by providing their location to the caregiver.[34] The GPS Locator Watch* is designed to track children, but its features apply as well to persons with dementia. The watch has a wireless transmitter/receiver that transmits the location of the person and allows transmission of information to the watch. The watch has an electronically activated lock to keep it in place in order to prevent individuals (whose disability makes it difficult to understand the purpose of the watch) from trying to remove it. The lock can be remotely released for removal of the watch. The device also has a built-in pager, clock, and emergency call function.

Because these individuals often try to remove unfamiliar objects (such as bracelets, leg bands, etc.) that are often used for attaching GPS-based monitoring devices, the effectiveness of GPS systems can be limited. However, procedural memory is often preserved in patients with dementia and these individuals typically get dressed as part of their daily routine. The GPS Shoe† takes advantage of these characteristics by installing a GPS receiver and transmitter in the patient's shoes. The GPS signal can be monitored from a smart phone or from the Internet. The patient's travel is superimposed on a map for display to family or other care providers.

An iPhone application called Community Sidekick‡ sends automated e-mail messages containing Google Map links that show the user's location. This allows the care provider or family to track the person's travels in the community. When the user starts a trip and launches the program, automated location information is sent via e-mail every few minutes. The user can also send simple stored messages by pressing one key. Sample messages include "I am OK" or "Please contact me" if the person has a question, needs assistance, or wants to speak with someone directly. Sidekick is intended to support parents of children with autism, spouses of people with traumatic brain injuries or other cognitive injuries, and support staff for people with intellectual and developmental disabilities.

The concept of a **Smart House** (Figure 10-10) has been used to denote living environments in which automatic functions are provided including monitoring, communication, household functions (lights, air conditioning/heating, door locks), physiological measurements, and medication alerts.[34] Smart houses have the potential to allow individuals with cognitive limitations greater independence and, in the case of elderly individuals, a chance to stay in their homes rather than move to group living facilities. Mann (2005) describes levels of smart houses from basic communications (Internet, phone) through complex monitoring and tracking of the resident's health, behavior, and needs.[34] The core of the smart house is a processing and communication system linked to a sensory array. One example of a monitoring application is described in the Case Study "Dementia: Assistive Technology to Allow Staying at Home." The system aids a user in performing common tasks of daily living by assessing the person's current physiological state and the state of various utilities throughout the home and then providing the user with feedback should they become disoriented or confused on a given task.[24] Mann describes several smart house projects.[34]

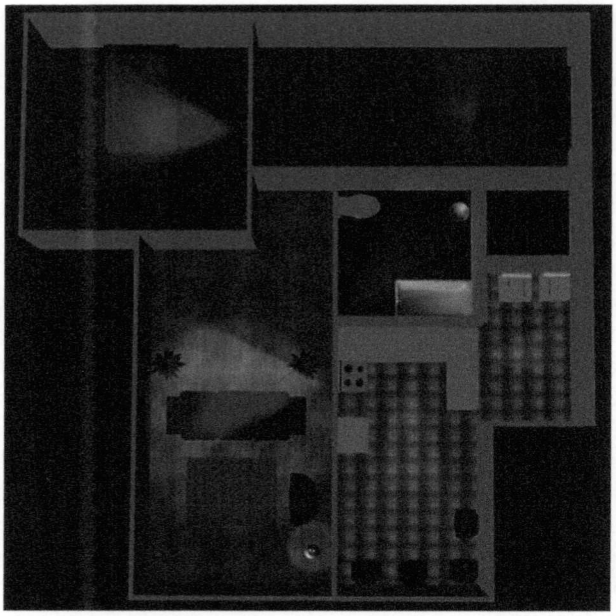

Figure 10-10 Smart House conceptualization. Light areas represent sensor field for detecting movement by room. (Courtesy Medical Automation Research Center, University of Virginia, http://www.modeltech.com/smh.htm.)

CASE STUDY – DEMENTIA: ASSISTIVE TECHNOLOGY TO ALLOW STAYING AT HOME*

Eighty-six-year-old Emily has lived in her own home for many years. She and her husband (deceased) raised their family in this home and her daughter still lives nearby. Emily now lives alone in the home. She has had difficulty remembering things and occasionally gets confused since she sustained a series of mini-strokes a few years ago. While her daughter helps out as much as she can, her own family and full-time job limit her availability. Emily's confusion and memory loss have resulted in her leaving a gas stove knob in her house turned on but not lit. Several possible solutions were proposed by the local assistive technology clinic. Because Emily still enjoyed cooking her own meals, turning off the gas permanently was ruled out. An electric stove was suggested, but Emily had spent her life cooking on a gas stove and didn't want to "learn how to cook all over again." A microwave oven

*Wherify (www.childlocator.com/)
†http://www.gpsshoe.com
‡http://itunes.apple.com/us/app/community-sidekick/id413107872?mt=8

CASE STUDY – DEMENTIA: ASSISTIVE TECHNOLOGY TO ALLOW STAYING AT HOME*—cont'd

was ruled out for the same reason. The solution that was implemented involved using a gas sensor connected to a shut-off valve. The sensor was originally connected to an audible alarm, and modification was now required to use the sensor to control the shut-off valve. The system was also set-up to notify a central home monitoring system that a gas leak had been detected. The home monitoring center then notified Emily's daughter, who was able to go to the home and turn the gas back on. This approach allowed Emily to remain at home and to continue preparing her own meals. In the past year or so, her daughter has only had to reconnect the gas about four times in total.

*Safe Home Project

Another method of tracking is home monitoring systems that can keep track of the status of a person with cognitive disabilities. These systems include monitoring of the environment within a house (e.g., gas or smoke detectors), cardiac parameters (heart rate, arrhythmias), objects and people (e.g., sensors that determine if a person has left their bed by monitoring the weight applied to a pressure sensor placed under the bed frame), and emergency call (a button that is pushed and automatically dials a central station). There is typically a charge for the equipment (a central station and pendant or other link worn by the individual) and a monthly service fee. Funding may be from private health insurance, government agencies, or private pay by the individual.

CASE STUDY – DEMENTIA AND WANDERING

Tito is 70 years old and has recently been diagnosed with Alzheimer's dementia. He lives with his wife Betsy in the small house in which he raised his family. His son comes by and checks up on his parents 3 to 4 times a week and is readily available should necessity arise. Due to Tito's condition, he has acquired a forgetfulness to turn things off that require vigilance and has been found taking "walks" late at night. Unfortunately, Tito has had problems finding his way home during his outings and his son has received calls from the local police on two occasions regarding this problem. Betsy helps him remember to take his medications and makes sure he doesn't forget the time of his weekly bingo game. Tito still has no problem remembering old friends' names or solving his morning crossword puzzles. Given this profile, what types of assistive technologies might benefit Tito?

The suppliers* of these systems describe many case examples on their Web sites that illustrate how these systems can make it possible for persons with memory loss, wandering, and other cognitive limitation to continue to live at home (See Case Study on "Dementia and Wandering"). These systems are often incorporated into the Smart House concept discussed in this chapter.

SUMMARY

Individuals who have cognitive disabilities of various types and severity can benefit from the use of assistive technologies. Cognitive disabilities represent a wide variety of skill levels and severity, but there are an equally wide range of types of assistive technologies available to ameliorate these conditions and increase functional performance in ADLs. The implementation of these assistive technologies and strategies is based on the augmentation of or substitution for cognitive skills that are required for the completion of specific functional tasks. A successful application of cognitive assistive technology depends on support provided by caregivers and families.

STUDY QUESTIONS

1. How do assistive technology approaches differ for congenital and acquired cognitive disabilities?
2. Pick a specific disorder and describe both the cognitive skills that are likely to be available for use of an assistive device and those that may need to be replaced or augmented by such a device. How would this affect your training and support of a person who has this disability?
3. What characteristics of mild cognitive disabilities are the most important to consider when training and supporting someone to use assistive technologies.
4. What characteristics of intellectual disabilities are the most important to consider when training and supporting someone to use assistive technologies?
5. What characteristics of dementia are the most important to consider when training and supporting someone to use assistive technologies?
6. In terms of providing training and support for assistive technologies, how do CVA and TBI differ?
7. What are the characteristics of mobile time management systems that make them useful for persons with intellectual disabilities?
8. Describe the general characteristics of memory aids.
9. What differences would you encounter in training someone to use a memory aid if they had an intellectual disability, dementia, or a TBI?

*For example, in Canada: www.lifeline.ca/; in the UK: http://www.tunstall.co.uk/home.asp and in the US: http://www.lifestation.com/?ASK=Medical-Alert

10. Systems designed to provide prompting, cueing, or coaching are available to assist persons with intellectual disabilities. What steps would you take to train someone to use such a system?
11. List several factors that can be used to make Web pages more accessible to individuals who have cognitive disabilities.
12. How would you explain the special features of a cognitively accessible Web browser to a family?
13. How would you teach someone to use a cognitively accessible Web browser?
14. If you are working with an individual who has dementia, what challenges are you likely to encounter in helping them learn to use an assistive technology device to aid memory?
15. How can word completion and word prediction benefit students and adults who have learning disabilities? What are the limitations of these applications?
16. What alternatives would you suggest to the family of a person who is having difficulty accessing printed text in books and magazines?
17. How would you introduce a time management device to a stroke patient?
18. What are the major factors that make tracking systems useful for individuals who may wander?
19. What characteristics of tracking systems may make it difficult for them to be accepted by individuals with dementia?
20. What is a Smart House and how are its features meant to support aging in place?

REFERENCES

1. American Psychiatric Association: *Diagnostic and statistical manual of mental disorders, DSM-IV*, ed 4, Washington DC, 2000, American Psychiatric Association.
2. Anderson JR: *Cognitive psychology and its implications*, New York, 2000, Worth Publishers.
3. Ashcraft MH: *Fundamentals of cognition, New York*, 1998, Addison-Wesley-Longman.
4. Ashton TM: Students with learning disabilities using assistive technology in the inclusive classroom. In Edyburn DL, Higgins K, Boone R, editors: *Handbook of special education technology research and practice*, Whitefish Bay, Wisconsin, 2005, Knowledge by Design, pp 229–238.
5. Bergman MM: The benefits of a cognitive orthotic in brain injury rehabilitation, *J Head Trauma Rehabil* 17(5):431–445, 2002.
6. Bower B: Mind-expanding machines: artificial intelligence meets good old-fashioned human thought, *Sci News* 164(9): 136–138, 2003. Retrieved on May 5, 2005 from http://www.findarticles.com/p/articles/mi_m1200/is_9_164/ai_108050570.
7. Braddock D, Rizzolo MC, Thompson M, et al: Emerging technologies and cognitive disability, *J Spec Educ Tech* 19(4): 49–56, 2004.
8. Bruno-Petrina AA: Motor recovery in stroke, 2004. Retrieved April 6, 2005, from http://www.emedicine.com/pmr/topic234.htm.
9. Cicerone KD, Dahlberg C, Malec JF, et al: Evidence-based cognitive rehabilitation: updated review of the literature from 1998 through 2002, *Arch Phys Med Rehabil* 86(8):1681–1692, 2005.
10. Cole E, Matthews MK: Cognitive Prosthetics and Telerehabilitation: Approaches for the Rehabilitation of Mild Brain Injuries. In *Proceedings of Basil Therapy Congress*, Basel, Switzerland, June 1999, pp 111–120 retrieved July 27, 2006 from http://www.brain-rehab.com/pdf/cpt1999.pdf.
11. Cole E, Dehdashti P: Computer-based cognitive prosthetics: assistive technology for the treatment of cognitive disabilities. In *Proceedings of the Third International ACM Conference on Assistive Technologies*, Marina del Rey, CA, April 15-17 1998, *ACM SIGCAPH*.
12. Daley D: Attention deficit hyperactivity disorder: a review of the essential facts, *Child Care Health Dev* 32(2):193–204, 2006.
13. Davies DK, Stock SE, Wehmeyer ML: Enhancing independent Internet access for individuals with mental retardation through use of a specialized web browser: a pilot study, *Educ Train Ment Retard Dev Disabil* 36(1):107–113, 2001.
14. Davies DK, Stock SE, Wehmeyer ML: Enhancing independent time-management skills of individuals with mental retardation using a palmtop personal computer, *Ment Retard* 40(5):358–365, 2002.
15. Davies DK, Stock SE, Wehmeyer ML: A palmtop computer-based intelligent aid for individuals with intellectual disabilities to increase independent decision making, *Res Pract Persons Severe Disabl* 28(4):182–193, 2003.
16. Davies D: Personal correspondence, March 4 2011.
17. Dawodu ST: Traumatic brain injury (TBI): definition, epidemiology, pathophysiology, *Web MD*. Retrieved August 27, 2006 from http://www.emedicine.com/pmr/topic212.htm#top.
18. Demaerschalk B, Hachinski V: Stroke (brain attack), In *Griffith's 5-minute clinical consult*, from http://www.5mcc.com/Assets/SUMMARY/TP0175.html. Accessed August 27, 2006.
19. Edyburn DL: Assistive technology and students with mild disabilities: from consideration to outcome measurement. In Edyburn D, Higgins K, Boone R, editors: *Handbook of Special Education Technology Research and Practice*, Whitefish Bay, Wisconsin, 2005, Knowledge by Design, Inc, pp 239–270.
20. Erlandson RF, Sant D: Poka-yoke process controller: designed for individuals with cognitive impairments, *Assist Technol* 10(2):102–112, 1998.
21. Golisz KM, Toglia JP: Perception and cognition. In Blesedell Crepeau E, Cohn ES, Boyt Schell BA, editors: *Willard and Spackman's Occupational Therapy*, ed 10, Philadelphia, PA, 2003, Lippincott Williams and Wilkins, pp 395–416.
22. Gorman P, Dayle R, Hood CA, et al: Effectiveness of the ISAAC cognitive prosthetic system for improving rehabilitation outcomes with neurofunctional impairment, *NeuroRehabilitation* 18(1):57–67, 2003.
23. Granlund M, Bond A, Linstrom E, et al: Assistive technology for cognitive disability, *Technol Disabil* 4:205–214, 1995.
24. Haigh KZ, Kiff LM, Ho G: The independent lifestyle assistant: lessons learned, *Assist Technol* 18(1):87–106, 2006.
25. Heart and Stroke Foundation of Canada: *What is a stroke?* (n.d.) Retrieved April 06, 2005, from http://ww2.heartandstroke.ca/Page.asp?PageID=33&ArticleID=431&Src=stroke&From=SubCategory.

26. Hunt RR, Ellis HC: *Fundamentals of cognitive psychology*, ed 6, Boston, 1999, McGraw-Hill College.
27. Johnson E, Mellard DF, Byrd SE: Alternative models of learning disabilities identification: considerations and initial conclusions, *J Learn Disabil* 38(6):569–572, 2005.
28. Kautz H, Patterson D, Fox D, et al: *Opportunity knocks: a community navigation aid*, 2004, University of Washington. retrieved July 27, 2006 from http://www.cs.washington.edu/homes/kautz/talks/access-symposium-2004.ppt.
29. Kim HJ, Burke DT, Dowds MM, et al: Utility of a microcomputer as an external memory aid for a memory-impaired head injury patient during in-patient rehabilitation, *Brain Inj* 13(2):147–150, 1999.
30. Lewis RB: Classroom technology for students with learning disabilities. In Edyburn DL, Higgins K, Boone R, editors: *Handbook of Special Education Technology Research and Practice*, Whitefish Bay, Wisconsin, 2005, Knowledge by Design, pp 325–334.
31. Levinson RL: The planning and execution assistant and trainer (PEAT), *J Head Trauma Rehabil* 12(2):769–775, 1997.
32. LoPresti EF, Mihailidis A, Kirsch N: Assistive technology for cognitive rehabilitation: state of the art, *Neuropsychol Rehabil* 14(1):5–39, 2004.
33. LoPresti EF, Bodine C, Lewis C: Assistive technology for cognition, *IEEE Eng Med Biol Mag* 5:29–39, 2008.
34. Mann WC, editor: *Smart technology for aging, disability and independence: the state of the science*, 2005, John Wiley and Sons.
35. Mihailidis A, Barbenel JC, Fernie G: The efficiency of an intelligent cognitive orthosis to facilitate handwashing by persons with moderate to severe dementia, *Neuropsychol Rehabil* 14(1):135–171, 2004.
36. Mihailidis A, Fernie GR, Barbenel JC: The use of artificial intelligence in the design of an intelligent cognitive orthosis for people with dementia, *Assist Technol* 13(1):23–29, 2001.
37. Novack T: What to expect after traumatic brain injury and rehabilitation, *Presented at the Recovery after TBI Conference, September, 1999*, Retrieved October 31, 2006 from http://images.main.uab.edu/spinalcord/pdffiles/tbi3pdf.pdf.
38. O'Sullivan SB, Schmitz TJ: *Physical rehabilitation: assessment and treatment*, Philadelphia, 1994, FA Davis.
39. Rabins PV, Lyketsos CG, Steele CD: *Practical dementia care*, ed 2, 2006, Oxford Press.
40. RESNA: *Clinical application of assistive technology*, 1998, Retrieved April 06, 2005 from http://www.rehabtool.com/forum/discussions/94.html.
41. Schuck SEB, Crinella FM: Why children with ADHD do not have low IQs, *J Learn Disabil* 38(3):262–280, 2005.
42. Sitko MC, Laine CJ, Sitko CJ: Writing tools: technology and strategies for the struggling writer. In Edyburn DL, Higgins K, Boone R, editors: *Handbook of Special Education Technology Research and Practice*, Whitefish Bay, Wisconsin, 2005, Knowledge by Design, Inc, pp 571–598.
43. Sternberg RJ: *Cognitive Psychology*, ed 3, Belmont, CA, 2003, Wadsworth.
44. Sturm JM, Rankin-Erickson JL: Effects of hand-drawn and computer-generated concept mapping on the expository writing of middle school students with learning disabilities, *Learn Disabil Res Pract* 17(2):124–139, 2002.
45. Szymkowiak A, Morrison K, Gregor P, et al: A memory aid with remote communication: preliminary findings, *Technol Disab* 17(4):217–225, 2005.
46. Van Hulle A, Hux K: Improvement patterns among survivors of brain injury: three case examples documenting the effectiveness of memory compensation strategies, *Brain Inj* 20(1):101–109, 2006.
47. Wehmeyer ML, Smith SJ, Davies DK: Technology use and students with intellectual disability: universal design for all students. In Edyburn DL, Higgins K, Boone R, editors: *Handbook of Special Education Technology Research and Practice*, Whitefish Bay, Wisconsin, 2005, Knowledge by Design, Inc, pp 309–323.
48. Wehmeyer ML, Smith SJ, Palmer SB, et al: Technology use and people with mental retardation, *Int Rev Res Ment Retard* 29:291–337, 2004.
49. WHO: *World Health Organization: International Classification of Functioning, Disability and Health (ICF)*, Geneva, Switzerland, 2001.
50. Willingham DB: *Cognition: the thinking animal*, New Jersey, 2001, Prentice-Hall.

CHAPTER 11

Augmentative and Alternative Communication

CHAPTER OUTLINE

LEARNING OBJECTIVES

Upon completing this chapter, you will be able to do the following:

1. Describe the different communicative needs of persons with disabilities
2. Discuss the basic approaches to meeting these differing needs
3. Describe the major characteristics of alternative and augmentative communication devices
4. Describe current approaches to speech output in assistive technologies
5. List and describe the major approaches to rate enhancement and vocabulary expansion
6. Discuss the major goals for, and the significance of, training in AAC device use and communicative competence
7. Describe the steps and procedures involved in implementing an augmentative and alternative communication device for an individual consumer
8. Carry out an implementation plan

KEY TERMS

AAC Systems
Access Barriers
Apraxia
Aphasia
Augmentative and Alternative Communication (AAC)
Capability Assessment
Complex Communication Needs (CCN)
Context-Dependent Communicators
Coverage Vocabulary
Digitized Speech
Dynamic Communication Displays
Dysarthria
Emergent Communicators
Human/Technology Interfaces

Icon Prediction
Independent Communicators
Opportunity Barriers
Participation Model
Rate Enhancement
Selection Set
Semantic Encoding
Social Networks Inventory
Speech
Speech Generating Devices (SGDs)
Synthesized Speech
Traditional Orthography
Visual Scene Displays (VSDs)
Vocalization

Augmentative and alternative communication (AAC) is an area of clinical practice that deals with communication problems of people who have **complex communication needs (CCN).** These problems may occur at any point across the life span. Communication is the very essence of being human, and when someone is not developing speech and language skills, or has lost the ability to speak and/or understand spoken or written language, then AAC intervention approaches are required to meet their complex communication needs (CCN). People communicate differently with different partners, under different conditions, and by using a variety of tools, techniques, and strategies. AAC involves a wide range of techniques, strategies, and technologies to support the communication needs of individuals with CCN (see Figure 11-1). The focus of AAC must be on augmenting communication in ways the person values.

Infants, toddlers, and preschoolers with CCN require AAC interventions that support the development of language, communication, and emerging literacy (reading and writing) skills. School-aged children with CCN need AAC interventions that enhance participation in their education, enable them to make friends, develop literacy and other academic skills, and engage with family members

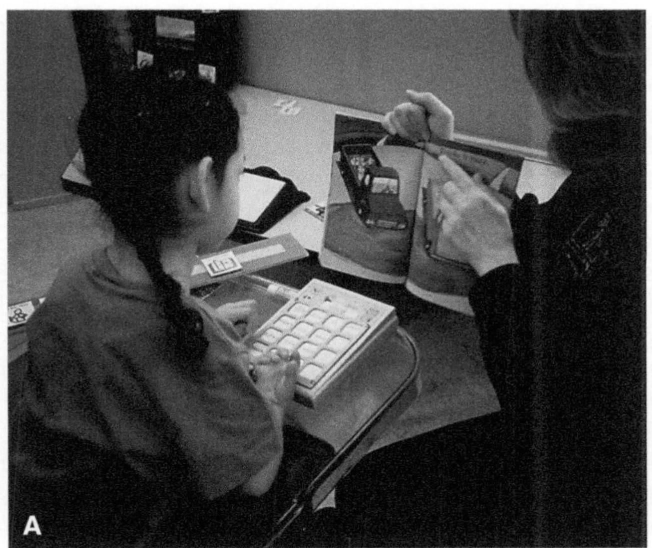

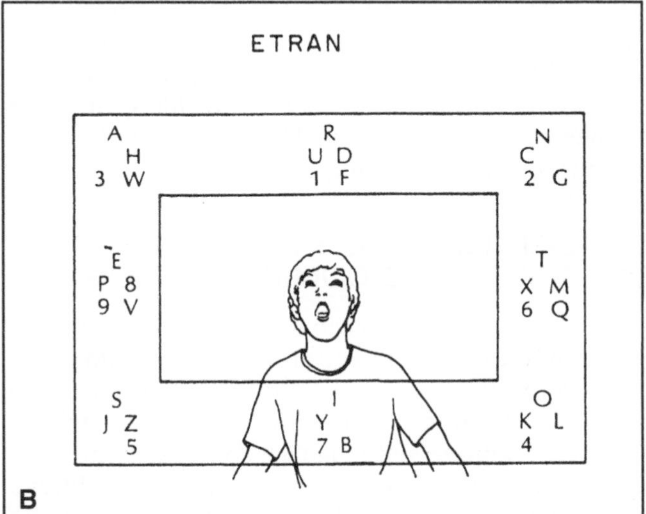

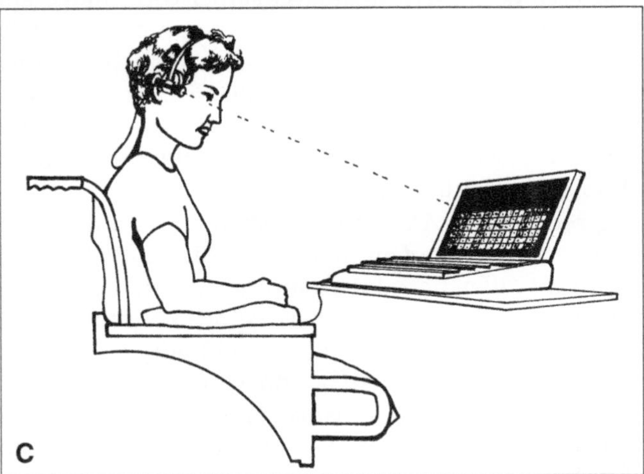

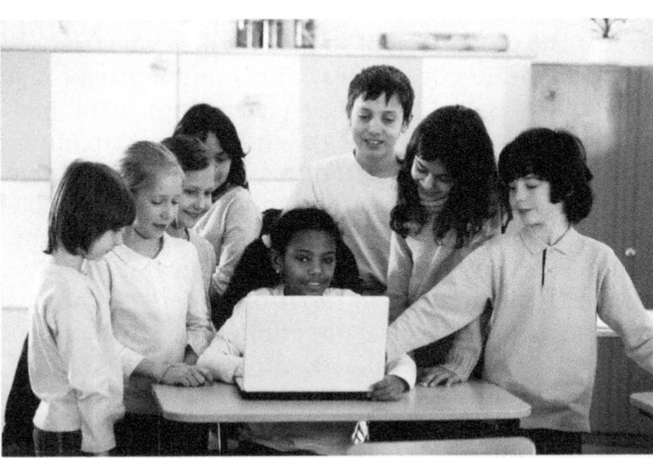

Figure 11-1 There are a variety of approaches and needs for augmentative and alternative communication systems. **A,** Conversations about a story. **B,** An eye transfer communication device (ETRAN). Eye gaze is used to indicate the choice. **C,** Head pointing is often used to make choices from a communication device. **D,** AAC systems with focused vocabulary are used in classrooms. (**B** and **C** from Blackstone S: *Augmentative communication,* Rockville, Md., 1986, American Speech-Language-Hearing Association.)

and people in their communities. For all children and adolescents, AAC can assist in meeting age-appropriate psychological and social development milestones. Individuals who acquire disabilities later in life need AAC to help them sustain employment and maintain their relationships and social networks, independence, and dignity. As Daniel Webster said in 1822,

> "If all my possessions were taken from me with one exception, I would choose to keep the power of communication, for by it I would soon regain all the rest."

Today, people with CCN are using AAC to attend schools and universities, work, carry on chats, participate in computer list serves and social networks, shop, order in restaurants, talk on the phone, and generally participate fully in society. People with CCN who have severe disabilities and who are able to obtain speech generating devices (SGDs) are living independently, getting married, and are active members of their communities. Individuals with CCN who do not gain access to AAC interventions may have limited social networks, have difficulty in reporting abuse, and be limited in their access to employment.[21,25]

This chapter is devoted to a discussion of the major aspects of AAC that are important in enabling individuals with CCN to communicate across the life span, while recognizing that each individual has unique needs, goals, preferences, skills, and abilities.

DISABILITIES AFFECTING SPEECH, LANGUAGE, AND COMMUNICATION

There are many disabilities that can affect an individual's communication skills and abilities. Communication disorders can be categorized into those that affect the production of sounds and intelligible speech and those that affect cognitive and language abilities. Some individuals cannot produce speech because of conditions present at birth or acquired later in life. For some, the problem is in making sounds, although many individuals can produce sounds without being able to produce speech. The production of sounds is called **vocalization** and it can be an effective way of communicating some things like yes and no, anger (screaming), happiness (laughing), sadness (crying), and getting attention. Even if sounds can be produced, an individual may have limitations that interfere with his ability to make sounds or control the muscles of the chest, diaphragm, mouth, tongue, and throat to produce intelligible speech. **Dysarthria** is a disorder of motor speech control resulting from central or peripheral nervous system damage that causes weakness, slowness, and a lack of coordination of the muscles necessary for speech production.[1] Verbal **apraxia** is a disorder affecting the coordination of motor movements involved in producing speech caused by a central nervous system dysfunction.[1] Written communication is also important and limb apraxia may impair the ability to write. When speech and/or writing are severely impaired, AAC approaches are indicated.

There is a difference between speech disorders and language disorders. Cognitive and language abilities are necessary in order to understand the speech of others and to express thoughts. A language is a set of symbols and the rules for organizing them. Each symbol represents a concept or concepts with expressive meaning. The symbols may be the familiar alphabetic written language (referred to as traditional orthography) or it may be a set of pictographic symbols conveying meaning (such as hieroglyphics or other special symbols) or a set of hand movements (sign language) or gestures. **Speech** is the oral expression of language.

Children who have severe language delays or disorders need **AAC systems** that will support the development of receptive and expressive language and literacy (reading and writing) skills. The AAC system can aid them in meeting age-appropriate psychological and social development milestones. **Aphasia** is a language disorder that can affect both the ability to formulate concepts for expression and the understanding of spoken and/or written language. For example, some people may lose the ability to recall names, places, or events and others may lose the ability to understand spoken language. Others may not be able to organize language into meaningful utterances to speak and/or write meaningful utterances. The degree to which various language functions are impaired is variable. AAC interventions for severe aphasia often focus on strategies that help individuals compensate for a severe loss of language function in ways that support functional communication.

Many individuals with disabilities affecting their communication benefit from AAC interventions. Developmental conditions such as cerebral palsy (CP), intellectual disabilities, and autism spectrum disorder (ASD) affect children and adults. Acquired conditions such as traumatic brain injury (TBI), stroke/cerebral vascular accident (CVA), high-level spinal cord injury, and degenerative diseases such as amyotrophic lateral sclerosis (ALS), progressive aphasia, and multiple sclerosis can affect older children and adults. Estimates indicate that approximately 2 million people in the United States and from 0.3% to 1.0% of the total world population of school-aged children have a need for AAC.[8]

Approaches to AAC differ depending upon the severity, type, and onset of an individual's disability. There are significant differences, for example, between meeting the needs of children who have never spoken or used written language (congenital disabilities) and adults who have developed language, speech, and writing and then lost these skills because of a disease or injury. Conventional means of communication (i.e., speaking and using a pencil or pen) are unavailable to young children who have severe motor impairments and CCN. They must use AAC approaches to learn language at the same time they are learning to "talk" and "write" with AAC devices. These children also have few, if any, opportunities to interact with competent AAC users who might serve as role models and help them learn how to communicate using AAC. Someone who develops ALS at age 46 years typically has years of experience using multiple forms of communication and their language skills are intact. AAC interventions for this person are likely to focus on providing technologies and strategies so they can continue to communicate effectively with preferred partners. The challenge for these individuals is that communication via AAC is very different than communication via speech and they must learn new ways of expressing themselves.

What Is Augmentative and Alternative Communication?

There are many ways of looking at augmentative and alternative communication (AAC) systems. *Unaided communication* or *body-based modes* describe communication behaviors that require only the person's own body, such as pointing and other gestures, pantomime, facial expressions, eye gaze and manual signing, or finger spelling. These modes are often used together and may be combined with any available speech. A person's disability affects interpretation of unaided modes of communication. For example, individuals with some physical disabilities have difficulty controlling facial muscles as well as their limbs. This lack of control can lead to unintended "communication" such as inadvertent smiling or unintended limb movements that could be interpreted as a meaningful gesture. When this happens, communication partners frequently misinterpret the nonverbal behaviors because eye gaze, facial expression, body movements, posture, traditional head nods, and pointing or reaching may be incongruent with the intended meaning or tone.[41] Rush (1986)[59] gives an example when he describes the difficulty his cerebral palsy causes him in delivering his line (a yell) in a play: "When a person with cerebral palsy wants to do something, he can't and when he wants not to do something, he involuntarily does it. So getting my vocal cords to cooperate with the cue was as hard as memorizing a Shakespearean play [for a non-disabled person]." (p 21)

Aided AAC components may include a pen or pencil, a letter or picture communication board, a computer, a cell phone, or a speech generating device (SGD). Aided AAC may be either electronic or non-electronic. While a paper letter board (non-electronic) differs from a computer-based SGD (electronic), both non-electronic and electronic devices require the person to use a symbol system and have a way of selecting messages. All forms of AAC require consideration of how communication partners will participate in the communication process.

Approaches to Alternative and Augmentative Communication

We all use a variety of communication modes (e.g., phones, e-mail, or computers) to interact with others and accomplish our activities of daily living. In order to meet all of their needs, people with complex communication needs require multiple communication methods and devices. Many communicators use "no-technology" or body-centered methods such as speech, gestures, facial expressions, and vocalizations (non-speech sounds). They also use "low-technology" systems such as paper communication boards and books (where their choices are indicating by pointing) or paper and pencil for writing messages. Some individuals who have CCN use "high-technology" electronic devices including talking picture frames, smart phones and computers that have speech outputs, and devices specially designed for AAC use called **Speech Generating Devices (SGDs).** AAC systems can take on many forms. Not everyone uses all of these approaches, but many people do.

No-Tech AAC Approaches

Gestures, facial expressions, and body movements help display emotional states, regulate and maintain a conversation, and support information exchange. Gestural codes (e.g., Amer-Ind* or Tadoma†) and formal manual sign systems (e.g., American Sign Language, Signing Exact English) are examples of more formal approaches.[8]

Low-Tech AAC Systems

In Chapter 1 we defined low technology as inexpensive devices that are simple to make and easy to obtain. Many types of AAC approaches fit into this category. Examples of low technology approaches are shown in Figure 11-2. The communication cards shown in Figure 11-2, *A*, are on a chain worn around the neck of the person. The communication book shown in Figure 11-2, *B*, and the board or display shown in Figure 11-2, *C*, are based on letters/words/phrases or graphic symbols, respectively. The communication display in Figure 11-2, *D*, is an example of an activity-specific communication display that is placed by the door to facilitate the choosing of a recess activity. Other low-tech approaches, as described later in this chapter, may include placing symbols on items around a room to develop labeling skills, or using miniature objects as labels and formal systems such as the Picture Exchange System (PECS) to teach requesting.

High-Tech AAC Systems

The term "high-technology AAC" refers to devices that have electronic components. Figure 11-3 illustrates some examples of high-tech AAC devices. There are two broad categories that are discussed in Chapter 5: direct selection and scanning. Some devices with limited functions are called "lite" technologies. The light pointer in Figure 11-3, *C*, is an example of a direct selection lite technology that has greater range and is easier to use than a mechanical head pointer. The lite technology devices in Figure 11-3, *B* and *C*, use scanning to choose between a few items

* American Indian sign language

† The deaf-blind method used by Helen Keller

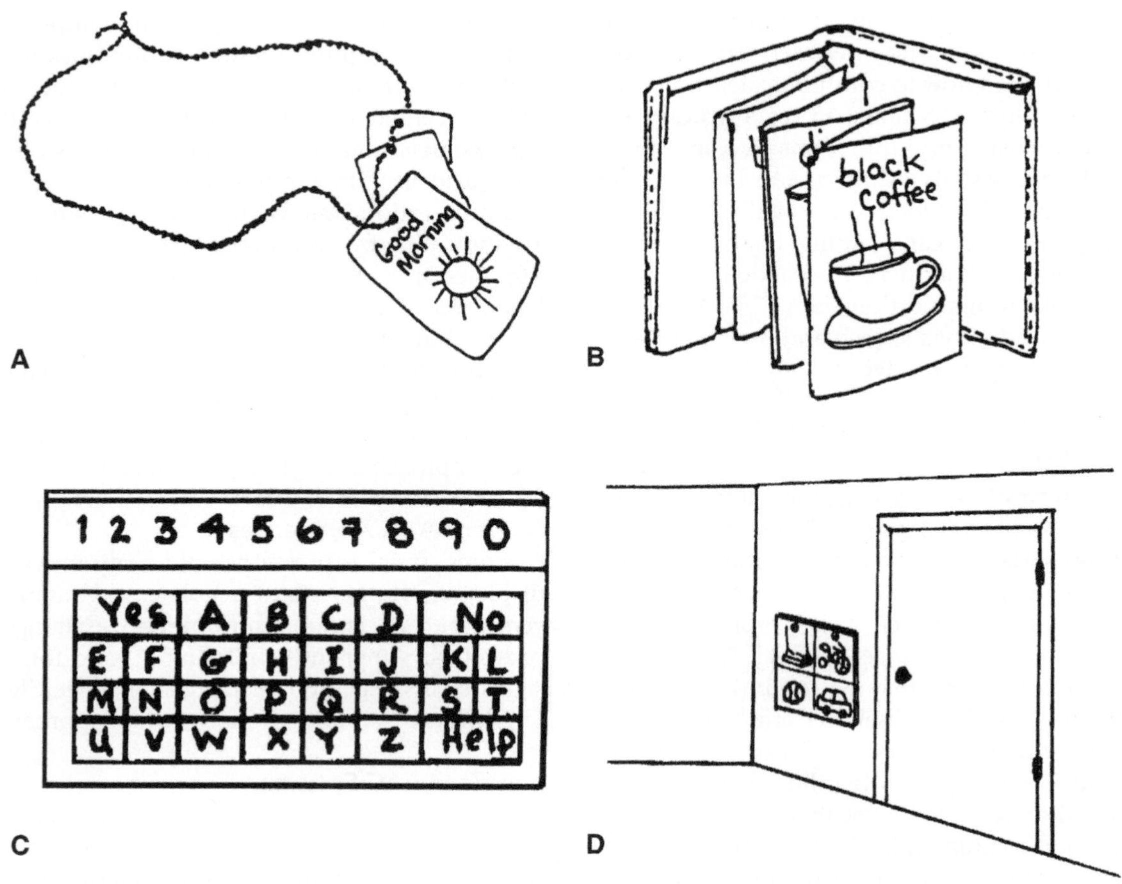

Figure 11-2 Low-tech communication aids.

using a single switch. "High technology" devices have many choices and typically provide speech output. They can use either direct selection (Figure 11-3, *E*) or scanning (Figure 11-3, *F*). Some AAC devices use mainstream technologies (e.g., computers and cell phones) with special software. These can use direct selection (Figure 11-3, *G*) or scanning (Figure 11-3, *H*).

The AAC Team

Finding the right AAC system for an individual requires a team approach. Each member of the AAC team has important roles and responsibilities: The *client and family* have the greatest knowledge of the daily communication needs of the person who has CCN. Family members are often the individual's primary communication partners and serve as advocates and facilitators. The *speech-language pathologist* typically has the greatest general understanding of communication in general and can assess language and communication needs, abilities, and skills; select AAC materials and technologies; and develop a training program for the individual, caregivers, and family. The *speech assistant* may be responsible for programming the device with vocabulary for the individual and implementing the training program to teach the individual, family, and staff to use AAC system components effectively. The *teacher* sets educational goals and oversees classroom implementation of each child's AAC system and has knowledge of literacy, social interaction, and education. The *PT* and/or *OT* carry out the motor evaluation, address seating and positioning needs, evaluate physical access to the AAC system, and have knowledge of how to support writing, drawing, and other activities of daily living. The positioning of the communication device for use (e.g., mounting to a wheelchair, locating on a table, or attaching it to the person for walking), the positioning of the control interface (see Chapter 6), and ensuring that the person is properly positioned to access the AAC system are often the responsibilities of a *PT-assistant* and *OT assistant*. In a classroom setting, an *educational assistant* may take on the roles of programming specific vocabulary into the device to meet educational goals and training the individual to use the device effectively for school work. In a work setting, programming and training may fall to a *job coach*. Family members may also be involved in programming and helping the individual learn to use the device effectively. These individuals support the person in the development of skill in using AAC to meet the person's communication needs. They also may receive instruction that allows them to add vocabulary, set up the AAC system for daily use by the person, and take care of maintenance tasks such as charging batteries and cleaning the device. Key team members such as family, friends, co-workers, fellow students, residents living in the same group home, and employers are often referred to as "natural supports"

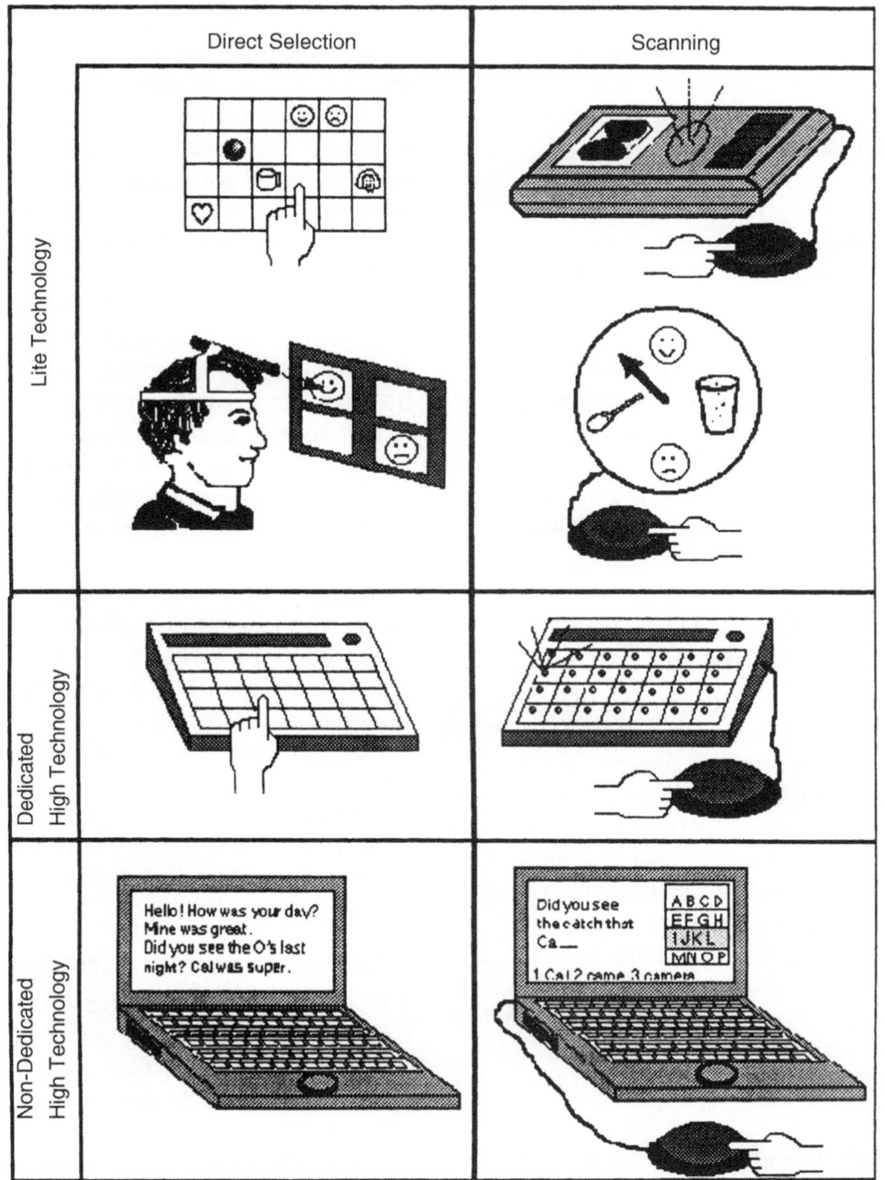

Figure 11-3 A variety of high-tech AAC systems. (From Glennen SL, DeCoste DC: *The handbook of augmentative and alternative communication,* 1997, San Diego, Singular Publishing.)

because they have an ongoing relationship with the individual. Occasionally physicians, psychologists, vision specialists, and other professionals also play a role on AAC teams.

The Importance of Augmentative Communication in the Lives of People with Complex Communication Needs (CCN)

First person accounts of AAC users provide an important perspective. Christopher Nolan,[57] a man with cerebral palsy, wrote in the third person (as Joseph) about the importance of attentive and responsive communication partners. "Such were Joseph's teachers and such was their imagination that the mute boy became constantly amazed at the almost telepathic degree of certainty with which they read his facial expression, eye movements, and body language. Many a good laugh was had by teacher and pupil as they deciphered his code. It was moments such as these that Joseph recognized the face of God in human form. It glimmered in their kindness to him, it glowed in their keenness, it hinted in their caring, indeed it caressed in their gaze." (p 11)

AAC systems can enhance interaction, but they can also become the center of attention, detracting from the real goal of interpersonal interaction, as William Rush[59] noted:

> "My new friend (Wendy) was good looking. She was just over five feet tall and had brown eyes that matched the color of her shoulder length hair. Her skin showed a summer tan and she had a dynamite smile. 'Did he show ya all his electronic stuff?' one of my dorm mates asked her. "Go on, Bill, show her." So I demonstrated the controls for my lights and clock radio. I showed off my

door opener, which I could control via a radio transmitter attached to the Plexiglas tray on my wheelchair. She was impressed with the space-age technology. 'Hey, show her your wheelchair and how it works. I'll never understand how it works. It baffles me,' another dorm mate said. So, wondering if I should sell tickets, I wheeled about the room. I demonstrated how I went straight, reverse, and turned left and right. I was angry at my dorm mates because I was a man, not a side show freak. My wheelchair was a tool for my mobility, not a novelty. Why couldn't they see that? And why couldn't they see that I was trying to get to know Wendy. Why didn't they understand I had a right to my privacy just as they did? As I was wheeling around the room, I noticed that Wendy was typing something. I was disappointed in her. I thought she knew that I could hear and that she didn't have to write things to me. Apparently I was wrong. When I was done showing my electric marvels to her and the guys, I rolled back to my typewriter to read, "I wish they would go, so we could talk by ourselves." They finally left and we finally got to talk. Our friendship had started." (p 137)

The loss of speech can also occur later in life. Doreen Joseph[38] lost her speech following an accident. She described her situation: "I woke up one morning and I wasn't me. There was somebody else in my bed. And all I had left was my head. Speech is the most important thing we have. It makes us a person and not a thing. No one should ever have to be a 'thing.'" (p 8) Sue Simpson[64] lost her speech after a stroke at age 36. She wrote: "So you can't talk, and it's boring and frustrating and nobody quite understands how bad it really is. If you sit around and think about all the things you used to be able to do, that you can't do now, you'll be a miserable wreck and no one will want to hang around you for long." (p 11)

Partners of People with CCN Who Rely on AAC

Communication almost always involves a partner who may be in the room, on the phone, or a continent away on e-mail. Some "partners" may be merely imagined, as when someone writes a story. The "Circle of Communication Partners" (Figure 11-4) is helpful in

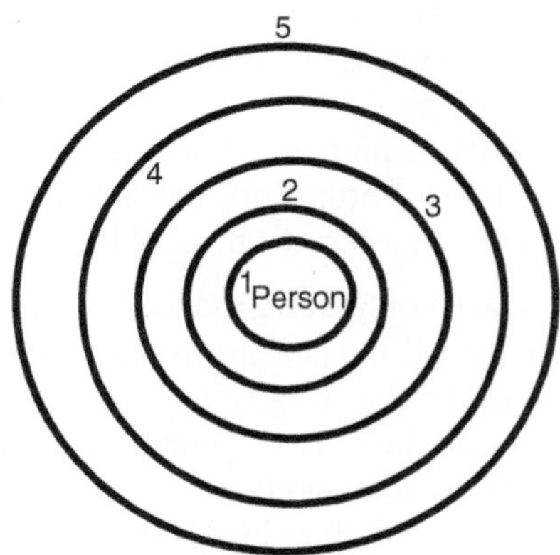

Figure 11-4 Circle of communication partners.

defining the range of partners that a person with Complex Communication Needs who relies on AAC might encounter.[13] The first circle represents the person's life-long communication partners. This is primarily immediate family members. The second circle includes close friends (e.g., the people you tell your secrets to). These are often not family members. Acquaintances such as neighbors, schoolmates, co-workers, distant relatives such as aunts and cousins, the bus driver, and shopkeepers are included in the third circle. The fourth circle is used to represent paid workers such as a doctor, speech-language pathologist (SLP) or a physical therapist (PT), occupational therapist (OT), occupational therapy assistant (OTA), physical therapy assistant (PTA), speech assistant, teacher, educational assistant, or babysitter. Finally, the fifth circle is used to represent those unfamiliar partners with whom the person has occasional interactions. This circle includes everyone who doesn't fit in the first four circles.

Table 11-1 shows that as we move from circle 1 to circle 5 the modes of communication required to communicate with people in each circle vary.[17] For example, gestures and speech (even if it difficult to understand) are often preferred modes in circles 1 and 2. Circle 2 also includes some non-electronic communication boards as well as telephone and e-mail. Circle 4 reflects the school, work, and professional provider partners and therefore a wide range of modes are used. Circle 5 relies primarily on non-electronic communication boards, books, and SGDs of various types.

Attitudes About and Acceptance of AAC

McCarthy and Light[51] reviewed 13 research studies on partners' attitudes toward individuals who rely on SGDs. They identified several factors affecting attitudes: (1) characteristics of typically developing individuals, (2) characteristics of the person using AAC, and (3) characteristics of the AAC system. These are elements of the social context of the HAAT model (see Chapter 2). Attitudes toward individuals who use AAC vary across the parameters of gender, type of disability, age, experience of the user of AAC, experience and familiarity with the disability and AAC by the partner, and social context. Attitudes appear to be formed by the interaction of many of these factors. Some of these attitudes are summarized in Box 11-1.

COMMUNICATION NEEDS THAT CAN BE SERVED BY AAC

We as humans communicate in a myriad of ways depending upon the circumstances. If speaking and/or writing are not possible, we search for (and find) other ways of communicating. People with complex communication needs (CCN) are often unable to speak and write so that others can understand them. This can impact performance of the activities of daily living even if assistance from an attendant is available. AAC approaches help with face-to-face communication, as well as with communication

TABLE 11-1 Each of the Circles in Figure 11-4 Has Different Partners and Modes of Communication

Circle	Partners	Commonly Used AAC Modes and Techniques*
1	Life-long communication partners, immediate family members	Facial expressions, gestures, vocalizations, speech, and manual signs
2	Close friends (i.e., people who you tell your secrets to), often not family member	Facial expressions, gestures, vocalizations, non-electronic communication boards and books, telephone, and e-mail
3	Acquaintances such as neighbors, schoolmates, co-workers, distant relatives (such as aunts and cousins), regular shop keeper or bus driver	Facial expressions, gestures, vocalizations, low-tech and high-tech dedicated SGDs, telephone, and e-mail
4	Paid workers such as a speech-language pathologist (SLP) or a PT, OT, OTA, PTA, speech assistant, teacher, teacher assistant, or babysitter	Facial expressions, gestures, vocalizations, manual signs, non-electronic communication boards and books, writing, low-tech and high-tech dedicated SGDs, and mainstream-based SGDs
5	Unfamiliar partners with whom the person has occasional interactions (e.g., a bus driver and seldom-visited or new shop keepers)	Facial expressions, gestures, non-electronic communication boards and books, low-tech and high-tech dedicated SGDs, and mainstream-based SGDs

*Blackstone SW and Hunt Berg M: Social networks: a communication inventory for individuals with complex communication needs and their communication partners – Inventory Booklet, Monterey, Calif.: Augmentative Communication, Inc., 2003.

BOX 11-1 Attitudes of Partners Influence AAC Effectiveness

WHAT THE RESEARCH TELLS US:

Attitudes about and acceptance of AAC

Children

- The attitudes of children who do not have disabilities toward children who do and who use AAC is influenced by their familiarity with children who have disabilities (i.e., whether the non-disabled students had a classmate with a disability) and by age (older children are less positive than are younger children).[4]
- In general girls are more positive toward disabled peers than boys.[5]
- Children who use AAC communicate mostly through responses and their typically developing peers initiate almost all of the requests.[24]
- The longer the messages produced (2-word vs. 4-word utterances), the more positive are peers' attitudes toward the child using AAC. Much of the interaction among peers involves expressions of humor and intimacy (e.g., laughing, joking, teasing, tickling, etc.).[4]
- Attitudes of peers toward an AAC user do not appear to be affected by the type of AAC system used.[5]
- The use of voice output led to more positive peer attitudes than when the output was only visual (letters on a display).[49]

School settings:[39]

- Unequal status with classmates and dissimilar interests lead to social exclusion for students who rely on AAC.
- Often peers speak to the teacher or teacher's assistant rather than directly to the student.
- Teachers are concerned about lack of academic gain.
- Some device features (e.g., speech synthesis) are perceived as disruptive to other students.
- Teachers require time to adjust to the idea of having students with disabilities in class.

Employment:[53]

- Employers and co-workers are influenced by workers who use AAC.
- Benefits for the worker are social interaction, personal enjoyment, and financial gain.
- Benefits to the employer include positive impacts on other employees, high quality of work performance, and loyalty of the employee.
- Employment challenges:
  - Finding a good job match to individual skills
  - Communication challenges (e.g., noisy AAC device, speaker phone use)
  - Difficulty with typical office tasks (e.g., manipulation of paper, telephone use)
  - Education or vocational skill level too low
  - Lack of knowledge of work culture and physical challenges necessitating assistance from other workers
  - Financial (e.g., insurance costs to company)

on the phone and across the Internet. Writing includes such activities as drawing, plotting graphs, and mathematics. These are all the things that we normally do using a pencil and paper, computer, calculator, and other similar tools.

Light (1988)[43] describes four goals of communicative interaction: (1) expression of needs and wants, (2) information transfer, (3) social closeness, and (4) social etiquette. Expression of needs and wants allows people to make requests for objects or actions. Information transfer allows expression of ideas, discussion, and meaningful dialogue. Social closeness serves to connect individuals to each other, regardless of the content of the conversation. Social etiquette is used to describe those cultural formalities that are inherent in communication. For example, students will speak differently to their peers than to their teachers.

Dowden and Cook (2002)[28] defined three types of AAC communicators. **Emergent communicators** have no reliable method of symbolic expression and they are restricted to communicating about here and now concepts. **Context-dependent communicators** have reliable symbolic communication, but they are limited to specific contexts because they are either only intelligible to familiar partners, have insufficient vocabulary, or both. For example, a child may have symbols and understanding for specific school activities such as circle time or for interacting with their friends, but lack general vocabulary for going shopping or ordering at a restaurant or other typical activities of daily living. **Independent communicators** are able to communicate with unfamiliar and familiar partners on any topic. Each of these communicators has different needs and goals.

In this chapter communication needs are discussed for three major types of disorders that affect speech and language: (1) individuals with developmental disorders, (2) individuals with acquired conditions, and (3) individuals with degenerative conditions. While acknowledging that the focus of AAC interventions may vary across these groups, there is also substantial overlap in the issues we face when communication is severely limited, no matter what the causes may be.

AAC for Individuals with Developmental Disabilities

Because the development of speech, language, and communication begins at birth, early intervention is important. Effective AAC interventions for children with developmental disabilities require that AAC be integrated into the child's daily experiences and interactions, and that it take into account what we know about child development.[48] For example, many young children do not have the physical or cognitive skills to learn to use current AAC selection techniques (e.g., scanning or encoding), and thus are unable to access some AAC systems. Also, the design of current hi-tech AAC technologies often requires a child to stop playing in order to use a communication device. A more desirable approach is to design AAC technologies and strategies that incorporate the use of AAC into the child's play activities so the child can talk about her play or interact with peers while engaged in the activity. In short, to be effective the design, type, and layout of the AAC system components should match the desires, preferences, abilities, and skills of those who rely on AAC systems. This is often called "feature matching."

A major concern for parents is whether the use of AAC will impede their child's development of speech. Research data puts all such fears to rest.[17] In fact, research has shown that the use of AAC does not interfere with speech development and may enhance the development or return of speech. There are a number of possible explanations for this, including increased acoustic feedback (from voice output SGD); increased experience with conversational turns and other communicative functions; reduced pressure to speak, which releases motor stress; and the development of an internal phonology due to AAC systems use.[18] Research shows that children with a broad range of developmental disabilities can benefit from AAC interventions. Developmental disabilities include children with cerebral palsy, intellectual disability, Down syndrome, other genetic disorders, and autism spectrum disorder (ASD).

Cerebral Palsy

Cerebral palsy is a non-progressive motor impairment due to a lesion or anomalies of the brain arising in the early stages of its development.[66] Cerebral palsy syndromes describe motor disorders characterized by impaired voluntary movement resulting from prenatal developmental abnormalities or perinatal or postnatal central nervous system (CNS) damage. It is primarily a disorder of muscle tone and postural control. Individuals who have cerebral palsy will often exhibit apraxia, which is the inability to perform motor activities even though sensory motor function is intact and the individual understands the requirements of the task.[23] Primitive reflexes, characterized by immediate and automatic movement performed at a subconscious level, also accompany cerebral palsy.[36] Typically these reflexes are inhibited or (more often) integrated into volitional movements in order to control posture and perform basic movement patterns as the infant develops. Cerebral palsy may affect the degree to which these reflexes are integrated and some reflex patterns persist into adulthood for those with CP. The primitive reflexes that most commonly influence AT use are the asymmetrical tonic neck reflex (ATNR) and the symmetrical tonic neck reflex (STNR). The impact of these on AAC use is shown in Figure 11-5.[8]

CP is also characterized by variation in muscle tone ranging from increased tone (referred to as hypertonicity or spasticity) to low tone (referred to as hypotonicity). In an individual child the tone may be mixed, may vary over the course of the day, or vary depending on the

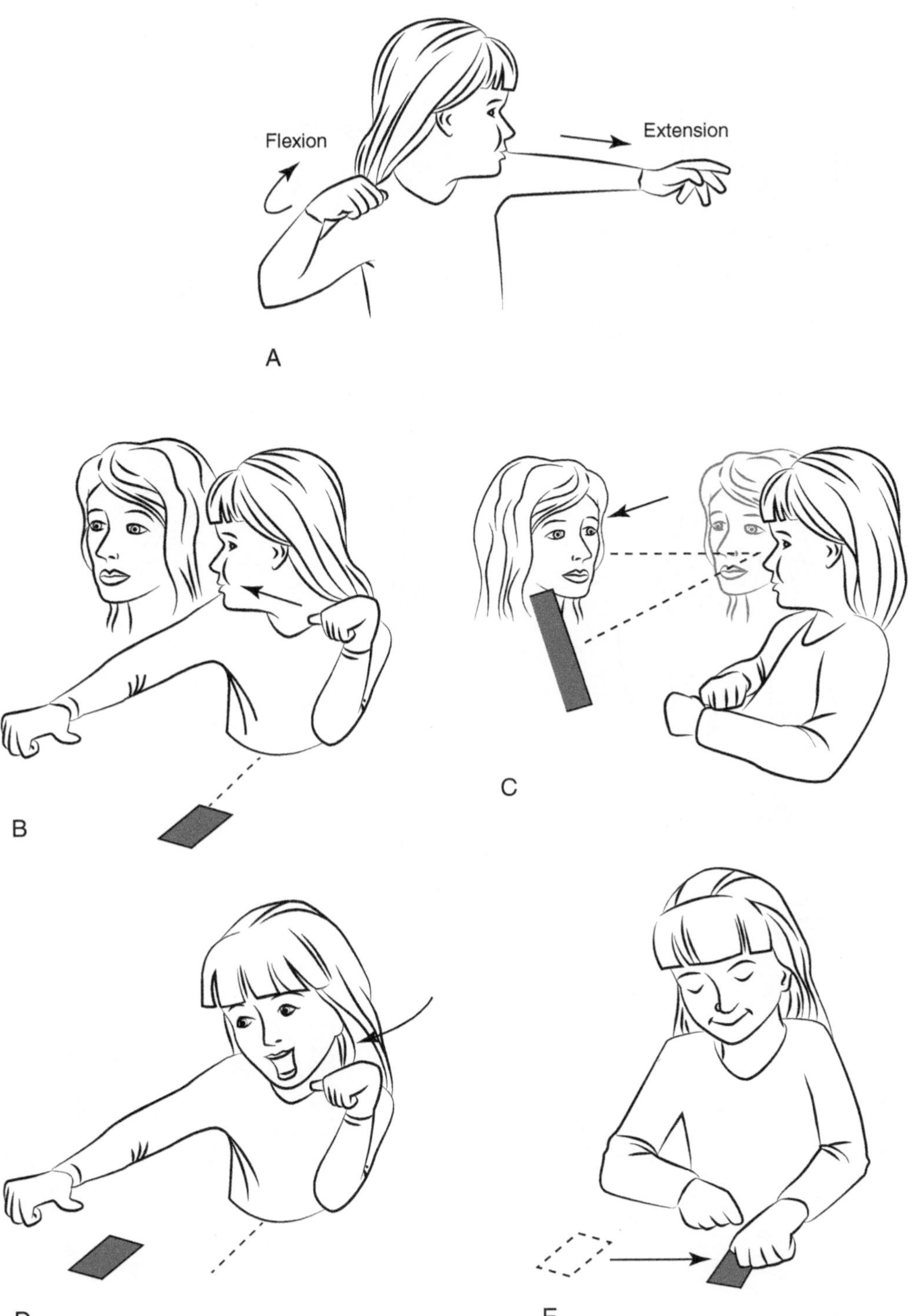

Figure 11-5 The asymmetric tonic neck reflex (ATNR) (left) and symmetric tonic neck reflex (STNR) (right) reflexes can impact AAC system use. (From Beukelman DR, Mirenda P: *Augmentative and alternative communication: management of severe communication disorders in children and adults,* ed 3, Baltimore, 2005, Paul H. Brookes.)

child's position.[66] This altered muscle tone has an impact on motor control required for the use of AAC devices. Oculomotor function is also abnormal (problems with eye movements) in many children with CP. Duckman (1979)[29] found that 92% of the children with CP had oculomotor dysfunction of some type. This finding has direct bearing on tasks that require frequent redirection of gaze, such as looking at a keyboard to find the desired character and then looking at a display or screen to monitor the selections.

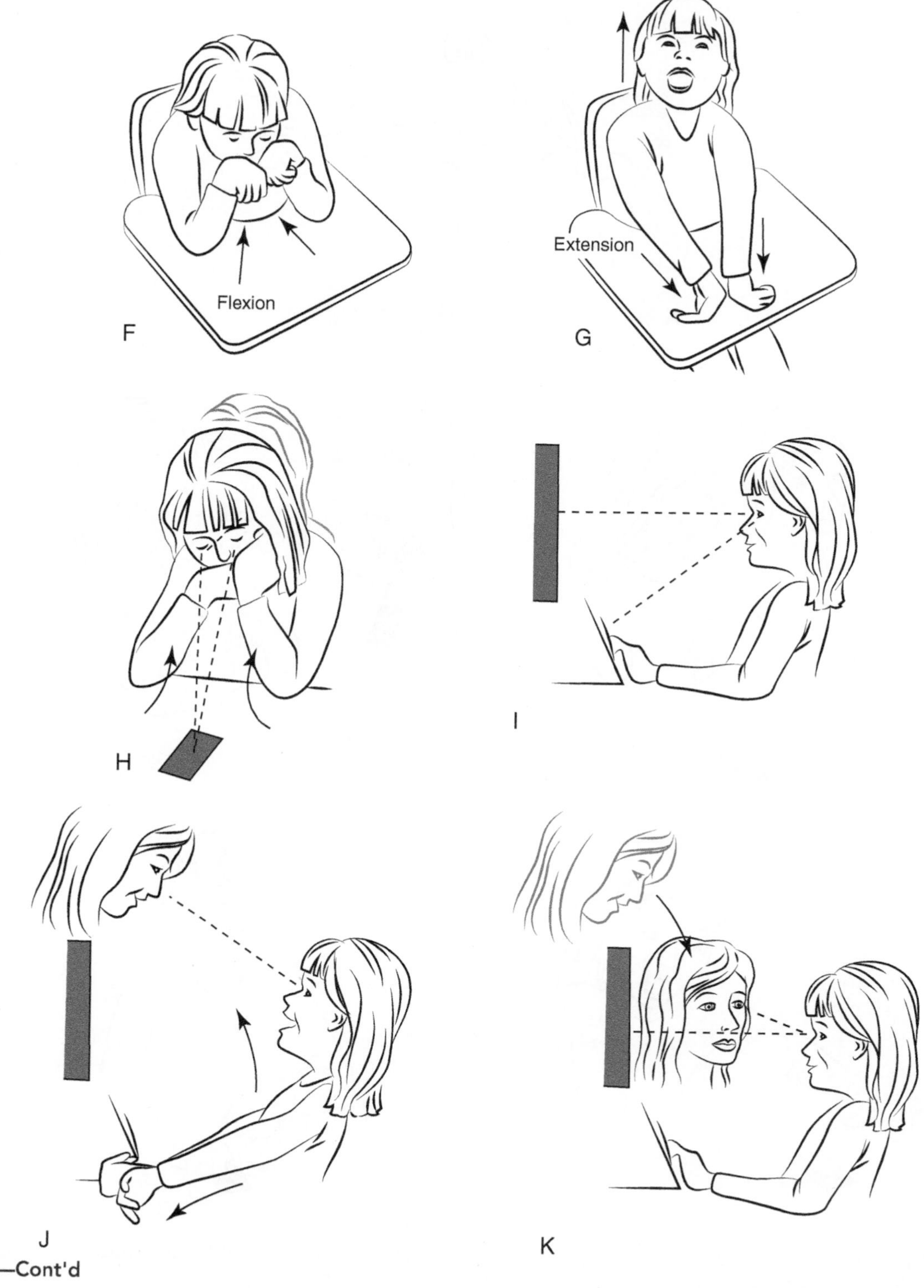

Figure 11-5—Cont'd

As Scherer (1998)[61] points out, the person who is born with cerebral palsy is likely to have adjusted to the disability and developed strategies that help accommodate for the lack of coordinated motor control. For example, some individuals are able to use a primitive reflex to initiate a movement. Others have learned to position equipment and materials in order to maximize the motor control they have. These individuals are inclined to view assistive technology as opening up new opportunities for them and they often apply their developed strategies to the control of these devices.

CASE STUDY 11-1 – MEETING A CONGENITAL NEED FOR AAC

Joyce is 39 years old. She has cerebral palsy and she currently lives with her parents. Her speech is dysarthric and she is unable to use a pen or pencil for writing. Unaided communication modes include head nods and eye gaze. Joyce currently uses a switch mounted near her knee to control her scanning communication device, which has synthesized speech output and a small word-processing program for writing. To meet Joyce's need to activate a call device for emergency help over the telephone, she uses an alarm tied into a 24-hour surveillance company and activated by a separate switch using her left arm. She uses her left arm for the emergency call device because this movement is less limited by being supine in bed than is knee movement. Also, when she is seated in her wheelchair, left arm use does not interfere with either her powered mobility or her communication, since they use other control sites.

List the steps you would take to evaluate Joyce's success with these systems.

Autism Spectrum Disorder (ASD)

Autism Spectrum Disorder (ASD) is characterized by significant social communication challenges throughout life that reflect impairments in social interaction and in verbal and non-verbal communication as well as restricted, repetitive, stereotypical patterns of behavior, interests, and activities.[14] Early intervention (starting as young as two years) improves outcomes for children with ASD. These children often have difficulty with joint attention (i.e., coordinating attention between people and objects) and with understanding and using symbols. Approximately one-third to one-half of children with ASD do not use speech functionally.[14] The learning styles of children with ASD show a strong preference for static information (e.g., visual information that doesn't change). As a result, they often benefit from the use of "visual supports" (e.g., printed guides that provide cues such as a list of common phrases). Because speech and other elements of conversation are transient, AAC devices and communication displays that utilize static visual symbols provide possible assistance for the child with ASD. Also, because of their dependence on rote or episodic memory, children with ASD often benefit from contextual clues and prompts. However, this can lead to them becoming prompt or context dependent and can decrease the carryover of skills. Thus, AAC interventions that extend the use of language and appropriate communication behaviors across different contexts and partners are needed. Blackstone (2003)[14] argues that AAC can be effective for children with ASD because it addresses both their unique learning styles and communication needs.

Children with ASD can use no-tech (e.g., manual signs) and high- and low-technology approaches to AAC.[54] At this time, there is no clear evidence that one approach is superior to any other. The use of total communication (speech and manual signing) provides advantages because there is no need to care for or operate a device and because it promotes more natural forms of communication. However, not all children (or their partners) do equally well with this approach.

Some children develop more functional communication using low-tech–aided systems. The Picture Exchange Communication System (PECS)* is one widely used example. Voice-output communication aids can also support interactions. For example, Schlosser and Blischak (2001)[62] suggested that electronically generated speech may be beneficial for children with ASD who have difficulty processing natural speech. Also, computer-aided instruction may help children with ASD attend to instructions and prompts when provided via electronic speech output. There are many considerations in choosing between the many available AAC approaches, including an individual's preferences, ease of learning, effect on the development of speech and language, ability to use the approach functionally across partners, and the communication tasks the person needs to accomplish and contexts in which they take place. Finally, the degree of partner support and responsiveness is considered. Current best practices rely on clinician judgment as much as evidence because current research on the use of AAC approaches for individuals with ASD is promising, but inconclusive, in each of these areas.

AAC for Individuals with Acquired Disabilities

Adults with acquired disabilities such as traumatic brain injury (TBI), aphasia, and other static conditions may require the use of AAC interventions as part of the rehabilitation process.[7] Persons with recovering conditions (e.g., traumatic brain injury or stroke) often experience changing levels of motor, sensory, and/or cognitive/linguistic capability. This group of users may benefit from the use of AAC to help them adapt. While many people may be unable to speak or write directly after a severe head injury or brain stem or cortical stroke, most will recover some abilities over a period of months or years. However, over the long-term, some individuals continue to benefit from the use of AAC if speech is unintelligible. In this section traumatic brain injury (TBI) and aphasia are discussed as examples of individuals with acquired AAC needs.

Traumatic Brain Injury (TBI)

TBI can result in the loss of speech and often causes physical, cognitive, and language impairments.[6,46] The motor impairment is often severe in TBI and the

*Pyramid Educational Consultants, Newark, Del. (http://www.pecsproducts.com/catalog/)

sequelae include problems with cognition (thinking, memory, and reasoning); sensory processing (sight, hearing, touch, taste, and smell); communication (expression and understanding); and behavior or mental health (depression, anxiety, personality changes, aggression, acting out, and social inappropriateness). These factors frequently hamper function and often are long-term outcomes that effect communication and other functions in very subtle ways, limiting the ability to access AAC.[22] While the long-term recovery of speech is variable, immediately following the injury many individuals benefit from AAC interventions to support functional communication.

Beukelman et al. (2007)[9] carried out a study of AAC use by individuals who had sustained a TBI. The individuals with TBI in this study generally accepted AAC recommendations, and none of the participants rejected AAC after receiving a low-tech or high-tech AAC option. When it did occur, AAC technology abandonment usually reflected the loss of a facilitator (a soft technology loss; see Chapter 1), not rejection of the technology (Box 11-2). Participants in this study relied predominantly on letter-by-letter spelling strategies primarily due to the interference of cognitive limitations with the ability to encode messages or utilize other message-formulation strategies. Beukelman et al. attempted to teach the use of encoding and/or word retrieval to several individuals with TBI who spelled their messages using AAC technology. Some were able to learn the encoding or prediction strategy in the intervention setting, but none used the strategy in their everyday communication, reporting that it was "too much work."

BOX 11-2 AAC and TBI

WHAT THE RESEARCH TELLS US

TBI and AAC

- 68% of this sample was advised to utilize high-technology AAC devices.
- 94% of these individuals and their decision makers accepted the recommendations.
- After 3 years, 81% continued to use their AAC technology, 6% had not received the technology because of funding problems, and 12% had discontinued AAC device use because they did not have appropriate AAC facilitator support.
- 87% used letter-by-letter spelling, while the remaining 13% relied on symbols and drawings.
- Low-technology AAC options were recommended for 32% of the total group.
- 100% accepted the recommendation.
- After 3 years, 63% continued to use their low-technology AAC strategies at least part time.
- 37% discontinued use because they regained sufficient natural speech to meet their communication needs.

Aphasia

Persons who sustain a stroke often experience language difficulties that we collectively call *aphasia*. One lasting problem these individuals have is vocabulary retrieval or word-finding difficulties. There are several AAC-related approaches with potential for aphasia rehabilitation.[37] For example, individuals who can recall first letters and recognize a desired word from a list may use word prediction devices or software. The individual begins typing a letter and then the device predicts several words from which to choose (see Figure 5-11). There are many factors that must be considered when applying AAC in aphasia rehabilitation. Research supporting aphasia intervention using AAC is described in Box 11-3. Some people with severe aphasia learn to augment their speech and communication efforts by relying on gestures and an alternative symbol system.[37] However, while persons with aphasia may be able to use graphic symbols, many find it difficult to apply them socially or to generalize their use.

CASE STUDY 11-2 – AAC FOLLOWING STROKE

Eileen is a 62-year-old woman who has sustained a brainstem stroke and now requires maximal assistance for daily living. Eileen's unaided communication modalities include isolated words, facial expressions, yes/no responses, and inflectional vocalizations. She also has two AAC devices. The first of these is a letter board, accessed by her eye gaze that she uses to indicate her needs and choices (Figure 11-2). The unaided systems and letter board have limitations. The unaided systems require significant amounts of interpretation by the partner, and the manual eye gaze device is slow because it relies on spelling and interpretation by her partner. These limitations are partially overcome by Eileen's electronic AAC device, which she accesses using head movements to make selections with a head pointer using a reflective dot on her forehead (see Chapter 6). This device includes vocabulary storage so she can use whole words and phrases, and it provides synthesized speech output. These features allow Eileen to converse with more people, and they make it easier on the communication partner. Each of these devices contributes to the quantity and quality of her communication interactions.

Eileen's daughter has just gotten engaged and is bringing her fiance to meet Eileen. How would you help her prepare for the visit?

One commercial device designed specifically for persons with aphasia is the Lingraphica™, which organizes symbols by semantic categories (e.g., places, foods, and clothing) and includes synthetic speech output and animation of verbs (e.g., "walk" or "give").* Lingraphica

* http://www.aphasia.com/

BOX 11-3 AAC Can Provide Assistance for Individuals with Aphasia

WHAT THE RESEARCH TELLS US

Aphasia and AAC

Speech feedback can provide additional monitoring of written work, which helps the person to identify and correct mistakes. King and Hux (1995)[40] describe the use of a talking word processor to increase writing accuracy for individuals with aphasia.

Garrett and Beukelman (1992)[32] present a classification system for aphasic individuals that is useful in planning AAC interventions. This scheme guides intervention planning by describing five types of aphasic communicators: basic choice, controlled situation, augmented, comprehensive, and specific need. For each of these categories, the authors identify residual skills, intervention goals, and AAC skills and suggest AAC activities for both partners and the individual with aphasia.

Fox and Fried-Oken (1996)[31] propose questions related to effectiveness, efficiency, and generalization in AAC aphasiology research.

One area of concern for future development in AAC is how best to represent meaning on AAC technologies for persons with aphasia.[7]

provides graphic building blocks which are called icons (small pictures, sometimes animated). The icons can be manipulated to generate messages using a cursor. Lingraphica also has applications that allow favorite icons, phrases, and videos selected on the Lingraphica to be transferred to the iPhone and iPod touch. The mobile accessory can be used as an AAC device for communication or for self-cueing and scaffolding (i.e., helping to generate expressive language by providing prompts). Other technological interventions for aphasia are focused on supporting specific communication tasks such as answering the phone, calling for help, ordering in restaurants or stores, giving speeches, saying prayers, or engaging in scripted conversations. These may be either paper-based systems or electronic devices.

Portraits (static pictures or other symbols) contain limited, usually decontextualized information (e.g., a picture of a person with a plain background), and additional information about the person(s) or object in a portrait must be generated by the individual with aphasia or speculated on by the communication partner.[9] This spontaneous generation of additional specific and detailed information is difficult for individuals with severe chronic aphasia. An alternative approach uses Visual Scene Displays (VSDs) (see Figure 11-6 and discussion later in this chapter). VSDs

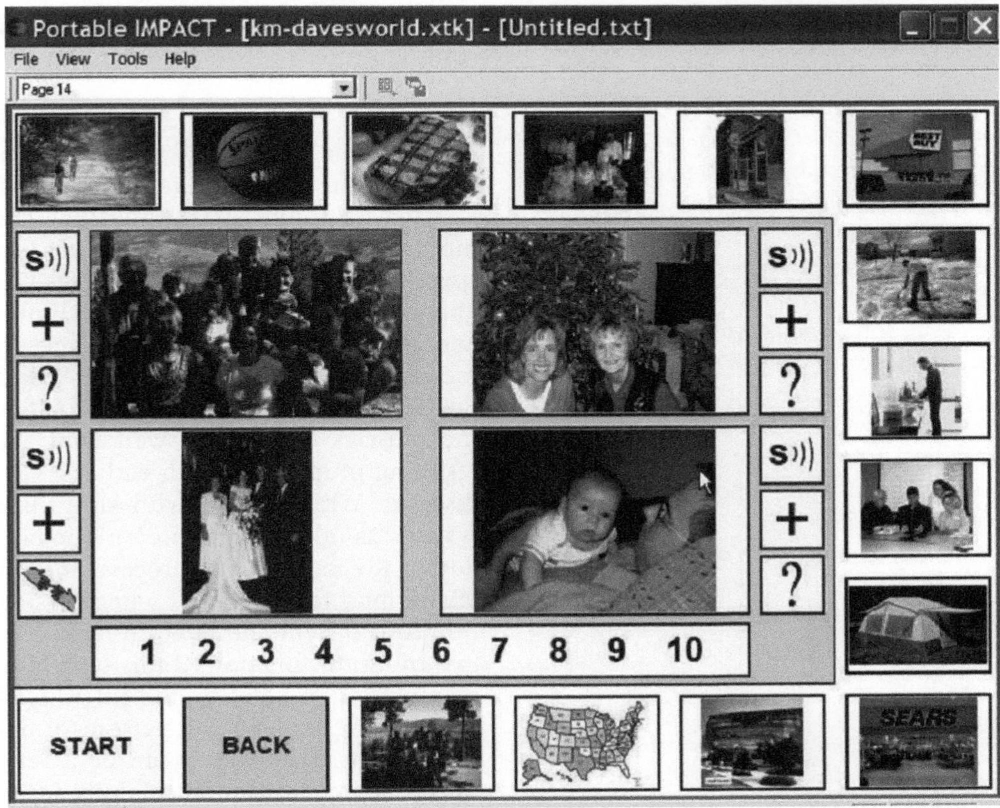

Figure 11-6 VSD layout for family outing or wedding (personalized). (From Blackstone S: Visual scene displays, *Augment Commun News*, 16(2):1–5, 2004.)

use personalized digital photos of scenes and arrange these on a dynamic display device (these devices are described later in this chapter). Each element in a visual scene is pictured in its natural relationship and position to all other elements in the scene.[52] The meaning of all elements and semantic associations are integrally tied together, creating a holistic context.

VSDs enable individuals with severe aphasia to use familiar photographs to engage partners in interactions about multiple topics. In addition, the design of the technology makes it relatively easy for partners to provide conversational supports such as prompting with familiar reminders. The individual with aphasia and the communication partner co-construct "the gist" of the visual scene. Contextualized pictures are paired with text and voice output to communicate specific messages, ask questions, and/or provide support for the communication partner. Because of the dynamic nature of the display, the user is continually prompted regarding the available choices, reducing the individual's need to rely on recall memory. It is also possible to use the same approach with paper-based displays. There is a template provided by the University of Nebraska at http://aac.unl.edu/intervention.html.

CASE STUDY 11-3 – AAC IN AN ADULT DAY CARE CENTER

You work as a member of the transdisciplinary rehabilitation team in an adult day healthcare program. The program has participants with a variety of disabilities and needs, and some have difficulty speaking. The center offers nursing, social work, physical therapy, speech-language pathology, occupational therapy, a variety of activities, and meals. There is an Individual Program Plan (IPP) in place for each participant. Some participate in the program's art activities in small groups with an instructor or aide; others are in supported employment for half days and in the center for the other half of the days. Other participants are in the center all day and they have occasional community outings with care staff to recreational sites, stores, and physical activity venues (e.g., swimming). You have been asked to help address the communication needs of four of these participants:

- A 25-year-old man with TBI living in an apartment with supported living services and a roommate.
- A 40-year-old man with severe intellectual disability and good fine motor control, who is ambulatory and living in a group home with other adults functioning at about the same level.
- A 19-year-old woman with cerebral palsy that limits her fine and gross motor abilities in all four limbs, who lives with her primary caregiver, her sister.
- A 67-year-old woman with aphasia secondary to a CVA, living at a rehab facility.

CASE STUDY 11-3 – AAC IN AN ADULT DAY CARE CENTER—cont'd

None of these individuals has functional speech that is consistently understood by either strangers or even their caregivers, who know them well.

What things are important to know as you prepare to attend the interdisciplinary team meeting to discuss these participants' augmentative communication assessment needs and as you prepare to consult with the participants' family members and/or caregiving staff?

AAC for Individuals with Progressive Neurological Conditions

A degenerative medical condition in which speech and/or language functions are gradually lost presents a different set of challenges for the person with complex communication needs (CCN) and for AAC interventions. For many conditions, multiple AAC modes are necessary as the disease progresses and motor skills and cognition decline. Persons with degenerative conditions often experience changing levels of motor, sensory, and/or cognitive/linguistic capability that require the adaptation of the **human/technology interfaces** to accommodate their changing motor and cognitive skills. In this section ALS is discussed as an example of a degenerative condition that significantly impacts communication.

ALS

Amyotrophic Lateral Sclerosis (ALS), also referred to as one of the motor neuron diseases, is a rapidly progressing neuromuscular disease that gradually reduces motor control until total paralysis results. It affects speech in the majority of cases (see Case Study 11-4). The spinal form of ALS affects one limb asymmetrically and spreads to other limbs and eventually to upper motor neurons and respiration.[33] Speech is affected in the later stages. The bulbar form of ALS primarily affects the muscles of speech, swallowing, and respiration, resulting in loss of speech earlier in the course of the disease.[33] While persons with ALS utilize the same AAC systems as others, there are unique factors considered during the intervention process. For example, it is not uncommon for someone to begin using a direct selection AAC system and later on require scanning due to loss of motor function. If this type of transition is not planned for initially by the interdisciplinary team, it can be very hard for the person to maintain effective interactions. However, it can be a very difficult topic for both the clinician and family to discuss. Families differ in their desire and ability to deal with the longer term implications of physical decline.[11] Some families prefer to "plan ahead" and consider future needs while others prefer to take things as they come. Some Speech Generating Devices (SGDs) can accommodate direct selection and a variety of indirect selection modes, so these are often recommended. ALS patients tend to use high-tech aids with strangers for conversation.[11] No-tech approaches, including "20 questions" (the person can answer *yes* or *no* by head nod, eye blink, or other means) or gestures may be most effective with family communication and to express basic needs. Because the no-tech approaches are only understood by family members, low-tech approaches such as letter boards are more often used with strangers.

CASE STUDY 11-4 – AAC AND ALS: CHANGING NEEDS

Mr. Webster was assessed for an AAC device shortly after he began to lose the ability to speak as a result of ALS. He received a direct selection spelling device, which he accessed using his right index finger. This device was highly effective for him, and he was fond of making lists of tasks to be done around the house, planning menus, and creating shopping lists for his wife and son, which allowed him to maintain his role as head of the household. Unfortunately, Mr. Webster eventually lost the ability to use his finger to type and was again referred for an AAC assessment.

A new device was recommended and purchased for him. This device utilized single-switch scanning accessed through eyebrow movement. This system was not effective for Mr. Webster. Several factors led to the difference in results between the two systems. First, there was an 11-month period between when he was unable to use the first system and the delivery of the second system. This time without a functional communication system probably contributed to a much more dependent role in the family for Mr. Webster, and he told us that he had "nothing to say" when we asked about his nonuse of the new system. His dependent role in communication also changed his role as head of the household. The new system was also more complicated to set up and to operate. It required his wife and attendant to learn more about the system, and he had to wait for one of them to set it up for him. The effort involved on everybody's part seems overwhelming.

What steps would you take to try to re-establish a role for Mr. Webster in the family?

Individuals with ALS use their technology until within a few weeks of their deaths. In one study those with primary bulbar ALS used their AAC technology an average of 24.9 months, and those with spinal ALS used their AAC technology for an average of 31.1 months.[52] This means that they will require support for AAC throughout the later stages of the disease.

It is important that clinicians provide information regarding the speech-language characteristics of ALS at the outset of intervention. There is a relationship between speaking rate and intelligibility, with 80% intelligibility occurring at about 130 wpm.[3] Speech rate continually drops as ALS progresses, and this measure is used to determine the timing of AAC interventions. It is recommended that individuals with ALS be referred for AAC assessment when their speaking rate reaches 100 to 125 words per minute on the Sentence Intelligibility Test (the mean speaking rate on this test for adults without disability is 190 words per minute).[52]

Families need to remain aware of AAC service intervention opportunities and the need for ongoing training. Flexible AAC devices and strategies that will accommodate for changes over the course of the disease are important. Acceptance of AAC by persons who have ALS is high. In one four-year study, over 96% of those given the choice of AAC accepted that choice.[3] A key reason for acceptance of AAC by persons with ALS is their desire to continue interacting with communication partners in a variety of contexts. As the disease progresses it is increasingly important for the individual with ALS to have a reliable method to make their needs known. Establishing a reliable no-tech communication method, such as eye gaze or eye-blink *yes* or *no*, is important so that the individual retains some means of communication when all other motor functions are no longer available.

Dementia

Dementia is a syndrome, or pattern of clinical symptoms and signs, that can be defined by: (1) a decline of cognitive capacity with some effect on day-to-day functioning; (2) impairment in multiple areas of cognition (global); and (3) a normal level of consciousness.[58] The incidence of dementia is expected to grow. Currently 10% of people aged 65 years and older and 47% of people 85 years and older have been diagnosed with Alzheimer's disease.[52] This percentage translates into about 4 million people in the United States, a number that is expected to increase to 14 million by the year 2050. A major characteristic of dementia is difficulty in communicating, both receptively and expressively.

The aim of AAC intervention in dementia is to maximize communicative and memory functioning, to maintain (or increase) activities that increase participation/engagement, and maintain (or increase) quality of life for people with dementia across the disease progression.[52] Successful AAC intervention may also increase the quality of life and decrease the stress of family and professional caregivers of individuals with dementia.

AAC interventions for dementia are designed to maintain function, compensate for lost function, and/or counsel the individual or family regarding conditions and options for managing the symptoms of dementia. There are several forms of compensatory support typically used.

Low-technology communication cards and books, pictures, drawings, and printed reminders can be designed to support those with dementia to remind them of temporal or semantic information. High-technology support such as computerized memory aids for visual or auditory information is also available (see Chapter 10). AAC in dementia intervention is typically designed to support the individual, rather than to support his or her communication interactions, per se.[52]

AAC interventions for dementia are relatively new, but there is mounting evidence of their effectiveness. Investigation of the use of AAC and cognitive support technology by persons with dementia is encouraging. Most approaches involve low-technology memory and communication books and high-technology displays that are positioned within the individual's living space. Additional techniques include modifications of the communication partner's behavior during communicative interactions by:

- Reducing distractions
- Using short, simple sentences
- Reducing questions to the yes/no format
- Allowing time for the individual with dementia to respond
- Assisting with word-finding strategies, such as word description, if a word cannot be retrieved

Other AT interventions for dementia are discussed in Chapter 10. Case Study 11-3 illustrates the application of AAC for each of these major disorders discussed above.

OVERVIEW OF THE AAC ASSESSMENT

The goals of AAC intervention are to: (1) document communication needs; (2) determine how many needs can be met through current communication methods, including speech; and (3) reduce the number of unmet communication needs through systematic AAC intervention.[8] When reviewing the effectiveness of an AAC system, an OTA, PTA, or speech assistant should determine if the system is meeting as many communication needs as possible for the individual.

Initial AAC assessment and evaluation of system effectiveness require systematic consideration of many factors.[8,26,50] There are two models that are useful in collecting and analyzing required information through an AAC assessment: the Social Networks Inventory and the Participation Model. Each of these can be used as a guide when developing and evaluating AAC systems.

The Social Networks Inventory: Who Are the Partners?

The **Social Networks Inventory,*** based on the circle of partners described earlier, provides a systematic approach to identifying key communication partners and the goals to be achieved and current communication methods in use with each group of partners.[13] It enables the perceptions of many individuals to be considered when planning an intervention and it provides a structure for the gathering of information. The Social Networks Inventory is administered by a speech-language pathologist or other person with expertise in AAC. The key informants are people in the individual's 1st circle and 4th circle and, if at all possible, the individual with CCN. The inventory is meant to be re-administered over time to track progress. Sections on demographic and diagnostic information and the individual's skills and abilities in motor, sensory, language, speech, and cognitive areas are included.

For each circle, the inventory identifies key partners (e.g., favorite partner, partner who understands the person best, etc.), the primary communication modes a person uses in each circle (facial expressions/body language, gestures, vocalizations, manual signs, speech writing, non-electronic communication display, and electronic communication devices) as well as all current use of AT. Information is also collected about the size of the vocabulary the person can access and the effectiveness, efficiency, and intelligibility of the person's current means of communication.

Representational strategies (e.g., object, photograph, pictographic, manual sign language, auditory) and selection techniques (e.g., direct selection, scanning, coding using icons, alphanumeric coding) are also identified, as are topics the individual can (or would like to) talk about. The inventory also helps document which strategies communication partners rely on to support the individual's comprehension (e.g., aided language simulation, modeling AAC use, visual prompts, pictured sequences of tasks, social stories) and expression (e.g., gesture dictionaries, asking for repeat of utterance, suggesting slower speed, prompting for conversational repair strategy use). Summary sheets are included for clinicians to use for intervention planning. This model is very useful for ensuring that all of the important current and future communication partners are considered.

The Participation Model: Identifying Barriers and Opportunities

AAC must be effective in a variety of contexts (i.e., environments and social settings). The **Participation Model** provides a systematic method for understanding these *contexts* by defining communication opportunities and barriers.[8] **Opportunity barriers** are those that involve the *policies, practices, attitudes, knowledge,* and *skills* of those who support the person with CCN. As an illustration, consider the situation where a school district purchases an SGD for a child, but the child is required to leave it at school at all times for fear that it will be lost or damaged if taken off school property. This practice is a barrier to the child's full societal participation and academic

*Social networks: a communication inventory for individuals with complex communication needs and their communication partners. (www.augcominc.com/index.cfm/social_networks.htm)

success because the device is not available to her outside of school. Another example of an opportunity barrier is the employer who is resistant to a worker using an AAC device because the artificial-sounding voice output is distracting to other workers. Opportunity barriers are part of the social or institutional contexts of the HAAT model (Chapter 2). **Access barriers,** described by the human component of the HAAT model, are those that make it difficult for a person with CCN to communicate using an AAC device or technique. Access barriers include motor limitations (speech and fine and gross movement), and hearing, vision, and cognitive ability (including language deficiencies).

Policies are formal rules put in place by an agency (e.g., the funder of rehabilitation services) or institution (e.g., a group home), or by a government agency or private company. These are hard to change and it may be necessary to work around them. *Practices* are less formal and are established within a facility to meet local demands. These may involve how time is allocated to various tasks, such as supporting an individual who uses an SGD, and there may be insufficient time for training and programming due to constraints placed on staff. These barriers can be reduced or removed more easily than formal policies, but they may still require creativity and thoughtful consideration of local circumstances. *Attitudes* are also informal opinions, but they are generally specific to one individual or possibly a few people in the same facility. These might involve resistance to the use of technology or lack of willingness to devote the time necessary to support the user. For example, a teacher with 30 students in her class may not be willing or able to devote a large amount of time to one student who has CCN. Because attitudes are subjective, they can be changed through negotiation rather than a formal policy change process. Alternative approaches can be developed by the interdisciplinary team members and the family. *Knowledge* of AAC by the people who are supporting the person may be lacking due to lack of familiarity with the technologies or with AAC in general, leading to a fear of the technology due to its complexity. In-service education can help in this regard. Weakness in *skills* is usually the product of lack of direct experience, which is most easily dealt with by on-the-job training by a more experienced person.

An assessment of access barriers is also included in the Participation Model. An "activity standards inventory" is developed in which desired communication-related activities of the person with CCN (termed "target person") are listed and then compared to the performance of a non-disabled peer doing the same activity.[8] In a school the peer would be a student in the same classroom. In a group home it might be an adult without a disability. The level of participation of the target person is then rated as: (1) independent; (2) independent with set-up (i.e., someone else needs to arrange the device so the person can use it); (3) requires verbal (e.g., prompting) or physical assistance cues (e.g., hand over hand); or (4) unable to participate. Any difference between the peer and the target person is determined to be either an opportunity or access barrier.

Once the type of barrier is determined, then a plan to reduce or remove that barrier is developed. The plan includes the possibility of: (1) increasing natural abilities (e.g., using speech-language pathology to improve motor speech function); (2) making environmental adaptations (e.g., moving a child to the front of the class to encourage greater participation, or adjusting dining room arrangements to allow greater participation by an AAC user in a skilled nursing facility); and (3) making use of AAC systems and/or devices to avoid or overcome barriers. If the third choice is included in the plan, then it is necessary to assess the skills and abilities of the target person in order to select appropriate AAC systems and devices. The Participation Model refers to this as a **capability assessment.** An important component of the capability assessment involves documenting the individual's speech, language, motor, sensory, cognitive, and social communication skills. When used in combination, the HAAT model (Chapter 2), the Social Networks Inventory, and the Participation Model provide a comprehensive approach for ensuring that all information needed for successful AAC implementation is obtained during the assessment process.

Gathering the Data

The most effective AAC assessments are planned by an interdisciplinary team consisting of the OT, PT, and SLP.[26] Once the assessment has been planned the OTA, PTA, and speech assistant may participate in the gathering of data. If a low- or high-tech AAC system component (e.g., SGD or computer) is required to meet the goals and needs of the individual, then the assistive technology characteristics can be chosen to match the person's physical, motor, sensory, and cognitive abilities and skills.

As in many areas of assistive technology, the assessment process is not a one-time event. Not everything that is planned as result of the initial assessment will be successful, and needs may change over time. For example, children may progress from emergent to context-dependent communicators, and adults with progressive diseases may lose motor and/or cognitive abilities. Technologies available to meet AAC needs will also continue to evolve, and it may be desirable to consider changes in the individual's AAC system. As the front-line contact with the individual and family, the OTA, PTA, or speech assistant may be the first to notice that changes might be needed. In the following sections we provide suggestions for carrying out this type of monitoring of on-going performance.

Relating Goals and Skills to AAC System Characteristics: Developing the Implementation Plan

The AAC assessment process results in an intervention plan that is unique for a specific person. Development of the plan should involve the person with CCN, his or her family, and the entire team. A key element of this plan is the definition of a set of AAC system characteristics that meets the needs of the person with CCN, is consistent with his or her skills, and will support communication across multiple partners and contexts. This is often called "feature matching." All modes of communication (speech, gestures, sign language, vocalizations, facial expressions, and AAC) must be included in the implementation plan. Skills to be developed as part of a training plan as well as strategies that might be helpful should be identified at this time.

When an SGD is a part of the recommended AAC implementation plan for the individual with CCN, it is important to determine a match between the needs and goals of the person and the characteristics of the SGD.[26] Table 11-2 lists the most important characteristics of a speech generating device (SGD) that need to be identified in the assessment. Input features, message characteristics, output features, and accessories are all specified based on the assessment results. In the United States these features are also used as part of the justification for funding of an SGD. Blackstone (2001)[12] includes several case studies that illustrate the application of this matching process for the selection of an AAC device and the preparation of a funding justification.

COMPONENTS OF CURRENT ASSISTIVE TECHNOLOGIES FOR AAC

The HAAT model (Figure 2-1) can be used to describe the major parts of an AAC system. All three of the HAAT activities in Figure 2-2 (self care, productivity, and leisure) may involve communication at various times, and communication occurs in all of the contexts described in Figure 2-4. The person controls the AAC technology through a keyboard (including touch screens) or through an on-screen keyboard accessed with a pointing interface (mouse, trackball, or head pointer) for direct selection. For indirect selection either a single or dual switch is used. This is the *input* to the device from the user. In the HAAT model these controls are referred to as the **human-technology interface** (Figure 2-5, *B*).

Ways of Representing Language in AAC

AAC systems can use a variety of symbol systems that are understood by an individual and used to communicate. The most flexible symbols are letters and words (called **traditional orthography**). However, the use of traditional orthography depends on spelling ability and literacy (reading and writing) skills. Spontaneous spelling requires the person to spell the requested word letter-by-letter like the typical spelling test for children in school. This is the most flexible and versatile capability, and it allows traditional orthography to portray any concept about which the user wishes to communicate. Sixth grade spelling is generally recognized as the minimal level for general communication. Even if spontaneous spelling is weak, the individual may be able to choose the first letter of the desired word and recognize the completed word from a list presented

TABLE 11-2 Features Typically Included in an SGD

Input Features/Selection Techniques (also see Chapter 5)	Message Characteristics	Auditory Output Features	Additional Features	Accessory Features
Direct Selection: *Keyboards/display*: Dynamic/static, size and number of keys/ locations *Activation type*: Touch or pressure sensitive, adjustable *Indirect contact*: Head pointing, eye gaze	**Types of symbols:** Words, phrase, letters, tactile, pictures (color/ B&W), pictographic **Vocabulary size:** Number of words, phrases, etc., needed	**Type:** Digitized speech Synthesized speech Other sounds	**Outputs:** **Electronic Aids to Daily Living (EADL)** – also see Chapter 14 **Infrared** **Bluetooth** **Computer access:** **USB** **Bluetooth** (also see Chapter 7)	**Mounts:** Position of switches Position of device **Portability** Size, weight, transport/mount, case/carrier requirements
Scanning: *Display*: Number of elements, dynamic/static *Mode*: Visual/auditory *Type of scan*: Linear, row/ column, group row/ column, directed	**Organization of messages:** Message length, files of messages, number of different messages stored or formulated	**Vocabulary expansion:** Rate enhancement, prediction (word/ icon), coding strategies, screens/levels	**General computer-based:** Laptop Tablet Palm PDA	**Switches** Type, pressure, feedback **Pointing devices** Type (infrared, ultrasonic) **Feedback** Visual, tactile, auditory

by the Speech Generating Device (SGD) word completion function (see Chapter 5). Even without first letter spelling, *recognition spelling,* which requires the individual to pick the correct entry from a list of options, can be used with a paper communication board or SGD that presents word lists or other stored vocabulary choices and relies on recognition memory. If the person has a large word recognition vocabulary, the AAC system vocabulary choices for the user should be based on words with possible "carrier phrases" that are filled in with limited spelling (e.g., "I would like a drink of ____").

When spelling or word recognition is not possible, alternative symbol systems are used. A variety of symbol types are shown in Figure 11-7. Perhaps the most concrete type of symbol is the use of real objects (full size or miniature). However, to a person with cognitive disabilities, a miniature object may not appear to represent the full-sized version, and care must be taken to ensure that the concrete association between the two different-sized objects is made by the user.[50] Real objects and photographs have the disadvantage that many communicative concepts (e.g., "good," "more," "go," and "hurt") are difficult to portray using these symbols. Pictographic symbols include provisions for more abstract concepts and allow much greater flexibility in developing vocabulary usage. Figure 11-8 illustrates the use of line drawings, words, and photographs to portray similar concepts. As can be seen, photographs can sometimes be less clear than line drawings.

There are a number of ways to determine if an individual understands the association between the symbol and its meaning.[8] Visual matching of a single stimulus to one item from a multiple symbol array, or vice versa, presents an object and two symbols, one of which represents the object, or two different objects, one of which matches a single symbol presented. The individual is asked "Look at the different one" or "Look at the one that is the same" to match the symbol to the correct object or the correct object to the symbol. Confirmation of the choice can be via any controllable movement (e.g., eye gaze, head nod, or pointing). The functional object approach asks the person to "Show me what you do with this." Yes/no validation asks, "Is this a ______?" A question and answer approach asks, "Can you show me

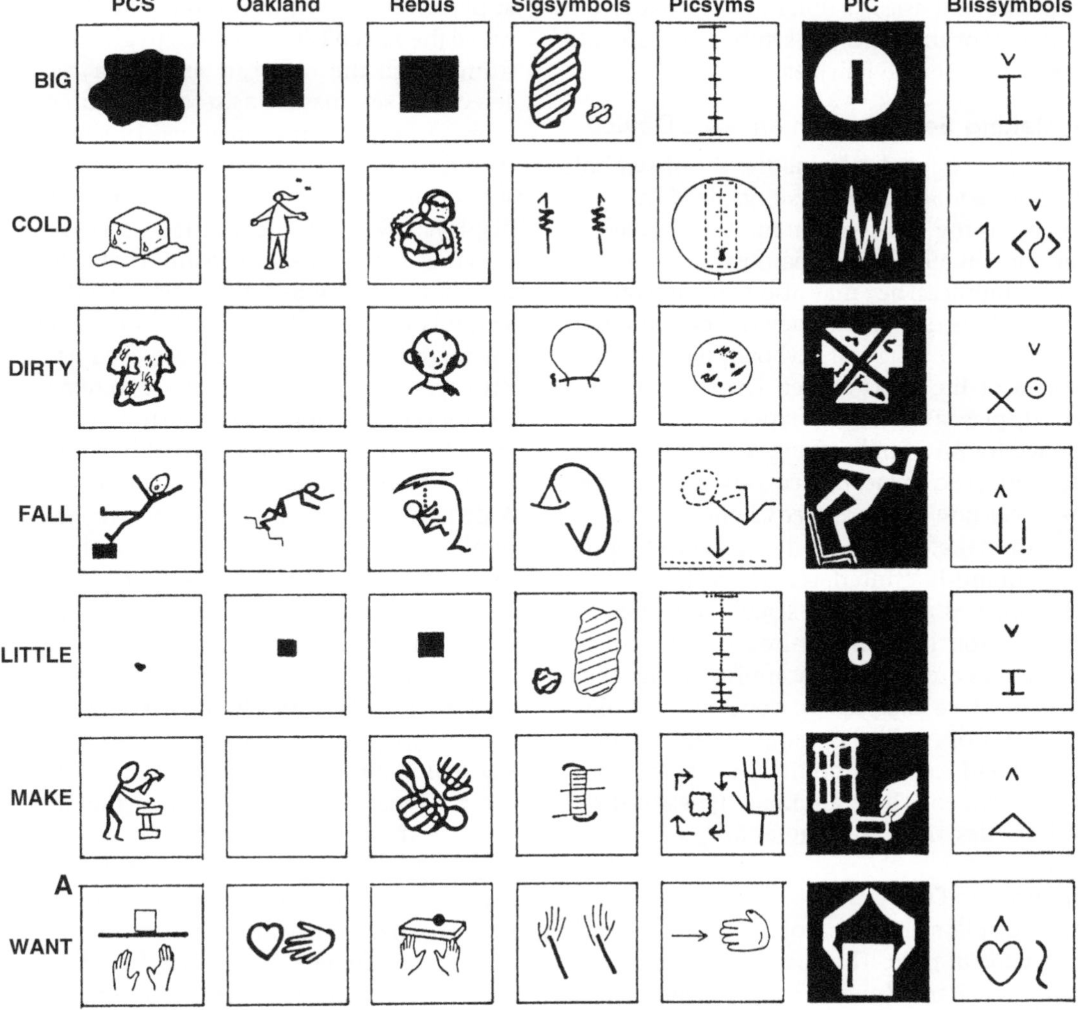

Figure 11-7 Examples of the variety of symbol systems that have been developed for AAC use. (From Blackstone S: *Augmentative communication,* Rockville, Md., 1986, American Speech-Language-Hearing Association.)

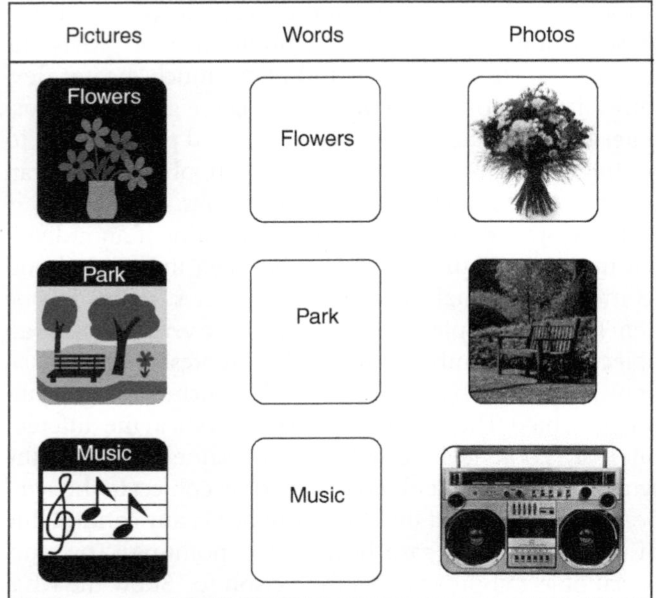

Figure 11-8 A comparison of drawings, words, and photographs to describe the same topic. (Photographs from istockphotos.com)

the _______ that does ______?" Finally, a requesting format presents two choices and asks, "I don't know what to do. Can you help me?" For this case, the symbol object could be a cup (drink), brush (brush hair), etc.

Options for Making Selections in an AAC Device

There are many options for displaying the set of symbols so they can be selected. Static displays organized in a grid or matrix format are the most common. The displays or keyboards may contain all of the alpha-numeric characters like on a laptop computer. They may also contain words or non-alphabetic symbols or a small array of keys on a portable device. These may be physical keyboard-like panels or on-screen displays of the selection set. Dynamic displays and visual scene displays are two other types of input devices that are well suited for AAC applications. All of these different ways of presenting vocabulary choices can be accessed by direct or indirect selection methods (see Chapter 5).

The person can make choices by directly selecting the item using a keyboard-like interface. Often the vocabulary items are displayed on a touch screen, and they are selected by directly touching the desired item. For indirect selection, choices are made by scanning using a single or dual switches (see Chapter 6). Vocabulary choices can also be selected from a display using a pointing interface (mouse, trackball, or head pointer) to move a cursor around on the screen. There are many types of input device or interfaces described in Chapter 6.

Static Communication Displays

Communication displays that do not change with each entry are called *static displays*. The size of a static display can range from a few items (one to four, or eight) up to 128 or more items. Considerations for selecting the most appropriate configurations for an individual are discussed in Chapter 7. Because static displays do not change, they are ideal for developing motor patterns that can dramatically increase the rate of selection and therefore the rate of communication. The key to motor patterns is that the individual items (symbols, letters, and icons) always remain in the same position. Thus a sequence of symbols always uses the same pattern of motor actions. Eventually this pattern becomes automatic. To get a sense of this think about those cases in which you tried to remember a phone number, but you couldn't until you pretended to enter it on the telephone keypad. The number was still in memory, but it was stored as a motor pattern. When the number of symbols or vocabulary is small, static display can work well. When the communication depends on the entry of sequences of symbols (e.g., iconic representations*) to generate large vocabularies, then static displays also work well. Static displays may also be indicated for cases in which the cognitive demands of dynamic displays are not present.

Dynamic Communication Displays

Dynamic communication displays change the selection set displayed when a choice is made. They are often used on smart phones, Web sites, and many other mainstream applications as well as on many SGDs. When a choice is made the screen is reformatted to give a new set of options from which the user can select. For example, a general **selection set** may consist of categories such as work, home, food, clothing, greetings, or similar classifications. If one of these is chosen, either by touching the display surface directly or by scanning, then a new selection set is displayed. For example, a variety of food-related items and activities (eat, drink, ice cream, pasta, etc.) would follow the choice of "foods" from the general selection set. The symbols on the display can be varied, and this changes the targets for the user. Because each new selection set is displayed, the user does not have to remember what is on each level. This approach, illustrated in Figure 11-9, also avoids having to squeeze several pictures into one square (of ½" × ½" dimensions) on a traditional grid display. A dynamic display also relies on recognition rather than recall memory for identification of the selection set elements, which can make it easier to use. Once an item is selected, the dynamic display automatically branches to the selected new page and displays it.

Blackstone (1994)[10] describes a number of key features of dynamic displays. The nature of these devices allows the user to quickly change the screen and to configure the size, color, and arrangement of the symbols to match the topic. Dynamic displays reduce memory requirements because the user is prompted by the display after each choice. The constant vigilance to the screen requires a high level of visual attention and constant decision making. The user must also have mastered the concept of object permanence. These may be challenging for some individuals who have cognitive limitations.

* Prentke Romich Company (http://store.prentrom.com/)

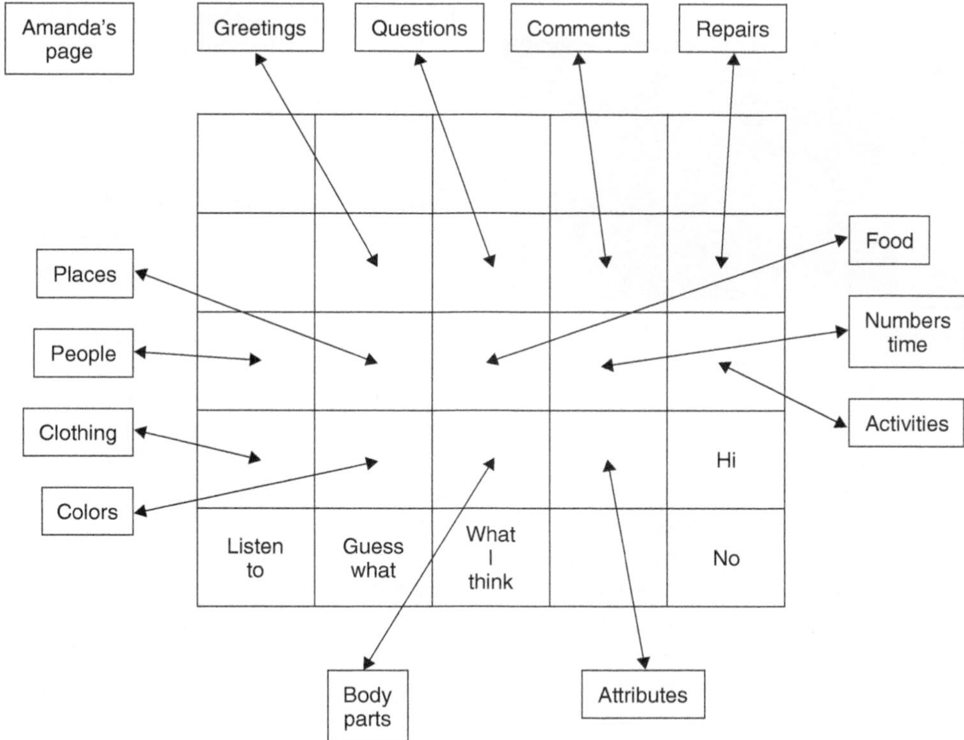

Figure 11-9 Dynamic display devices change the selection set presented to the user each time an entry is made.

Visual Scene Displays (VSDs)

Visual Scene Displays (VSDs) create displays that capture events in a person's life on the screen with "hot spots" that can be accessed to retrieve information (Blackstone, 2004).[16] A hot spot is a region of a picture on the screen that the user can choose by pointing to it with a finger, a mouse, or a scanning cursor. VSDs may represent either a generic or personalized context. Generic context includes drawings of places (e.g., a house or schoolroom), whereas a personalized context is specific to one person (e.g., a picture of his house or a family outing). The images can be personal digital photographs of an event (e.g., a marriage or birthday party) or important people (e.g., family or friends or teacher). The images can also be more generic photographs or other graphical representations that portray an area (e.g., a child's room or a kitchen) or event (e.g., going to the circus). Visual scene displays offer the user of AAC and her partner a greater degree of contextual information to support interaction. The richness of the display and the information content can also enable communication partners to participate more actively in a conversation.

Table 11-3 describes the difference between a traditional AAC display (referred to as a grid) and a VSD.[16] The traditional grid supports communication of needs and wants and information exchange well. However, this type of display is usually restricted to symbols, text, or static drawings (although some animation is used with dynamic display items) and the vocabulary items are separated from any context in order to maximize their versatility. Personalization is also limited. Traditional grid displays present symbols out of context (i.e., language is presented in a box, isolated from the context in which it occurs).[45] The grid display also does not preserve conceptual or visual relationships between elements in the grid display. In a traditional grid display, the line drawing of the apple used to represent *apple* may be as big as the head of the boy used to represent the concept *boy*, which in turn may be as big as the entire person used to represent the concept *run*.

TABLE 11-3 Comparison of Traditional Grid Displays and Visual Scene Displays

Variable	Typical AAC Grid	VSD
Type of representation	Symbols, traditional orthography, line drawings	Digital photos, line drawings
Personalization	Limited	High
Amount of context	Low	High
Layout	Grid	Full or partial screen, grid
Display management	Menu, pages	Menu pages, navigation bars
Concept retrieval	Select gird space, pop ups	Hot spots, speech key, select grid space

Figure 11-10 illustrates the differences between a typical static grid display and a VSD.[16] The VSD is developed for conversational support as a shared activity. Since it utilizes a range of information media including video and family pictures in addition to text, symbols, and line drawings, it can be highly personalized, as shown in Figure 11-6.[16]

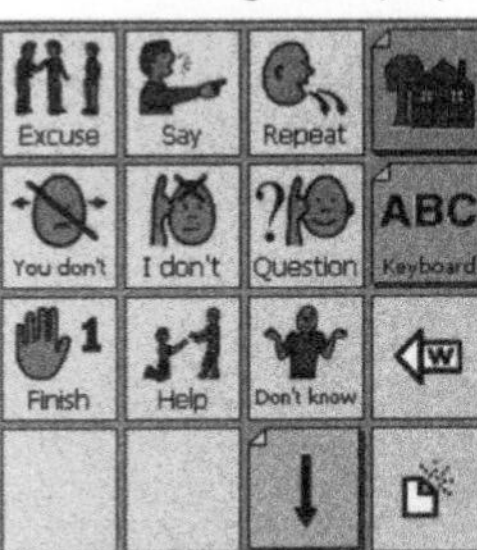

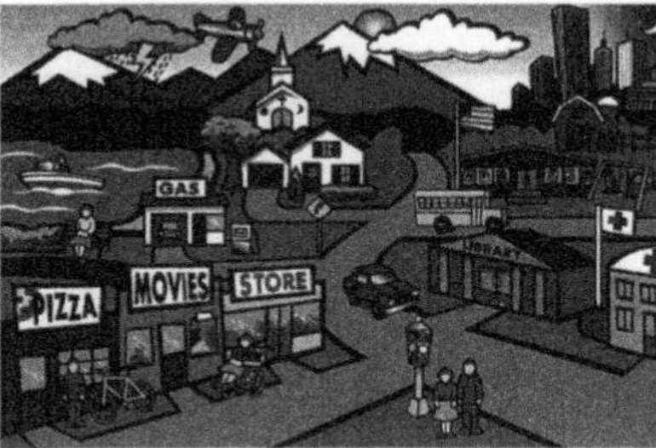

Figure 11-10 A comparison of a grid display (left) and a Visual Scene Display (VSD) (right). (From Blackstone S: Visual scene displays, *Augment Commun News,* 16(2):1–5, 2004.)

In addition to communication of needs, wants, and information exchange, VSDs also support social closeness. Due to the dynamic nature of the VSD approach it can also serve as a learning environment providing instruction, specific information, or prompts to help the user interact effectively. VSDs can be useful to individuals with cognitive limitations (e.g., Down syndrome) or language limitations (e.g., aphasia or autism) and young children. Research on the use of VSDs with children is summarized in Box 11-4.

VSDs can stimulate conversations in which the communication partners play, share experiences, and tell stories. The dynamic nature of VSDs facilitates active participation of partners during these shared activities. For example, the topic of play could be illustrated both in the VSD and on the grid by a digital photograph of the child's room that includes the toy box as a symbol for play. Clicking on the hot spot associated with the toy box in the VSD or on the grid element for play resulted in branching in both formats to more detailed information.

Outputs from AAC Devices

SGDs or other AAC devices can produce a variety of *communication outputs.* Since AAC often involves conversation, electronic devices commonly produce speech as an output. Printed output is important for communication in written form. Often AAC devices also have outputs that control appliances or connect to other communication devices, such as computers and cell phones, and the Internet. Finally, AAC devices can be used to control power wheelchairs. These various outputs are discussed in this section.

Speech Output

The two major types of speech output used in SGDs are digitized and synthesized. **Digitized speech** is like a recording that is played back. **Synthesized speech** is electronically generated and can produce speech without it being pre-recorded. The quality of these speech outputs is quite variable. Both types of speech output are described in Chapter 7. Speech is, of course, the main form of human-to-human communicative interaction. In comparison to devices with only visual displays, or manual systems where the output is indicated by pointing at words or symbols, speech allows communication

BOX 11-4 VSDs and Children: What the Research Tells Us

VISUAL SCENE DISPLAYS (VSDS) AND CHILDREN

Use of VSDs by typically developing children (as young as 2½ years old) for a birthday party communication task (Drager, 2003)[27]

- Did significantly better when using a schematic VSD layout (based on activities) than when using a grid layout (schematic or taxonomic).
- One explanation is that the provision of a more meaningful context in the VSD reduced the language demand on the child.
- The VSD was organized around scenes of rooms: living room (arrival of children for party), kitchen (eating cake), family room (opening presents), and playroom (playing games).
- This reduces the demands on the child's working memory since the location of the item required fewer demands in the VSD.
- The grid layout was organized around the activities, which required more language processing by the child (e.g., categorizing, remembering the symbols).

CRITICAL ASPECTS OF LAYOUT AND ORGANIZATION AND IMPACT ON LEARNING AND USE[45]

- Youngest children (age 2.5 years) were most accurate locating vocabulary using the visual scene displays compared to the grid layouts, even though the displays were not personalized to the experiences of the children.
- By ages 4 and 5, the children located vocabulary with the visual scene displays and the grid layouts with similar levels of accuracy, but they had significant difficulty learning to use iconic encoding.

VISUAL SCENE DISPLAYS USED WITH YOUNG CHILDREN[45]

- Intervention with children who have developmental disabilities (ages 1 to 3).
- All of the children were able to use the visual scene displays to participate in social interactions, upon initial introduction in the first session, once their use had been modeled.
- The children demonstrated significant increases in turn taking immediately upon introduction of the AAC technologies utilizing visual scenes.
- The children sustained these gains in turn taking over the long term.
- All of the children also learned to use other types of displays over time, including traditional grid displays and hybrid displays.
- Similar results in a study of preschoolers with autism (ages 3 to 5).

with partners who cannot read (e.g., small children or persons with cognitive impairments). It is also the only type of output that can be used conveniently for speaking to groups (including use in classroom discussions) or for speaking over the telephone. Key factors in making speech output successful are (1) ensuring that it is appropriate to the gender and age of the person using it and (2) ensuring that the speech is intelligible to the person and his or her communication partners. When using digitally recorded speech it is important that the speaker who is recorded be age and gender appropriate for the person who will use the device. It is not a good idea to use family members since they will also be the communication partners.

Written Output

Written output requires a printer. Most often people with complex communication needs (CCN) use computer word processors and printers to generate written output. The AAC device may be connected to the computer (see Chapter 7) so that the stored vocabulary and other features such as indirect selection can be used by the person. Alternatively, the individual may use the computer directly with some of the built-in accessibility features (see Table 7-1 in Chapter 7). Some SGDs allow connection of a printer via a USB port.

Outputs to Control Assistive Technologies

Specialized assistive technologies, such as Electronic Aids to Daily Living (EADL) (e.g., remote controls for lights, television, other appliances, covered in Chapter 14) and powered wheelchairs (discussed in Chapter 12) are also often of use to individuals with CCN. Many SGDs either provide the functions of EADLs or interface with them through wireless remote connections. The real power in connecting people with CCN to the rest of the "information society" lies in granting them access to mainstream technologies. In addition to access to EADLs, SGDs allow connection to electronic games (e.g., PlayStation®, Wii™) and other electronic devices. The most common types of wireless connection to external devices use infrared or Bluetooth signals. The infrared signals are often used for appliances or toys. Bluetooth control of appliances is increasing and this is the most common wireless connection to cell phones, computers, and other mainstream applications. Many SGDs have built-in infrared outputs and an increasing number, especially those based on standard computers, also have Bluetooth signals available.

Access to Mainstream Technologies

The Internet provides significant information resources from the computer desktop. Through the use of e-mail, quick, easy, and low-cost communication with individuals around the world is possible. Many people who have disabilities use e-mail to communicate with friends, business associates, and organizations (see Case Study 11-4). When someone with CCN uses their SGD to access the Internet, all of the special features of the device are available to them for use while on-line. These features include any stored vocabulary that can be accessed quickly, word prediction, abbreviations, and their optimal method of making selections. Some commercial SGDs are based on portable computers with AAC software, and they can also access the Internet.

CASE STUDY 11-5 – AAC IN POST-SECONDARY EDUCATION

Heidi is a doctoral student studying English at a major university. She has cerebral palsy, which limits her ability to speak and use her hands for writing. She uses her computer to complete writing assignments and has written two plays (one for her master's degree thesis) and one book for teenagers who have cerebral palsy. She uses her notebook computer with a speech synthesizer for conversation and a word processor for writing. She also uses e-mail to communicate with her PhD thesis advisor, colleagues, students, and friends. This technology allows her to keep in touch with people without the use of the telephone, which is difficult with her AAC device. Her computer system allows her several modes of communication and also provides her the opportunity to work at home much of the time and avoid the hassles of special transportation arrangements. Her e-mail contacts also prevent her from being isolated in her home environment.

The Internet also provides access to information through company, organization, and individual Web sites. By accessing this information, AAC users can learn about new technologies, conduct business independently, carry out research for academic pursuits, book airline reservations, and many other activities. Access to the Internet provides many opportunities for reading and writing, and this practice can help improve literacy skills for AAC users.[15] Temple University provides mentoring programs for individuals who rely on AAC.* The course consists of two weeks of intensive training on site and one year follow-up via the Internet. Program graduates mentor new students in the program.

E-mail allows composition at a slower speed, because the recipient reads it at a later time as opposed to a live chat where there's back and forth exchange in real time.[15] E-mail also allows an AAC user to communicate with another person without someone else being present, allowing for increased independence. Because the person's disability is not immediately visible, AAC users report that they enjoy establishing relationships with people who experience them first as a person and then learn of their disability.

---

* http://disabilities.temple.edu/programs/assistive/aces/index.htm

Using social media (e.g., Facebook, Twitter), people not only obtain information from the Web, but they can also upload and exchange information in real time and communicate with more people at once. For non-disabled people, smart phones allow people to interact and get information much easier. Skype and other conferencing software can also be useful in connecting people with disabilities to family and friends. Listservs, which consist of a group of individuals with common interests but are more like bulletin boards, also provide rich sources of information and friendly interaction. A popular AAC listserv is ACOLUG* hosted by Temple University.

Unfortunately, the benefits of using the Internet are not available to everyone. Those without an Internet connection or the ability to use an SGD and those who are not literate can still depend on friends or family to support their participation by reading Internet content (e-mails, Web sites) and typing responses based on input from the AAC user (e.g., using symbols or pictures). However, this strategy has implications for the privacy of the user as all content must be fully shared in the process of getting assistance.

Features that were developed for people with disabilities (e.g., word completion/prediction, voice recognition, and abbreviation expansion) are now built into cell phones and general-purpose computers; these formerly specialized features are now available to individuals with CCN at low cost due to the mass production of cell phones. Digital photography built into cell phones also increases utility for persons with CCN. In addition to the mainstream uses (e.g., photography for recording family events, business, or school) the camera features can also be used to develop custom communication displays. For example, pictures can be integrated into Visual Scene Displays and used as input devices. Pictures can also be used as vocabulary elements for non-literate individuals or to enhance message generation for young children or others who have limited literacy skills, thereby reducing the descriptive information required to convey a message.

People with CCN can download applications (often called "apps") from the Internet as needed. Many of the available applications are for smart phones using the Android† and the Apple iOS‡ operating systems. Many applications function like a full-featured SGD. Features include text-to-speech, voice personalization, a built-in default vocabulary of over 7000 items organized by category, and the availability of a variety of symbol systems. The cost is less than 10% of a stand-alone SGD. However, the individual must be able to access the smart phone or pad computer both physically and visually. As with most SGD applications, there is a set of individuals for whom this device is well suited but there are many for whom other choices would be more successful. The number of smart phone applications is growing rapidly, and there are many for people with disabilities. Gosnell has provided a feature-mapping tool for evaluating the suitability of AAC apps for individual users of AAC.*

There are a number of potential barriers to the use of smart phone applications to meet basic AAC needs. The first, as discussed earlier, is accessibility and some apps address alternative accessibility, including scanning. As with all choices of technology, the primary consideration must be whether the application will really meet needs and not just whether it is inexpensive. The applications must be robust. Apps are software programs, and, like any software, they can crash. When they do the person may be left with a bare smart phone with no way to access it. A robust application will have ways for the person to recover from a software crash built into the program. There is also generally a lack of support for the individual using an application, especially if it is purchased online and downloaded into the individual's phone.

Vocabulary Storage and Retrieval Techniques

Speech allows communication at a rapid rate, between 150 and 175 words per minute.[1] For an individual using an augmentative communication device to generate unlimited vocabulary, some form of letter or symbol selection is required. In many cases, persons who are unable to speak use a keyboard to type their messages, which are then spoken by an AAC device. This can result in significantly lower rates of communication than for speech. Many people who have disabilities must rely on single-finger typing for conversation. Using this mode, a person with a disability may only be able to type at a maximal rate of 10 to 12 words per minute. For individuals who use scanning (see Chapter 5), the maximal rates can be as low as three to five words per minute. Although there are several methods of increasing communication rates, the great disparity in rates of communication between a speaking person and an AAC system user often results in the speaking person's dominating a conversation with a non-speaking person. Thus one of the goals in the design of augmentative communication devices is to reduce the magnitude of this disparity in communication rates. Many SGDs use the approaches to increase input rate that are discussed in Chapter 5 (i.e., abbreviation expansion, word prediction, and word completion). In addition, there are several methods for storing and retrieving vocabulary that are designed specifically for SGDs.

Instant phrases are those used frequently for greetings, conversational repairs (e.g., "that's not what I meant"), or similar actions. These are often included as single keystroke entries in an "activity row" or in a row of the scanning matrix, near the beginning of the scan. They can also serve

* http://disabilities.temple.edu/programs/aac/acolug/
† For examples for Android phones, see http://www.androidzoom.com/android_applications/augmentative%20communication
‡ For iPhone, iPod Touch, and iPad apps, see http://store.apple.com/us

* Gosnell, J, Costello, J, & Shane, H (2011) Using a clinical approach to answer "what communication apps should we use?" Perspectives on Augmentative and Alternative Communication. 20, 87–96. www.childrenshospital.org/acp

as "floor holders" as in "having the floor" in a conversation (e.g., "please wait while I type my question/answer").

The coding of words, sentences, and phrases on the basis of their meanings is also known as **Semantic Encoding** or Minspeak.[2] This approach utilizes pictorial representations that can have multiple meanings as codes, making recall easier. For example, if I use a picture of an apple for "food," and a sun rising for "morning," then selecting "apple" and "sunrise" could be a code for "What's for breakfast?" Icons can have multiple meanings. Thus the apple symbol can take on the meaning of "eat" or "red" or "fruit" rather than simply "food."

With practice, these sequences of icons can be developed as motor patterns that can be generated at a more automatic, subconscious level. This has led to an approach that relies on motor planning and natural consequences for learning symbols. "Children learning to communicate with LAMP (Language Acquisition through Motor Planning) learn how to say the target words without initially learning the symbol or the association of the symbol to the word." (p 13)[35]

Unity® is a family of Minspeak® application programs included with Prentke Romich* AAC devices. It includes 4-, 8-, 15-, 32-, 45-, 60-, 84-, and 128-element displays of symbols. The larger numbers of elements require finer and finer pointing resolution for direct selection. They can also be selected using scanning. Sequences of icons and their locations on the keyboard are kept as consistent as possible among the overlays in order to maximize the development of motor patterns. Versions of Unity® vary from a few hundred to over 4000 words intended to address the core vocabulary that is responsible for the majority of conversational utterances.

When large numbers of sentences, words, and phrases are stored, the icon sequences can become difficult to remember. **Icon prediction** initially displays each symbol that forms the beginning of an icon sequence. When one of these icons is selected, only those icons that are part of a sequence beginning with the first selected icon are displayed. This continues until a complete icon sequence has been selected. This feature can aid recall and increase speed of selection because the device limits the number of icons that must be visually scanned for each selection.

Vocabulary Programs for Language Development

The *Gateway*† series is an approach to vocabulary organization that is based on language development in typically developing children. The levels of Gateway are designated by the number of elements in the selection set, from 12 through 75. These are intended for six distinct target user groups, beginning with the 12 to 24 month language development level, progressing to two formats for mild/moderate cognitive disability for children or adults, arrays for children and adolescents/adults with typical cognitive/language development and physical limitations, and a high-end array for augmented communicators who have well-developed syntactical skills. Pop-up menus with frequently used items (word, phrases, or sentences) are available on the larger arrays.

WordPower™* combines a core vocabulary of 100 words that represent about 50% of spoken communication. It includes approximately 100 single hit (single selection) words, hundreds of two- or three-hit words (those requiring require 2 or 3 selections), a core dictionary for word prediction of 30,000 words, automatic grammatical endings (-ed, -ing, and -s), and a QWERTY keyboard for spelling. For literate users, this approach is intuitive and leads to efficient communication. There are both direct and indirect (scanning) versions available. *Picture WordPower* uses labeled symbols as word cues. The same basic core vocabulary is available.

TALK[65] is based on the perspective of a typical conversation: person (me/you); queries (where, what, how, who, when, and why); and tense (present, past, or future). Figure 11-11 shows a typical TALK board with "where me/where/past" perspectives selected. This leads to the display of a particular set of phrases that can be chosen and spoken with one switch selection. There are also a set of comments, repair phrases along the right side, and the conversation sections (initiation, greeting, response to greeting, small talk, wrap up, farewells) along the top. Using TALK and similar systems, the AAC user can obtain conversational rates of 30 to 60 wpm. One version of TALK is available with Speaking Dynamically Pro.† When individuals who have limited experience with conversations are introduced to systems such as TALK, significant training specifically oriented toward conversational flow is required.[65]

The decision as to which of these approaches is best for an individual person is based on a thorough assessment. The OTA, PTA, or speech assistant may participate in the assessment process as described earlier, but their major role will be in the implementation of the developed AAC intervention plan. It is important to realize

* Prentke Romich Company, Wooster, Ohio (www.prentrom.com)
† Dynavox Systems, Inc., Pittsburgh, Pa. (www.dynavoxtech.com/)

* Inman Innovations, available on several commercial AAC systems
† Mayer Johnson, Solana Beach, Calif. (www.mayer-johnson.com)

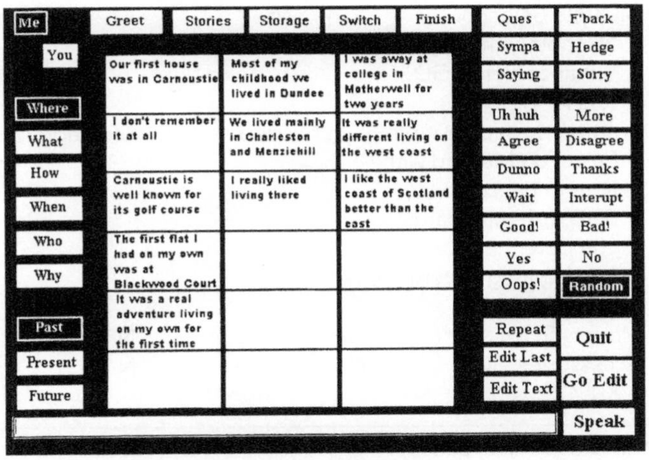

Figure 11-11 TALK board. (Courtesy Mayer-Johnson.)

that there are many approaches, and that no one vendor has all the answers for all of the people that you may need to support.

The rehab assistant (OTA, PTA, or speech assistant) is the person who has the most day-to-day contact with the person using the AAC system, and she is in the best position to determine if the system is meeting the agreed-upon goals and is effective for the person. By using the Social Networks Inventory, a rehab assistant can identify the key communication partners and determine if the needs of the person to communicate with each group of partners is being met. Careful consideration of the Participation Model can help to identify barriers to effective communication and possible approaches to removing the barriers. Throughout this process of reevaluation, it is essential that family members and other close contacts be involved to ensure the maximum possibility of success.

Configurations of Commercial SGDs

In order to describe current SGDs, we have created seven categories of the major commercially available devices, as shown in Table 11-4. The categories reflect different groupings of the characteristics discussed earlier in the section on AAC characteristics as well as the funding codes and categories for Medicare reimbursement of SGDs in the United States.[12] Table 11-4 also includes accessories and mounting systems for AAC devices. We have opted for a few large categories based on the most essential features, resulting in variability within each category. The format in Table 11-4 appropriately groups devices serving distinct populations. Within each category there is still significant opportunity for decision making based on a thorough assessment of skills and needs. Each category has many commercial devices available. Table 11-5 is a partial listing of manufacturers of AAC devices. The Appendix contains Web links to resources that can provide up-to-date information.

Simple Scanners, the first category in Table 11-4, are generally operated by a single switch, although some can have dual-switch scanning and others allow four- or five-switch–directed scanning. The devices in this category are distinguished by the use of a light to indicate the output selection, very limited vocabularies (32 items or less), no **rate enhancement** or vocabulary, and the general absence of voice output as a standard feature.

The devices categorized as *Simple Speech Output* are further delineated by length of the recorded digital speech. They were all developed to provide a limited-vocabulary, easy-to-use output for very young children

TABLE 11-4 Feature Categories Commonly Combined in Commercial AAC Systems

Category	Speech Output**	Message Type**	Message Formulation Techniques**	Access Method**
Simple Scanners	None	Pre-stored	NA	1, 2, 4, or 5 switch scanning
Simple Speech Output (8 minutes or less) SGD, K0541**	Digitized	Pre-stored coverage vocabulary only	NA	Scan or direct selection, multiple methods
Simple Speech Output (greater than 8 min) SGD, K0542**	Digitized	Pre-stored coverage vocabulary only	Minimal rate enhancement or vocabulary expansion	Scan or direct selection, multiple methods
Direct Selection, Writing Only	No speech output	Message formulation	Spelling, rate enhancement	Direct selection
Spelling Only SGD, K0543**	Synthesized	Message formulation	Spelling	Direct selection
Multiple Selection Method with Rate Enhancement SGD, K0544**	Synthesized	Message formulation	Spelling and rate enhancement	Variety of selection methods and control interfaces
Software-based Multiple Selection Method with Rate Enhancement SGD, uses standard computer hardware as operating system, K0545**	Synthesized	Message formulation	Spelling and rate enhancement	Variety of selection methods and control interfaces
Mounts SGD, K0546**	NA	NA	NA	NA
Accessories, SGD K0547**	NA	NA	NA	NA

**Medicare Billing Codes

TABLE 11-5 Major Manufacturers of AAC Devices

Company	Web Site
Adaptivation, Inc.	www.adaptivation.com
Alexicom Tech	www.alexicomtech.com
Attainment Company	www.attainmentcompany.com
Augmentative Resources	www.augresources.com
CaDan Computers dba Technology for Education	www.tfeinc.com
DynaVox Mayer-Johnson	www.dynavoxsys.com
FRS Custom Solutions	www.frs-solutions.com
Jabbla	www.jabbla.com
LC Technologies	www.eyegaze.com
Madentec Limited	www.madentec.com
Possum, LTD	www.possum.co.uk
Prentke Romich Company	www.prentrom.com
Saltillo Corporation	www.saltillo.com
Therapy Box	www.tboxapps.com
Words+, Inc.	www.words-plus.com
Zygo Industries, Inc.	http://zygo-usa.com/

or for individuals with limited language abilities. In general they require direct selection, but some also allow scanning. Rate enhancement in this category is primarily related to the use of different pages for different vocabulary categories. Stored vocabulary capacity varies from a low of a few seconds of speech to several minutes.

The devices in the *Direct Selection, Writing Only* category are distinguished by their small size and focus on features that support writing. Some may have a built-in printer. Several devices in this category provide direct file transfer to a desktop computer, and several also have rate enhancements such as abbreviation expansion, instant phrases, or word completion.

The devices in the *Spelling Only SGD* category are primarily distinguished by their dependence on spelling for message formulation. Generally, they are of a small size and use direct selection through a keyboard or touch screen. They may include word completion and instant phrases.

The *Multiple Selection Method with Rate Enhancement* category in Table 11-4 represents the highest level of sophistication in currently available devices. They incorporate all the rate enhancement approaches discussed in Chapter 5. Devices in this category are based on SGD hardware that is specifically designed for AAC. Vocabulary storage capacity varies from a few hundred utterances to thousands of utterances. Interaction with other devices (e.g., computers [Chapter 8], power wheelchairs [Chapter 12], or EADLs [Chapter 14]) and peripherals such as printers is possible for most of the devices in this group by using USB ports as the primary means of interconnecting these other devices with the SGD devices. SGD devices in this category can meet the needs of a variety of consumers from very young children who cannot spell to quantum physicists who make full use of sophisticated rate enhancement techniques. In some cases the same device can serve a wide range of needs because the software and stored vocabulary can be customized. In other cases the devices are targeted to a smaller range of potential users and are relatively inflexible.

Devices in the *Multiple Selection Method with Rate Enhancement* category provide great flexibility in control interfaces and selection methods. Several of the direct selection types allow both standard size and expanded or contracted keyboards as control interfaces. Several devices in this category allow scanning with single-switch or four- or five-switch–directed scanning. Some also provide both one- and two-switch Morse code, and some provide direct selection via head pointing. Options for head pointing are discussed further in Chapter 6.

The flexibility provided by devices in this category is particularly useful when compensating for progressive loss of function with degenerative diseases such as ALS. Initially a person may use direct selection with his hand. As he loses this ability, direct selection using head control is feasible. However, because the device has not changed, the stored vocabulary, rate enhancement strategies, and operational characteristics of the device remain the same. If direct selection via head control becomes impossible, scanning or Morse code can be used (see Chapter 5). Once again the device is not changed, and the vocabulary, rate enhancement, and operational features remain the same. This is a great advantage over having to learn a new device at each stage of the disease.

Another way to characterize AAC devices is by the hardware "platform" that is used. All of the categories of devices in Table 11-4 are available as specially designed and packaged electronic devices. In some cases these are computers, but the computer is hidden from the user. All of the categories of devices in Table 11-4 can also be implemented using mainstream technologies (laptops, tablet computers, PDAs, pad computers, or smart phones). In these cases the AAC features are captured in a software program, called an "application" or an "app," that is loaded into the device.

In summary, the categories shown in Table 11-4 are intended to provide a rough framework in which to view SGDs. It is important for those working with individuals using AAC to remain current regarding technologies. One of the easiest ways to do this is to attend conferences (see Appendix) that feature assistive technologies. Most SGD manufacturers maintain home pages on the Internet (see Table 11-5). Product Web sites typically offer product specifications, comparative data on devices offered, training programs or materials, funding, support, case studies, software downloads, and similar accessories. These are useful resources if you will be charged with setting up AAC systems, programming devices, and implementing training programs.

PUTTING AUGMENTATIVE COMMUNICATION SYSTEMS INTO USE—THE IMPLEMENTATION PROCESS

Once the SGD is obtained, the implementation of the AAC system begins. At this time, the OTA, PTA, and speech assistant may be tasked with making the system work for the individual. There are a number of steps that may be required to make the AAC device usable. Box 11-5 lists some important questions to answer in managing the implementation process. Sometimes it is necessary to integrate components from different manufacturers (e.g., a communication device from one manufacturer and a switch or mounting system from others). Almost always it will be necessary to program (and plan on re-programming) a device to add the specific vocabulary that the individual user will need.

In order to gain more insight into this process, there are also frequent case studies presented in journals such as *Augmentative and Alternative Communication,* newsletters such as *Communication Matters* and *Augmentative Communication News,* and on-line resources including YouTube and other video sites. These case studies vary from anecdotal reports written by individuals who use AAC devices or work with them to formal case studies and single-subject research designs. In this section we discuss the most basic considerations related to training and follow-up. Things do not always progress smoothly when a new AAC system is being set up for an individual. Fields (1991)[30] presents a case study indicating the steps that one family went through to implement an AAC system for their son. There is also a listserv for those who rely on AAC at http://listserv.temple.edu/archives/acolug.html. Many practical considerations related to the setup and use of SGDs are discussed on this list, as are strategies for using devices and for augmented communication in general and related topics,.

Best practices suggest that the individual or family go through a trial period with the SGD as a means of obtaining valuable information. For example, the person's interest in using the SGD may increase when she sees how effective it is in meeting her needs. Or, conversely, their interest in using the SGD may decrease as she may not like how it sounds, how her friends react to it, or how difficult it is to use. A trial period can also help the multidisciplinary team to identify specific short- and long-term training goals for the person and her communication partners so she can develop communicative competencies that enable her to interact effectively and efficiently. If there are special features that require learning new skills (such as storing and retrieving information), these may be assessed during the trial. For individuals who prefer a longer trial period, many companies will lease a device for a one- to three-month period. The outcomes of an SGD assessment should include recommendations for the SGD, any accessories or mounts, and the instructional strategies that are required to meet the person's unique needs and goals.

BOX 11-5 Managing the AAC Implementation Process

1. Who will monitor the overall program of use of this system?
2. How much direct supervision does the individual require when using the system?
3. Who will provide supervision and assist in the day-to-day operation of the system?
4. Who should be called if the system does not work properly?

Vocabulary Selection

When a person needs an augmentative communication device it is because they cannot rely exclusively on speech. In order for them to benefit from an augmentative communication device, it must have a stored vocabulary that they can access. Determining what that vocabulary should be can be very challenging.

The vocabulary is often not "built-in" or pre-programmed by the manufacturer (or if it is, it is so generic that it is useful only as a starting point), and once an AAC system is selected for an individual, it is necessary to create an initial vocabulary set that can be programmed into an electronic device or used with a non-electronic system. Some dedicated SGDs have many pre-programmed vocabulary sets provided from the manufacturer, albeit not customized. The challenge is to determine a good fit between the individual using AAC and the vocabulary sets. Mobile communication apps (e.g., for smart phones and pad computers) offer a mix of some pre-programmed vocabulary and some generic, limited vocabulary.

There are several categories of messages that are used by people who rely on AAC.[8] The conversational categories shown in Table 11-6 provide a useful framework for initial vocabulary selections. Conversational messages begin with greetings and then often involve "small talk" as a transition between the greeting and information sharing. Small talk often utilizes scripts for initiating and maintaining conversations. In general, SGDs do not support small talk well because it is spontaneous and unpredictable. Small talk may be generic and usable in different conversations with different people. Specific small talk is more focused. Examples of both types of small talk are shown in Table 11-7.

A common form of conversational interaction for adults, particularly older adults, is storytelling. Stories entertain, teach, and establish social closeness. An important role for those who support people using AAC systems is to help them remember and describe stories (often by interviewing family and friends as well as the AAC user or obtaining photographs, journals, or other records of past experiences). Once the stories are described, then the person will need assistance with programming the story into the device. The person can then retell/"playback" the story over and over for different audiences (individuals or groups). Devices typically allow playing back a stored

TABLE 11-6 Categories to Be Included in Conversational AAC Systems

Category	Sample Vocabulary
Initiating and interaction	Hey, I've got something to say. Check this out. Come talk to me. May I help you?
Greetings	Hello, I'm pleased to meet you. I'm (name) and you are? Where have you been? I've been waiting forever. What's happening?
Response to greetings	I'm fine. Great, how are you? Not so hot, and you? I've had better days. Hanging in there.
Requests	I'd like a ___________. (object, event) I'd like to go to _________. (place, event)
Information exchange	What time is it? I have a question. The concert begins at 8:00 pm.
Commenting	I agree (disagree). What a great idea! Uh-huh. OK.
Wrap-up/farewell	Well, gotta go. See you later. Bye, nice talking to you.
Conversational repair	Let's start over. That's not what I meant. You misunderstood me.

TABLE 11-7 Generic and Specific Small Talk

Generic	Specific
How is your family?	How is your wife?
What's happening?	What are you doing?
Isn't that beautiful!	That is a beautiful flower.
Good story!	Good story about your vacation.
She is great.	She is a great teacher.

message one sentence at a time by the individual pressing a key or hitting a switch to allow the pace of the story to be controlled.

Vocabulary needs vary by the context (e.g., school, home, or shopping mall), communication mode (SGD, communication board, or gesture), and individual characteristics. *Emerging communicators* are often preliterate (those who cannot read or spell) and they need to communicate essential messages. This is called a **coverage vocabulary.** Since generation of novel utterances by spelling isn't possible, the AAC team must ensure that as many messages as possible are stored in the device for easy retrieval. The specific vocabulary is highly dependent on the individual's needs. Most often the coverage vocabulary is organized by context with separate displays or pages for different activities. An example is a trip to the zoo or circus. A child's system could be programmed with things that she would want to do during the activity. Box 11-6 has vocabulary suggestions for a zoo activity.

BOX 11-6 Some Vocabulary Suggestions for a Zoo Outing:

- Look at the poop!
- I want to see the _________.
- Monkeys
- Giraffe
- Lions
- Birds
- I'm hungry.
- Can we buy an ice cream?
- Let's ride the carousel.
- Look at the snake.

Emerging and context-dependent communicators also need a *developmental vocabulary* that includes words and concepts that are not yet understood. These are selected based on their educational value, not for functional purposes, and they encourage language and vocabulary growth. New words can be added around special events or activities, especially when an activity is to be experienced for the first time.

Required vocabulary resources include a core vocabulary that is used with a variety of situations and partners and occurs frequently. A limited basic core vocabulary of high-frequency words can serve as a coverage and development vocabulary for emergent and context-dependent communicators. Words and messages that are unique to the individual are included in a *fringe vocabulary* that includes names of people, places, activities, and preferred expressions. This approach personalizes the AAC system by complimenting the core vocabulary list. The fringe vocabulary content is often identified by family and friends as well as by the individual herself. The initial items are those that are of high interest to the user and have the potential for frequent use. It is important to include items that denote a range of topics. It is also important to include conversational functions such as those shown in Table 11-6. The vocabulary should be easy for the user to select and for the partner to understand.

There are a number of ways of determining what specific vocabulary is needed by an individual. One useful resource is the *Hearing Them Into Voice** inventory that can be used by families and other informants to identify current language usage as well as identified communication needs. A nice feature of this form is that it poses questions in a functional way that makes it easy for families to respond. The Web site also contains sample filled-in forms to guide families in completing the actual form. While the form as presented on the Web site is for children, it can easily be adapted for use with adults. Since it captures the specific things an individual needs to say as well as how they currently communicate, the *Hearing Them Into Voice* form is useful for group settings to ensure that a variety of communication partners communicate in a consistent way. The various partners can also identify a greater range of needs than any one respondent is likely to identify alone.

Environmental inventories document the individual's experiences by recording precipitating events and subsequent consequences.[8] For example, if a resident of a group home hits another resident, it is important to note what caused the hitting (the precursor) and then to determine if vocabulary such as "I don't like what you did" might have provided an alternative for the person rather than hitting. The documentation includes words that might have been used by peers with and without disabilities. The identified pool of vocabulary items is reduced to a list of the most critical words or concepts that the individual needs and can effectively use. *Communication diaries and checklists* are records of words and phrases needed by an individual for AAC that are kept by informants such as family members.

Participants in adult programs (daycare and residential) who have intellectual disabilities have unique needs for vocabulary that differ from those of typical adults or children (with or without disabilities).[34] Using diaries compiled by staff working with adults who needed AAC, over 80% of the conversational topics were functional (e.g., physical needs and daily activities) for those with the most severe disabilities. For individuals with more moderate disabilities, the percentage of functional topics was twice that of physical needs topics. Emotional (feelings of anger, anxiety, fear, or love) topics amounted to only 3.4% of all topics. Possible reasons for this low response may relate to cognitive difficulties in expressing feelings and to cultural factors that limit the degree to which staff are able to provide emotional support to residents. These results differ from standard vocabulary lists in content and emphasis, and they reinforce the need for care in applying standardized vocabulary lists to AAC vocabulary selection.

Because most AAC devices are programmable, it is possible to continually add or change vocabulary as needs change for adults or children or as children's language skills develop. The choice of which additional vocabulary items to include is generally based on needs that occur frequently but are not part of the stored vocabulary. These needs may be identified by family, care providers, and other communication partners. Another reason for adding vocabulary is that new situations arise. For example, a grandchild may have been born recently and is being brought to his grandmother for the first time. Vocabulary about "proud parents," "he's adorable," "he has your grandfather's eyes," and "is he a good eater?" would be added to allow her to talk about her grandchild during the visit and afterwards.

Beukelman and his colleagues and students at the University of Nebraska at Lincoln have compiled a large number of resources relating to vocabulary selection and messaging in AAC. This information can be accessed through their Web site (http://aac.unl.edu/vbstudy). Included in this resource are core vocabulary lists (consisting of high-frequency words) for preschool and school-age children, young adults, and older adults. They also include unabridged vocabulary lists (with use statistics) both for nondisabled persons (20- to 30-year-old adults, older adults, and preschool children) and AAC users (four separate volumes). Vocabulary lists of small talk for children and adults, as well as context-specific messages suggested by AAC specialists, are also included. This site also provides vocabulary lists for school settings (preschool activities and classroom activities). Finally, vocabulary lists for use as initial recommendations in AAC are reported, as well as references for AAC messaging and vocabulary selection. This site is a rich source of information for those charged with developing vocabulary for individuals who use AAC.

Motor Skill Development

AAC devices require the physical skills to control a switch, keyboard, or mouse for effective operation. This applies to both direct selection and scanning. It takes practice to develop these skills, and it can be useful to separate the physical skills required for the use of an augmentative

* Available from http://www.drsharonrogers.com/

communication device from the communication skills required. This aspect of training is described in more detail in Chapter 5

If the individual has insufficient motor skill to make reliable selections but is expected to develop the necessary motor control, it is important that this *physical competence* be developed separately from the *use* of the physical skill for communication. If we attempt to teach motor skill using the communication device, it is possible that errors in selection caused by lack of motor skill will be misinterpreted as lack of communicative skill. For example, an adult with left field neglect may make repeated errors when asked to spell his street address (e.g., "MacKenzie" Drive may be typed as "MscKenxie"). The first assumption may be that he has a cognitive limitation and can't spell correctly. Another might be that he can't reach the far edge of the keyboard. However, if the keyboard is moved to the left, he suddenly can correctly type "MacKenzie." He can still reach the far right side of the keyboard, so the conclusion is that his errors were due to his left field visual neglect and not physical or cognitive limitations.

Setting Up an AAC System for Use

Mounting SGDs to Wheelchairs

It is often necessary to attach the AAC device to a wheelchair and mount a switch or other control interface where the individual can easily access it. This is a critical step in the implementation process. In order for the SGD to be accessible by the user it must be mounted so he can use it. If a switch or other interface is required to control the SGD, it must also be placed where it is accessible. Other changes need to be considered and their impact anticipated. For example, if the person is getting a new wheelchair and the assessment and recommendation were based on the old chair, then things may not all fit together properly. The mounting of switches and other control interfaces for ease of use is discussed in Chapter 6. If the AAC user has a wheelchair, the SGD must be appropriately mounted to the wheelchair in a manner that is both sturdy and flexible. As shown in Table 11-4, mounting systems are considered accessories that are typically funded as part of the total AAC system. There are some companies that specialize in mounting systems,* and there are other mounting systems that are available from manufacturers of SGDs.† The complexity and need for flexibility in location varies by person. There is a concept from prosthetics called "gadget tolerance" that refers to how much "stuff" a person can stand to have around them in their personal space. Some people are happy to have many different gadgets available to them while others are overwhelmed by only one. When mounting an SGD and associated switches to a wheelchair, this concept must be taken into account. The mounting for a switch may be a part of the seating and positioning system (e.g., switches attached to a head rest or to the lap tray).

Once the SGD is mounted it may create a physical distance between the individual and their communication partners (see Figure 11-12). The location of the device when mounted on the chair needs to take this factor into consideration. The device must also be mounted with the option to move the device out of the way for transfers or for times when it is not in use. Ease of removal from the wheelchair is also important for transportation on a bus or in a van (see Chapter 13). There are a lot of factors at play in Figure 11-12. The mounting of the communication device is set so the child using it can see the display for scanning access, but this location for the display can block face-to- face interaction. Her mother is sitting next to her and this helps to see the display, but this location also limits face-to-face interaction and results in a close physical relationship between the person using AAC and their communication partner. This may not always be comfortable for one or both of the participants in the communication interaction.

Mounting systems that are specifically designed to mount SGDs to wheelchairs have several advantages. They are generally more stable because they are matched to the individual client's needs. These devices have a fixed orientation and position that do not change when they are moved out of the way for transfer or taken off of the wheelchair, so they do not need to be readjusted. Most of these systems swing away so that the individuals can perform their activities of daily living or be taken out of the wheelchair without changing the position of the SGD on the mounting system. Commercial mounting systems generally have a main structure that provides support and a variety of mounting plates that are matched to the most common SGDs. They also provide mounting brackets for attaching the system to a wheelchair. Various types of

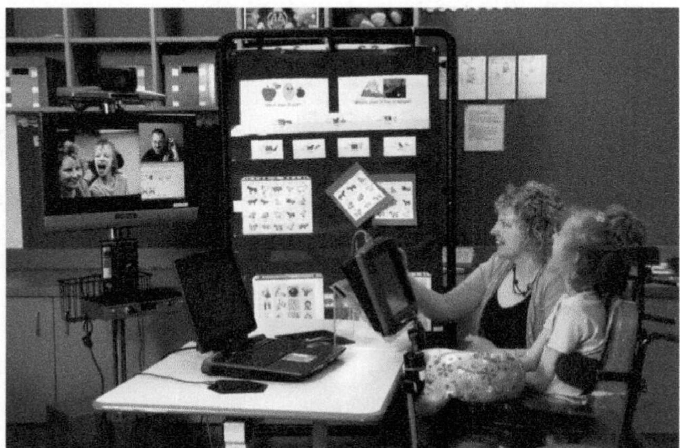

Figure 11-12 An AAC device can change the dynamics of interpersonal interaction.

* For example, Daedelus Technologies, Inc. (http://www.daessy.com/); Blue Sky Designs, Inc. (www.mountnmover.com). Also see http://www.abledata.com/abledata.cfm?pageid=19327&top=10857&trail=22,10825,10837

† E.g., Words+ (http://www.words-plus.com/website/products/accs/wheelmts.htm); Prentke Romich Company (http://www.liberator.net.au/index.php/products/mounting-systems)

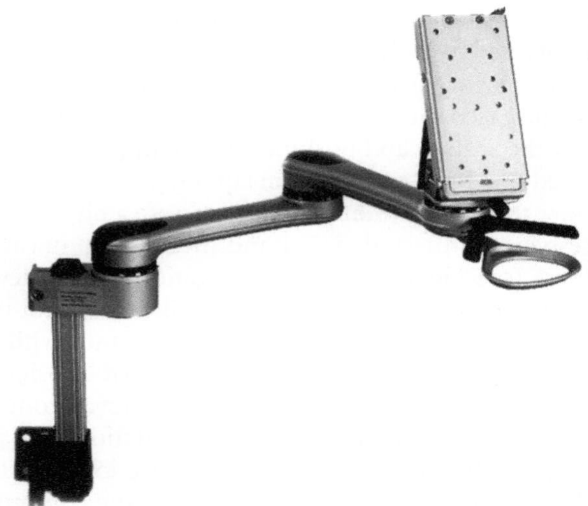

Figure 11-13 The user of this mounting system can move it out of the way by gripping and pressing on the silver ring. (Courtesy of Blue Sky Designs, Minneapolis, MN www.mountnmover.com.)

wheelchair tubing are accommodated in these systems. For most mounting systems the user is dependent on someone else to move the device out of the way and then move it back for use. If the other person isn't paying attention, the user may be without access to a means of communication. The *Mountnmover* from Blue Sky Designs* (Figure 11-13) has provision for the user to move the SGD out of the way independently.

How to Choose Parts for a Mounting System†

Providing a stabilized and accessible custom mounting system involves many considerations. There are many different component parts and mechanisms available. The creation of a mounting system may include Velcro, glue, duct tape, carpet, pipe, rods, clamps, knobs, wood, fabric, paper clips, foam, corrugated cartons, or any other handy material as well as commercially available parts or complete systems. When designing a mounting system for an individual, it is often useful to obtain assistance from the SGD manufacturer or an assistive technology center or one of the companies specializing in mounting systems. This may require that digital photographs of the client in a variety of locations where the SGD will be used (the easy chair in the living room, a bed, the wheelchair, at work, and at school) together with the SGD to be mounted. These digital photographs can then be e-mailed to share the physical information and get help and suggestions on how to proceed. Box 11-7 contains a step-by-step approach to selecting an SGD mounting system for a wheelchair. Figure 11-14 shows an example of how a completed installation of an SGD will look. The OTA or PTA may be responsible for ensuring that all of the mounting components are adjusted for maximum efficiency and minimal effort by the person using AAC. Mounting systems also need to be checked frequently to make certain that the connections are tight and secure. Nuts and bolts can loosen from vibration during use.

BOX 11-7 Suggestions for Developing a Mounting System for an SGD on a Wheelchair

Determine where in space the device needs to be when it's mounted:

- With a digital camera, take pictures of the user in the wheelchair from different vantage points. If possible, have someone hold the device in position for the photos. Otherwise, sketch on the pictures where the device should be.
- Determine where on the wheelchair the mount needs to attach and measure the diameter of the wheelchair tubing or note the cross-section configuration and dimensions (e.g., round, square, or rectangular), and look for mounting holes on the frame under the seat cushion sides.
- Decide how the mount and/or the device are to be removed from the wheelchair. Does the device need to swing out of the way for transfer or when getting close to tables? Does the device need to be placed flat on a table or desk when it's removed from the wheelchair? Does the device need to be moved from one mount to another?
- Determine the required strength of the mount: heavy duty mounts for heavy devices or for forceful users, medium strength or light weight for lighter, more protected units.

Decide on the mounting components required:

- Select the wheelchair clamp from the wheelchair tubing diameter or frame configuration.
- Check to see if the vertical mount tubing can clear the parts of the wheelchair between the clamp and its supporting end.
- Is there a wheelchair lap tray to clear? Is there a joystick on the chair? If so, make sure that the mounting system will not interfere with these components.
- Select the style of the mount: fixed, right angle tubing; straight tubing with a right-angle joint; folding, etc.
- Choose the device mounting tray or plate and tube clamp to secure it to the mounting tubing.

(Courtesy ZYGO-USA, Fremont, California www.ZYGO-USA.com)

Training System Use: Developing Communicative Competence

When the installation is completed, the individual and those working with him (e.g., care providers, family, teachers, employers, therapists, and speech-language pathologists) can begin the process of learning to use the device. Depending on the complexity of the device and the sophistication of the features included, this process can take from a few hours to several months.

*www.mountnmover.com

†Courtesy of Zygo Industries.

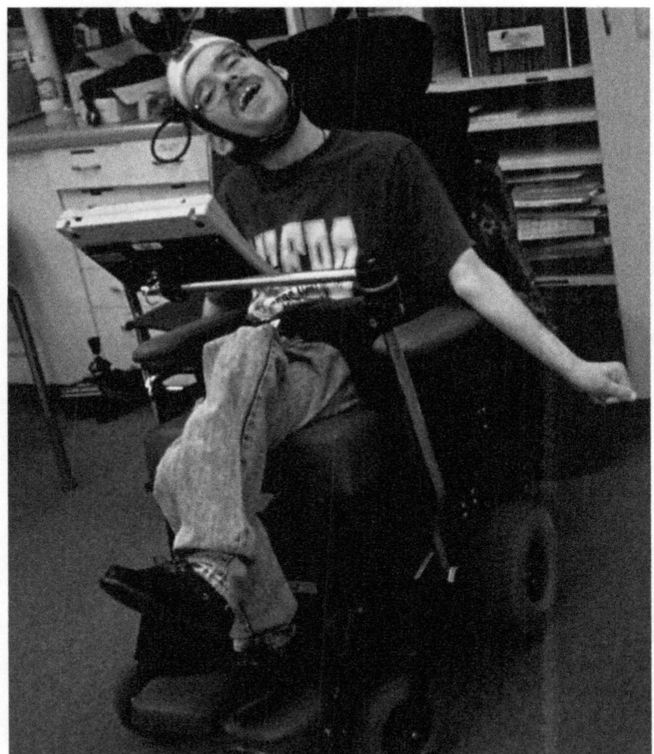

Figure 11-14 Implementation of an AAC system includes proper mounting of the AAC device and control interface to the wheelchair if necessary. Here is a completed installation ready for checkout. See text for explanation of numbers.

The development of communicative competence is most effective when a comprehensive program is employed. One such approach is the System for Augmenting Language (SAL).[63] SAL involves a multimodal approach to training of the individuals who rely on AAC and their partners. It also includes ongoing follow-up. Sevick, Romski and Adamson (2004)[63] illustrate the application of SAL through a case study of a pre-school child who used both an SGD and a manual display consisting of Picture Communication Symbols (PCS).* For young children with cognitive and language disabilities, the development of both expressive and receptive vocabulary can be developed using an SGD in an exercise to teach requesting.[19] Children were taught to request objects using PCS symbols on an SGD. After learning these symbols, the children's comprehension was evaluated. The use of an SGD during the labeling instruction appeared to increase later comprehension of the symbols.

Scripts that are programmed into an AAC device can be used in a training paradigm. One formal approach is called "Script Builder."† The scripts are a way of training individuals to achieve greater social competence and more effective interactions. The scripts are co-planned and oriented toward the development of social closeness by encouraging social purpose and a sense of belonging. Typical topics of trivia, sports, gossip, hanging out, and "who's cute?" allow the individual to display aspects of her personality through humor, teasing, whining, and joke telling. Scripts change perceptions of individuals who use AAC because greater social competence is evident. Some scripts focus on information content, others on conversation (new information plus social closeness). Example scripts are shown in Box 11-8. There are three roles in the training: the individual who is developing AAC skills, his partner, and a "prompter" who

* www.mayer-johnson.com/

† Linda J. Burkhart, Eldersberg, Md. (www.lburkhart.com)

BOX 11-8 Scripts

THE SURPRISE	THE PROM – GETTING READY
Hey, come here.	Hey, Mom
Want to know a secret?	Come here!
It's here in my bag.	Oh no!
It's one of my favorites.	I've got to do my make-up for the Prom!
I don't think you've seen this before.	It's getting late.
Take a guess.	Hurry, Mom!
Want to see it now?	Remember, my dress is blue.
Naw - take another guess.	Let's do lipstick first.
Oh, you've waited long enough.	Please . . . not purple!
Oops – can't get it out.	Keep my lipstick on my lips.
Oh all right – here it is.	Don't get it on my teeth.
Have you ever seen anything like this before?	I don't want to look like Bozo.
I've got a ton of things in this bag.	I have that red hair!
Let's tell everyone but the teacher!	I want to look like Britney Spears.
	She's beautiful.
	Could I have a little more mascara, please?
	Thanks!
	I can't wait to get to the Prom!
	Mom, you did a great job.
	I don't want to miss the dance.
	Let's go!

prompts in an unobtrusive way and only when necessary. The partner's role is communicating as naturally as possible, pausing when necessary, and not prompting at all. All *social scripts* start with a greeting and include a range of communicative functions such as positive and negative comments, teasing, and questioning. They provide for multiple turns and use topic maintainers such as "tell me more." They need to be designed to ensure that the conversation can be retrieved if it gets off course. For example, the AAC user may be slower than a speaking conversational partner. If an AAC utterance is misunderstood, then it may take the conversation in a totally different direction before the AAC user can correct the misinterpretation. If there is a quick phrase such as "That is not what I meant," then things might get back on track before the AAC user gets "backed into a corner." The vocabulary chosen must be appropriate to the individual's age, setting, and personality.

Communicative competence depends on many factors.[44] The *context* in the HAAT model affects competence in several ways. The partner and her skill in listening, the environment of use, and cultural factors all contribute to or detract from communicative competence. The degree of competence can also vary, and complete mastery of an AAC device is not necessary to have functional communication interactions. Light (1989)[44] describes four areas of competence required for successful use of AAC devices: (1) operational, (2) linguistic, (3) social, and (4) strategic.

Operational competence requires the skills and understanding of the technical operation of the AAC device that are described in Table 11-8. The degree of operational competence can be quite variable, ranging from very

TABLE 11-8 Developing Competence in the Use of AAC Devices

Type	Description	Training Topics and Approaches
Operational	Physical skills to make selections Technical device operation Varies from basic to advanced Cognitive demands dictated by device features	User: Making a selection Opportunities for practice in their use Storage of new vocabulary Input acceleration techniques and vocabulary manipulation features such as text editing and reformatting the output Facilitators: Connecting the device to the control interface and to a wheelchair Charging batteries Adding vocabulary Troubleshooting Cleaning device safely Providing written instructions in bullet form attached to the device for settings in which facilitators change or there are a number of staff who support the individual Approaches: Group training sessions One-on-one training Practice using the device in simulated or actual communication settings
Linguistic	Understanding of the symbol system meaning and how it is used by the individual using the AAC system	Development of competence in this area may require many hours of practice Practice based on functional tasks Prompt-free strategy to avoid drill and practice fatigue (Mirenda and Santogrossi, 1985)
Social	The use of AAC devices for social discourse is different than using speech New skills are required The perception of the AAC user by communication partners changes	Rules of conversation (e.g., turn taking, initiating a conversation, and conversational repair) Understanding of how people interact Developing a positive self-image Showing interest in communication partner and putting partner at ease Developing skill at drawing others into the conversation, and actively participating in the conversation Use scripts (Box 11-3)
Strategic	Developing ways to make AAC system use more effective Degree to which the person is able to develop adaptive strategies to make the most of the system	Examples: Letting the partner guess the next letter on a spelling board Using gestures (e.g., waving to indicate that a misunderstanding has occurred) with an electronic device A child whose speech may be better understood at home than at school, relies on SGD more in school, but develops strategies to make maximal use of both systems See Table 11-1 for different AAC use with different partners

basic operation to advanced features. An AAC device is like a musical instrument that can be played by an accomplished AAC communicator. This means that basic operation needs to be practiced (like musical scales) until it is automatic. Training operational competence requires a systematic introduction of technical features. For example, the first thing to learn is how to make a selection. After this is well understood and mastered, then other techniques such as rate enhancement and unique vocabulary retrieval techniques can be learned. As with a musical instrument, AAC device competence only comes with practice, and there should be lots of opportunities to practice using the device. The best practice will come in simulated or actual use situations in which the individual is communicating with others by using the device, as shown in Figure 11-15. Those people supporting or facilitating the individual's training will also need to be trained in certain operational features of the device (e.g., battery charging and connecting control interfaces).

Basic operation of the AAC system includes some things that a support person (including family) would be required to learn, such as how to connect the device to the control interface, how to charge batteries, how to attach the device to a wheelchair, how to add vocabulary using rate enhancement techniques (e.g., codes), and how to conduct basic troubleshooting in case the device fails to operate properly. The manufacturer's Web site can be helpful in solving problems that arise. After these basic features and operations are mastered, those characteristics related to storage of new vocabulary, input acceleration techniques, and vocabulary manipulation features such as text editing and reformatting the output can be introduced. Often the first two phases are accomplished in one session. However, in some cases, they may require multiple training sessions, and the process is often a lengthy one that may be integrated with the other aspects of training in communicative competence. Other factors need to be taken into account too. For example, technical proficiency varies by generation. For many individuals English is a second language and explanations need to take that into account. As described in Chapter 2, cultural factors can influence how people react to assistive technologies and how they approach the use of them in social contexts.

Linguistic competence requires that the meanings of the symbols used and how they can be combined or used in multiple ways be understood by the individual using the AAC system. As Light (1989)[44] points out, the individual often must be competent in two languages: the spoken language of the community and the language of her AAC device. It is likely that the individual also lacks models of proficient use in the language of her device. Development of competence in this area may require many hours of practice. Often this practice is built around a functional task such as that shown in Figure 11-16.

In contrast to the typical "drill and practice" approach to developing vocabulary and AAC use, Mirenda and Santogrossi (1985)[55] used a prompt-free strategy to teach a young child to use a picture-based communication board. The approach involved a four-step process, which began with a picture of a soft drink being available to the child during her regular therapy session. A drink was visible to her, as was the picture of the drink. The child was not told that touching the picture would result in her getting a drink, nor was she prompted in any way to touch the picture. If she touched the drink directly, she was told that she could have some later. If she accidentally or deliberately

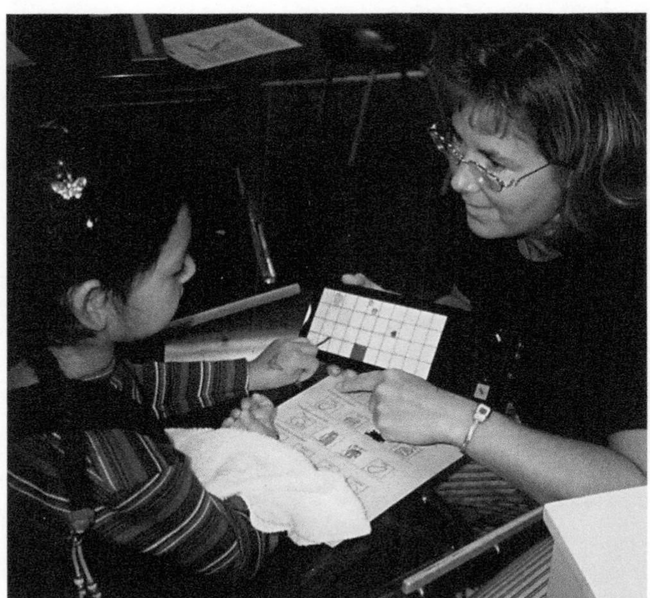

Figure 11-15 Development of operational competence with an AAC device requires a structured training program in which the device features are carefully explained and skill in their use is developed.

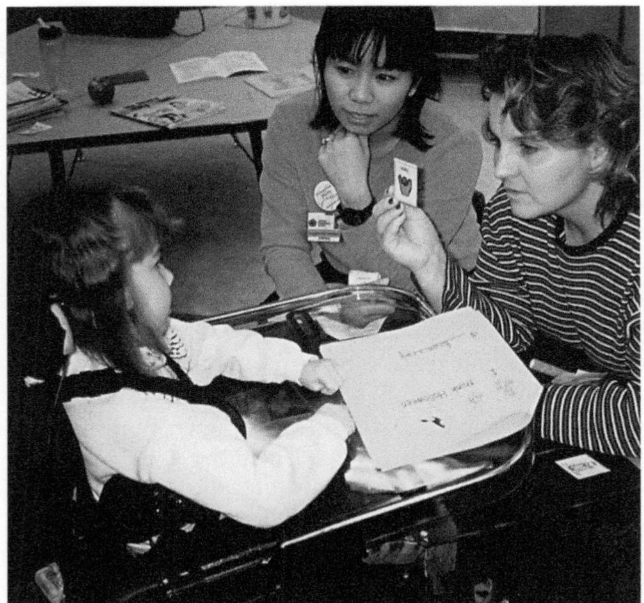

Figure 11-16 AAC users need to learn about conversational conventions and strategies. Training of these skills is often done in simulated situations. Here an aide is teaching the child how to use her AAC tools to interact with another adult partner.

touched the picture, she was immediately given the drink with the explanation, "Yes, if you touch the picture, you may have the drink." Once the deliberate response had been established over several sessions, Mirenda and Santogrossi proceed to shape the pointing behavior by progressively moving the picture farther away, until it was out of sight and the child had to actively find it. As the child became proficient in this task, the number of pictures was increased to four and the process repeated for the other choices. Eventually the child was able to generalize to a language board of 120 pictures. The advantage of this approach is that the child learns the meaning and significance of the symbolic representation by discovery rather than by drill, which leads to greater generalization and more functional use of the AAC system.

Many people who use AAC devices have little or no experience in social interaction. For example, a child who has never spoken will have to be taught how to interact, how to participate in a conversation, and how to interact with others who generate communication exchange. Even adults who have used natural language for communication prior to sustaining a disease or injury are faced with a very different mode of interaction when an AAC device is used. Rules of conversation are altered and the perception of the individual by their communication partners is different. In order to be socially competent, the individual must have knowledge, judgment, and skills in both *sociolinguistic* (e.g., turn taking, initiating a conversation, and conversational repair) and *sociorelational* areas.[44] The latter term describes the understanding of interactions between individuals. The effective communication device user is described[43] as having a positive self-image, interest in her partner, skill at drawing others into the conversation, the ability to put a partner at ease, and an active participation in the conversation. These are sociorelational skills, and the degree to which they are understood and used is one measure of social competence. These skills are best taught in the contexts in which they are to be used. One example of such training is shown in Figure 11-16, in which the child is being taught strategies for interacting with an adult partner.

Self-determination is difficult for people who rely on AAC.[25] They must know what they want, know how to get it, and have a sense of self-worth. In order to achieve these goals they need the "language of negotiation" and negotiation skills that require both transactional language to supplement requesting and information exchange, as well as conversational control vocabulary. Without these skills, individuals who rely on AAC are dependent on others for the determination of their life goals, direction, and other important matters such as medical decisions. They also need these skills to avoid abuse and harassment by caregivers and others and to report such incidents if they do occur.

Every person who uses an AAC system develops strategies to make the use of that system more effective. Examples include letting the partner guess the next letter on a spelling board and using gestures (e.g., waving to indicate that a misunderstanding has occurred, or shaking their head "no") in conjunction with an electronic device. Strategic competence describes the degree to which the person is able to develop adaptive strategies to make the most of the system. These may differ in different contexts. For example, a child's speech may be better understood at home than at school. He will rely on the electronic SGD more in school, but he will also develop strategies to make maximal use of both systems.

Just as the individual using the AAC system must develop several types of competencies, there are many ways of carrying out the training. One approach, shown in Figure 11-17, is to simulate a situation, model the types of interaction likely to occur, and have the user "practice" the strategies and skills necessary to make it a success. This step can be followed by an actual situation in which the trainer accompanies the user as she encounters the situation. The trainer can then prompt the user at appropriate times, add encouragement, and help to clarify when necessary. This combination of clinic-based practice and community-based skill development is often very effective and provides feedback on training areas to be explored further.

In order for training to be effective, staff must have sufficient skill and experience to assist the AAC user. This requires training for those who are supporting AAC use. Schepis and Reid (2003)[60] identified five basic steps in competency- and performance-based training for staff. These include (1) specifying desired outcomes, (2) specifying

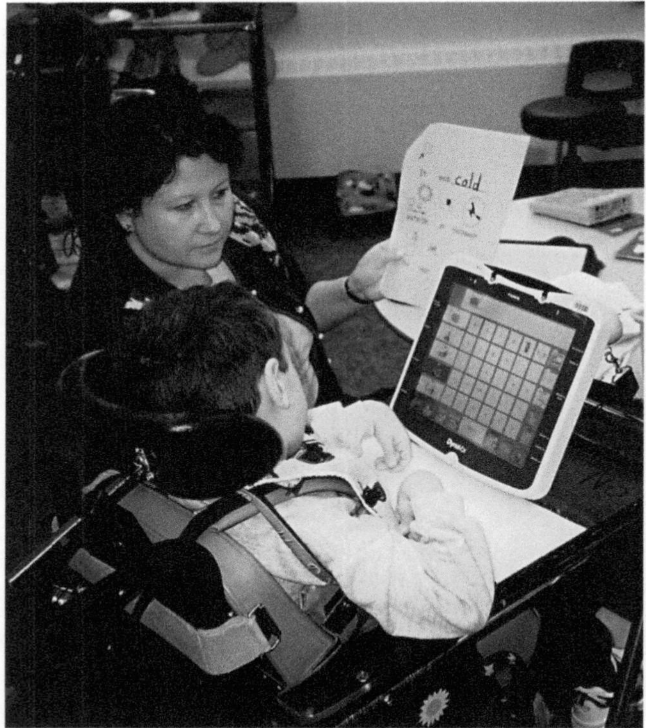

Figure 11-17 Development of linguistic competence is often taught in conjunction with other functional tasks such as the one shown here.

roles for staff to support individuals in achieving these outcomes, (3) providing both written and oral expectations and instructions to staff, (4) demonstration of how to perform duties, and (5) observation of staff performing the duties with corrective feedback as necessary.

Training of the individual who relies on AAC is only effective if communication partners are also trained. It is important to get as many individuals involved with training as possible, so that no one single person is responsible to do it all. For children, the training of parents to recognize communication attempts and to understand the child's operational, linguistic, strategic, and social competencies is also important. Bruno and Dribbon (1998)[20] evaluated a parent training program conducted as part of an AAC summer camp experience where parents attended the camp with their children. Parents reported making positive changes in both operational and interactional skills during the camp.[20] These changes were reflected in gains made by the children in skills related to the use of pragmatic functions (e.g., giving and requesting information, requesting assistance, and responding and protesting) over the course of the camp. The areas of social exchange and giving of information continued to increase at the 6-month follow-up evaluation.

AAC training can be both complicated and lengthy.[8] Light and Binger (1998)[47] have developed the seven-step process for developing AAC communication competence shown in Box 11-9. Light and Binger provide data collection and assessment forms, as well as strategies, for implementing this program. The ACETS (Augmentative Communication Employment Training and Supports)* has been developed specifically to assist those who rely on AAC in seeking employment. A formal training manual is available for this program that is based on three principles: (1) immersion in the workplace culture, (2) acquiring a broad base of employment-related skills and experience, and (3) support of individualized goals.

* Institute on Disabilities, Temple University, Philadelphia, Pa. (http://disabilities.temple.edu)

BOX 11-9 Developing AAC Communication Competence*

(1) Specify the goal, do baseline observations.
(2) Select vocabulary.
(3) Teach the facilitators how to support development of the target skill.
(4) Teach the skill to the target individual.
(5) Check for generalization.
(6) Evaluate outcomes.
(7) Complete maintenance checks.

*Light and Binger[47]

Follow-up: Measuring Short- and Long-Term Outcomes

The evaluation of communicative competence in the four domains (operational, linguistic, social, and strategic) will identify areas in which the AAC system is and is not adequately meeting the individual's needs. Periodic reevaluation of the individual's skills and needs may also result in changes in the training or the AAC system(s). The reevaluation may lead to new training goals in one or more of the four areas of communicative competence. In other cases the caregivers, family, or other support staff may require additional training in order to facilitate the use of the AAC device. There can be frequent staff changes in many settings (e.g., group home, day program, or long-term care). Providing ongoing training for new front line staff needs to be included in any AAC implementation plan.

The AAC device as it is configured may also be inadequate to meet the individual's needs. It may be possible to adjust some of the features (e.g., scanning rate or stored vocabulary) or it may be necessary to consider a completely new device. The magnitude of the changes in the device dictates the amount of additional operational training required. In some cases the individual's skills may decrease (e.g., degenerative disease) or increase (e.g., a young child who develops greater language skills). In either case a reevaluation and adjustments in the AAC system (i.e., device plus training and support) will be required. Murphy et al. (1996)[56] identified obstacles to effective AAC system use (see Box 11-10).

The variety of formal partners also reinforces the need for inclusion of both useful vocabulary and multiple modes of communication. The development of strategic competence is vital to increase the likelihood that an AAC user will be able to independently carry out conversations in a variety of settings and with a variety of partners. Availability and accessibility of AAC systems can be addressed by both appropriate mounting of systems on wheelchairs and training to ensure that care providers understand the need to have the system available to the user at all times. The results reported by Murphy et al. also emphasize the importance of basic vocabulary required by AAC users.

The MPT model (Chapter 3) has been adapted to AAC use as the *AAC Acceptance Model*.[42] This model focuses on the prediction of acceptance of AAC by adults with acquired communication impairments. While the technology may play a small role in acceptance or non-acceptance, other factors are more important. Among these other factors are: (1) the communication partners acceptance of the technology; (2) the rate (sudden or gradual) of onset of the communication impairment; (3) affective, behavioral, and cognitive components of a user's attitude toward AAC technology; (4) perception of the user and other people toward the device; and (5) how other people view the person using the device. At this time, the measure has not been studied for use with other populations (e.g., children with disabilities).

BOX 11-10 Obstacles to AAC Use for Adults

WHAT THE RESEARCH TELLS US

Obstacles to AAC System Use in Adult Programs

- 93 users of AAC systems and 186 partners (93 formal and 93 informal).
- Formal partners: speech-language pathologists (80%) and teachers.
- Informal partners: care providers in the day or living program (62%), family, friends, and others.
- The majority of low- and high-tech AAC system use was in the day placement (90%), residential (70%), and leisure (60%) settings.
- Use was limited to organized therapy sessions in general.
- AAC availability:
  - 48% of the users while shopping,
  - 62% during outings such as day trips during their program,
  - 66% where they lived.
- Independent use of AAC: Only 57% of the low-tech and 59.4% of the high-tech AAC users.
- Knowledge of the AAC system sufficient enough to interact with the AAC user was reported in less than half of the formal partners and one third of the informal partners.
- Training:
  - 88 % of users received training from their formal partners.
  - 60 minutes or less (or 40 hours per year based on sessions conducted).
  - Basic vocabulary required for daily interactions (see Table 11-5) was not included in the AAC systems.

Murphy et al.[56]

We can relate meaningful AAC outcomes to the three central categories of the WHO ICF classification system (see Chapter 2).[8] At the level of body structures and functions, we can determine the degree to which AAC intervention compensates for lost or absent speech and/or language function. Evaluations related to activity focus on the quality and quantity of communication interactions and the degree to which these meet the goals and needs of the individual. Evaluation related to participation relates to existence of socially defined role and tasks within a sociocultural and physical environment. Some "Big Picture" AAC outcomes are shown in Box 11-11.[8] There are several types of measures for AAC system outcomes. Operational measures evaluate the user's ability to interact with the system itself (operational competence), while representational measures evaluate the AAC user's symbol and grammatical capabilities.[8]

The most important result of the follow-up phase is to evaluate the outcomes of the AAC intervention to determine their effectiveness (including both the hard and soft technologies), as well as to determine the appropriateness of the match between the originally specified needs and the resulting system. The principles of outcome measurement discussed in Chapter 3 apply to AAC system evaluation as well.

BOX 11-11 Big Picture Outcomes for AAC Intervention (after Beukelman and Mirenda[8])

Has the AAC system resulted in increased:
Self-determination for the user?
Inclusion of the user in social groups?
Independence, to the degree the AAC user wants it?
Participation in the community?
Gainful employment?
Academic achievement?
Social connectedness?
Educational inclusion or decreased special class placement?

SUMMARY

Augmentative and alternative communication systems serve needs for both writing and conversation for individuals who have difficulties in these areas. Low-tech AAC systems provide quick and easy help for meeting communication needs, whereas high-tech devices offer great sophistication in available vocabulary, speed of communication, and flexibility of access. The latter features allow persons who have very limited physical skills to utilize AAC systems. AAC systems also have great flexibility in required user cognitive, sensory, and perceptual skills, allowing for persons with a diversity of intellectual abilities to benefit from AAC. The OTA, PTA, and speech assistant can play a major role in the successful implementation of AAC systems.

STUDY QUESTIONS

1. What are the four major communicative goals normally addressed by augmentative communication systems?
2. Distinguish between aided and unaided communication.
3. Do mothers and fathers have different needs for AAC for their nonspeaking children?
4. Describe differences in the conversational rules that apply between two speaking persons and those between one speaking person and one user of augmentative communication.
5. Describe the relationship between the Social Networks Model and the Participation Model. How do each of these relate to the HAAT model described in this text?
6. Pick two of the circles in the Social Networks Model and describe the types of AAC that would be expected in each one.
7. What factors influence the attitudes of children toward their peers who use AAC?
8. What features distinguish competent augmentative communicators from those who are not successful?
9. What are the major approaches used to increase conversational rate when the individual is using scanning?

10. What are dynamic displays, and what advantages do they provide?
11. What are Visual Scene Displays and what unique features do they have?
12. What populations might benefit most from Visual Scene Displays? Why?
13. Describe the major challenges and approaches for an AAC intervention for an individual whose primary disorder is language or cognitively based. How does this compare to individuals whose primary disorder is motor or physical?
14. List and discuss three advantages that the Internet provides for communication by AAC users.
15. What are the four types of competencies acquired in AAC training? Pick an AAC system for an individual and design the training. You must make assumptions regarding the person's skills, her needs, and other people available to help facilitate the training.
16. What is a "feature matching" process?
17. List three factors to be considered when mounting an SGD to a wheelchair.
18. What are the key steps in training staff to support a user of AAC?
19. Why do we separate motor from cognitive/language training in AAC?
20. What is the "prompt free" strategy? Why is it useful?
21. What are the seven steps to build communication competence through training?
22. What are scripts and how are they used in AAC training?
23. List three advantages and three disadvantages of mainstream technologies when used as AAC devices.
24. List three ways of determining what vocabulary to include in an AAC system.
25. Describe two different ways of representing language in AAC systems.

REFERENCES

1. Anderson NB, Shames GH: *Human communication disorders: an introduction*, Boston, 2006, Allyn and Bacon.
2. Baker B: Minspeak™: a semantic compaction system that makes self-expression easier for communicatively disabled individuals, *Byte* 7(9):186–202, 1982.
3. Ball LJ, Beukelman DR, Patee GL: Acceptance of augmentative and alternative communication technology by persons with amyotrophic lateral sclerosis, *Augment Altern Commun* 20(2):113–122, 2004.
4. Beck AR, Bock S, Thompson JR, et al: Influence of communicative competence and augmentative and alternative communication technique on children's attitudes toward a peer who uses AAC, *Augment Altern Commun* 18(4):217–227, 2002.
5. Beck AR, Dennis M: Attitudes of children toward a similar-aged child who uses augmentative communication, *Augment Altern Commun* 12(2):78–87, 1996.
6. Beukelman D, Garrett K: Augmentative and alternative communication for adults with acquired severe communication disorders, *Augment Altern Commun* 4(2):104–121, 1988.
7. Beukelman DR, Ball LJ: Improving AAC use for persons with acquired neurogenic disorders: understanding human and engineering factors, *Assist Technol* 14(1):33–44, 2002.
8. Beukelman DR, Mirenda P: *Augmentative and alternative communication: management of severe communication disorders in children and adults*, ed 3, Baltimore, 2005, Paul H. Brookes.
9. Beukelman DR, Fager S, Ball L, et al: AAC for adults with acquired neurological conditions: a review, *Augment Altern Commun* 23(3):230–242, 2007.
10. Blackstone S: Dynamic displays: an option for accessing language, *Augment Commun News* 7(2):1–6, 1994.
11. Blackstone S: Amyotrophic Lateral Sclerosis, *Augment Commun News* 11(1/2):1–15, 1998.
12. Blackstone S: Assessment protocol for SGDs, *Augment Commun News* 13(6):1–16, 2001.
13. Blackstone S: Social networks: What is it? Why use it? *Augment Commun News* 15(2):1–16, 2003a.
14. Blackstone S: Autism Spectrum Disorders, *Augment Commun News* 15(4):1–6, 2003b.
15. Blackstone S: The Internet and its offspring, *Augment Commun News* 15(3):1–3, 2003c.
16. Blackstone S: Visual scene displays, *Augment Commun News* 16(2):1–5, 2004.
17. Blackstone SW, Hunt Berg M: *Social Networks: A communication inventory for individuals with complex communication needs and their communication partners – inventory booklet*, Monterey, Calif, 2003, Augmentative Communication, Inc.
18. Blischak DM, Lombardino LJ, Dyson AT: Use of speech-generating devices: in support of natural speech, *Augment Altern Commun* 19(1):29–35, 2003.
19. Brady NC: Improved comprehension of object names following voice output communication aid use: two case studies, *Augment Altern Commun* 16(3):197–204, 2000.
20. Bruno J, Dribbon M: Outcomes in AAC: evaluating the effectiveness of a parent training program, *Augment Altern Commun* 14(2):59–70, 1998.
21. Bryen DN, Cohen KJ, Carey A: Augmentative communication employment training and supports (ACETS): some employment-related outcomes, *J Rehabil* 70(1):10–18, 2004.
22. Carlisle Ladtkow M, Culp D: Augmentative communication with traumatic brain injury. In Yorkston KM, editor: *Augmentative communication in the medical setting*, Arizona, 1992, Communication Skill Builders, pp 139–244.
23. Crepeau EB, Cohn ES, Schell BAB, editors: *Willard and Spackman's occupational therapy*, ed 11, Philadelphia, 2009, Lippincott Williams & Wilkins, p 1154.
24. Clarke M, Kirton A: Patterns of interaction between children with physical disabilities using augmentative and alternative communication systems and their peers, *Child Lang Teach Ther* 19(2):135–151, 2003.
25. Collier B: When I grow up ... supporting youth who use augmentative communication for adulthood, In *Proceedings 2005 Alberta Rehabilitative and Assistive Technology Consortium Conference*, Edmonton AB, Canada, 2005, www.acrat.ca.
26. Cook AM, Polgar JM: *Cook & Hussey's assistive technologies: principles and practice*, ed 3, St Louis, 2008, Mosby.
27. Drager KDR: Light technologies with different system layouts and language organizations, *J. Speech hear. Res* 46(2): 289–312, 2003.
28. Dowden P, Cook AM: Choosing effective selection techniques for beginning communicators. In Reichle J, Beukelman DR, Light JC, editors: *Exemplary practices for beginning communicators*, 2002, Paul H. Brookes, pp 395–432.
29. Duckman R: The incidence of visual anomalies in a population of cerebral palsied children, *J Am Optom Assoc* 50(9):1013–1016, 1979.

30. Fields C: Finding a voice for Daniel, *Team Rehabil Rep* 2(3):16–19, 1991.
31. Fox LE, Fried-Oken M: AAC aphasiology: partnership for future research, *Augment Altern Commun* 12:257–271, 1996.
32. Garrett K, Beukelman D: Augmentative communication approaches for persons with severe aphasia. In Yorkston K, editor: *Augmentative communication in the medical setting,* Tucson, 1992, Communication Skill Builders.
33. Gilman S: *Neurobiology of disease,* New York, 2007, Academic Press.
34. Graves J: Vocabulary needs in augmentative and alternative communication: a sample of conversational topics between staff providing services to adults with learning difficulties and their service users, *Br J Learn Disabilities* 28(3):113–119, 2000.
35. Halloran J, Emerson M: *LAMP: language acquisition through motor planning,* Wooster, Ohio, 2010, The Center for AAC and Autism.
36. Hopkins HL, Smith HD, editors: *Willard and Spackman's occupational therapy,* ed 8, Philadelphia, 1993, JB Lippincott.
37. Jacobs B, Drew R, Ogletree BT, et al: Augmentative and alternative communication (AAC) for adults with severe aphasia: where we stand and how we can go further, *Disabil Rehabil* 26(21/22):1231–1240, 2004.
38. Joseph D: The morning, *Comm Outlook* 8(2):8, 1986.
39. Kent-Walsh JE, Light JC: General education teachers' experiences with inclusion of students who use augmentative and alternative communication, *Augment Altern Commun* 19(2):102–124, 2003.
40. King JM, Hux K: Intervention using talking word processor software: an aphasia case study, *Augment Altern Commun* 11(3):187–192, 1995.
41. Kraat AW: Developing intervention goals. In Blackstone S, Bruskin DM, editors: *Augmentative communication: an introduction,* Rockville, Md, 1986, American Speech-Language-Hearing Association.
42. Lasker J, Bedrosian J: Promoting acceptance of augmentative and alternative communication by adults with acquired communication disorders, *Augment Altern Commun* 17(3): 141–153, 2001.
43. Light J: Interaction involving individuals using augmentative and alternative communication systems: state of the art and future directions, *Augment Altern Commun* 4(2):66–82, 1988.
44. Light J: Toward a definition of communicative competence for individuals using augmentative and alternative communication systems, *Augment Altern Commun* 5(2):137–144, 1989.
45. Light J, Drager K: AAC technologies for young children with complex communication needs: State of the science and future research directions, *Augment Altern Commun* 23(3):204–216, 2007.
46. Light J, Beesley M, Collier B: Transition through multiple augmentative and alternative communication systems: A three year case study of a head injured adolescent, *Augment Altern Commun* 4(1):2–14, 1988.
47. Light JC, Binger C: *Building communicative competence with individuals who use augmentative and alternative communication,* Baltimore, 1998, Paul H. Brookes.
48. Light JC, Drager KDR: Improving the design of augmentative and alternative technologies for young children, *Assist Technol* 14(1):17–32, 2002.
49. Lilienfeld M, Alant E: Attitudes toward an unfamiliar peer using an AAC device with and without voice output, *Augment Altern Commun* 18:91–101, 2002.
50. Lloyd LL, Fuller DR, Arvidson HH: *Augmentative and alternative communications: a handbook of principles and practices,* Boston, 1997, Allyn and Bacon.
51. McCarthy J, Light J: Attitudes toward individuals who use augmentative and alternative communication: research review, *Augment Altern Commun* 21(1):41–55, 2005.
52. McKelvey ML, Dietz AR, Hux K, et al: Performance of a person with chronic aphasia using a visual scene display prototype, *J Med SpeechLang Pathol* 15(3):305–317, 2007.
53. McNaughton D, Light J, Gulla S: Opening up a 'whole new world': employer and co-worker perspectives on working with individuals who use augmentative and alternative communication, *Augment Altern Commun* 19(4):235–253, 2003.
54. Mirenda P: Toward functional augmentative and alternative communication for students with autism: manual signs, graphic symbols, and voice output communication aids, *Lang Speech Hear Serv Sch* 34(3):203–216, 2003.
55. Mirenda P, Santogrossi J: A prompt-free strategy to teach pictorial communication system use, *Augment Altern Commun* 1(4):143–150, 1985.
56. Murphy J, et al: AAC systems: obstacles to effective use, *Eur J Disord Commun* 31(1):31–44, 1996.
57. Nolan C: *Dam-burst of dreams,* New York, 1981, St. Martin's Press, p 11.
58. Rabins PV, Lyketsos CG, Steele CD: *Practical dementia care,* ed 2, 2006, Oxford Press.
59. Rush WL: *Journey out of silence,* Lincoln, Neb, 1986, Media Productions and Marketing.
60. Schepis M, Reid D: Issues affecting staff enhancement of speech-generating device use among people with severe cognitive disabilities, *Augment Altern Commun* 19(1):59–65, 2003.
61. Scherer MJ: *Matching Person and Technology: a series of assessments for evaluating predispositions to and outcomes of technology use in rehabilitation, education, the workplace and other settings,* Webster, NY, 1998, The Institute for Matching Person & Technology.
62. Schlosser RW, Blischak DM: Is there a role for speech output in interventions for persons with autism? A review, *Focus Autism Other Dev Stud* 16(3):170–178, 2001.
63. Sevcik RA, Romski MA, Adamson LB: Research directions in augmentative and alternative communication for preschool children, *Disabil Rehabil* 26(21/22):1323–1329, 2004.
64. Simpson S: If only I could tell them, *Communication Outlook* 9(4):9–11, 1988.
65. Todman J: Rate and quality of conversations using a text-storage AAC system: single-case training study, *Augment Altern Commun* 16(3):164–179, 2000.
66. Winter S: Cerebral palsy. In Jacobson JW, Mulick JA, Rojahn J, editors: *Handbook of intellectual and developmental disabilities,* New York, NY, 2007, Springer.

CHAPTER 12

Technologies That Enable Mobility

CHAPTER OUTLINE

LEARNING OBJECTIVES

Upon completing this chapter, you will be able to do the following:

1. Discuss needs underlying evaluation of the consumer for a mobility system
2. Describe the three categories of mobility systems based on the need served by each
3. Describe the two primary structures of wheelchairs
4. Identify the major characteristics of manual wheelchairs
5. Identify the major types of powered mobility systems and their characteristics
6. Understand the influence of the relationship between the center of gravity of the user and the center of mass of the wheelchair on the function of the wheelchair
7. Describe the implementation phases for personal mobility systems

KEY TERMS

Alignment
Anti-tip Devices
Armrests
Bariatrics
Bariatric Chair
Camber
Center of Gravity
Center of Mass
Dependent Mobility System
Electrically Powered Wheelchair
Footplate
Front Rigging
Independent Manual Mobility
Independent Powered Mobility
Leg Rest
Lightweight Wheelchair
Lightweight High-Strength Wheelchair
Low-Shear Systems
Manual Wheelchair
Nonproportional Control
Propelling Structure
Proportional Control
Push Handles
Recline
Rigid Sport Ultra Lightweight Wheelchair
Scooter
Shear
Standard Wheelchair

Standing Frame
Standing Wheelchair
Supporting Structure
Tilt
Ultra Lightweight Wheelchair
Wheel Lock

Mobility is fundamental to each individual's quality of life and is necessary for functioning in each of the performance areas: self-care, work or school, and play or leisure. As we have described for other activity outputs, limitations to functional mobility can be either augmented or replaced with assistive technologies. The activity output of ambulation can be augmented with low-tech aids such as canes, walkers, or crutches or replaced by wheeled mobility systems of various types. In addition to the functional gain of increased independence in mobility, other goals such as positive self-image, social interaction, and health maintenance are achieved. In this chapter we focus on manual and powered wheelchair systems to enhance an individual's mobility. Our emphasis is on the total process of delivering these systems to those who need them, from initial need and goal setting, through assessment and recommendation, to implementation and training.

MOBILITY NEEDS SERVED BY WHEELCHAIRS

There has been a significant increase in the number of individuals using mobility systems related to three different trends: (1) the increasing proportion of older adults in many countries, (2) rising rates of obesity, and (3) accessibility legislation. The population of most developing countries is aging, with the proportion of older individuals (65 years and older) expected to reach over 20% of the population in the United States by 2030[9] and earlier in Canada.[5] Age-related physical changes, such as arthritis, result in mobility impairments that require the use of mobility devices. The proportion of morbidly obese individuals is rising, particularly in North America, which has resulted in the development of mobility devices that are specifically designed to support the increased size and weight of these individuals. **Bariatric chairs** are now available for those individuals whose mobility is impaired by obesity and related chronic diseases. Accessibility legislation in many countries has reduced the physical and institutional barriers to community participation of individuals with disabilities, with the result that more people are using mobility devices for instrumental activities of daily living.

Data collected in the 2000 U.S. Census indicates that 20.9 million families in the United States have at least one individual with a disability living in their household.[60] Of these, 16.6% report a physical disability that results in a functional limitation. *A Profile of Disability in Canada, 2001* indicates that 13.7% of the Canadian population report a mobility impairment.[15]

Kaye, Kang, and LePlante (2002)[30] provide information on the number of Americans who use mobility devices. These data are derived from the 1994–1995 National Health Interview Survey on Disability (NHIS-D). The survey indicated that 1.6 million Americans who live outside of an institutional setting use a mobility device. The vast majority of these individuals (1.5 million) use a manual wheelchair.[30] Elderly individuals (65 years of age or older) have the highest rate of mobility use, accounting for 57.5% of manual wheelchair users and 69.7% of power wheelchair users.[30]

Disorders Resulting in Mobility Impairments

There are many causes of mobility impairment. Disorders that result in mobility impairment may be neurological, musculoskeletal, or cognitive in nature. Bear in mind that not all individuals with a given diagnosis experience a similar impairment in mobility. The onset of the disorder, whether it was acquired or congenital, also affects the individual's mobility needs.

Kaye et al. (2002)[30] present the top 10 conditions in the United States that result in use of a wheelchair or scooter. Individuals who have had a stroke are the leading group of mobility device users (11.1%).[30] Additional neurological disorders that may result in mobility impairment include cerebral palsy, Guillain-Barré syndrome, Huntington's chorea, traumatic brain injury, muscular dystrophy, Parkinson's disease, poliomyelitis, spinal cord injury, spina bifida, and multiple sclerosis. Symptoms commonly seen in these neurological disorders are muscle weakness or paralysis, sensory deficits, and abnormal muscle tone. All these disorders can lead to limitations with joint range of motion, postural control, and mobility. The individual may also have cognitive and behavioral problems as a result of the disorder.

Orthopedic and rheumatological conditions account for another large group of mobility device users. Some of the symptoms commonly seen in individuals with arthritis include painful, swollen, and stiff joints (particularly in hand and wrist); muscle weakness, muscle wasting around the affected joints, complaints of feeling fatigued, and, in later stages, joint contractures resulting in range-of-motion limitations. Other disorders that affect the musculoskeletal system and may result in mobility impairments include ankylosing spondylitis, osteogenesis imperfecta, osteoporosis, Paget's disease, and scoliosis. Individuals with an amputation may also use a mobility device.

Diabetes, cardio-respiratory conditions, and obesity are chronic conditions that may require the use of a mobility device. Frequently, fatigue or restrictions related to energy expenditure are the reasons for use of a mobility device with these populations. Amputations resulting from complications due to diabetes may also lead to the use of a mobility device.

Disorders that affect an individual's cognitive functioning and ability to learn, such as Alzheimer's disease and cognitive impairment, can also be associated with mobility impairments. In the first instance, dementia, the adult wheelchair user may require special consideration of safety measures if he has limited memory or insight concerning safe mobility. For example, as the cognitive impairment progresses, judgment can become impaired. A client at this stage may not recognize unsafe situations such as a stairwell and may attempt to propel the chair down the stairs, or the client may not be able to control anger and may use the wheelchair as a weapon and propel it into another person. In situations where cognitive impairment limits safe mobility, modifications are required to wheelchair skills training to simplify instructions and provide additional way finding cues in familiar environments. Measures such as use of seat belts may be used for safety, and consideration should be given to the ability of the caregiver to push the chair and lift and stow it when this assistance is required. A wheelchair seat belt may be considered a restraint in some jurisdictions. A summary of best practices for use of restraints is provided in Chapter 4.

Functional Limitations of Mobility

The World Health Organization's *International Classification of Functioning, Disability and Health (ICF)*[64] identifies mobility as an activity, rather than an impairment of a body structure or function. This system categorizes the source of the mobility impairment. For example, strength, range of motion (ROM), and endurance all have the potential to limit mobility. Another useful categorization scheme describes different abilities to ambulate.[61] The degree of limitation in mobility varies across a broad scope, as shown in Box 12-1. At one end of the range are individuals who are considered *marginal ambulators*. At the opposite end of the range are those individuals who have severe mobility limitations and are dependent in manual mobility, with powered mobility being their only option for independence.

Warren (1990)[61] describes marginal ambulators as able to move independently in their environment but functional only at a slow rate or for short distances. Persons who have marginal ambulating skills can benefit from part-time use of a powered mobility device such as a **scooter**, which allows them to walk inside the home using a walker or cane and use a powered device outside the home to augment ambulation. Next are individuals who are exclusive users of manual wheelchairs. They may rely on a caregiver to propel the wheelchair or they propel a manual wheelchair using one of three methods: (1) using both upper extremities, (2) using both lower extremities, or (3) using an upper and lower extremity on the same side of the body (e.g., a person who has had a stroke). *Marginal manual wheelchair users* are able to propel a wheelchair manually but have upper body weakness, respiratory problems, or postural asymmetry as a result of pushing that limits their ability to propel a manual chair for a prolonged time.[61] Marginal manual wheelchair users may also include individuals who formerly used a manual wheelchair for their mobility needs and have sustained an overuse injury from propelling the chair. Propelling a wheelchair for any length of time depletes the energy of these individuals and compromises their productivity in other areas of life. Marginal manual wheelchair users can benefit from powered mobility on a full-time or part-time basis.

When an individual has a severe mobility limitation, powered mobility may be the best option to gain functional mobility. These individuals typically have a manual wheelchair, propelled by a caregiver, as a back-up chair. Powered mobility devices have the potential to enable the user's participation in school, work, leisure, and other community-based activities. The control interfaces (see Chapter 6) that are available today make it possible for someone with only one or two movements (e.g., lateral flexion of the head or shoulder rotation) to operate a powered wheelchair; however, perceptual, cognitive, and behavioral impairments may prevent individuals from using a powered wheelchair even if they have the necessary motor skills. For example, a client with a visual-spatial impairment may have difficulty navigating a cluttered environment if she cannot maintain a safe distance from people or objects in the environment. When the individual also uses an augmentative communication system or an adapted van, integration of all of these devices is considered at the time of selection of the most appropriate mobility device. All mobility device users will require a system to support their seating needs (see Chapter 4).

BOX 12-1 Scope of Mobility Limitations

Full ambulator: no mobility impairment.
Marginal ambulator: can walk short distances; may need wheelchair at times, particularly outside the home.
Manual wheelchair user: has some method of propelling a manual wheelchair, whether it is with both upper extremities, both lower extremities, or one upper and one lower extremity.
Marginal manual wheelchair user: may have upper extremity injury caused by overuse, or manual wheelchair mobility may not be the most efficient means of mobility for the person; manual wheelchair is used part of the time and powered wheelchair part of the time.
Totally/severely mobility-impaired user: unable to propel self independently in a manual wheelchair; needs dependent mobility base; powered mobility base the only option for independent mobility.

Mobility Issues Across the Lifespan

Mobility needs differ across the lifespan. In this section, we focus on three issues that warrant special attention: (1) powered mobility for young children, (2) mobility for older adults, and (3) obesity, which is not strictly a lifespan issue, but is becoming a more prevalent reason for mobility device use after childhood.

The use of powered mobility by young children is an area that has received a great deal of attention in the last decade. In the past, powered mobility was deemed inappropriate for young children for a number of reasons. These concerns were related to (1) the ability of children to operate a powered wheelchair safely, (2) the initial cost of the wheelchair and cost of replacing it as the child grows, and (3) possible detrimental effects on physical development if the child depends on a powered system instead of his own locomotion.[32] Recent literature supports the provision of powered mobility to young children.[25,50] Opportunities for early mobility have widespread benefits to the child, not only physically, but also cognitively and socially.[17,50] Children who are able to move independently in their environment can initiate interactions with others; they don't need to wait for another person to take them where they want to go. Most current literature suggests that affording the opportunity for mobility should occur at an appropriate developmental time. The goal of such mobility is not to learn how to control a chair, but to experience movement within the environment and to engage in relevant functional tasks, supported by mobility. As with any young child, it is the responsibility of the parent, caregiver, or rehabilitation assistant to ensure a safe environment in which the child can explore and experience mobility.[50]

Some needs that are specific to the older adult wheelchair user have been identified in the literature. Comfort, safety, increased function, and a feeling of security when moving in their environment have been identified as important needs related to seating and mobility for residents of long-term care facilities.[40,43,44] The older adult wheelchair user may depend on another person to push the wheelchair. Therefore a mobility device that can be used easily by an attendant is important.[27,58] Safety and security were deemed important for the user of the wheelchair, as well as for the care provider. For instance, it is important that the care provider be able to transfer a person in and out of the wheelchair safely. Both the user and the care provider will be more inclined to use a wheelchair that is comfortable, safe, secure, and easy to use. Wheelchairs that target the bariatric client are a recent development in wheelchair design. **Bariatrics** is a term that describes the practice of medicine concerning individuals who are significantly overweight. It is derived from the Greek *baros*, meaning weight, and *iatrics*, meaning medical treatment. In some situations, the client's obesity is the cause of their mobility impairment. Obesity has become a major health problem in North America. The Center for Disease Control data[10] report a growing trend in the prevalence of obesity (generally defined as a BMI of 30 or over). In 1995, the prevalence of obesity was less than 20% in all states. In 2000, 28% of states reported obesity prevalence of less than 20% and by 2005 this incidence had dropped to only 4 states. The 2005 figures further indicate that 17 states report a prevalence of obesity of equal to or greater than 25% and 3 states report a prevalence rate of equal to or greater than 30%.[10] Diabetes is a serious chronic health condition that is associated with obesity. Mobility in this population is restricted by excessive weight, low physical endurance, cardio-respiratory complications, and complications arising from diabetes including vision impairment, circulatory and sensory impairments, and amputation. Typical wheelchairs have standard weight limits up to 300 pounds. Chairs for bariatric clients are capable of supporting weights up to 600 pounds and in some cases up to 1000 pounds. Examples of these chairs will be described later in this chapter. Clients who are morbidly obese present specific challenges when measuring for a wheelchair, as will be discussed later.

EVALUATION FOR WHEELED MOBILITY

Needs Assessment

The goal of wheeled mobility intervention is to support the user's ability to move in his environments (i.e., the mobility output of the activity component of the HAAT model). Consistent with the HAAT model described in Chapter 2, the evaluation to determine the most appropriate wheeled mobility base starts with an assessment of the activities in which the individual wishes to engage while using mobility technology. Will the mobility device be used primarily to move from one place to another in the community, or will the individual use it as his primary means of mobility and consequently perform most activities (i.e., ADL and work and leisure occupations) while seated in the device? The rehabilitation assistant frequently interacts with an individual in the school, home, and long-term care (LTC) context. She has excellent opportunities in these settings to observe the activities in which the user wants and needs to engage. Further, the rehabilitation assistant is able to provide information on how an individual completes their activities, including the level of assistance required. For example, will the user complete these activities on his own, with the assistance of another person, and/or by using other technology such as an augmentative communication system?

Evaluation of the Human Factors

Box 12-2 identifies the factors that should be considered when selecting a mobility base for a consumer. Some of this information is available through the client's chart or background information. The rehabilitation assistant provides information on the day-to-day function in other areas. For example, the daily interaction with the client by the OTA gives her a sound understanding of the client's interaction with caregivers, behavior in different situations, impulsivity, skin integrity, and daily activities. The *consumer profile* provides background information about the client. Knowing whether an impairment is acute or long-term and relatively stable or progressive influences the choice of wheeled mobility. A client who has a progressive

BOX 12-2 Factors to Consider When Selecting a Wheelchair

Consumer profile: disability, date of onset, prognosis, size, and weight
Consumer needs: activities, contexts of use (e.g., accessibility, indoor/outdoor), preferences, transportation, reliability, durability, cost
Physical and sensory skills: range of motion, motor control, strength, vision, perception
Functional skills: transfers and ability to propel (manual or powered)

impairment such as amyotrophic lateral sclerosis (ALS) will lose function over time, so the rehabilitation assistant should be alert to signs that the wheelchair is no longer meeting the client's needs. For example, a client whose motor function is declining may show fatigue when propelling a manual wheelchair over a distance that was easy for him to travel earlier. Alternately, a client who uses a joystick to control a power wheelchair may show loss of ability to reliably stop the chair or control its speed. Clients whose cognitive abilities are declining may become lost in familiar surroundings, use their chairs inappropriately to run into people or objects, or forget how to control the chair.

Noting changes in a client's weight or posture will also provide clues that the wheeled mobility device (and seating system) is no longer adequate. The individual's *physical and sensory skills* are evaluated for range of motion, strength, motor control, skin integrity, vision, and perception. This assessment also includes determining the user's optimal control site and interface for propelling the wheelchair. Information on the person's weight and size is gathered in order to determine the size and capacity of the wheelchair. Measurements of the person's leg length, thigh length, back height to base of scapula, back height to top of shoulder, and hip breadth are taken while the person is sitting. An obese person will need a bariatric wheelchair. Clients who are obese should be measured while sitting, as adipose tissue spreads when they lie down, resulting in an inaccurate measurement.[16] If the consumer is a child and is expected to grow, that expected change needs to be reflected in the decision making as well.

The person's functional abilities are also evaluated. Two elements are important. The first is evaluation of different ADLs and Instrumental Activities of Daily Living (IADLs). IADL refers to those daily tasks that a person does to manager her life, for example banking, grocery shopping and use of transportation. In addition to identifying in which occupations the individual wishes to engage, this evaluation will determine how they complete those activities. The second element involves evaluation of wheelchair skills. The Wheelchair Skills Test (WST)* is a well-developed, standardized measure of various wheelchair skills.[34,35] This test assesses the individual's ability to perform basic wheelchair skills ranging from removal of an armrest and application of the brakes to more complex, advanced skills such as performing a wheelie in order to negotiate a curb. This test is one of the few that has had extensive research in all phases of its development. In addition to the evaluation, a training program has also been developed and evaluated. Information about this test and the training program are available at: www.wheelchairskillsprogram.ca.

Environmental Factors

Physical Context

The *physical contexts* in which the mobility device is used influence the selection. Will the device be used both indoors and outdoors? How accessible are these environments? Width of doorways, floor surfaces, bathroom layout, and access to the structure (e.g., ramp, stairs) all need to be considered. On what type of surfaces will the consumer travel when using the device outdoors? Does the user expect or need to transport the device between different locations such as home, school, or work? How will the user and his mobility device travel (i.e., will he use a private vehicle or public transportation)? Does the user access other modes of transportation such as trains, airplanes, or school buses?

Just as the climate was a factor in the recommendation concerning a seating system, it also influences the recommendation of a mobility device. A different mobility device recommendation may be made for a consumer who lives in a climate where snow is a typical part of winter and who expects to use his device outdoors than would be made for a consumer who lives in a climate where snow and cold temperatures are not a routine expectation.

Social Context

Family members, peers, and others in the social environment can influence the choice of a mobility device. Peers with experience with various mobility devices can be a great source of information and can share their knowledge of what works and what does not work. Conversely, peers and families may exert pressure in the choice of a manual versus a power wheelchair. The individual may prefer to use a power chair because it allows her to conserve energy for other occupations but may be viewed as lazy by others if she chooses this technology. The willingness or ability of decision makers in the school, workplace, and other community environments to accommodate various types of mobility devices also needs to be considered. Lack of knowledge of necessary accommodations by an employer may result in a work environment that is not physically accessible to the client. In this instance, what is limiting is the employer's lack of information rather than the actual physical barriers.

Institutional Context

Institutional regulations and policies influence the recommendation of a mobility device. While the ATP is typically responsible for making a recommendation for

* WheelchairSkillsTest 4.1 Manual (http://www.wheelchairskillsprogram.ca/eng/manual.htm)

a mobility device, the rehabilitation assistant is often responsible for the use of the mobility device in the institutional (e.g., rehabilitation facility or LTC) context. The rehabilitation assistant may be responsible for monitoring the client's ability to use the chair safely, follow the policies and procedures of the institution regarding maintenance of the mobility device, and receive long-term training in device use (frequently with supervision of the ATP or other clinicians). Policies are established or being developed in some long-term care facilities that will limit the resident's ability to use a wheelchair if they have repeatedly demonstrated use of the chair in a manner that threatens the safety of themselves or others in the environment.[40] The rehabilitation assistant's regular interaction with the client puts her in an excellent position to provide feedback on the client's use of the chair and his potential to benefit from further training in wheelchair skills or from modification to the chair in order to promote its safe use.

CHARACTERISTICS AND CURRENT TECHNOLOGIES OF WHEELED MOBILITY SYSTEMS

In this section we discuss the major characteristics of manual and powered mobility systems. Table 12-1 lists the major manufacturers of personal mobility systems. Modern mobility systems are more flexible and capable

TABLE 12-1 Major Wheelchair Manufacturers

Manufacturer	Type of Wheelchairs	Web Address
Altimate Medical, Inc. 800-342-8968	Standing systems	www.easystand.com
Amigo Mobility International, Inc. 800-692-6446	Scooters	www.myamigo.com
Bruno Independent Living Aids 800-882-8183	Adult and pediatric scooters, sedan and van wheelchair lifts	www.bruno.com
Columbia Medical 800-454-6612	Dependent mobility bases	www.columbiamedical.com
Convaid, Inc.	Dependent mobility bases, transport chairs	www.convaid.com
ConvaQuip	Bariatric wheelchairs	www.convaquip.com
Etac (in the USA) Balder USA, Inc. 888-422-5337	Independent manual wheelchairs for children and adults	www.etac.com
Freedom Designs 800-554-8044	Pediatric wheelchairs, tilt-in-space wheelchairs	www.freedomdesigns.com
Invacare 800-333-6900	Manual, power, and sports wheelchairs	www.invacare.com
Levo USA, Inc. 888-538-6872	Manual and powered stand-up wheelchairs for adults and children	www.levo.com
Mulholland Positioning Systems, Inc. 800-543-4769	A variety of standing systems, pediatric wheeled bases and tilt bases	www.mulhollandinc.com
Otto Bock 800-328-4058	Pediatric seating and positioning, adult positioning, manual and power wheelchairs	www.ottobockus.com
PDG 888-858-4422	Wheelchairs for individuals with special needs, such as bariatric chairs, high agitation, and manual tilt wheelchairs	www.pdgmobility.com
Permobil, Inc. 800-736-0925	Stand-up powered wheelchairs; powered wheelchair with elevating seat; sports wheelchairs, lightweight manual wheelchairs	www.permobil.com
Pride Mobility Products Corp. USA: 800-800-8586 Canada: 888-570-1113	Manual and electrically powered wheelchairs, scooters	www.pridemobility.com
Snug Seat 800-336-7684	Specialty bases for children and adults, car seats, dependent and independent mobility bases, pediatric wheelchairs	www.snugseat.com
Sunrise Medical 800-333-4000	Dependent and independent manual bases, sports wheelchairs, lightweight manual wheelchairs, powered wheelchairs, add-on power unit; adult and pediatric wheelchairs, tilt wheelchairs and scooters	www.sunrisemedical.com
TiLite 800-545-2266	Adult and pediatric titanium wheelchairs; manual wheelchair; sports wheelchair	www.tilite.com

of being adapted to a variety of functional tasks. These adaptations may include height, tilt, recline, and axle-position adjustments, or combinations of any of these. The selection of a wheelchair is based on the evaluation discussed in the previous section and is a process of matching wheelchair characteristics to the consumer's needs and skills.[53] To meet the varied needs of individuals with mobility impairments, there are three broad categories of wheeled mobility systems: (1) dependent mobility, (2) independent manual mobility, and (3) independent powered mobility. **Dependent mobility systems** are propelled by an attendant and include strollers and transport chairs as well as a manual chair that is propelled by an attendant. A dependent mobility system is chosen when (1) the individual is not fully capable of independently propelling a wheelchair or (2) a secondary system is needed that is lightweight and easily transported. An **independent manual mobility** system is for those individuals who have the ability to propel a wheelchair manually. These bases have two large wheels in the back that allow the user to propel independently and two smaller front wheels. **Independent powered mobility** systems are required when the user has difficulty propelling a **manual wheelchair**. These are **electrically powered wheelchairs** that are driven by the user. There are many commercial options available within each of these categories to meet the needs of the individual user. In this section we discuss the characteristics of mobility systems, starting with the wheelchair's two basic structures: a supporting structure and a propelling structure. Figure 12-1 shows the anatomy of a folding manual wheelchair. Figure 12-2 shows the anatomy of a rigid frame manual wheelchair.

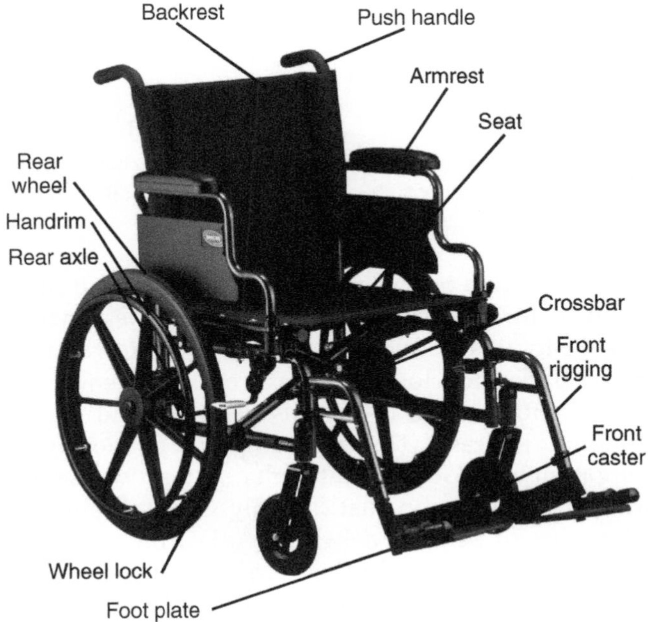

Figure 12-1 Manual wheelchair showing the major parts of the supporting and propelling structures. (Courtesy Invacare Canada.)

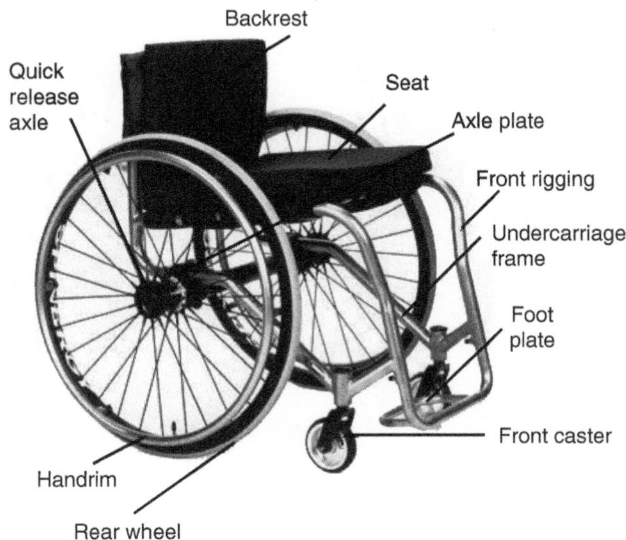

Figure 12-2 Rigid frame wheelchair showing the major parts of the supporting and propelling structures. (Courtesy Invacare Canada.)

Supporting Structure

The **supporting structure** of the wheelchair consists of the frame and attachments to it. Specialized seating and positioning (see Chapter 4) is often considered part of the supporting structure. Accessories to the frame (e.g., armrests, footrests) are also a part of the supporting structure. In some wheelchairs these accessories are manufactured as part of the frame. Some supporting structures are unique in that they are adjustable to allow for changes in the orientation of the user in space, including systems that provide tilt or support in a standing position.

Frame Types

Three underlying factors will be discussed before describing different classifications of manual wheelchairs: (1) type of frame (rigid or folding), (2) adjustability of the position of the axle of the rear wheels, and (3) material used to construct the wheelchair frame.

Frames may be either folding or rigid, and there are three common frame styles.[11] Rigid frames are available in a box, cantilever, or *T*- or *I*-frame style. Typically the box frame construction (see Figure 12-3) has a rectangular shape that provides a strong and durable base to which the seat and wheels are attached. Lighter-weight designs are accomplished by replacing the box with a single bar extending between the wheels, forming a cantilever structure. Upright tubes from this main support are used to attach the seat and back. The footrests are extensions of the seat rails. As shown in Figure 12-3, the *T* construction uses a bar similar to the cantilever design but has a single bar attached to the center of the cantilever that connects to a single front caster. This configuration forms a *T* shape under the seat. If two front casters are used, then the *T* shape becomes an *I* shape. For transportation, the wheels on all these chairs are removed, and in some cases the back folds down. The choice between a rigid or

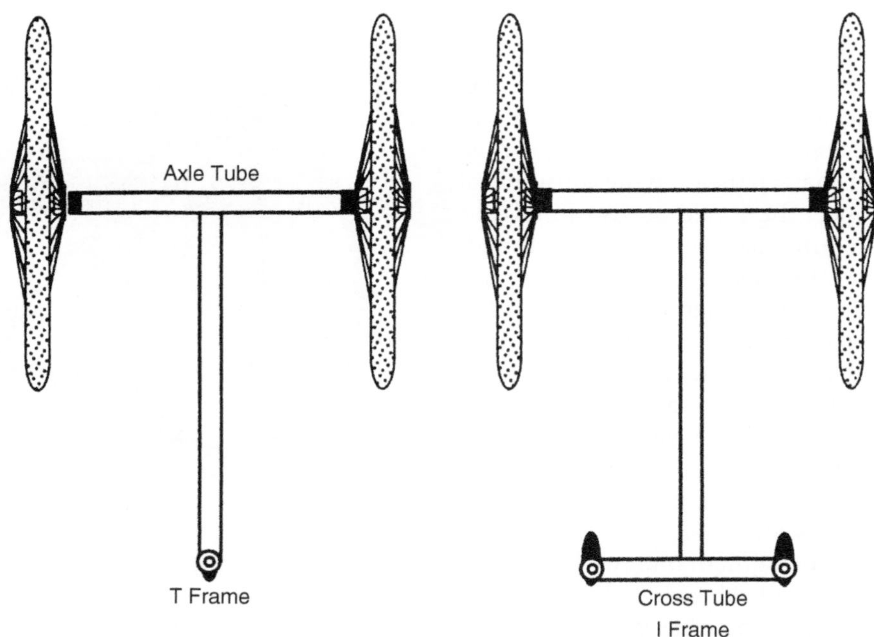

Figure 12-3 *T* and *I* frame styles. (From Cooper RA: *Wheelchair selection and configuration,* New York, 1998, Demos Medical Publishing.)

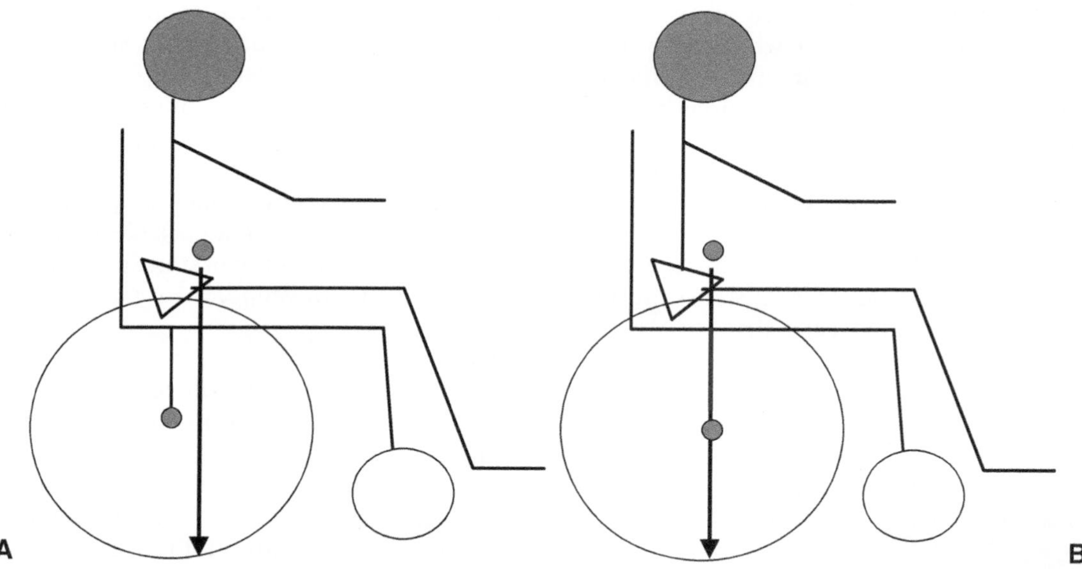

Figure 12-4 Relationship of the center of mass of the user to the axle of the wheel affects the mobility and stability of the chair. **A,** When the user is seated with his center of mass ahead of the axle of the wheelchair, the chair is more stable; **B,** When the user is seated with his center of mass directly above the axle of the wheelchair, the chair is more mobile.

box frame and folding frame styles involves a number of factors including the consumer's needs, functional ability, method of transfer, and level of activity.[11]

The position of the axle of the drive wheel relative to the user's **center of gravity** affects the stability and maneuverability of the wheelchair. Figure 12-4 displays this relationship. The **center of mass** of an empty wheelchair is located under the seat, in front of the drive wheels.[21] When the user is seated in the wheelchair, the center of mass moves above the seat and forward or backward depending on the seated position of the individual relative to the drive wheels. When the center of mass is forward of the axis of the drive wheels, more weight is placed on the castors, making it more difficult to lift them.[21] The chair is more stable but less maneuverable in this configuration. As the center of mass moves backward, closer to the axis of the drive wheel or even slightly behind it, stability decreases and maneuverability increases. Understanding this relationship is important when setting up the chair. An active user will want a configuration that is easily maneuverable and allows her to perform a "wheelie" (i.e., lift the castors up) to clear curbs and other barriers. A less-confident wheelchair user will be most comfortable with a chair that does not tip backward easily, allowing them to feel secure in their chair.

Another fairly recent advancement in the wheelchair industry is the material used to form the chair frame. Much of the advancement in materials comes from the cycling industry. Wheelchair frames are made from many different materials including steel, aluminum, steel/aluminum alloys, titanium, and carbon fiber composites. These materials vary in their weight, strength, cost, how they conduct vibration, method of attaching components together, and how they are formed. Wheelchairs are classified according to a number of parameters including weight, adjustability, and available options. **Standard wheelchairs** are generally useful for very short-term use such as rentals at an airport or shopping mall.[54] They are folding chairs, with very limited adjustment; in particular, the axle of the rear wheel is fixed. Features such as footrests and armrests may be fixed or detachable. There is limited choice of seat width and depth. They are the heaviest of the manual wheelchairs and therefore are not useful for long-term use as they require a great deal of energy to propel on a regular basis.

Lightweight wheelchairs or **lightweight high-strength wheelchairs**[54] weigh less than the standard chair, as their name would suggest. Otherwise, they tend to have similar features. These chairs offer more flexibility in choice of seat width and adjustment of back height. Both the standard and lightweight chairs are available with a lower seat to floor height that allows the user to propel with their feet.

An **ultra lightweight chair** is substantially lighter than the standard chair. Schmeler and Buning[54] suggest that the chairs in the standard and lightweight categories are not suitable for use over the long term. The ultra lightweight chair is one they consider useful for an individual who uses a manual wheelchair as her primary means of mobility. It retains the folding frame and is available with a lower seat to floor height for individuals who propel with their feet. The axle of the rear wheel is adjustable relative to the center of gravity of the user.

Rigid sport ultralightweight wheelchairs[54] are a huge growth area for the wheelchair industry. The primary difference between these and the previous categories is the rigid frame. These chairs have quick-release rear wheels and most have backs that fold down to facilitate transfer and storage of the chair in a vehicle. The axle of the rear wheel of these chairs can be adjusted relative to the center of gravity of the user. The implication of the position of the rear wheel axle relative to the user's center of gravity for the stability and maneuverability of the chair will be discussed shortly.

A final comment will be made about the seat-to-floor height of the chair. This dimension is important for two reasons: (1) access to tables, counters, and other structures and (2) access to the floor for users who propel the chair with their feet. In the first instance, the height of the chair should allow the user to roll her chair to a table or desk, permitting her knees to be under the table or desk. In the second instance, so-called "hemi-chairs" are available that provide a seat-to-floor height that allows the person to "walk" her feet on the floor, thus propelling the chair.

Accessories

Armrests on conventional wheelchairs may be manufactured as a fixed part of the frame, flip back out of the way, or be completely removable. Nonremovable armrests decrease the width of the wheelchair slightly, and do not get lost because they cannot be removed. In general it is advantageous to have armrests that flip back or are removable in order to facilitate transfers and other activities. Two lengths of armrests are available. Desk-length armrests are shorter in the front to allow the consumer to move close to a desk or table. Full-length armrests, which provide more support, extend to the front of the seat rails. Armrests may be fixed or adjustable in height. Armrests that are height adjustable can be moved up or down to accommodate the length of the user's trunk and provide the proper amount of support for the arms. A clothing guard on the armrests prevents clothing and body parts from rubbing against the wheels.

Leg rests and **footplates** support the legs and feet. Taken together, these two components are often called the **front rigging** of the wheelchair. Angle options are often available for the leg rests with either 90° or 70° hangers. These options increase the comfort of the user by accommodating his preferred knee flexion angle, but they can also add to the turning radius, which may be a factor for mobility in some environments. Leg rests may be fixed (built into the frame) or removable (swing away). Styles that swing away make it easier to transfer in and out of the wheelchair. Footplates are attached to the leg rests and are available as a single plate to support both feet or as two separate units, with individual height adjustment. The height of the footplate should support the desired position of the lower extremities. The angle of the footplate can also be adjusted to accommodate ankle flexion or extension. Heel loops can be attached to the back of the footplate to prevent the foot from sliding backward (see Figure 12-1).

Wheel locks are the devices that prevent the wheels from moving during transfers and other stationary activities. They are available in a number of configurations, such as push or pull to lock, with lever extensions for individuals with limited reach; under-the-seat mounts; hill holders (devices that "hold" the wheelchair on an incline, preventing it from rolling downhill); and attendant controlled. Figure 12-5 (*A–C*) shows some of the various brake styles. The client's preferred method of transfer and ability to access the wheel lock, the most reliable method available to manipulate the wheel lock, and the ability of the user or caregiver to maintain the wheel lock influence the selection of this component. As with the brakes of a motor vehicle, proper maintenance of the wheel locks is an important safety consideration. Wheel locks that are improperly maintained may not be in secure contact with

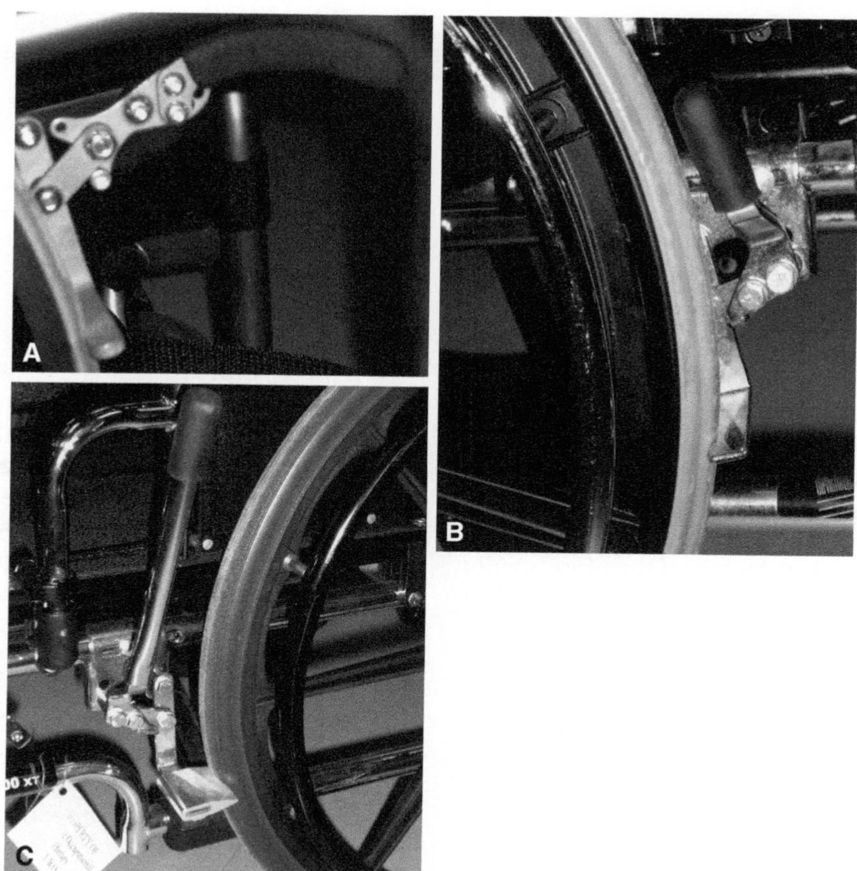

Figure 12-5 Wheel locks. **A,** Example of push-to-lock wheel lock. **B,** Example of pull-to-lock wheel lock. **C,** A wheel lock with an extended handle.

the tire, causing instability, particularly during transfers or when holding the chair on an incline/decline.

Anti-tip devices are small wheels, attached to a rod and mounted at the back of the chair. These devices prevent the chair from tipping backwards. When the drive wheels are located forward on the chair, anti-tip devices are recommended, particularly when the individual cannot safely perform a wheelie. Since these devices limit backward tipping of the chair, they can interfere with travel over some obstacles such as curbs. Anti-tip devices can be removed or rotated so they do not interfere with such travel when an attendant is pushing the chair. However, they should be returned to their original position when the user resumes propelling the chair.[21] Anti-tipping devices can be seen on the back of the chair in Figure 12-9, which shows a composite mag wheel.

Push handles are another option on a manual chair. These are the handles used by an attendant or caregiver to maneuver the chair. Some of these are height adjustable to accommodate the different heights of individuals who push the chair. Extended handles are available for pediatric chairs to avoid low back strain for the individual pushing the chair. Push handles have different shapes and are of different materials to assist with grip and handling in difficult situations such as inclement weather or traveling up or down a hill.

The upholstery of most wheelchairs that are intended for regular, long-term use is designed to be used with a seating system. The option exists for most chairs to remove the upholstery completely and replace with a back or seat that is attached directly to the frame of the chair. Generally, only those chairs that are for occasional use come with hammock-style upholstery attached to the frame.

Frames for Recline and Tilt

Tilt and **recline** features are available on both manual frames and power bases. Figure 12-6 (*A* and *B*) shows examples of these systems. These features recognize that sitting is not a static activity and that we need to provide the opportunity to change position for individuals who cannot do so independently. Tilt refers to the ability to rotate a specific seating position around a fixed axis, thus changing the orientation in space. Recline refers to changing the seat-to-back angle, resulting in a seat-to-back angle greater than 90°.[37] The seat-to-back angle typically ranges from upright to nearly horizontal. Tilt and recline have some common benefits to the user. Both provide a change of position and improved circulation, thus bringing pressure relief and greater comfort.[37,55,63] They have the potential to improve head and postural control, provide an improved functional position, and influence muscle tone.[21,36,37,55] Clients

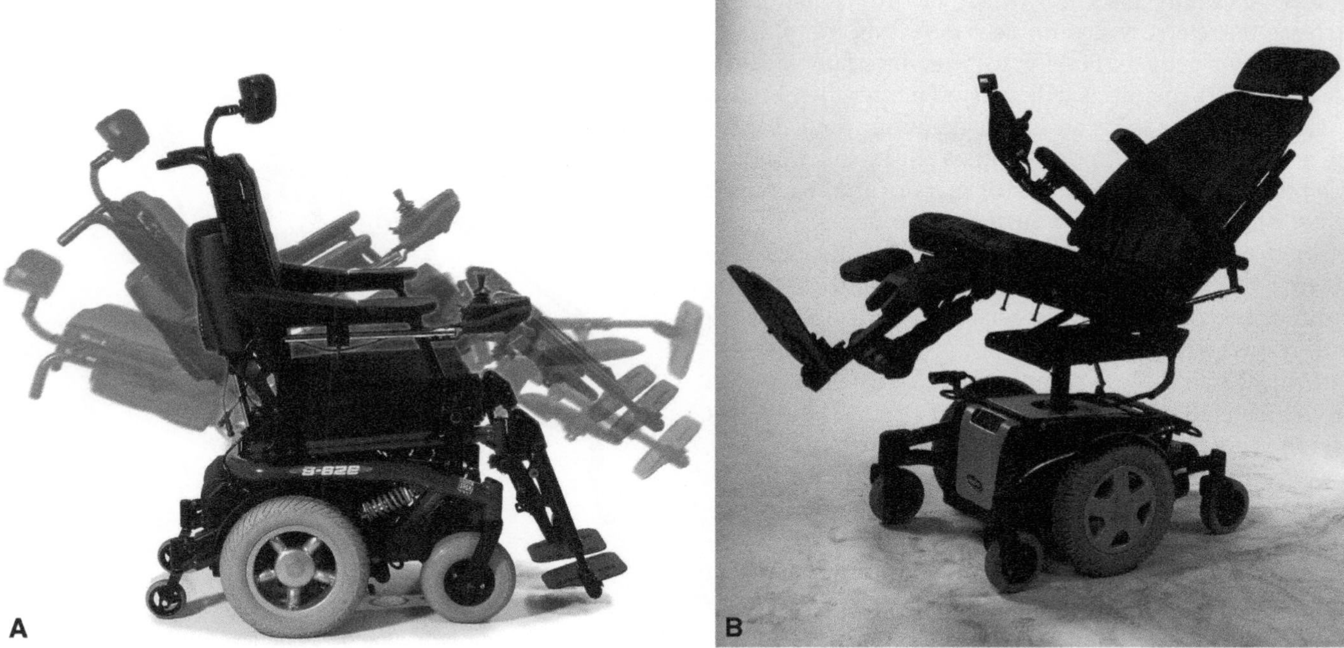

Figure 12-6 Tilt-and-recline wheelchair supporting structures. **A,** Supporting structure with tilt feature. **B,** Supporting structure with recline feature. (**A** courtesy Sunrise Medical; **B** courtesy Motion Concepts.)

with neurological problems may have difficulty maintaining postural control (see Chapter 4) in an upright position. Moderate tilt and recline positions may reduce the effects of gravity, allowing a more upright posture, thus aiding function. They have the potential to improve respiratory function, provide a better visual field, regulate blood pressure, ease transfers, and allow rest during the day.[36,37] Recline or tilt can be used to achieve a more typical spinal alignment, for example, to reduce a thoracic kyphosis.[21]

Recline is also useful for individuals who become fatigued when sitting upright for a length of time. A chair with a recline feature allows rest without the need to transfer to bed. Clients with a hip deformity that limits their ability to flex the hip will benefit from recline to achieve a comfortable seating position. It can alleviate orthostatic hypotension[36,37] and improve bowel and bladder function. Recline may be preferred to tilt in a work or social environment since it is considered by the user to be less obtrusive.[37] Recline does not raise the knees during the position change, which allows the use of this position while continuing to work at a desk or table. Recline is not a good option for some consumers. Opening the hip angle will cause excessive extensor tone in some individuals, particularly children with cerebral palsy or individuals who have sustained a head injury. Obviously, it is not useful when the user has limited hip extension range of motion. Individuals who use a custom contoured seating system should not use a recline system due to the shear forces that are inevitably present when changing the seat-to-back angle.

Shear is of concern when changing the seat-to-back angle. Recall from Chapter 6 that shear is defined as the friction that occurs when two surfaces slide across each other. Shear has the potential to tear skin, which can lead to a pressure ulcer. Most recline systems are designed to minimize shear and are referred to as **low-shear systems**. These systems follow the user as the system reclines, resulting in a reduction of shear but not its elimination.[55] Low-shear systems are available in both manual and power options.

Tilt systems are recommended when it is desirable to maintain the seating position for function or for control of other devices mounted to the wheelchair, such as augmentative and alternative communication devices.[37] Because the whole seat pivots around an axis, shear is not as significant a concern as it is with a recline system. In addition to rearward tilt, some systems also provide lateral tilt, which again maintains the seating position but tilts the user in the saggital plane. The combination of anterior-posterior and lateral tilt gives users control to change their positions as they wish.

Tilt systems do pose disadvantages that recline systems do not. Most tilt systems increase the seat-to-floor height. In addition, when the user is in the tilt position, their knees are raised, sometimes higher than the level of their head. The seat-to-floor height and position may interfere with the ability to work at a table or desk and may pose a risk for injury if the user attempts to move into a tilt position while seated at a desk or table. As the seat tilts and the knees are raised, the lower extremity may be impinged between a desk and the system.[37] Since tilt maintains the hip angle (typically 90°), bladder constriction may occur, causing problems with fully emptying the bladder.[36] Extreme degrees of tilt may cause the user to feel posturally insecure, which has the potential to increase muscle contraction, thus defeating the purpose of alleviating fatigue. Finally, tilt may interfere with the use of a tray (i.e., objects will slide off a tray when in tilt).

Center of mass shifts are a consideration when evaluating a wheelchair that incorporates a tilt-in-space option. The relationship of the center of mass of the seat to the center of mass of the base must be considered. The center of mass moves posterially as the seat tilts on some systems. This movement can cause rearward instability if the center of mass of the seat is shifted too far back with respect to the center of mass of the base. Most current wheelchair designs compensate for this concern with mechanisms that maintain the center of mass of the seat over the center of mass of the base.

Consumers who use either a tilt-in-space or a recline system frequently also have other assistive technologies whose use must be integrated with these positioning options. These specifically include control of a power wheelchair with a head array, use of a ventilator, and use of an adapted van. Head array controls should be turned off when the user is in the tilt or recline position so that she can fully rest her head. When a ventilator is mounted on the wheelchair, care must be taken to ensure that the tilt or recline mechanism does not impinge on the unit and that the ventilator retains its proper position.[38] Finally, evaluation of the user's method of transportation must be considered when tilt and recline options are used. Tilt increases the seat-to-floor height, which may prevent the user from transferring into an adapted van. Both have the potential to increase the overall length of the system, which may limit the maneuverability of the user and her chair once in a van.[37,46] Integration of wheelchairs with adapted vans will be considered in Chapter 13 when transportation is discussed.

Frames for Standing

We normally think of mobility in terms of wheelchairs; that is, the user is seated. There are, however, many advantages to placing an individual in a standing position.[19,42] Among the positive effects of standing are physiological improvement in bladder and bowel function, alleviation of orthostatic hypotension, prevention of decubitus ulcers (see Chapter 4), reduction in muscle contractures and osteoporosis, and improved circulation. In addition, there are psychological benefits from being able to interact face to face with other people. For example, the height differential between someone seated and someone standing may imply an adult-child relationship, whereas standing and interacting face to face implies a relationship among peers. Standing frames and standing wheelchairs are two different types of supporting structures that allow the individual to stand.

Standing frames are categorized as prone standers, supine standers, upright standers, and mobile standers.[42] Prone standers, such as the one shown in Figure 12-7, are the most common type. They provide support on the anterior side of the body. Weight bearing on the long bones and lower extremity joints is a major benefit. Weight bearing strengthens bones and can limit advancement of osteoporosis (loss of bone density) that results from prolonged immobility and lack of weight bearing. Often a lap tray is added to the stander, which serves two purposes. First, it provides a supporting surface for the upper extremities as the user leans on it. Second, it provides a work surface for activities such as writing, playing with toys, or using a communication device. Prone standers are generally tilted forward to use gravity to assist maintenance of an upright position in the stander. Some types have fixed angles and others are adjustable. Adjustment for growth is incorporated into some designs. This type of standing frame does not give the individual the option of moving into a seated position, as does the stand-up wheelchair discussed below.

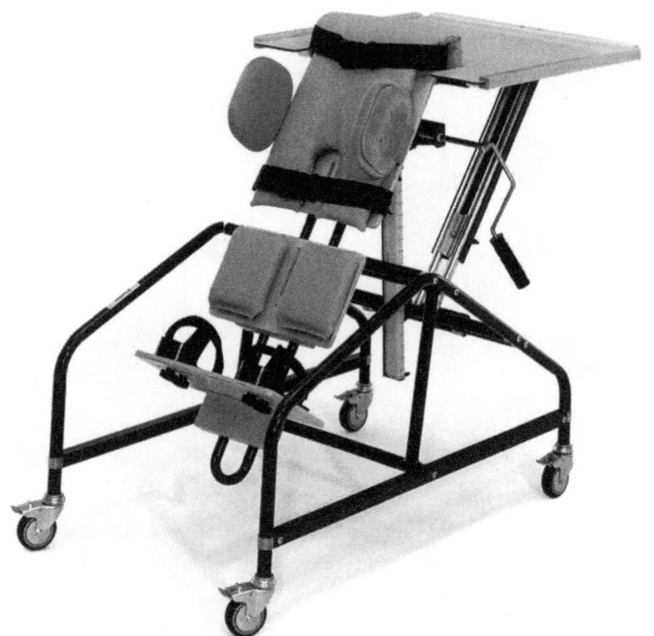

Figure 12-7 Large prone stander (Courtesy Rifton.)

Supine standers are less common, and there are fewer options. This type of stander provides support for the posterior surfaces of the body. Because the user is leaning back, it is more difficult for her to use her hands. Line of sight will also be affected. This type of stander is useful for persons who do not have good head control, since the stander supports the head and neck. *Upright standers* provide for complete weight bearing on the lower extremities. People who have good upper-body strength can use stationary models. Mobile versions are often sit-to-stand wheelchairs that allow changes in position from sitting to standing throughout the day. The change from sitting to standing and vice versa can be either powered or manual. When in a vertical position, these units generally function like a prone stander.

Standing wheelchairs have both functional and social benefits. Many tasks of daily living, such as cooking, are simplified with the use of a standing wheelchair. Additionally, the use of a standing wheelchair may make it possible to avoid modifications to a home or work setting. For example, a person cooking dinner while using a standing wheelchair is able to reach items in upper cabinets and reach the surface of cabinets and stoves without requiring modifications. Individuals who use a standing wheelchair report positive psychological benefits when they are at the same level as others.[20]

Standing wheelchairs (Figure 12-8) are available in three basic configurations: manual driven with a manual lifting mechanism, manual driven with a power lifting mechanism, and power driven with a power lifting mechanism. Standing wheelchairs with manual lifting mechanisms consist of a hydraulic system that uses either a pump or a lever to raise the person to the standing position. With a powered system, the person activates a button to move into the upright position. When standing, the person is supported by padded bars at the knees and torso. Stability in the upright position is a concern with standing wheelchairs since movement into the standing position moves the client's center of gravity forward in the chair, ahead of the center of mass of the base. For this reason not all standing wheelchairs are mobile while in the upright position. Those that are designed to be mobile in the standing position have a wider-than-normal base of support or adjust the center of mass of the user so that it remains over the center of the drive wheels. Typically, those chairs that are not meant to be mobile in the standing position have a drive lock out.

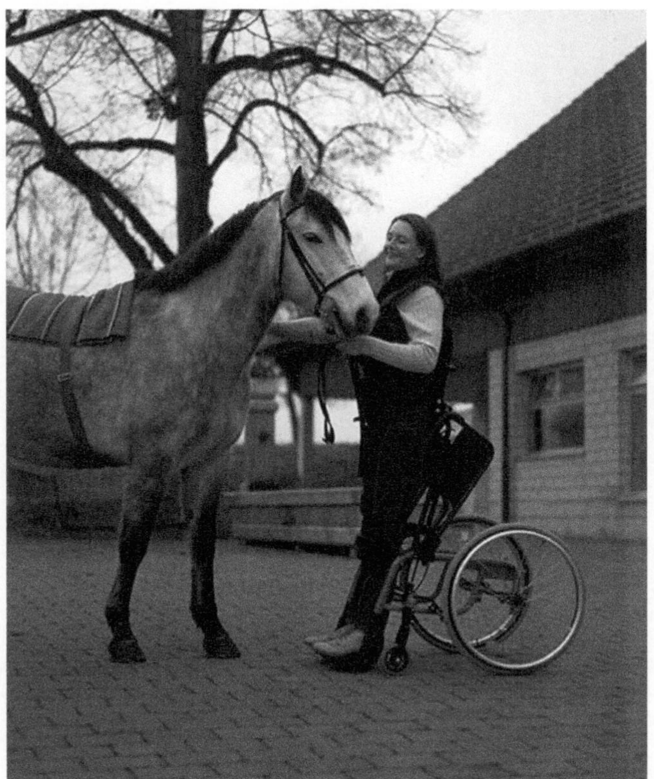

Figure 12-8 Stand-up wheelchair. (Courtesy Levo AG.)

Frames That Provide Variable Seat Height

Another available option on powered wheelchair frames is an elevating seat. The person remains in a seated position, and when the mechanism is activated, the wheelchair seat raises and lowers within a given range. A seat that lowers near the floor is particularly useful for small children. Being at floor level allows the child to play on the floor and interact at a level with children his age. There are also benefits to raising the height of a seat. As with a standing wheelchair, a seat elevator can make it easier for the individual to participate in certain self-care, work, and educational activities by reducing the need for environmental accommodations. As with standing wheelchairs and tilt-in-space and recline systems, the location of the center of mass has implications for safety. Some systems have a power lockout that prevents the chair from moving when the seat is raised to a certain height. Stability when traveling around corners may be compromised if the center of mass is too high relative to the footprint of the chair.

Frames that Accommodate Growth

A major requirement of the supporting structures of wheelchairs for children is that they accommodate growth. Two approaches are commonly used to accommodate growth (including clients with weight gain). The first of these is to design the supporting structure so that it can be adjusted directly. Kits are provided for the second option that allow replacement of various tubes on the frame and increasing seat width and length, seat-to-floor height, and access to the wheels. Wheelchairs that are adjustable are now more common.

Access to the drive wheels is another consideration when recommending pediatric chairs. One strategy to improve this access is to set the drive wheels in slight camber. A second approach, for very young children, is to reverse the configuration of the drive wheels, placing them at the front of the chair with the casters at the back. Rearward stability of the chair must be carefully assessed with this configuration.

Push handles are a final consideration for a pediatric frame. Extended handles are available so that the caregiver does not need to lean or bend forward to grasp the push handles. This configuration greatly reduces the load placed on the caregiver's lower back by allowing her to maintain an upright position during this activity.

Propelling Structure: Manual

For manual wheelchairs, the **propelling structure** consists of two main parts: (1) wheels (including tires and casters) and (2) an interface that the consumer uses to move the wheelchair.[47] We discuss each of these components in this section.

Tires

There are three main types of wheelchair tires: solid, semi-pneumatic, and pneumatic.[49] Solid tires require less maintenance than other types but are the least versatile.

They generally perform well on smooth indoor surfaces but are less efficient when used on carpeted surfaces or other rough, uneven terrain. Solid tires typically have a smooth surface.

Pneumatic tires may have an inner tube or a flat-free insert. Although they are useful over more varied terrain than solid tires, they require maintenance to maintain proper tire pressure and can be punctured, resulting in a flat. Sawatzky et al. (2004)[50] found that rolling resistance and energy expenditure were significantly decreased when tires were inflated to 50% of their recommended pressure. They report clinical evidence that wheelchair tires are commonly found to be inflated to only 25% of their recommended pressure. In addition to maintaining tire pressure, the user should inspect the tires regularly for any cracks or imperfections that may lead to a flat. These tires are available with different tread depths; deeper treads are useful on rough terrain but create more rolling resistance when used on smoother surfaces.

Wheels

Rear wheels are of two basic types: composite or spoke, as shown in Figure 12-9.[49] Composite wheels tend to be more economical than spoke wheels and require less maintenance. There is less risk of the user getting his hand caught in the wheel. These wheels tend to be more rigid than spoke wheels and thus may make for a more uncomfortable ride.[49] Spoke wheels typically require maintenance as it is more difficult to clean them and the spokes should be re-adjusted. These wheels tend to transmit less vibration from the surface to the user than more rigid composite wheels.[49] They are lighter in weight than composite wheels. High performance wheels, such as the *Spinergy* wheel, are available for active users (e.g., individuals who use their chairs to travel long distances regularly; use a wheelie to change heights, as in climbing a curb; or use their chairs most of the day as they move around their environment). These wheels use lightweight materials that provide better strength and greater shock absorption. Wheels range in size from 18 to 26 inches in diameter. Power wheelchairs typically have 18-inch wheels and conventional manual types have 24-inch wheels.

Many wheelchairs allow adjustment of the location of the drive wheels forward or rearward on the chair. Figure 12-10 shows an axle mounting plate that allows adjustments of the position of the drive wheels. The location of the wheels relative to the center of gravity of the user affects the mobility and stability of the chair. When the axle of the wheel is located either directly under the user's center of gravity or anterior to it, the result is a more maneuverable, responsive chair, which is what the active user desires. More novice wheelchair users or those with less control will feel most comfortable with the axis of the

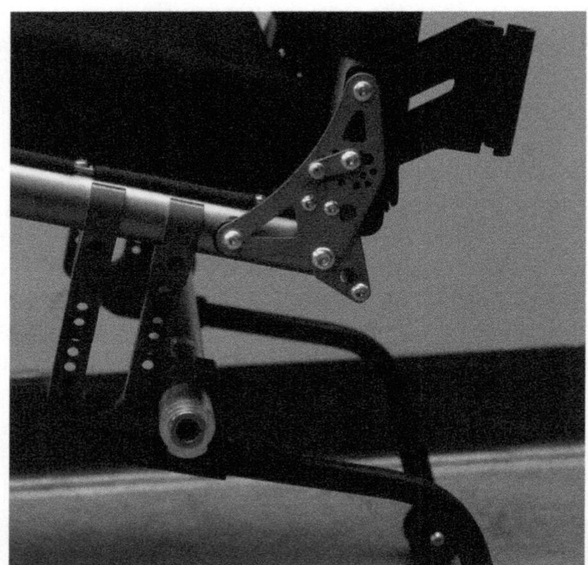

Figure 12-10 Axle plate of manual wheelchair that allows adjustability of the position of the rear wheels.

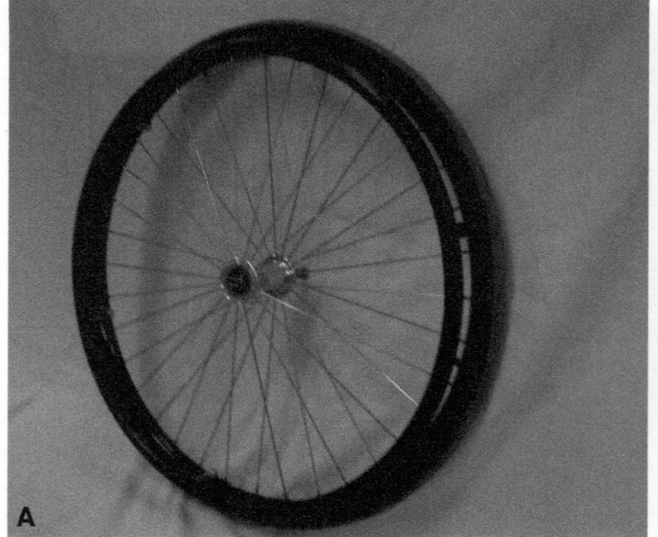

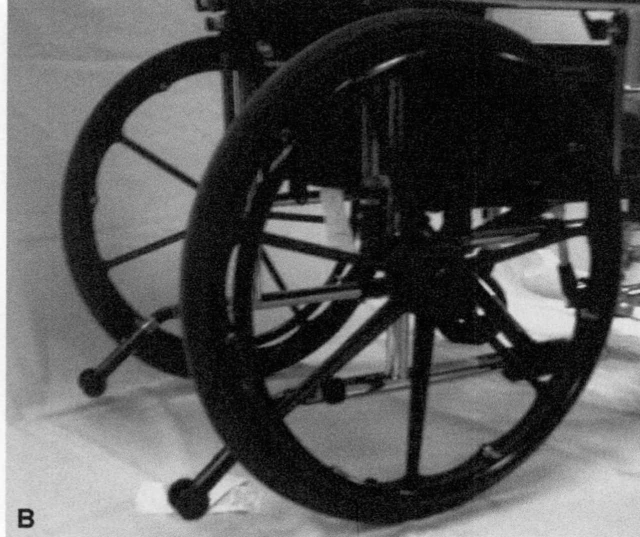

Figure 12-9 Types of rear wheels for a manual wheelchair. **A,** Spoked wheel. **B,** Composite mag wheel.

wheel located behind their center of gravity, resulting in a more stable chair.[21] Wheel camber affects the responsiveness of the chair. **Camber** refers to the degree to which the wheel is mounted off vertical, usually 1–4 degrees. Camber tips the wheel so the top is closer to the user's body. When the wheels are set this way the wheelchair becomes more stable and propulsion is more efficient. There is greater access to the wheels. Camber increases the overall width of the chair and lowers the rear seat to floor height.[49] Wheel alignment also affects the ease with which the chair can be propelled. **Alignment** refers to the degree to which the two wheels are parallel to each other. If they are not parallel and at equal distance from each other, there is greater rolling resistance for the wheelchair.

Casters

The front wheels on wheelchairs are referred to as *casters*. They range in diameter from 2¾ to 8¼ inches.[23] Larger casters give a smoother ride but are less responsive and can interfere with foot placement.[49] Smaller casters are more responsive, contribute to more efficient propulsion, and allow more flexibility in the position of the feet, but these benefits are compromised by a rougher ride.[21,49] Solid, semi-pneumatic casters are available. The relationship of the user's center of gravity to the chair's center of mass is important here. If the user is seated too far forward in the chair, excess weight is placed on the casters (i.e., front loading the casters), making it more difficult to propel as the force required to overcome inertia is greater.[21] This situation may also result in loss of forward stability with an added risk of the chair tipping forward.

Attention to the function of the casters is important as they contribute to the overall function of the chair. Shimmy is one of the major problems with casters.[23] This term refers to the rapid vibration that is often experienced when pushing a shopping cart. Smaller casters tend to have less shimmy than larger ones. Shimmy can result from the position of the caster fork and stem, uneven wear of the caster wheel, and the tension in the caster axle and swivel mechanism where they attach to the frame. *Caster float* occurs when one of the casters does not touch the floor when the wheelchair is on level ground,[11] which can result in reduced stability and performance. If the rehabilitation assistant observes caster shimmy, it is an indication that maintenance of the chair is needed. Excessive wear on one caster or unequal camber in the rear wheels will bring about caster float. Replacing the caster, adjusting the rear wheel camber, or lowering the caster that floats with a spacer can eliminate the problem.[11]

Hand Rims

The human/technology interface for a manual wheelchair is most commonly a ring attached to the wheel, called a *hand rim*. Hand rims are made from a variety of materials including titanium, aluminum, and stainless steel. They may have a vinyl coating. Knobs or extensions can be added for individuals who have difficulty gripping hand rims (Figure 12-11). Ergonomically designed hand rims use a material that spans the space between the wheel rim and the hand rim, thus allowing a natural fit with the user's palm. If an individual has the use of only one arm and hand for propelling the wheelchair, two hand

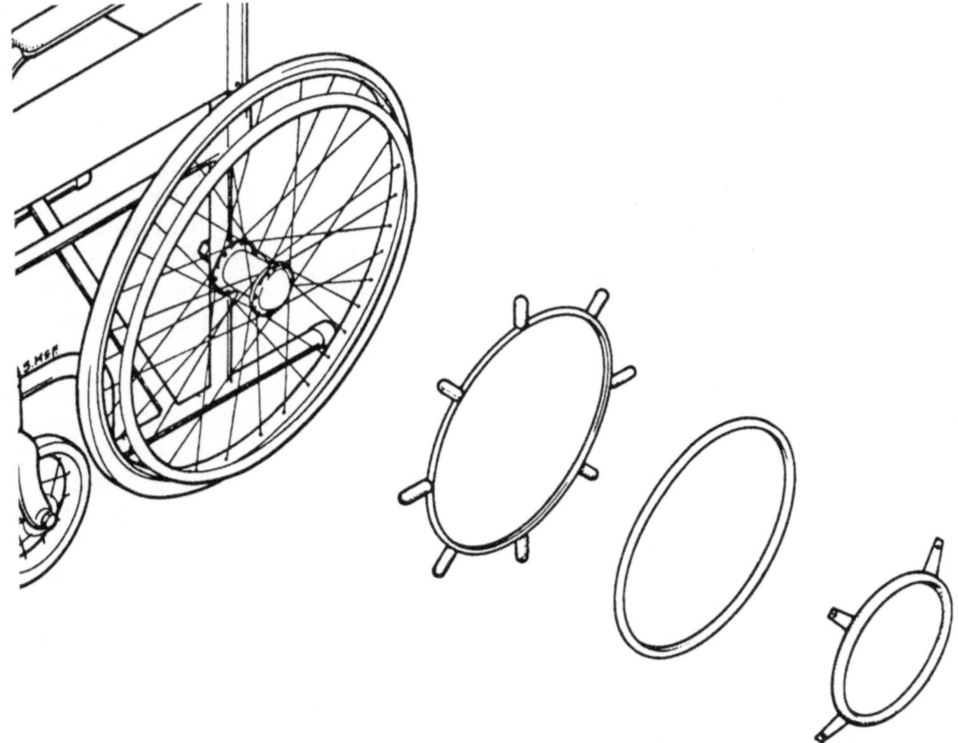

Figure 12-11 Examples of hand rims. (From Wilson B, McFarland S: Types of wheelchairs, *J Rehabil Res Dev Clin Suppl* 27:104–116, 1990.)

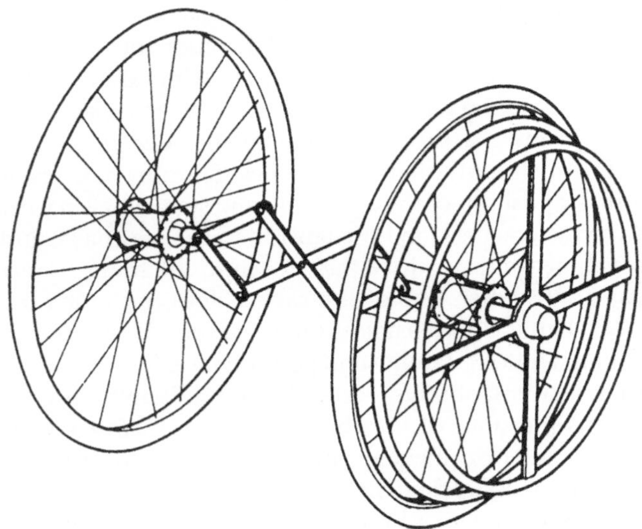

Figure 12-12 One-hand drive mechanism. (From Wilson B, McFarland S: Types of wheelchairs, *J Rehabil Res Dev Clin Suppl* 27:104–116, 1990.)

rims are put on the intact side and a linkage is attached between the inner hand rim and the opposite wheel, as shown in Figure 12-12[8]. By grasping both hand rims, the user can move forward. Turning is possible using one hand rim at a time. Often the person who uses this hand rim configuration will also use at least one leg to propel the chair.

Propelling Structure: Powered

The propelling structure of powered wheelchairs has more variability than do manual systems. The major components are a wheeled mobility base with a power drive to the wheels, a control interface that the consumer uses to direct the movement of the wheelchair, an electronic controller, and powered accessories (e.g., recline, tilt). In this section we discuss current approaches.

Drive Wheels

Electrically powered wheelchairs have undergone a tremendous change in the last decade. The development of micro-processing capabilities enables developers of power mobility technology to include a wide range of functions in these devices. One of the most significant developments is the change in the location of the drive wheels. Power is delivered to one pair of wheels in mobility technology with additional sets of wheels providing stability. Direct drive systems also often provide dynamic or active braking of the wheelchair by providing a voltage that stops the motor. This action offers more control than the common situation of letting the chair coast to a stop after the voltage is turned off to the motor. Electrically powered wheelchairs are generally classified as rear-, mid-, or front-wheel drive depending on the location of the wheels that propel the chair. Rear- and mid-wheel drive chairs are the most common. In addition to castors, anti-tipping devices may also be present on a power chair.

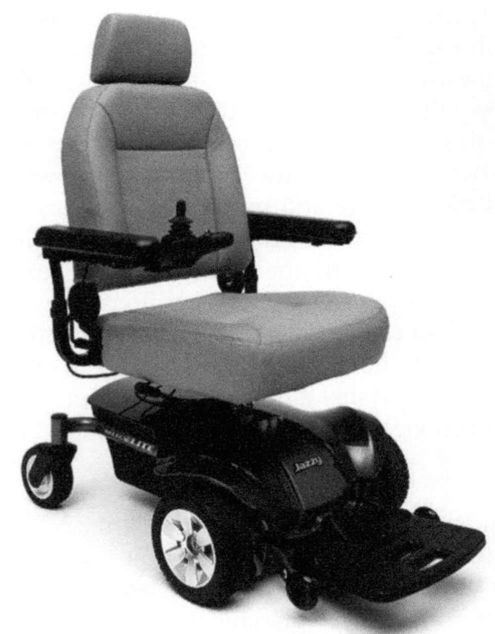

Figure 12-13 Electrically powered wheelchair with mid-wheel drive system. (Courtesy of Pride Mobility Products Corporation.)

Figure 12-13 shows a mid-wheel drive electrically powered wheelchair, with the housing for the motor and batteries located underneath the seat.

Denison (2001)[18] proposed an additional drive classification based on the relationship of the drive wheel to the center of gravity of the user as well as the ratio of the weight on the drive wheels to that on the castors. The drive wheels of a rear-wheel drive chair are located behind the center of gravity of the user. These are well behind the center of gravity in a low-ratio rear-wheel drive. The front wheels are castors and anti-tipping wheels may or may not be present. The drive wheels of a high-ratio rear-wheel drive are closer to the user's center of gravity. In addition to front castors, anti-tipping wheels are located behind the drive wheels. The drive wheels of a mid-wheel drive chair are located directly under the user's center of gravity. Castors are located both in front of and behind the drive wheels. These castors are intended to be in contact with the surface when the chair is in motion. The drive wheels of a front-wheel drive chair are located ahead of the user's center of gravity, with the high-ratio front-wheel drive wheels being closer to the center of gravity than the low ratio. The location of the drive wheels affects the performance of the chair, making it an important consideration when recommending a chair to a client.

Evaluation of the client's physical and cognitive abilities and examination of their mobility needs are important steps in determining which type of power wheelchair is most suited to their needs and lifestyle. There is limited literature that evaluates the function of power wheelchairs to assist the client and clinician in making a power mobility decision. Rentschler and colleagues from the Rehabilitation Engineering Research Center on Wheeled

Mobility at the University of Pittsburgh used the ANSI/RESNA standards to evaluate five power chairs that were commonly recommended for clients in the Veterans Affairs health care system.[48] They examined two rear-wheel drive chairs, two mid-wheel drive chairs and one front-wheel drive chair. While their results did not point conclusively to the benefits of one chair over another, they do give a good initial foundation with which to compare a chair's performance to the consumer's needs.

Control Interfaces for Powered Mobility Systems

There are a number of ways in which a powered wheelchair can be controlled. Two control distinctions need to be made first before discussing the various technologies: proportional versus non-proportional control. **Proportional control** with 360-degree directionality means that the chair moves in whichever direction the joystick is displaced. The greater the displacement, the faster the chair moves.[39] The joystick controls fewer degrees of movement with **non-proportional control**. Regardless of the displacement, the chair travels at a preselected speed. If the user wishes to change direction she must release the joystick in one direction and activate it in the direction of the change.[39]

Many options exist that provide access to powered wheelchair controls. The initial assessment by the rehabilitation assistant and ATP includes the determination of movements that the client is able to make reliably. A similar process can be used to determine the most appropriate method of access as was described in Chapter 7 regarding computer and AAC access. An important difference between assessment for computer access versus power wheelchair control is that the rehabilitation assistant/ATP needs to determine that the movement used to control the powered wheelchair is safe as well as reliable (i.e., the user must be able to initiate or cease a movement as required because they are controlling a moving vehicle). The rehabilitation assistant plays a key monitoring role to assist with the determination that the user's preferred method of accessing the controller continues to be both reliable and safe.

Many of the types of switches that are described in Chapter 7 are also useful for powered mobility control. These switches can be mechanical or electronic.[39] Mechanical switches must be physically activated to initiate a control command. For example, they must be moved, depressed, touched, or released. Electronic switches do not require physical contact from the user. Proximity switches activate when the user is close to the switch, but not necessarily touching it. Fiber-optic switches emit an invisible beam that initiates an action when interrupted.[39]

The most common method of control of a powered wheelchair is direct selection through the use of a four-direction joystick. Typically, a joystick can be positioned on either side of the chair or in midline to be controlled with the hand or forearm. It can also be fixed or mounted on a swing-away plate that facilitates transfers. It can be positioned to be used with the chin, foot, leg, or head. When a chin joystick is used, an additional switch (often activated by a shoulder shrug) can be used to control a powered arm that moves the joystick into position for use and swings it out of the way for eating, talking, or mouthstick use.

Most joysticks have a ball on top. However, many different types of tops are available for users with different grasping abilities.[39] For example, a U-shaped cuff that supports the person's hand on the sides may enhance his control of the joystick. Other variations include smaller or larger balls, a T-bar, and an extended joystick.

Sip and puff switches are a common control interface for individuals with a high spinal cord lesion. A small tube is placed in close proximity to the person's mouth. The user controls the switch with either a puff (blowing air out of the mouth) or sip (sucking air into the mouth). A hard puff causes the chair to move forward while a hard sip causes it to move in reverse. A soft puff turns the chair right; a soft sip turns it left. The forward direction is latched (i.e., once the user activates forward movement, the chair will continue to travel in that direction until reverse is activated). Good oral motor control is required to use a sip and puff system. Figure 12-14 shows a sip and puff system for controlling a wheelchair.

Various head control systems are available and are arranged in a head array in a headrest. Figure 12-15 shows an example of this type of control interface. These switches are electronic, not mechanical. Typically the user has access to three switches: (1) moving the head backwards causes the chair to move forward; (2) tilting it to the right moves the chair right, and the opposite initiates travel to the left; and (3) tilting the head forward stops the chair.[39] Control can be either proportional or non-proportional depending on the head control of the user. Individuals who tend to move into extension when their neck is extended may not be good candidates for this type of system, because they may not be able to reliably stop or reverse the chair if extensor tone inhibits forward flexion of the neck.

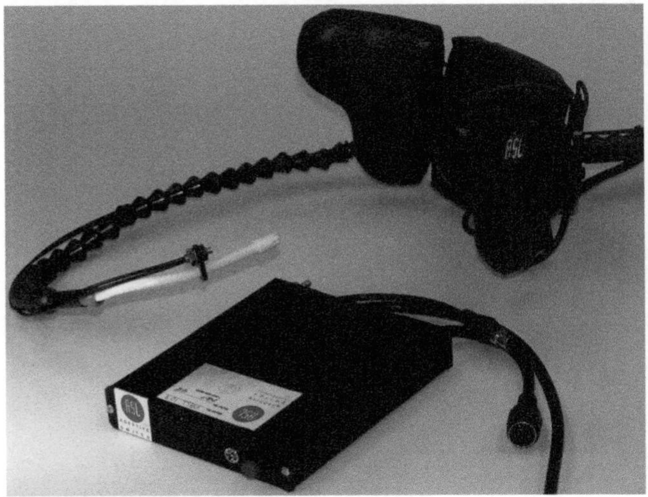

Figure 12-14 Sip-n-puff controller. (Courtesy Adaptive Switch Laboratories.)

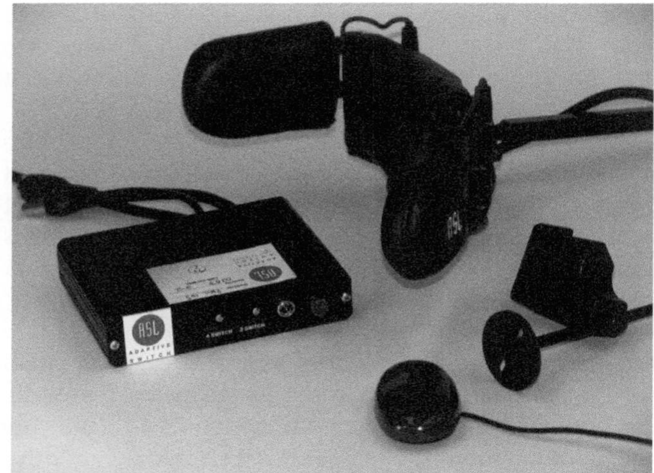

Figure 12-15 Head array, power wheelchair controller. (Courtesy Adaptive Switch Laboratories.)

Indirect selection using scanning is also available for consumers who can only use a single switch. In this case there are four lights, one for each direction, arranged in a cross pattern. The lights scan around the pattern until the user presses his switch. The wheelchair then moves in the direction selected. Other functions are also scanned. Single-switch scanning is time-consuming as well as cognitively demanding, and is typically considered only after other options have been excluded.

Controllers

A *powered wheelchair controller* connects the control interface to the drive system. This component is the processor in the assistive technology component of our Human Activity Assistive Technology (HAAT) model. Figure 12-16, *A*, shows a typical wheelchair controller with a joystick. Figure 12-16, *B*, shows a wheelchair controller with a T-bar joystick. In a proportional drive system the controller determines the amount of voltage supplied to the motor by the amount of deflection in the joystick. This voltage is directly related to motor speed. This type of proportionality is not obtained from a switched control interface. To allow the wheelchair to accelerate gradually (as the user with a proportional control would do), the controller provides a gradual acceleration when any direction is selected. In most controllers the rate of acceleration can be adjusted to meet the consumer's needs. For example, an expert powered-wheelchair user could have the acceleration set on the high end so that the chair is highly responsive, whereas a novice user could set the rate of acceleration lower to allow for a slower start. The rate of deceleration (braking) can also be adjusted. Deceleration is the swiftness with which the wheelchair comes to a stop once the control interface is deactivated. With these two features on a controller, it is possible to set one rate for acceleration and a different rate for braking.

Controllers also provide either momentary or latched switch control. In *momentary control* the motors are activated only while the switch is pressed, which provides the greatest control for the user. Some consumers are unable to maintain switch activation, but they can press and release quickly. In this case *latched control* is used. In this mode, when the switch is pressed once, the motors turn on and remain on. When the switch is pressed again, the motors turn off. It is important that the consumer be able to activate the switch reliably and rapidly when it is in the latched mode, so as to stop quickly when necessary. This feature is often used with sip-and-puff switches. It allows the user to give a hard puff once to latch the control for the wheelchair to move either forward or backward and then use soft sips and puffs to turn left or right.[57]

Most powered wheelchair controllers are programmable by the user to some extent, which gives them much more flexibility and adjustability. Forward and reverse maximal speeds can be independently adjusted. On some devices the ratio of forward to reverse speed is selected. It is more

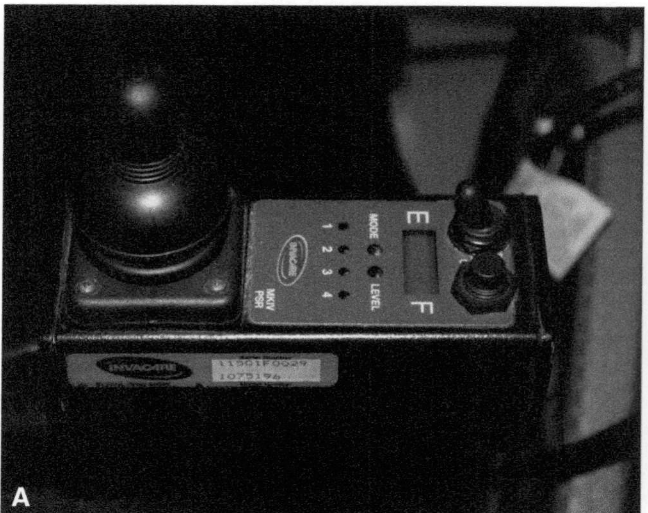

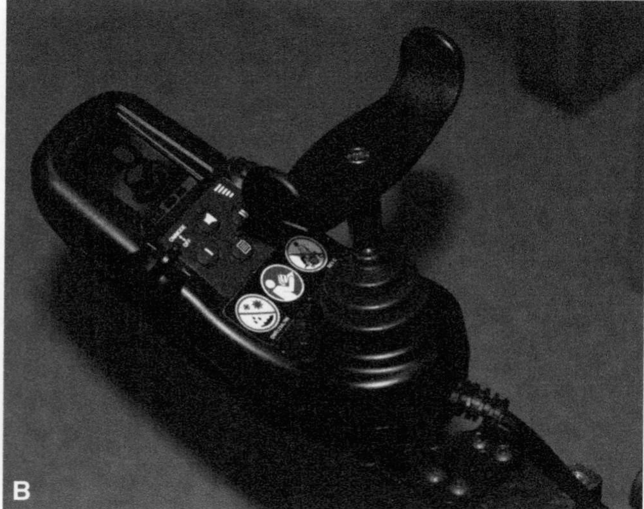

Figure 12-16 Electrically powered wheelchair controller with LED. **A,** Electrically powered wheelchair controller with joystick. **B,** Electrically powered wheelchair controller with T-bar joystick.

difficult to control the wheelchair when turning than when going straight, and the controller feature that allows turning speed to be set independently of (or as a function of) forward speed is useful.

Some consumers have difficulty controlling their movements because of tremor, which can make the use of a joystick or other wheelchair control interface difficult. To accommodate for tremor, an averaging feature is incorporated into some controllers. The averaging system effectively damps out the tremor by ignoring small rapid movements and responding only to larger, slower ones.[3] The disadvantage of this approach is that the system can become sluggish, resulting in reduced capability to respond to obstacles quickly. This feature is sometimes referred to as the *sensitivity* or *tremor dampening* of the controller.

Another adjustment allowed by the controller is the ability to alter the degree of range of motion required for an individual to operate a control interface. This feature is called the *short throw adjustment* and is most commonly used with joysticks. It is useful for consumers who have limited range of motion at the control site that is being used. Many controller models have an LED display that visually represents the different functions and the results of adjustments as they are made (Figure 12-16, *A* and *B*).

Computer-based controllers allow the storage of a set of values for parameters such as those described earlier. These parameters can then be recalled for use in a particular situation (e.g., outdoors on a hill or indoors on a smooth floor). A therapist working with a consumer to gradually develop driving skills can also store the setups and recall them when needed. Different configurations can be stored for each consumer in training or assessment settings where several consumers may use one powered wheelchair. Most powered wheelchair controllers also have provisions for the attachment of an "attendant control," which is very useful for training. This control can override the user's control interface in an emergency situation or during training.

Another feature of many controllers is the ability to operate different functions of the wheelchair or other devices with the same control interface. Generally an output from the controller is connected to the external device (e.g., an augmentative communication system or electronic aid to daily living [EADL]). These outputs may be called *auxiliary* or *ECU* on different commercial wheelchair controllers. Using a switch, the user is able to transfer the output of the controller from the motors to the external device. The control interface is then able to control the external device directly. A visual display identifies which function is being used. For example, if a joystick were being used for mobility, switching to the communication auxiliary mode would allow directed scanning (see Chapter 7) to be used for selections on an augmentative communication device. A switch allows the user to change between these two operations.

Batteries

The power for a powered wheelchair is supplied by a pair of batteries that are mounted under the seat of the chair. The batteries used are the rechargeable lead-acid type. Batteries differ in several ways. Automobile batteries require a high current for a short period to start the car. Wheelchair batteries, on the other hand, require smaller amounts of current for a longer time. This difference is reflected in the use of *deep-cycle* lead-acid batteries for power wheelchairs. These have thicker plates, which allow them to provide current for longer periods. The chemicals inside the battery may be in a liquid form, called a *wet cell*, or in a semisolid form, called a *gel*. Wet-cell batteries are less expensive and last longer; however, they are more hazardous and require more maintenance than gel batteries, so they are less commonly used for power wheelchairs. The fluid in wet cell batteries is subject to spilling and evaporation. Replacement of the fluid with distilled water is required at regular intervals. Gel (often called *sealed*) batteries will not spill, which makes them more desirable for transportation. They do not require any maintenance other than keeping them charged. These batteries are typically allowed on public transportation systems, whereas the wet cell batteries often are not. They do not need to be fully discharged before they require recharging. They do not have a "memory," which means that the battery capacity is not limited by previous recharges. Battery power between charges is determined by the capacity measured in ampere-hours. At room temperature, wheelchair batteries commonly have 30 to 90 ampere-hours capacity at 12 volts.[11] The type of motor, environmental conditions (e.g., extremes of temperature), and the amount of regular maintenance can all affect battery life and performance. Different batteries require different types of chargers, and it is imperative that the correct battery charger be used. The technology for wheelchair batteries has changed very little over the years. Smaller, lighter-weight batteries with an increase in capacity would help to decrease the weight of powered wheelchairs and increase the distance that the user can travel on one charge.

ANSI/RESNA standards identify a test method for determining the capacity of wheelchair batteries on a single charge. This test requires the chair to be driven at maximum speed around a 54.5 m track 10 times in each direction. Amperes per hour are measured and the theoretical maximum distance is calculated from this measurement.[2] Rentschler et al.[48] indicate that this test does not take into account, for example, the varying draw on battery power when the user travels uphill, in different weather conditions, or across different terrains. Information on the theoretical distance of a battery is vital information since serious injury or death could result from a power wheelchair user who is stranded by a dead battery.

Ventilators

Consideration must be given to the placement and movement of a ventilator when the power wheelchair user is dependent for respiratory support. Like many other products, ventilators have become much more compact and streamlined in recent years, yet they still affect the overall length, weight, and center of mass of the chair. Ventilators can be mounted low on the base of the chair or on a frame that is attached to the vertical uprights of the back. Mounts for ventilators can be fixed or articulating. The orientation of the ventilator is congruent with that of the wheelchair seat in a fixed mount. An articulating mount is required with a wheelchair frame that tilts or reclines. This option maintains the vertical orientation of the ventilator as the seat moves into tilt or recline modes. Further, it keeps the ventilator out of the way of the wheelchair batteries.

Specialized Bases for Manual Wheelchairs

Having described the major wheelchair characteristics, we can now look at dependent mobility bases that have unique structural and propelling characteristics. Because an attendant or care provider is responsible for pushing the consumer in a dependent-mobility wheelchair, special attention is given to the biomechanics of the caregiver during this activity. Items normally required for independent manual mobility (e.g., large rear wheels with hand rims) are often omitted in these systems. Bases for dependent mobility are commonly lighter in weight and lower priced than wheelchairs for independent manual mobility.[58]

Stroller Bases

Strollers, similar to those used for transporting very young children, are typically of two types: (1) umbrella folding with a sling seat and (2) full-sized units with solid seats.[58] Although originally designed for children, there are now strollers that accommodate consumers who weigh up to 200 pounds. The umbrella type generally does not provide good sitting support, but it folds easily for storage in a vehicle. Consumers who use strollers should not be transported in the stroller unless it has been crash tested.[31] In North America, stroller bases that have met crash testing standards will be identified in the WC19 category and will have attachment sites that are an integral part of the frame. A list of wheelchairs and seating products that are WC19 compliant can be found at: http://www.rercwts.org/RERC_WTS2_KT/RERC_WTS2_KT_Stand/RERC_WTS2_19_Chart.html. An attraction of stroller bases is that they resemble standard strollers in appearance, which can be appealing to parents. One feature that appeals to parents is the ease with which they can be transported. The small wheels and short wheelbase of most strollers make them easily maneuverable by an attendant. One disadvantage of the stroller is that the child or adult is often in a reclined position, which may limit his ability to carry out functional tasks. Strollers are sometimes purchased as a second wheelchair to facilitate transportation, with a standard wheelchair used for functional tasks. Figure 12-17 shows an example of a solid stroller base.

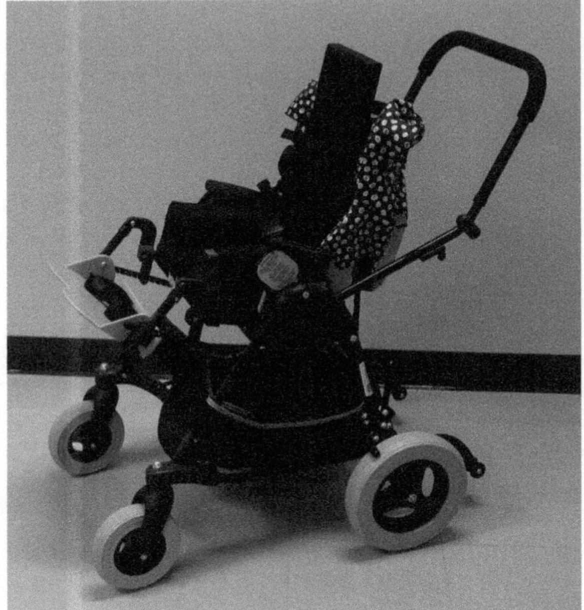

Figure 12-17 Firm stroller base.

Transport Wheelchairs

Transport wheelchairs are designed for occasional use and are often available for transporting patients in hospitals or in short-term situations such as traversing an airport or shopping mall. They typically have upholstery seating and four small wheels. They do not have any adjustability nor is it anticipated that seating systems will be used. They are lightweight, durable, and relatively maintenance-free. |These chairs provide a short term, dependent mobility option and are not intended to provide seating and positioning in the long term.

Wheelchairs for Use by Older Clients

The set up of a manual wheelchair for regular use by an older client is different from that of a younger, more active user. Age-related disabilities such as arthritis, osteoporosis (loss of bone density) and sarcopenia (loss of muscle fiber) contribute to reduced muscle strength and range of motion. Further, older clients may feel less secure in their movements. Age-related visual changes, including disorders such as age-related macular degeneration and glaucoma, are further considerations for setup of a chair for use by an older client. Care should be taken to ensure that the center of gravity ratio of the client to the axis of the drive wheel provides an optimal stability and mobility balance. Access to the drive wheels and hand rims relative to range of motion and strength in the upper extremities needs to be considered along with rolling resistance. Effects of visual-perceptual changes resulting from a cerebral vascular accident will affect the user's ability to navigate in his environment and will need to be considered when providing training in wheelchair skills. The rehabilitation assistant should be alert to changes in the user's function that affects their ability to use the mobility device.

Some manufacturers are producing chairs that have a rocking feature. Often these chairs have a tilt feature as well. A mechanism on the chair allows the user to rock the seat of the chair. This mechanism can be disengaged in some situations, such as transportation, when it is not desired. This feature is recommended for clients who become agitated, with the view that the rocking motion is calming for the client.

Wheelchairs for Bariatric Clients

Bariatric clients, those individuals with a BMI (Body Mass Index) of 30 or greater, are a population with an increasing prevalence in North America. These individuals require frames that are designed to accommodate their weight and their larger size. Most typical wheelchairs have a maximum weight capacity of 300 pounds. Chairs for bariatric clients accommodate a maximum weight of 600 pounds, with some manufacturers offering chairs that will accommodate up to 1000 pounds.[16] The location of the mechanics of electrically powered wheelchairs beneath the seat allows the use of a larger seat while still maintaining as narrow a width as possible. Some chairs provide user adjustable seat depth and width. Tilt is also an option that can be provided for the bariatric client. The Eclipse (Figure 12-18) is an example of a chair designed for bariatric clients.*

Fitting a wheelchair for a bariatric client has special considerations since soft tissue distribution and accumulation vary, resulting in different body sizes and shapes.[16] Measurement should be done in the seated position and on a firm surface. If there is significant soft tissue accumulation around the buttocks, the configuration of the seat back must be considered, since the buttocks may protrude further than the shoulders, requiring the individual to lean back if his upper back is to be in contact with the seat back. Some manufacturers produce a back that provides support along the entire back surface. A change in the width of the back from hip to shoulder to accommodate a different shape is another accommodation made by some manufacturers.

* PDG Mobility (www.pdgmobility.com).

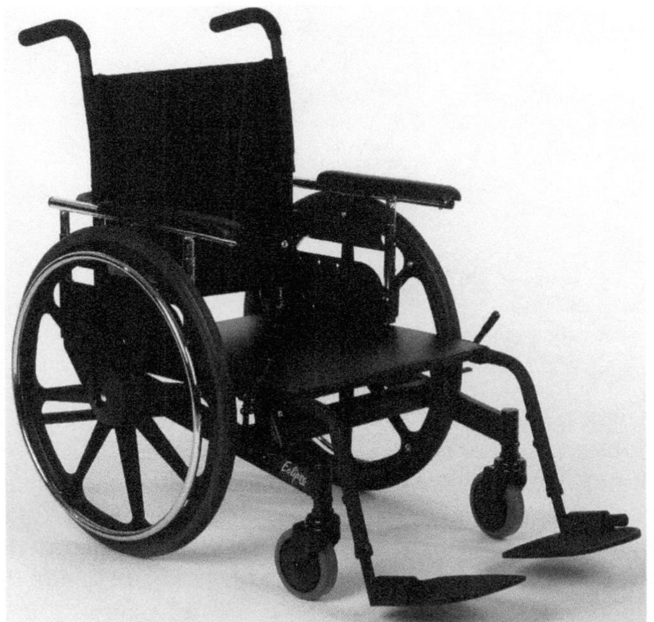

Figure 12-18 Eclipse wheelchair that allows rocking motion for bariatric client. (Courtesy PDG Mobility.)

Specialized Bases for Electrically Powered Wheelchairs

Customizable Electrically Powered Wheelchairs

The range and combinations of features available on electrically powered wheelchairs is rapidly increasing. Some of these features, such as tilt, recline, elevating seats, and footrests, have been mentioned already. The Attitude™ (Figure 12-19, *A*) and the Latitude™ (Figure 12-19, *B*) systems both provide power options to enable independent transfers. The Attitude™ has a foot platform that lowers to the ground and then rises up to seat height, allowing an individual to transfer independently. To transfer into the chair, the foot platform is lowered to the floor; the user transfers onto the foot platform, raises it to seat height, and then transfers onto the seat. The Latitude system is similar, but in this case the entire seat moves forward and down to the floor.*

Scooters

Scooter wheelchairs (Figure 12-20, *A*) comprise a large proportion of the electrically powered system market. Individuals who are marginal ambulators and need mobility assistance to conserve energy most often use the scooter. For this reason, it is most commonly used by the consumer outside the home. Grocery stores and shopping malls often provide scooters for customers who may need them. The propelling structure of the scooter includes the drive train, the tires, the tiller, and the battery. There are a number of models available in either three- or four-wheel versions with front-wheel drive or rear-wheel drive. Scooters with front-wheel drive do better on level terrain and are more maneuverable. For this reason, they perform better in small spaces. In rear-wheel drive scooters, the rider's weight is positioned over the motor so there is better traction and more power. The bases of rear-wheel drive scooters are wider and longer than the other powered chairs. These scooters are better able to handle inclines and uneven or rough terrain and therefore are preferable for outdoor use.

A tiller-type control is used to steer the wheelchair and acceleration is accomplished by either grasping a lever on the tiller with the fingers or pressing with the thumb. When the accelerator is released, the scooter eases to a stop. On some scooters the height and angle of the tiller

* From Motion Concepts (www.motionconcepts. com).

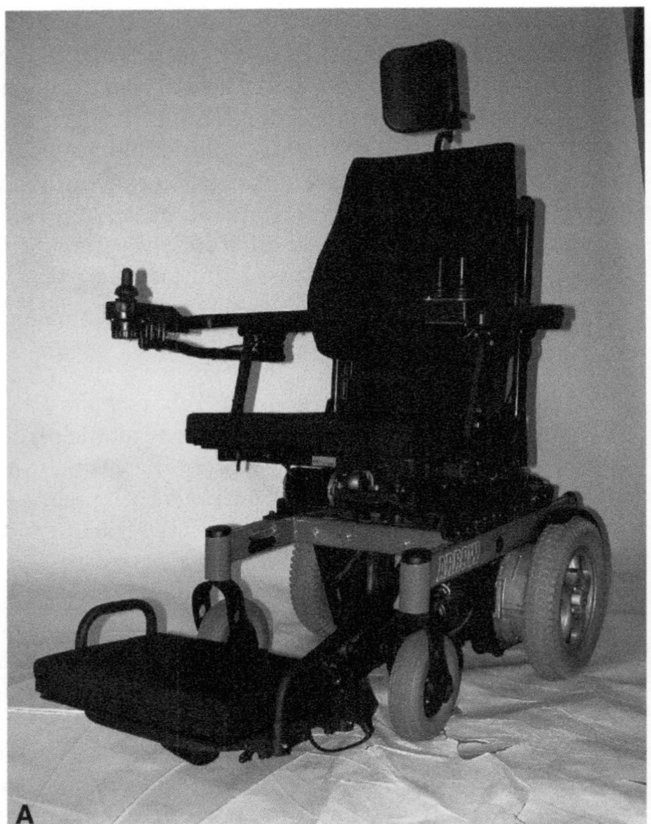
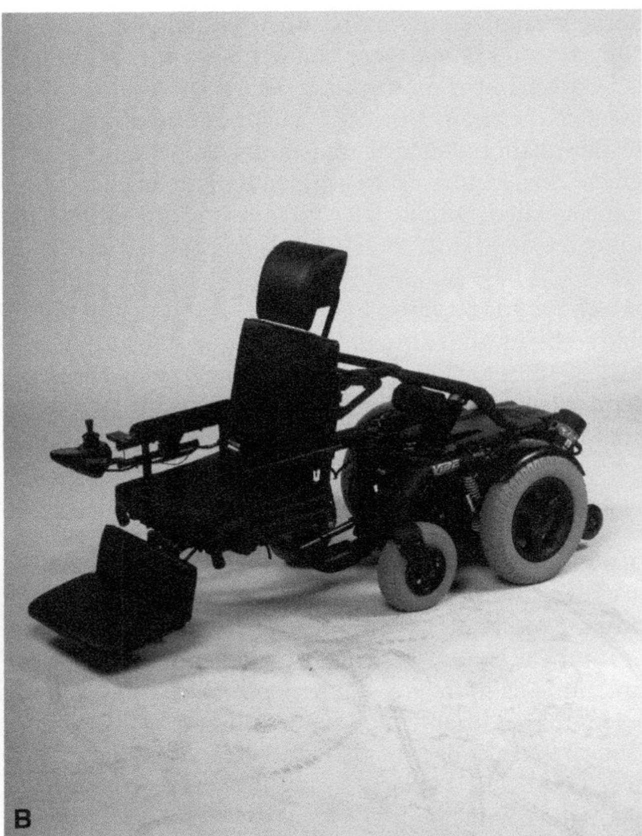

Figure 12-19 Attitude and Latitude electrically powered wheelchair systems that allow the user to transfer independently from the floor to the chair. **A,** Attitude. **B,** Latitude. (Courtesy Motion Concepts.)

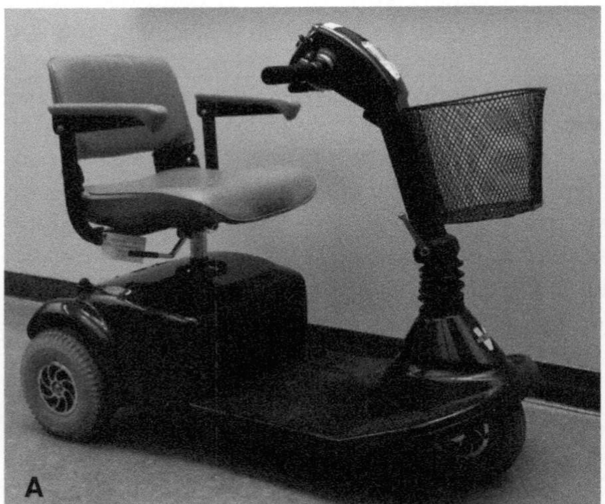
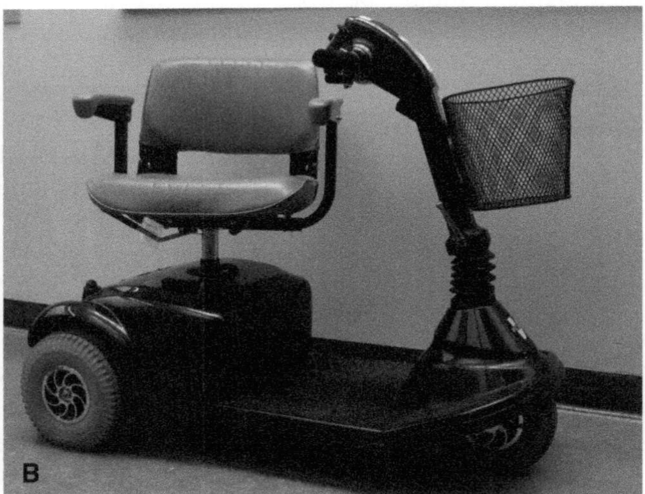

Figure 12-20 **A,** Electrically powered scooter; **B,** Electrically powered scooter with seat swiveled.

is adjustable. Depending on the model, scooters can have either proportional (variable-speed) control or switched (constant-speed) control. There is a separate control setting for adjusting the speed of the scooter. Some scooters have a dial that provides a range of settings, whereas others have a toggle switch for high and low.

The seat of the scooter is mounted to a single post coming up from the base. Typically the seat is a bucket type that has few options for seat width, depth, or back height[8]. The seats come in padded or unpadded versions and several types of armrest styles (fixed, flip-up, or none) are available. Most scooters have a mechanism that releases the seat so it can swivel to the side and then locks in place. This feature is helpful for transfers in and out of the seat and for accessing a table surface. Figure 12-20, *B*, shows a scooter with a swivel seat.

Some of the advantages of scooters are that they are lighter in weight, can be disassembled for transportation in a car, are easy to maneuver, are less costly than other powered wheelchairs, and are more acceptable than other types of powered wheelchairs. The primary disadvantage of scooters is that they do not provide flexibility in control interfaces. The consumer needs to have a fair amount of trunk and upper extremity control to operate the tiller of the scooter. Scooters also have very little flexibility in terms of speed, braking, or turning control. Finally, the seat of a scooter typically does not provide adequate postural support, and many types of seating systems needed by individuals with postural control problems cannot be interfaced to a scooter.

Power Assist Mechanisms

Considerable attention has been given to the shoulder injuries that result from prolonged propulsion of a manual wheelchair[5,6,14,52,59]. One option for individuals with shoulder pain that limits their ability to propel a manual wheelchair, but for whom an electrically powered wheelchair is not desirable, is pushrim-activated power-assist wheels. These wheels are interchanged with those of a manual wheelchair. A motor is located in the hub of the rear wheels that is linked to the hand rims.[1] These units supply power to the manual wheelchair as needed by the user. When the user applies force above a preset level to the hand rims, such as when going up an incline, the motors engage and help to propel the wheelchair. Propulsion and braking assistance are provided for both forward and rearward motion. The unit can also be turned off, which allows the manual wheelchair to function in the usual manner. These units add considerable weight to a manual chair, which is a consideration in their selection. Giesbrecht and colleagues (2009)[26] found that participation in daily activities and psychosocial aspects of device use were similar across power-assist wheels and a powered wheelchair, suggesting that the former are alternatives to a powered chair in some situations.

A new product on the market with a similar purpose is Magicwheels™, which provides geared technology for manual wheelchairs (Figure 12-21).* Magicwheels™ gives the user a selection of two gears, similar to the concept of bicycle gears, with the second gear providing a 2:1 mechanical advantage. The user selects the second gear by moving the housing of the gear, located on the hub of the wheel. Changing gears does not require grip or substantial strength. Magicwheels™ are most useful on inclines, where they provide assistance propelling upward and braking assistance when traveling downward. Finley et al. (2006)[24] completed a pilot study of the effect of Magicwheels™ use on shoulder pain, length of time the user was able to sustain uphill travel, and perceived exertion during this task. An A-B-A design was used, with baseline being use of the consumer's typical wheels. After four months of use, shoulder pain was stable or reduced and users were able to travel uphill for a longer time with no change in perceived exertion. Howarth and Colleagues[28,29] investigated muscle effort of healthy volunteers when ascending ramps of various grades, using both Magicwheels™ and non-geared wheels. Trunk muscle effort was lower with Magicwheels™ as the ramp grade increased, as was shoulder flexion. Overall, use of Magicwheels™ required more sustained muscle effort because of the longer time taken to ascend the ramp. Because this study used healthy volunteers, it needs to be repeated with wheelchair users to further investigate the effects of Magicwheels™ on propulsive efforts when ascending a ramp.

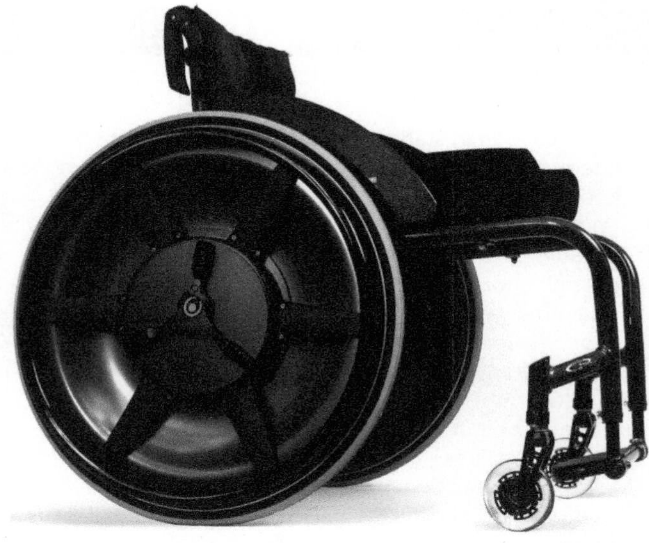

Figure 12-21 MagicWheels multigear wheels for manual wheelchair. (Courtesy Magic Wheels, Inc.)

Wheelchair Standards

As discussed in Chapter 1, *standards* can be used to provide manufacturing guidance to ensure product quality. One area of assistive technologies in which standards have been developed is for wheelchairs. Both the International Standards Organization (ISO) and the American National Standards Institute (ANSI) and Rehabilitation Engineering Society of North America (RESNA) have published standards for manual and power wheelchairs, seating systems, and wheelchair use during transportation. There is considerable overlap in these standards. A comparison of the ISO and ANSI/RESNA standards is shown in Box 12-3. Although these standards are voluntary, there are strong motivations for manufacturers to adhere to them. For example, the Department of Veterans Affairs (VA) has purchasing requirements for wheelchairs. As the largest purchaser of wheelchairs in the United States, the VA could significantly impact compliance with the standards shown in Box 12-3 by adopting them by reference rather than developing their own standards. Some published studies exist that have applied these standards to manual and electrically powered wheelchairs and seating cushions.[12,13,21,44,47,55]

* From Magic Wheels Inc. (www.magicwheels.com).

BOX 12-3 Comparison of ISO and ANSI/RESNA Wheelchair Standards

Standard	ISO	ANSI/RESNA
Nomenclature, terms, and definitions	X	X
Determination of static stability	X	X
Determination of overall dimensions, mass, and turning space	X	x
Determination of seating and wheel dimensions		X
Static, impact, and fatigue strengths	X	X
Test dummies		X
Determination of coefficient of friction of test surfaces	X	X
Requirements for information disclosures, documentation, and labeling	X	X
Determination of flammability	X	X
Wheelchairs used as seats in motor vehicles		X
Wheeled mobility devices for use in motor vehicles	X	
Determination of performance of stand-up wheelchairs		X
Setup procedures	X	X
Maximum overall dimensions	X	X
Determination of dynamic stability of electric wheelchairs	X	X
Determination of efficiency of brakes	X	X
Energy consumption of electric wheelchairs and scooters for determination of theoretical distance range (ISO)	X	X
Determination of maximum speed, acceleration, and retardation of electric wheelchair	X	X
Climatic tests for electric wheelchairs	X	X
Determination of obstacle climbing ability for electric wheelchairs	X	X
Testing of power and control systems for electric wheelchairs	X	X
Requirements and test methods for electromagnetic components of power wheelchairs and motorized scooters	X	X
Requirements and test methods for attendant-operated stair-climbing devices	X	
Requirements and test methods for user-operated stair-climbing devices	X	

IMPLEMENTATION AND TRAINING FOR MANUAL AND POWERED MOBILITY

As we have emphasized throughout this text, the assistive technology system includes much more than a piece of equipment. For the consumer to be satisfied and successful with an assistive device, proper implementation and training need to be part of the system. The same holds true in order to maximize the performance of consumers who use mobility systems.

Fitting of Mobility Systems

It is advisable that a fitting appointment be held with the consumer and caregiver. The purpose of this appointment is to make any adjustments needed to the wheelchair and to try out the chair and determine whether it meets the original objectives outlined during the assessment. During the initial fitting, time should also be spent demonstrating to the user and the care giver important features of the chair and going through instructions for maintenance. Box 12-4 shows a checklist of items to be covered during the fitting process for either a manual or powered wheelchair. Depending on the complexity of the wheelchair and whether seating components are involved, more than one fitting appointment may be necessary.

Because today's wheelchairs are often multifunctional, a number of components on the wheelchair are adjustable. Some adjustments and settings are made in the factory before shipping, but typically the provider of the wheelchair will need to make modifications to fit the chair to the user once it arrives from the factory. Adjustments to the wheelchair that can make a difference in user comfort, safety, and performance include axle position, wheel camber, and wheel alignment. Appropriate

BOX 12-4 Checklist for Wheelchair Fitting Process

Seating position
Position of control interface
Transfer method
Indoors: size, obstacles, doorways, turning circle
Outdoors: curbs, soft grass, rough ground, inclines
Distance required to travel
Maneuverability in community
Lights, horn
Care provider's training
Assembly and disassembly
Charging method
Battery life and maintenance
Transport in personal and public vehicles
Storage
Maintenance and repair

Modified from Ham R, Aldersea P, Porter D: *Wheelchair users and postural seating: a clinical approach,* New York, 1998, Churchill Livingstone, p 238.

adjustment of the seat angle, back height and angle, and height and angle of leg rests and footrests are also critical to user performance. Any adjustments to the chair should be made carefully and with the user's safety in mind. After adjustments are made, the user should be cautious in trying out the wheelchair until she gets acclimated to the changes.

Maintenance and Repair of Personal Mobility Systems

Wheelchairs are designed to be low maintenance and there are few items on a wheelchair, particularly a manual wheelchair, that require maintenance by the user.[11] The user is responsible for keeping the chair clean, the tires properly inflated, the brakes properly adjusted, and seeing that the wheelchair is inspected on a regular basis. The user of an electrically powered wheelchair needs to ensure that the correct battery for the wheelchair is used and that it is properly charged. A checklist of items that wheelchair users should monitor or have monitored regularly is shown in Box 12-5. The user manual for the wheelchair will also specify a schedule for periodic inspection and maintenance. Some of this maintenance may be the responsibility of the rehabilitation assistant. An ATP is responsible for maintenance beyond regular day-to-day monitoring.

Developing Mobility Skills for Manual and Powered Systems

Training in mobility skills can occur before and after the delivery of the final chair to the consumer. In situations where it is undetermined which chair is most suitable for the consumer or whether the consumer will be able to operate the wheelchair, a trial period takes place. During the trial period the consumer is loaned or leased a wheelchair, either manual or powered, which allows him to test the chair and determine if it is appropriate to meet his needs. Often, particularly with powered mobility, this trial involves a period of training to determine if the person can develop the skills

BOX 12-5 Checklist for Basic Wheelchair Maintenance

On receipt	Weekly	Monthly	Periodically	
				General
X			X	Wheelchair opens and folds easily
X	X			Wheelchair rolls straight with no excess drag or pull
X			X	Footrests flip up/down easily
X			X	Leg rests swing away and latch easily
X			X	Backrest folds and latches easily
X			X	Armrests easy to move and latch
X			X	All nuts and bolts are snug
				Wheels
X			X	Axle threads in easily or slides in and latches properly
X	X			No squeaking, binding, or excessive side motion while turning
X			X	All spokes and nipples are tight and not bent or nicked
X	X			Tire pressure is correct and equal on both sides
X		X		No cracks, looseness, or bulges in tires
				Casters
X		X		No cracks, looseness, or bulges in caster tires
X	X			No wobbling of caster wheel
X	X			No excessive play in the caster spindle
X	X			Caster housing is aligned vertically
				Wheel locks
X		X		Do not interfere with tire when rolling
X	X			Easily activated and released by operator
X	X			Hold tires firmly in place while activated
				Electrical system
X			X	Wires show no cracks, splits, or breaks
X	X			Indictors and horn work properly
X	X			Controls work smoothly and repeatedly
X		X		Battery cases are clean and free from fluids
X			X	Motor runs smoothly and quietly
				Upholstery
X			X	No tears, rips, burn marks, or excessive fraying
X		X		No excessive stretching (e.g., hammocking)
X	X			Upholstery is clean

(From Cooper RA: *Wheelchair selection and configuration,* New York, 1998, Demos Medical Publishing.)

to use the wheelchair. For example, powered mobility may be identified as a goal but the individual may not yet have the skills required to control a powered wheelchair safely. If there is any question, it is best to delay making an expensive equipment purchase and risking the safety of the user and others. It is important that the potential user develop these skills through a training program before permanently acquiring the device. Implementation should not always end with the consumer's acquisition of the device. In many cases, further training sessions are necessary. When developing either manual or powered mobility skills, it is important to set specific, measurable objectives for training.

For manual mobility, basic skills include maneuvering the wheelchair indoors on a level surface, in and around tight spaces, and over surfaces such as carpet, tile, or linoleum. For the active user of a manual wheelchair, preparation in advanced wheelchair mobility skills is suggested. These include the ability to negotiate rough, uneven terrain; propel up and down ramps and curbs independently; and execute "wheelies."

One well-researched training program is the Wheelchair Skills Program.[33,*] This program was developed in conjunction with the Wheelchair Skills Test.[34,35] The program teaches wheelchair users basic use of the wheelchair, such as applying and releasing the brakes, removing footrests, and folding the chair. It teaches basic propulsion such as rolling forward and backward and turning and maneuvering through doorways. More advanced skills include propulsion on an incline, level changes, performance of a wheelie, and various wheelie skills. Skills are classified as indoor, community, or advanced.[33] A version of the program for powered mobility devices has been developed as well, which requires users to demonstrate use of different features of the chair such as the controller, battery charger, and other functions.

Enabling the development of the ability to use a powered wheelchair for mobility in young children is different than that for adults. The great majority of adults who start to use a powered wheelchair have experience with mobility and likely experience driving a vehicle as well. Many young children do not. Rather than teaching the child how to use the chair, the goal of powered wheelchair provision is to enable the experience of movement.[40,50] Current practice regarding use of powered mobility by young children suggests that the only prerequisite to use is motivation on the part of the child to be mobile, rather than requiring a certain level of cognitive ability. When a young child is learning to walk, he is not aware of dangerous situations, so it is the responsibility of the parents or caregivers to ensure that the environment is a safe one in which he can learn. Similarly, children learning to use power mobility need to learn in a safe environment. It is the responsibility of the clinician, parents, or caregivers to shape the environment to provide a safe place for exploration of the control of a power wheelchair.[50]

Three phases of powered wheelchair use have been described in the literature: (1) exploration, (2) use of the wheelchair functions, and (3) use of the wheelchair for functional activities. Current practice guidelines recommend that a child who can benefit from powered mobility be given this opportunity as soon as they show an interest in movement. The exploration stage allows the child the opportunity to explore movement and to learn about moving about the environment. Play is the primary means of facilitating this exploration. Wherever possible, let the child move as they wish rather than directing the child to go right, go left, start, or stop (which requires understanding of these concepts). She stresses that the adult is responsible for the child's safety. As the child becomes more confident with movement, they are able to control the chair more directly, handling the joystick and appreciating the cause/effect relationship between their actions on the joystick and the movement of the chair. Ultimately, the control of the chair becomes a subskill[7] that enables the child to complete their daily activities while moving about their environment at will.

SUMMARY

Mobility is very important for participation in self-care, home, work, school, and leisure activities. Mobility needs for individuals with disabilities vary depending on the age and the disability status of the user. The ability to move about one's environment at will has physical, psychological, and social benefits. In this chapter we describe the general characteristics of personal mobility systems and the various types of mobility devices available to meet individual needs of the user. Personal mobility devices fall under the categories of independent manual, dependent manual, and powered mobility. Both manual and electrically powered wheelchair options were described. The rehabilitation assistant is frequently a key player in the training of wheelchair skills and the maintenance of the wheelchair. Because they often see the individual on a regular basis, they provide essential information that guides the selection of a wheelchair and its control, facilitating participation in daily activities for the wheelchair user. Case studies 12-1, 12-2, and 12-3 illustrate a typical situation in which a rehabilitation assistant interacts with a client who uses a mobility device. By reviewing and responding to the questions, you will be able to integrate the information that is presented in this chapter.

* Wheelchair Skills Program (www.wheelchairskillsprogram.ca).

CASE STUDY 12-1 CHANGE FROM MANUAL WHEELCHAIR TO POWER

Ted is a 53-year-old man who sustained a T12 incomplete spinal cord injury in a car crash 15 years ago. Ted is a businessman who commutes to work regularly using adapted public transit. His work and home are both fully accessible to support use of a manual wheelchair. Ted enjoys an active lifestyle, particularly getting out to visit friends, using his chair to travel on outdoor paths, and travelling with his wife. Ted has had increasing shoulder pain, resulting from many years of propelling his manual chair. For the past year, he finds that he is not able to do as much activity as he wishes because of the pain in his shoulder. He also finds that he becomes fatigued more easily when propelling his chair. Ted was recently admitted to a rehabilitation facility for a urinary tract infection. While in the facility, his wheelchair prescription is being reviewed. The seating and mobility team, with Ted, will decide if he should change to power-assist wheels or a power wheelchair. You are a rehabilitation assistant in the facility. Your observations will assist with this decision.

1. What observations would you make during your interactions with Ted that would contribute to this decision?
2. What factors or observations would indicate that power assist wheels are the best option?
3. What factors or observations would indicate that a powered wheelchair is the best option?

CASE STUDY 12-2 WHEELCHAIR SAFETY IN A LONG-TERM CARE FACILITY

Maude is an 83-year-old woman who lives in a long-term care facility. She has a diagnosis of mid-stage Alzheimer's disease. Two years ago, she sustained a stroke, followed immediately by a myocardial infarction. This combination of conditions resulted in the use of a powered wheelchair following the initial recovery from the stroke. In the past 6 months, staff and residents in the long-term care facility have expressed concerns about Maude's safe use of her powered wheelchair. She has had many collisions with doorframes and walls when travelling in the facility and several times has come close to colliding with staff or other residents. Last week Maude ran over the foot of one of the staff members. A family meeting will be held in two days to discuss these safety concerns and the plan to change to use of a manual chair. The staff members expect that the family will express concerns that this change will limit Maude's independence. You are an occupational therapy assistant in the long-term care facility and will participate in the family meeting because you interact with Maude on a regular basis.

1. What information is important for the occupational therapy assistant to provide in each of the following areas:
   a. Physical abilities
   b. Cognitive abilities
   c. Emotional state
   d. Environmental aspects
   e. The context in which incidents of unsafe use of the chair occur
2. What features of a manual wheelchair do you think will be important to include in order to minimize the effect this change will have on her mobility?

CASE STUDY 12-3 PEDIATRIC WHEELCHAIR TRAINING

Matthew is a 4-year-old boy who just started preschool. He has severe cerebral palsy, affecting upper and lower extremities, trunk, and head control. At rest his tone is low. When excited or when completing an activity, his tone increases. His head control is fair. He is unable to sit independently. He has a slight startle reflex to loud noises. Matthew has some right-hand function, as evidenced by his ability to play computer games using a four-position switch array. Matthew is nonverbal and communicates with facial expressions, gestures, sounds, yes/no signals, and a picture board. His communication is purposeful. He is able to express his needs and engage in a limited conversation with his picture board. His vocabulary is increasing rapidly now that he has some means to communicate. His functional vision appears to be intact.

Matthew's parents have used a solid-based stroller for mobility. They did not want to obtain a wheelchair as they wanted Matthew to walk. However, they recently realized that Matthew wants to be able to move about his environment independently and agreed to the purchase of a powered wheelchair. He recently received his powered wheelchair, with a four-position switch array embedded into the lap tray as a controller. You are the rehabilitation assistant who is responsible for conducting his powered wheelchair training.

QUESTIONS

1. Describe three stages in the training in use of a powered mobility device and give an example of an activity that you think would be beneficial at each stage.
2. How would you arrange the environment for Matthew in the initial stages of powered wheelchair training?
3. What opportunities would you use to help Matthew learn to control the chair, while at the same time ensuring his safety in the environment?
4. What skills do you think Matthew should demonstrate consistently before he uses his powered wheelchair in an environment with other children?

STUDY QUESTIONS

1. Describe the three broad categories of wheeled mobility systems.
2. Describe one aspect of a resident's cognitive, physical, and affective behavior or skill that a rehabilitation assistant may observe which provides useful information for a wheelchair assessment.
3. Describe one aspect of each of the physical, social, and institutional contexts that has the potential to affect a client's ability to use a manual wheelchair.
4. Describe three situations or behaviors that a rehabilitation assistant would observe that would suggest that a client should change from a manual to a power wheelchair.
5. What are the two major structures of a wheelchair?
6. Describe and contrast the advantages and disadvantages of tilt versus recline systems. What are the indications for the recommendation of each?
7. Discuss the relationship of the center of mass of the user to the center of mass of the wheelchair as it was described in the various sections of this chapter. What are the implications of this relationship to function?
8. What are the ways in which pediatric wheelchairs can accommodate growth?
9. List the four types of standing systems and give an advantage and disadvantage of each. What are the major benefits of these systems?
10. Define bariatrics and discuss the implications of wheelchair configuration and use for this population.
11. Discuss the considerations of wheelchair use and configuration for elderly clients.
12. Identify the different locations of the drive wheels of an electrically powered wheelchair and describe how each affects the function of the chair.
13. What types of control interfaces are typically used for powered wheelchairs?
14. What types of batteries are used in powered wheelchairs? How do they differ from automobile batteries? What is the difference between wet cell and gel batteries?

REFERENCES

1. Algood SD, Cooper RA, Fitzgerald SG, et al: Effect of a pushrim-activated power-assist wheelchair on the functional capabilities of persons with tetraplegia, *Arch Phys Med Rehabil* 86(3):380–386, 2005.
2. American National Standards Institute/Rehabilitation Engineering and Assistive Society of America: *American National Standard for Wheelchairs – volume 2: additional requirements for wheelchairs (including scooters) with electrical systems*, New York, 1998, ANSI/RESNA.
3. Aylor J, et al: Versatile wheelchair control system, *Med Biol Eng Comput* 17(1):110–114, 1979.
4. Belanger A, Martel L, Caron-Malenfant E: *Population projections for Canada, provinces and territories, 2005–2031*, Ottawa, ON, 2005, Ministry of Industry.
5. Boninger ML, Souza AL, Cooper RA, et al: Propulsion patterns and pushrim biomechanics in manual wheelchair propulsion, *Arch Phys Med Rehabil* 83(5):718–723, 2002.
6. Boninger M, Koontz AM, Sisto SA, et al: Pushrim biomechanics and injury prevention in spinal cord injury: recommendations based on CULP-SCI investigations, *J Rehabil Res Dev* 42(3):9–20, 2005.
7. Bruner JS: Organization of early skilled action, *Child Dev* 44(1):1–11, 1973.
8. Buck S: More than 4 wheels, Milton, ON, 2009, Therapy Now! Inc.
9. Bureau of the Census: *U.S. interim projections by age, sex, race, and Hispanic origin*, March 2004. Table 2a, "Projected population of the United States, by age and sex: 2000 to 2050", available at www.census.gov/ipc/www/usinterimproj/natprojtab02a.pdf.
10. Center for Disease Control: State-specific prevalence of obesity among adults—United States, 2005, *MMWR Morb Mortal Wkly Rep* 55(36):985–988, 2006.
11. Cooper RA: *Wheelchair selection and configuration*, New York, 1998, Demos Medical Publishing.
12. Cooper RA, Boninger ML, Rentschler A: Evaluation of selected ultralight manual wheelchairs using ANSI/RESNA standards, *Arch Phys Med Rehabil* 80(4):462–467, 1999.
13. Cooper RA, Gonzalez J, Lawrence B, et al: Performance of selected lightweight wheelchairs on ANSI/RESNA tests, *Arch Phys Med Rehabil* 78(10):1138–1144, 1997a.
14. Cooper RA, Robertson RN, VanSickle DP, et al: Methods for determining three-dimensional wheelchair pushrim forces and moments: a technical note, *J Rehabil Res Dev* 34(2):162–170, 1997b.
15. Cossette L: *A profile of disability in Canada, 2001*, Ottawa, ON, 2002, Ministry of Industry.
16. Daus C: *The right fit, Rehab Manag*, Aug./Sept. 2003, Available online: http://www.rehabpub.com/features/892003/4.asp. Downloaded October 31, 2006.
17. Deitz J, Swinth Y, White O: Power mobility and preschoolers with complex developmental delays, *Am J Occup Ther* 56(1):86–96, 2002.
18. Denison I, Gayton D: Redefining power wheelchair, *Proc 17th Int Seat Symp* 2001, pp 119–120.
19. Eng JJ: Use of prolonged standing for individuals with spinal cord injury, *Physical Therapy*, 81: 1392–1399, 2001.
20. Eng JJ: Getting up goals, *Rehab Manag* Jan./Feb. 2004. Available online: http://rehabpub.com/features/1022004/5.asp. Downloaded October 28, 2006.
21. Engstrom B: *Ergonomic seating: a true challenge*, Sweden, 2002, Posturalis Books.
22. Fass MV, et al: Durability, value, and reliability of selected electric powered wheelchairs, *Arch Phys Med Rehabil* 85(5):805–814, 2004.
23. Fields CD: Groundwork: casters, *Team Rehabil Rep* 3(2): 22–23, 33,1992.
24. Finley MA, Gordes KL, Meginniss S, et al: Effect of 2-speed manual wheelchair wheel on shoulder pain in wheelchair users: preliminary findings. In *Proc 22nd Int Seat Symp*, 2006.
25. Furumasu J, Guerette P, Tefft D: Relevance of the pediatric powered wheelchair screening test for children with cerebral palsy, Dev Med Child Neuro 46:468–472, 2004.
26. Giesbrecht EM, Ripat JD, Quanbury AO, et al: Participation in community-based activities of daily living: comparison of a pushrim-activated, power-assisted wheelchair and a power wheelchair, *Disabil Rehabil Assist Tech* 4(3): 198–207, 2009.

27. Ham R, Aldersea P, Porter D: *Wheelchair users and postural seating: a clinical approach,* New York, 1998, Churchill Livingstone.
28. Howarth S, Pronovost LM, Polgar JM, et al: Use of a geared wheelchair wheel to reduce propulsive muscular demand during ramp ascent: analysis of muscle activation and kinematics, *Clin Biomech (Bristol, Avon)* 25(1):21–28, 2010.
29. Howarth SJ, Polgar JM, Dickerson CR, et al: Trunk muscle activity during wheelchair ramp ascent and the influence of a geared wheel on the demands of postural control, *Arch Phys Med Rehabil* 91(3):436–442, 2010.
30. Kaye S, Kang T, LaPlante MP: Wheelchair use in the United States. In *Disability Statistics Abstract 23,* 2002.
31. Kemper K: Strollers: a growing alternative, *Team Rehabil Rep* 4(2):15–19, 1993.
32. Kermoian R: Locomotor experience facilitates psychological functioning: implications for assistive mobility for young children. In Gray DB, Quatrano LA, Lieberman ML, editors: *Designing and using assistive technology,* Baltimore, 1998, Paul H. Brookes.
33. Kirby RL: *Wheelchair Skills Program v. 3.2,* 2005. Available from: www.wheelchairskillsprogram.ca.
34. Kirby RL, Swuste J, Dupuis DJ, et al: The wheelchair skills test: a pilot study of a new outcome measure, *Arch Phys Med Rehabil* 83(1):10–18, 2002.
35. Kirby RL, et al: The wheelchair skills test (version 2.4): measurement properties, *Arch Phys Med Rehabil* 85(5):794–804, 2004.
36. Kreutz D: Power tilt, recline or both: looking at all aspects of the evaluation of a client for a tilt or recline system requires medical and environmental needs, *Team Rehab Rep* 29–32, March 1997.
37. Lange ML: Tilt in space versus recline: new trends in an old debate, *Tech Spec Int Sec Quart* 10:1–3, 2000.
38. Lange ML: Evaluating the options, *Rehab Manag,* Feb. 2002. Downloaded from www.rehabpub.com/features/22002/2.asp
39. Lange M: Power wheelchair access: assessment and alternative access methods. In *Proc 21st Int Seat Symp* January 2005, pp 87–88.
40. Livingstone R: A critical review of power mobility assessment and training for young children, *Disabil Rehabil Assist Technol* 5(6):392–400, 2010.
41. Mendoza RJ, Pittenger DJ, Savage FS, Weinstein CS: A protocol for assessment of risk in wheelchair driving within a healthcare facility, *Dis & Rehabil* 25, 520–526, 2003.
42. Mogul-Rotman B, Fisher K: Stand up and function, *Rehab Manag* Aug./Sept. 2002. Available online: http://www.rehabpub.com/features/892002/3.asp. Downloaded October 28, 2006.
43. Mortenson B, et al: Perceptions of power mobility use and safety within residential facilities, *Can J Occup Ther* 72(3):142–152, 2005.
44. Mortenson B, et al: Overarching principles and salient findings for inclusion in guidelines for power mobility use within residential care facilities, *J Rehabil Res Dev* 43(2):199–208, 2006.
45. Pearlman JL, Cooper RA, Karnawat J, et al: Evaluation of the safety and durability of low-cost nonprogrammable electric powered wheelchairs, *Arch Phys Med Rehabil* 86(12): 2361–2370, 2005.
46. Phillips K, Fisher K, Miller Polgar J: Thinking beyond the wheelchair, In *Proc 21st Int Seat Symp,* 2005, pp 97–98.
47. Ragnarsson KT: Prescription considerations and a comparison of conventional and lightweight wheelchairs, *J Rehabil Res Dev Clin Suppl* (2):8–16, 1990.
48. Rentschler AJ, et al: Evaluation of select electric-powered wheelchairs using the ANSI/RESNA standards, *Arch Phys Med Rehabil* 85(4):611–619, 2004.
49. Robson M: 25 Choices: Manual wheelchair configuration and new technology, In *Proc 20th Can Seat Mob Conf* 2005, p 113.
50. Rosen L, et al: RESNA position paper on the application of power wheelchairs for pediatric users, *Assist Tech* 21(4): 218–226, 2009.
51. Sawatzky BJ, Kim W, Denison I: Ergonomics of different tyres and tyre pressure during wheelchair propulsion, *Ergonomics* 47:1475–1483, 2004.
52. Sawatzky BJ, Slobogean GP, Reilly CW, et al: Prevalence of shoulder pain in adult- versus childhood-onset wheelchair users: a pilot study, *J Rehabil Res Dev* 42(3) Suppl 1:1–8, 2005.
53. Scherer MJ: Introduction. In Scherer MJ, editor: *Assistive technology: matching device and consumer for successful rehabilitation,* Washington, 2002, American Psychological Association, pp 3–13.
54. Schmeler M, Buning ME: Manual wheelchairs: set-up and propulsion biomechanics, 1999. http://www.wheelchairnet.org/wcn_wcu/SlideLectures/MS/5WCBiomech.pdf. Downloaded September 8, 2006.
55. Smith ME: The applications of tilt and recline, 2004. http://www.wheelchairjunkie.com/tiltandrecline.html. Downloaded October 28, 2006.
56. Sprigle S, Press L: Reliability of the ISO wheelchair cushion test for loaded contour depth, *Assist Technol* 15(2):145–150, 2003.
57. Taylor SJ, Kreutz D: Powered and manual wheelchair mobility. In Angelo J, editor: *Assistive technology for rehabilitation therapists,* Philadelphia, 1997, FA Davis.
58. Trefler E, et al: *Seating and mobility for persons with physical disabilities,* Tucson, Ariz, 1993, Therapy Skill Builders.
59. Veeger HE, Rozendaal LA, van der Helm FCT: Load on the shoulder in low intensity wheelchair propulsion, *Clin Biomech* 17(3):211–218, 2002.
60. Wang Q: *Disability and American families: 2000,* Washington, 2005, U.S. Census Bureau.
61. Warren CG: Powered mobility and its implications, *J Rehabil Res Dev Clin Suppl* (2):74–85, 1990.
62. Wilson B, McFarland SR: Types of wheelchairs, *J Rehabil Res Dev Clin Suppl* (2):104–116, 1990.
63. Wilson K, Miller Polgar J: The effects of wheelchair seat tilt on seated pressure distribution in adults without physical disabilities., In *Proc 21st Int Seat Symp,* 2005, pp 115–116.
64. World Health Organization: International classification of functioning, disability and health (ICF), Geneva, 2001, World Health Organization.

CHAPTER 13

Technologies for Transportation and Driving

KEY TERMS

Booster Seat
Child Vehicle Restraint System
Crashworthiness
Driving Evaluation
Forward-Facing Infant Seat
Large Accessible Transit Vehicles (LATVs)
Original Equipment Manufacturer (OEM)
Primary Driving Controls
Rear-Facing Infant Seat
Secondary Driving Controls
Vehicle Seat Belt Assembly
Wheelchair Tie-Down System
Wheelchair Tie-Down and Occupant Restraint System

CHAPTER OUTLINE

LEARNING OBJECTIVES

Upon completing this chapter, you will be able to do the following:

1. Describe correct use of child restraint systems for passenger safety
2. Describe correct use of child restraint systems designed for children with special needs
3. Understand basic features of standards for crashworthiness of wheelchairs and seating systems
4. Understand use and basic features of standards for wheelchair tie-downs and occupant restraint systems
5. Identify major components of driver evaluation
6. Discuss major design features to consider when making a vehicle purchase
7. Discuss vehicle access issues for individuals with disabilities
8. Describe vehicle modifications to promote access for individuals with disabilities
9. Describe primary and secondary driving controls

Robert Murphy, a social anthropologist who described his experience with a spinal tumor in a book called *The Body Silent,* eloquently describes how the loss of the ability to drive deprived him of the spontaneity to go places when he wanted to.

> The inability to drive was more than a retreat from mobility, for it was one step away from spontaneity and the free exercise of will. Whereas I could once act on whim and fancy, I now had to exercise planning and foresight. This was true of even the simplest of actions.[25]

Chapter 12 focused on personal mobility systems, specifically manual and electrically powered wheelchairs, that afford individuals the ability to move within their immediate environment and for short distances between local environments. In this chapter, we consider mobility systems that afford movement over longer distances, such as movement between home, school, work, and community sites such as shopping and leisure venues, as well as travel between communities. Our focus is on safe personal (car, van, etc.) and public transportation across the lifespan, including travel as a passenger or a driver. This chapter discusses technology that enables a person with a disability to ride safely in a vehicle (private or public) using devices provided by the original equipment manufacturer (OEM), infant/child restraint systems, or wheelchair occupant restraint systems. The chapter also describes devices that assist individuals to transfer into and out of the vehicle, including those devices that assist the caregiver. Box 13-1 lists a number of useful Web sites.

SAFE TRANSPORTATION FOR CHILDREN

Legislation exists in most jurisdictions that requires children of certain weights and heights to travel in a **child vehicle restraint system**. The majority of jurisdictions require children under 40 pounds to be properly secured in a vehicle restraint system. An increasing number

BOX 13-1 Suggested Web Sites for Further Information on Transportation Safety

GENERAL INFORMATION
- National Highway and Traffic Safety Administration: www.nhtsa.org
- Healthy Canadians (Health Canada): http://healthycanadians.gc.ca/index-eng.php
- University of Michigan Transportation Research Institute: www.umtri.umich.edu/news.php
- Monash University Accident Research Centre (Australia): www.monash.edu.au/muarc/

SAFE TRANSPORTATION FOR CHILDREN
- American Academy of Pediatrics: www.aap.org/healthtopics/carseatsafety.cfm
- Canadian: http://www.tc.gc.ca/eng/roadsafety/safedrivers-childsafety-index-53.htm
- Australian: http://www.rta.nsw.gov.au/roadsafety/children/childrestraints/index.html

OLDER DRIVER SAFETY
- Canadian Association of Occupational Therapists Older Driver Safety: www.olderdriversafety.ca
- American Occupational Therapy Association Older Driver Safety: www.aota.org/Older-Driver.aspx
- CanDrive: www.candrive.ca
- American Automobile Association Foundation: www.seniordrivers.org
- Rehabilitation Engineering Research Center on Wheelchair Transportation Safety: www.rercwts.org
- Vehicle Safety for People Who Use Wheelchairs: www.travelsafer.org

are also requiring the use of booster seats for children who weigh more than 40 pounds (e.g., the majority of the U.S. states, five provinces in Canada, the UK, and Australia). Many children with mild-to-moderate seating needs can safely sit in vehicle restraint systems that are produced for children who have no special seating needs. Our discussion begins with these products, including their proper use and installation. The array of products is vast and constantly changing. The following discussion is general, and readers should review specific requirements in their own jurisdictions, particularly those related to booster seats.

Vehicle Restraint Systems for Children

There are three main types of vehicle restraint systems for children: **rear-facing infant seats, forward-facing infant seats,** and **booster seats**. A number of Web sites provide access to up-to-date information on the proper use and installation of these devices for their specific jurisdiction (Box 13-2). The Co-operators Insurance and the Infant and Toddler Safety Association have the "Buckle up Bears" education program. Daimler-Chrysler and the U.S. National Highway Traffic Safety Administration (NHTSA) offer the "SeatCheck" program, which provides free car seat inspections and a determination of whether the vehicle restraint system is properly installed.* In the United States, the NHTSA maintains current information on vehicle restraint systems. The American Pediatric Association also provides current information on vehicle restraint systems, including those specifically for children with disabilities. Federal regulations exist that govern the structure and testing of vehicle restraint systems, including those for children with disabilities. In the United States, the Federal Motor Vehicle Safety Standards (FMVSS) group produces these regulations, and in Canada they are produced by the Canadian Motor Vehicle Safety Standards (CMVSS) organization. Restraint systems that meet these regulations are labeled with a sticker identifying either FMVSS or CMVSS and the specific standard that the system has met. These regulations can be found at http://www.nhtsa.dot.gov/cars/rules/rulings/ChildRestrSyst/Index.html or http://www.tc.gc.ca/eng/roadsafety/safedrivers-childsafety-index-53.htm for the U.S. or Canadian standards, respectively.

BOX 13-2 Web Sites Providing Information on Vehicle Restraint Systems for Children

INFANT AND TODDLER ASSOCIATION
http://www.infantandtoddlersafety.ca/

CO-OPERATORS' INSURANCE BUCKLE UP BEARS
http://www.cooperators.ca/en/About-Us/community/signature-safety-programs/car-safety-with-bub.aspx
http://www.seatcheck.org/

NATIONAL HIGHWAY TRAFFIC SAFETY ADMINISTRATION
www.nhtsa.org

AMERICAN ACADEMY OF PEDIATRICS
www.aap.org/healthtopics/carseatsafety.cfm

Rear-facing infant seats (Figure 13-1, *A*) are intended for use from the time the infant leaves the hospital after birth to the time they reach 12 months and 22 pounds (10 kg). While most vehicle restraint systems indicate a height and weight limit for the child, rear-facing infant vehicle restraint systems have an age and weight limit, which means that the child must be 12 months of age before they are turned to the forward-facing position. Infants younger than this age do not have sufficient head control and their bones are not sufficiently developed to withstand even a minor crash.[1] A common error on the part of parents is to move a child to the next type of child vehicle restraint system too early.[10,36,37,38] Many children reach the 22-pounds/10-kg weight limit well before their first birthday. In this instance, they should be moved to a vehicle restraint system that will accommodate their

* http://www.seatcheck.org/

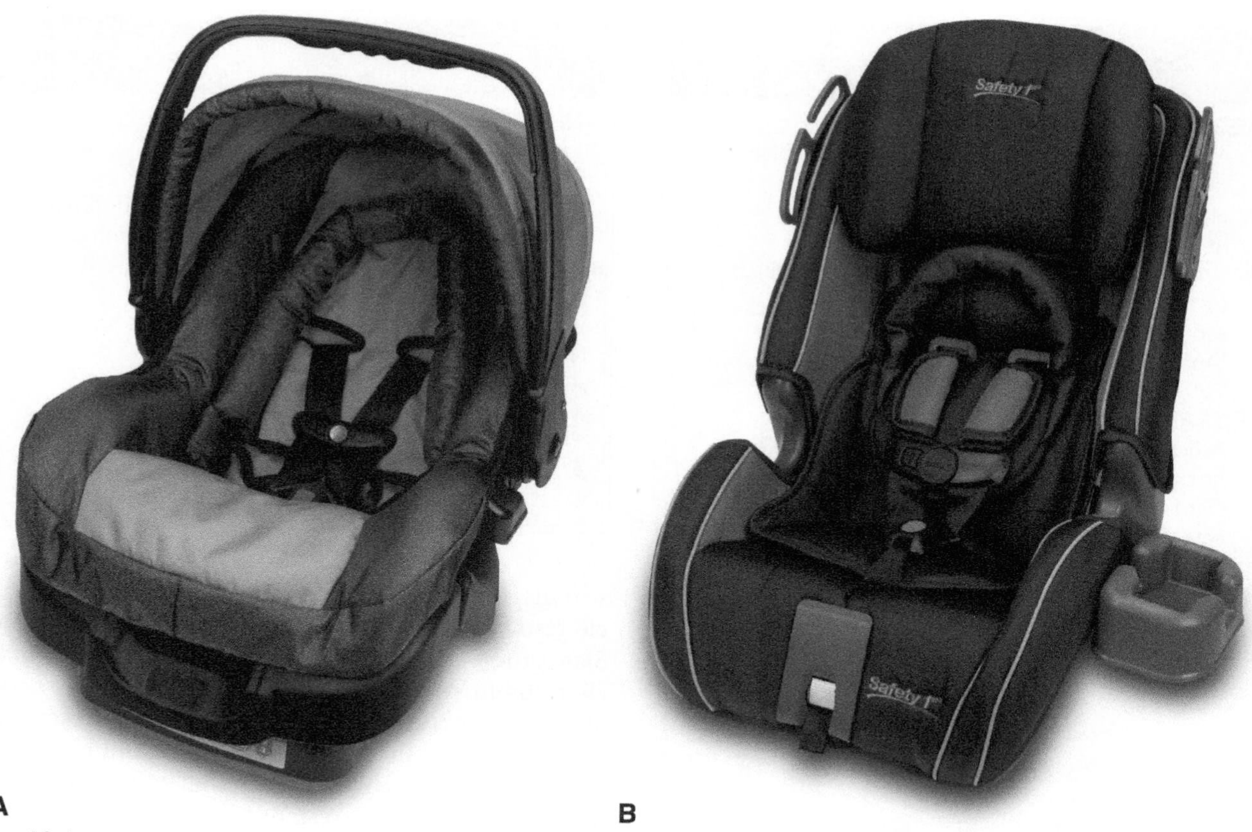

A B

Figure 13-1 A, Rear-facing infant restraint system. B, Forward facing child restraint system. (Courtesy of Dorel Juvenile Group: www.safety1st.com.)

heavier weight but will allow them to remain in the rear-facing position. Rear-facing infant seats are typically not left in the vehicle in the long term. Instead, the child is transported in the infant seat between the vehicle and destination. The car seat belt system provides restraint for the child and the seat inside the vehicle. Some seats secure into a base that remains installed in the vehicle over the long term.

Forward-facing vehicle restraint systems (Figure 13-1, *B*) are intended to be installed in a vehicle and remain for the long term. These systems typically accommodate children up to 40 pounds and 40 inches. This technology does change, so it is important to check your local area for the current law. Useful information can be found on the Web sites listed in Boxes 13-1 and 13-2, or check with your local jurisdiction.

Proper installation of these systems is critical. A biomechanical study of parents installing a forward-facing vehicle restraint system into a mock-up of the back seat of a sedan found that proper installation required efforts that were higher than the maximum that many participants were able to produce. Because the space in the back seat area is limited, parents were in postures that made it difficult to tighten straps so that the restraint system was properly secured. These postures put parents at risk for low back injury.[12,29]

Two errors are common when installing the forward-facing car seat: (1) nonuse or misuse of the tether strap, and (2) improper use of the strapping system of the restraint system.[20,22] These seats all fasten to the vehicle frame with a tether strap. All new vehicles in North America are equipped with tether anchors, which allow the seat to be fastened to a ring that is attached to the vehicle frame. The tether strap must be fastened and tightened so that an excursion of the restraint system of no more than ½ inch is allowed. The strapping component of the restraint system should be snug to the seat with the chest buckle about two fingers' width below the child's neck. Often, these straps are loose, allowing the child to wiggle free of them. Since 2002, vehicles have been equipped with Lower Anchor Tethers of Children (LATCH) (U.S. name) and Lower Universal Anchorage Systems (Canadian name) that make installation of forward-facing car seats simpler. Clasps attached to the restraint system are attached to anchors that are fixed at the level of the seat. These systems are tested to a weight of 48 pounds (21 kg). Box 13-3 summarizes the research on misuse of child safety restraint systems.

Once a child reaches 40 pounds and 40 inches, they can be moved to a booster seat. Again, this specification varies by jurisdiction and by product, so it is important to know the product specifications and to be up to date with legislation in your jurisdiction. These seats position the child so the vehicle seat belts fit properly. The vehicle seat belt provides restraint when a booster seat is used. Figure 13-2 shows the proper positioning of the seat belt,

BOX 13-3 What the Research Says—Common Misuses of Child Vehicle Restraint Systems

- Child is moved too early to another type of restraint system (e.g., child is moved to use of only a seat belt when they should still be restrained in a forward-facing restraint system).[10,36,37,38]
- Tether strap attaching child seat to vehicle seat is often too loose.[20,22]
- Tether strap attaching child seat to vehicle seat is not used.[20,22]
- Clip system that anchors child seat to vehicle seat is either not used properly or not used at all.[8]
- Child and restraint system are seated in front passenger seat.[9]
- Straps that hold the child in the restraint system are either too loose or not used at all.[20]
- Chest buckle is either too high or too low.[20,22]
- Pelvic straps are too loose or not used at all.[20,22]
- After market devices such as padding placed on straps that hold the child are added; these devices can change the effectiveness of the device in protecting the child in the event of a crash.[1]

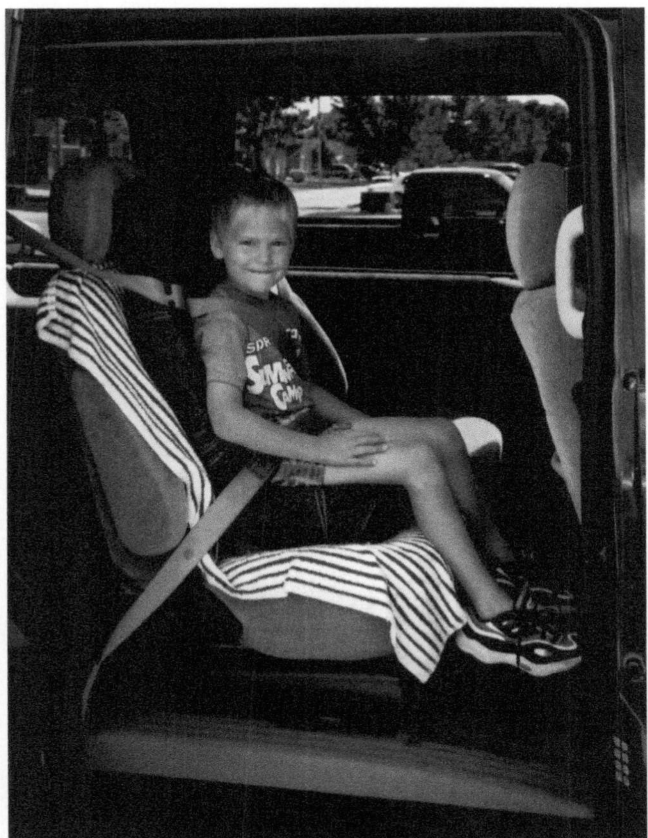

Figure 13-2 Proper positioning in a booster seat.

coming over the shoulder and not across the neck, and across the lap and not the abdomen. Booster seat laws are relatively recent and do not necessarily have the same provisions for when the child is ready to move to use the **vehicle seat belt assembly** alone. Usually, a child is ready to move to use of the vehicle seat belt only when they reach 80 pounds and are at least 4 feet 9 inches in height. Some booster seat laws specify an age at which a child can be moved to the vehicle seat belt assembly. However, given the variations of height and weight, some children will not be tall or heavy enough at the specified age to be safely restrained by the vehicle seat belt assembly, so they will benefit from remaining in the booster seat.

Location in the Motor Vehicle

The safest location for the child in a motor vehicle is the center rear seat.[1,2,9] When this position is not available, the right outboard seat (opposite side of the driver) is preferred because this seat is usually on the side of the lane that borders the road shoulder rather than the side that faces oncoming traffic (at least in jurisdictions where vehicles travel on the right side of the road). Booster seats require the use of a three-point seat belt assembly (i.e., one that has both a shoulder and lap portion), which sometimes precludes locating the child who uses a booster seat in the rear center seat because the restraint system in this location does not always include the shoulder portion. Children under the age of 12 should not travel in the front passenger seat of a vehicle that has passenger-side air bags. The air bags can seriously injure or kill a young child when they deploy. Some advances have been made, and there are "smart" air bags that sense the weight of the occupant of the front passenger seat and either adjust the force of the air bag deployment or turn it off.

Vehicle Restraint Systems for Children with Disabilities

As previously mentioned, some children with mild-to-moderate seating needs are able to use a car seat that is designed for children without disabilities. This option is preferred, when possible, due to the costs of vehicle restraint systems that are designed specifically for children with disabilities. In some cases, the child may be able to use the child restraint system without any modification. When modifications to these systems are required, elements of the system that are provided by the **Original Equipment Manufacturer (OEM)** cannot be altered or removed since the system was crash-tested with those elements present. Alteration or removal may limit the ability of the seat to protect the child in a crash. Similarly, nothing can be placed underneath the padding or the straps. In the case of the strapping system, placing something underneath alters the direction of the pull on the child's body and may cause him to be ejected from the seat in a crash. However, rolls can be placed alongside the child's legs, trunk, or head to help them maintain an upright position. A roll can also be placed under the child's knees to reduce extensor tone.[3]

Some children with disabilities cannot be safely transported in a child vehicle restraint system that is designed for children without disabilities, or they do not have sufficient postural control to be safely secured by the vehicle seat belt

BOX 13-4 Websites of Manufacturers of Safety Systems for Children with Disabilities

Britax	www.childseat.com
Besi	www.BESI-INC.com
Columbia Medical	www.columbiamedical.com
E-Z-On Products	www.ezonpro.com
Q-Straint	www.qstraint.com
Sammons Preston	www.tumbleforms.com
Snug Seat	www.snugseat.com

assembly once they become too heavy to safely use other restraint systems. Some indicators of the need for a vehicle restraint system that is specifically designed for children with disabilities are children with tracheostomies, children with either excessive high or low tone for whom the typical restraint system does not provide sufficient support, and children who have a spica cast following hip surgery.

Current commercial systems for children with disabilities can accommodate children up to 130 pounds and 56 inches/142 cm. The weight limit varies on these products so the ATP needs to check to determine that the child can be accommodated safely. In addition to accommodating children who are heavier than 100 pounds, these systems provide more postural support. In particular, these systems provide support to position the pelvis and trunk so that the child can maintain an upright position while seated. Postural control may be achieved by the form of the seat shell, providing contouring of the seat and more integral fit with the child's body, or by padding that is supplied by the manufacturer. Some of these products have the option for the addition of a pommel to maintain leg abduction. Tilt in the system helps maintain postural control in a similar manner as that provided in mobility systems described in Chapter 12. These systems must meet federal safety standards and be crash tested for use as a vehicle restraint system. Systems that meet federal requirements will have the FMVSS or CMVSS sticker or appropriate labeling from another jurisdiction. Transportation for children who are unable to maintain a sitting position is difficult. Federal regulations exist for car beds but the companies that manufactured or distributed these devices no longer produce them. The E-Z-ON Vest remains on the market as a product that will help restrain the child in the supine position. Box 13-4 lists Web sites of companies that manufacture child safety systems for children with disabilities.

SAFE TRANSPORTATION OF INDIVIDUALS USING WHEELCHAIRS

A person who routinely uses a wheelchair for mobility is safest in a motor vehicle when she is able to transfer into the vehicle seat and use the belt restraint systems that are supplied by the OEM. When transfers are not possible, the individual may travel in a motor vehicle while remaining seated in her wheelchair. Three factors collectively influence the increasing number of individuals who remain seated in their wheelchairs while riding in a motor vehicle: (1) legislation that promotes the rights of individuals with disabilities, (2) standards that are applied to wheelchairs and tie-down systems that relate to the design and testing of these devices for use in a motor vehicle, and (3) the increased availability of vehicle modifications that allow the wheelchair to be secured safely.

Crashworthiness of Wheelchairs and Seating Systems

Voluntary standards have been developed by ANSI/RESNA and the ISO that make provisions for the testing of wheelchairs and seating systems to determine their performance in a 21 g/48 km/h (30 mph) frontal impact crash simulation. These standards are: *ISO 7176-19: Wheeled Mobility Device for Use in Motor Vehicles,*[5,14] *ANSI/RESNA Wheelchairs/Volume 1: Requirements and Test Methods for Wheelchairs (including Scooters),*[4] and *ISO 16840: Seating Devices for Use in Motor Vehicles.*[17] See Box 13-5 for a summary of the ANSI/RESNA WC-19 standard. The first two standards identify crash test procedures and manufacturer requirements for labeling and provision of information for a wheelchair and its dedicated seating. The use of an after-market seating system invalidates the wheelchair crash testing. Because many consumers purchase a wheelchair from one manufacturer and a seating system from another, ISO 16840 makes provisions for testing of a

BOX 13-5 Summary of ANSI/RESNA WC-19 Standard

THE ANSI/RESNA WC-19 STANDARD

- Specifies general design requirements, test procedures, and performance requirements related to frontal impact performance for manual and powered wheelchairs.
- Applies to passengers in paratransit, public transit, school bus, over-the-road coaches, and personally licensed vehicles.
- Applies to securement of wheelchairs by four-point-strap–type tie-down systems that are occupied by children and adults.
- Applies to a wide range of wheelchairs, including manual, powerbase, three-wheeled scooters, tilt-in-space wheelchairs, and specialized mobile seating bases with removable seating inserts.
- Specifies strength and geometric requirements for wheelchair securement points and occupant restraint anchorage points on the wheelchair.
- Provides requirements and information for wheelchair accessory components, seat inserts, and postural support devices with regard to their design and use in motor vehicles.
- Applies primarily to wheelchairs that are retrofitted for use as a motor vehicle seat by the addition of after-market add-on components.

seating system independent of a specific wheeled mobility base. These standards are specific to a frontal impact crash; further development is required to test **crashworthiness** in side and rear impact crashes. Similar standards for wheelchair transportation exist or are being developed for Canada (Z605), Australia (AS-2942), and other parts of the world (ISO 10542, Parts 1 to 5). More information can be found on standards for wheelchair transportation on the Web site of the Rehabilitation Engineering Research Center on Wheelchair Transportation Safety (RERC WTS).* It is important to remember that the vehicle restraint system (i.e., the vehicle seat belt) provides restraint for the wheelchair occupant. The straps affixed to the wheelchair, which are intended to provide seating and positioning support to the user, will not protect the user in a crash.[6,31] The rating system that evaluates use of the vehicle restraint system considers the following factors: the size of the opening through which the vehicle restraint system is threaded, the contact of the system with the consumer's body and where that contact is made, the angle of the pelvic portion of the restraint system, and whether or not the vehicle restraint system comes into contact with any sharp surfaces.[5,14,17] As was described earlier for positioning of the vehicle restraint system for a child using a booster seat, the vehicle restraint system must sit across the pelvis, not the abdomen, and rest on the shoulder, not on the neck. Further, the vehicle restraint system must not be held away from the user's body by any part of the wheelchair or seating system. When assisting a person who uses a wheelchair, it is important to pay attention to these specifications in particular: that the seat belt strapping is not in contact with a sharp surface that can damage it, and that the seat belt is properly positioned on the individual and in contact with their body.

ISO 7176-19 and the corresponding ANSI/RESNA standard require manufacture of a frame that has four securement points for a **wheelchair tie-down system**. These standards apply to manual and electrically powered wheelchairs as well as scooters. Wheelchairs that have been successfully crash tested are commonly referred to as WC-19 chairs. As noted initially, these standards are voluntary, with the result that only a small percentage of wheelchairs have been crash tested. A number of reasons for this small proportion were identified at a recent "State of the Science Workshop on Wheelchair Transportation Safety."[19] These reasons included the concerns of manufacturers about assuming legal liability for marketing a wheelchair as conforming to WC-19 standards, the lack of knowledge of safe transportation requirements and issues on the part of many ATPs and consumers, the added expense of purchasing a WC-19 chair, the voluntary nature of the standards, and the fact that the standards are more rigorous and conflict with federal regulations for safe transportation in a public vehicle.[32]

* www.rercwts.org

The requirements for manufacturers to warn users of potential hazards provide useful information regarding safe transportation for persons who travel seated in their wheelchairs. The most protected position is for individuals to be seated forward facing, yet on many public transit vehicles, the configuration for securement of a wheelchair seats the individual sideways. In addition to being unsafe in a crash, the individual feels less secure as she is required to adjust to the acceleration and deceleration of the vehicle. Any peripheral devices such as a communication system or a laptray need to be removed from the chair and stored securely. Chest harnesses are recommended only when they have a quick release mechanism. While they may be useful in aiding proper positioning of the shoulder component of the vehicle restraint system, they do have the potential to restrict the user's airway if they come loose.[6] A head rest is also recommended.[6]

Wheelchair Tie-Down and Occupant Restraint Systems

The person with a disability is best protected from injury if she transfers to the vehicle seat and uses the standard OEM's restraint system. (See Box 13-6 for a summary.[28]) However, for many individuals with disabilities, transferring to the seat of a vehicle is not possible or practical. For these individuals, the wheelchair functions as the vehicle seat. Once the person is inside a personal or public vehicle, as either a passenger or a driver, both she and the wheelchair need to be properly restrained for safety. The four-point strap tie-down system with the three-point occupant restraint system is considered to be the standard means of securing a passenger who is seated in a wheelchair in a vehicle[35]. It is important to view **wheelchair tie-down and occupant restraint systems (WTORS)** as separate parts of a total system designed to protect the passenger or driver who uses a wheelchair.[34] The system that secures the wheelchair to the vehicle (wheelchair tie down) should be separate from the restraint that protects the occupant (i.e., the occupant restraint, which is the vehicle seat belt assembly as previously

BOX 13-6 Principal Elements of SAE Recommended Practice J2249:

1. Upper as well as lower torso restraint should be provided.
2. Restraint forces should be applied to the bony regions of the body and not the soft tissues.
3. Postural supports should not be relied upon as occupant restraints.
4. The occupant should face forward in the vehicle.
5. Adequate clear space should be provided around the occupants seated in wheelchairs.

From: ANSI/RESNA WC-18 / SAE J2249 - Wheelchair Tiedown and Occupant Restraint Systems for Use in Motor Vehicles, http://www.rercwts.org/RERC_WTS2_KT/RERC_WTS2_KT_Stand/Intro_WC18.html

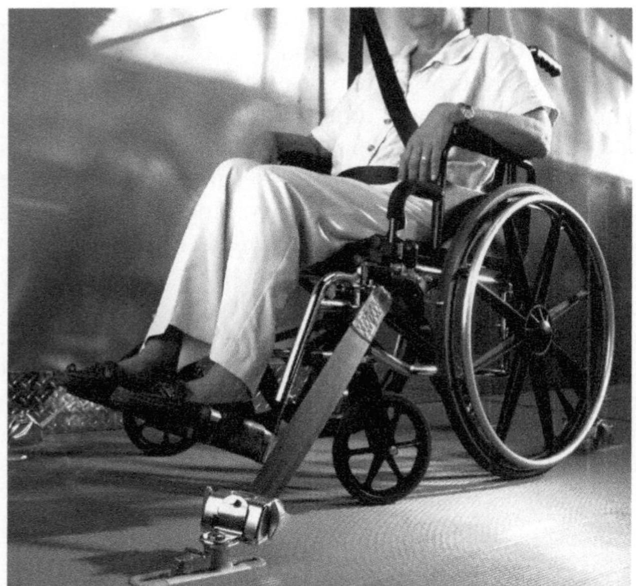

Figure 13-3 Wheelchair tie-down securement system for use of wheelchair in a vehicle. Q-Straint wheelchair tie-down system. (Courtesy of Q-Straint: www.qstraint.com.)

described). The standards that specify the design, testing, and manufacturer labeling and information are in *ISO 10542, Parts 1–5, Wheelchair tie-down and occupant restraint systems*. Tie-down systems secure the wheelchair to the vehicle floor (see Figure 13-3). There are two types of tie downs that have been crash tested: four-point strap and docking types.[13,18] The four-belt type of tie down, the most commonly used system in public transit vehicles, secures the wheelchair at each corner of the frame. In front the belts are attached to the frame (not the leg rests) just above the front caster pivot. WC-19 chairs have very obvious locations for the attachment of these straps. The strapping system and buckles are similar to those used in the aircraft industry for securing cargo. The major advantage of belt systems is their low cost and their ability to secure most types of wheelchair frames. Their disadvantage is that use is time consuming and cumbersome and cannot be done independently by the wheelchair rider. Dependence on the ability of the person providing assistance to properly fasten the belt systems is another disadvantage.

Docking systems have two components: a bracket that is secured to the vehicle floor and a component that is fixed to the lower portion of the wheelchair that couples with the bracket. These systems are specific to each model of wheelchair, thus limiting their use in public transit vehicles. Figure 13-4 shows the E-Z Lock system. Some of these devices have an auto-engage feature; all have some feedback mechanism that tells the user that the wheelchair is properly secured.[31] A switch control that is either activated by the wheelchair rider or by another vehicle occupant disengages the wheelchair from the docking component. The major advantages are quick and easy connection and independent use by the wheelchair rider. The disadvantage is that they require adding hardware to the wheelchair (which adds weight), they cannot be used in a public transit vehicle, and they are two to five times as expensive as belt systems.

For occupant restraint during transit on a public vehicle, variations of seat and shoulder belts, similar to those used in passenger cars, can be coupled with the four-belt and docking tie-downs to form a complete WTORS. These restraints are also regulated under ISO 10542. The occupant restraint systems used on a public transit vehicle can be attached either directly to the van floor or to a point that is common to the tie-down attachment point. It is less likely that the wheelchair and occupant will move different

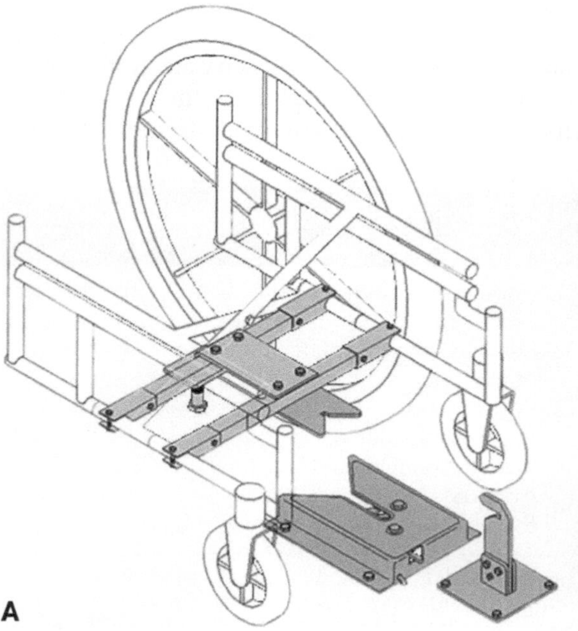

A

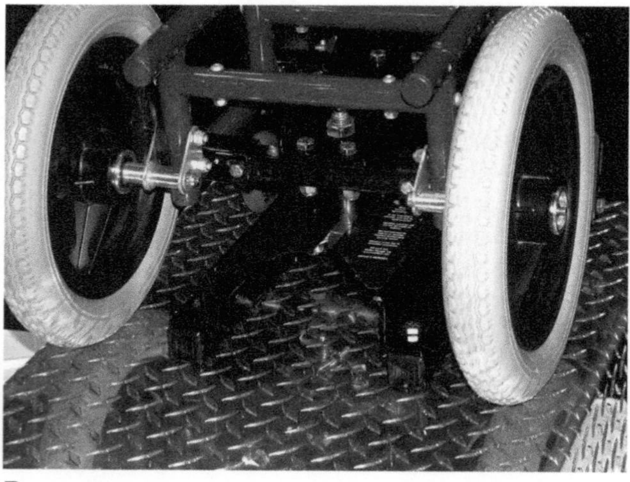

B

Figure 13-4 **A,** Schematic depicting the components of the E-Z Lock system; **B,** Wheelchair connected to E-Z Lock system in a vehicle. (Courtesy of EZ Lock: www.ezlock.net.)

distances during a collision if the occupant restraint is attached to the latter point. If they are not attached at the same point, it is likely that the wheelchair will move farther, forcing the occupant into the restraint and causing injury.[34] Another advancement in the technology for securing wheelchairs in a vehicle is a passive, rear-facing system that is being introduced in Canada, Australia, and Europe for **large accessible transit vehicles (LATVs)**. This technology uses a securement station based on external structures rather than straps to protect the passenger in the event of a crash. A padded structure that fits closely to the person's back and head protects in forward motion, the wall of the vehicle and a bar on the opposite side limit lateral movement, and the brakes of the wheelchair and the user's ability to grasp a bar limit rearward movement.[35] Wheelchair riders prefer this system because they can use it independently. However, problems remain, most notably the unreliability of many manual wheelchair brakes and the great variance in the ability of individuals to grasp and hold the barrier to stabilize themselves.[13] No industry standards exist for these stations.

EVALUATION AND TECHNOLOGIES FOR TRANSPORTATION AND DRIVING

Access to a private vehicle is an important enabler of daily activities, particularly in North America where people depend more on private vehicles than on public transportation. Further, public transportation that is accessible to individuals who use wheelchairs is limited, particularly in rural or remote areas. This section discusses technologies that assist drivers and passengers. Technologies that assist driving are often recommended by a driver rehabilitation specialist, who not only provides assessment but also training to ensure that the device is used safely.

Evaluation for Driving

An individual may require a **driving evaluation** for a variety of reasons including physical disability such as spinal cord injury, impairments resulting from a cerebral vascular accident or traumatic head injury, or age-related changes such as vision loss. A driving evaluation may be used to determine whether an individual whose license has been removed due to an illness such as a stroke is safe to return to driving or whether an individual who is currently driving remains safe to do so. The decision to recommend to a regulatory body that an individual is no longer safe to drive is a difficult one for two reasons: (1) the knowledge that removing a person's driver's license frequently results in withdrawal from social activities and depression[24] and (2) the concern that this conclusion is based on sound assessment procedures. Two consensus conferences on driving evaluation recently published their findings.[21,33] These conferences were prompted by concern that a common driving evaluation was not being used.

A driving evaluation usually has two components: an off-road assessment that is paper-based and/or computer-based, and an on-road component with a trained evaluator. In some situations, performance on the off-road assessment may indicate that the client is not safe to proceed with an on-road evaluation, or that the on-road evaluation should be conducted in a safer environment such as a closed-circuit course.

Both consensus groups recommended that the off-road assessment should include cognitive, physical, visual, and perceptual elements although these were not necessarily defined in the same way. The international group[33] also included cutaneous sensation as an element and the Canadian group[21] included behavior as a component. Both groups recommended that a medical history, driving history, and assessment of knowledge of rules of the road be completed. Box 13-7 provides a list of functions that are recommended for evaluation as part of a driving assessment.

Pre-driving Rehabilitation

The rehabilitation assistant may provide training to an individual on skills that support driving but are not specific to driving. These skills may be cognitive, motor,[11] perceptual, sensory, or functional. These skills parallel many of the components identified in Box 13-7. In the cognitive domain, the rehabilitation assistant may provide activities that promote attention, problem solving, and memory. Motor activities may promote range of motion, strength, balance and postural control, endurance, and reaction time. Perceptual skills include visual scanning, proprioception, spatial relations, and figure-ground distinction.

Important functional activities include transferring in and out of a vehicle, opening and closing the door, fastening/unfastening the seat belt, and stowing or removing items from the vehicle. Transferring into and out of the vehicle was an activity that was frequently noted by.[30] Participants frequently indicated concerns about balance when entering and exiting the vehicle as well as assisting others.

Vehicle Selection

A number of factors are important when selecting a vehicle for a person with a physical disability. Some of these include: whether the person will use the vehicle seat or a wheelchair, vehicle access, visual aspects, location and size of primary and secondary driving controls, and seat belt and air bag design. Resources are available to assist with the process of selecting a vehicle. Most of these are geared to the elderly population. Box 13-8 lists resources that are useful in guiding the choice of a vehicle.

Ingress and egress refer to getting into and out of the vehicle. Shaw, Miller Polgar, and colleagues conducted semi-structured interviews with seniors about their use of vehicle features.[30] Seniors reported a number of factors that made ingress and egress easier, including whether the

BOX 13-7 Common Assessment Components of Off-Road and On-Road Driving Evaluations

COGNITION
- Attention (sustained, divided, alternating)
- Memory
- Orientation
- Impulse control
- Judgment
- Insight
- Planning
- Problem solving

VISION*
- Acuity
- Useful field of view
- Contrast sensitivity
- Visual field
- Accommodation and adaptation
- Visual tracking

MOTOR
- Range of motion (neck, upper and lower extremities)
- Upper and lower extremity strength
- Coordination (fine and gross motor)
- Balance and postural control
- Endurance
- Reaction time

SOMATOSENSORY
- Proprioception
- Cutaneous sensation

VISUAL PERCEPTION
- Visual scanning
- Figure-ground
- Depth perception
- Spatial relations
- Form constancy

ON-ROAD EVALUATION
- Stop at stop sign or light
- Right- and left-hand turns
- Merge into ongoing traffic
- Lane change
- Driving on roads with different speed limits
- Acceleration/deceleration

*A licensed/registered vision care professional typically conducts the assessment of vision.

BOX 13-8 Resources for Selecting a Vehicle

- American Automobile Association Car Fit: Helping Mature Drivers Find the Perfect Fit: www.Car-Fit.org
- Canadian Association of Occupational Therapists Older Driver Safety Web Site: www.olderdriversafety.ca

height of the seat roughly matched their hip, a wide door opening, and some form of handle to help them steady themselves. Seats that have less bucketing also make transfers easier. The Handybar is a small after-market device that fits into the frame of the vehicle and provides a handle that is available to assist transfers. This device is readily available at many commercial health care outlets. Figure 13-5 shows an aftermarket modification of a passenger seat that pivots 90 degrees and then moves forward and down to come out of the vehicle to facilitate transfers. Seniors also reported that the weight of the door affected ingress and egress; a door that was too heavy was a concern because seniors felt less stable when they reached out to close it. Once in the vehicle, the driver should determine access to the steering wheel, pedals, and controls for secondary functions such as windshield wipers.

Visual aspects are another consideration when selecting a vehicle. The driver needs to determine the sightlines in the vehicle and whether she has clear visual access to the front, the side, and the mirrors. Further, the driver needs to determine whether she can read the information on the dashboard, both during the day and at night. A final aspect of vision relates to the location of various controls. Are controls for important features such as the temperature and wipers located in such a way that a quick glance away from the road is sufficient to guide a reach to use them?

The location and size of the controls have physical as well as visual implications. Consideration should be made of the range of motion required to reach vehicle controls for features such as wipers, turn indicators, temperature controls, and the window defroster. Are they of sufficient size that the driver or passenger can target them accurately when reaching? What force is required to activate them? What action is required to activate them? Modifications to these controls are discussed in a later section.

Seniors who participated in a study[30] overwhelmingly indicated that seat belts were problematic. They were difficult to reach, fasten, and unfasten. Participants had difficulty seeing the coupling mechanism. In some vehicles the location of the receiving part of the seat belt is very difficult to see. Seat belts did not fit properly (as described above), often sitting uncomfortably on the neck. Some after-market products are available that attempt to make seat belts more comfortable. These devices are not regulated, so there is the potential that they may invalidate any crash testing completed with the seat belt and limit the potential of the seat belt to protect the occupant in a crash. After-market devices should not alter the proper fit or the direction of travel of the seat belt.

Consideration should be made of the safe use of air bags. The driver should sit about 10 inches away from the steering wheel to avoid injury from an air bag that is

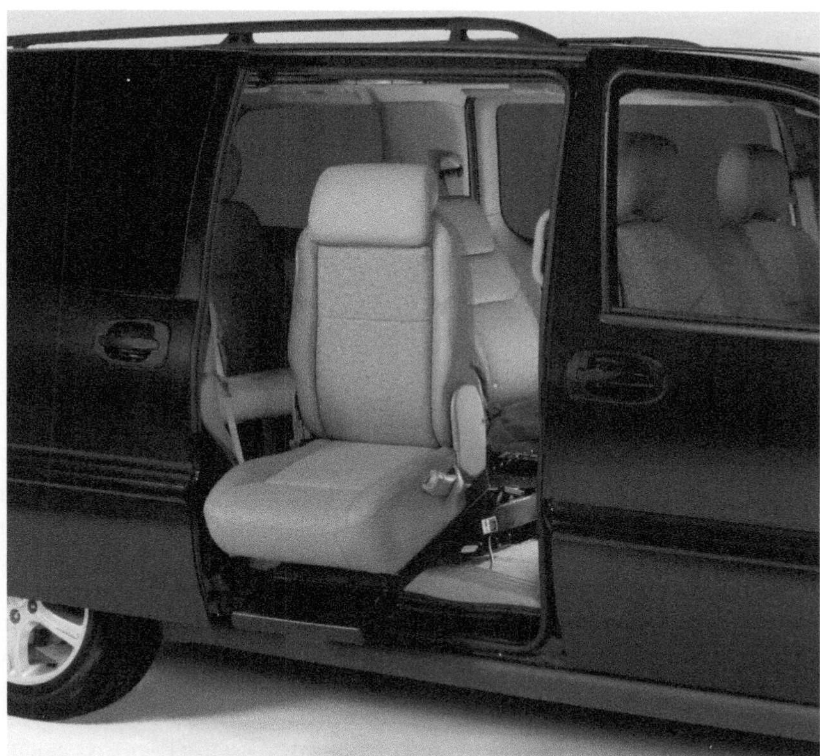

Figure 13-5 After-market seat modification that rotates seat 90 degrees and moves it toward outside of vehicle to facilitate transfer. (Courtesy of Braun Corporation: www.braunlift.com.)

activated at less than that distance. The height and weight of passengers is a further issue. Car manufacturers recommend that children under the age of 12 years should not occupy the front seat in a car equipped with passenger air bags due to the risk of serious injury or death. Adults who are the same height or weight as a typical 12 year old are at similar risk. Many new vehicles have sensors in the seat that vary the force with which the air bag activates or whether the air bag activates in a crash, based on the weight of the seat occupant.

Access to storage of a mobility device and any regularly transported equipment should be checked. If a vehicle occupant uses a wheelchair that is transported with them, it is important to determine whether the wheelchair will fit in the vehicle and how difficult it is to lift and position the device in the vehicle. This suggestion seems like a very obvious one, but it is one that can be neglected with a very frustrating outcome.

A final consideration is whether an individual who uses a wheelchair will transfer into the vehicle seat or whether they will be transported in their wheelchair. This discussion will focus on the driver, because of access issues to driving controls, but many of the comments will be applicable to a passenger who regularly uses a wheelchair. Transfer to the vehicle seat provides the most protection for the occupant because the OEM's seat belt provides the most effective protection in a crash.[31] The vehicle seat back and headrest also provide better protection than that of a wheelchair seating system. The vehicle seat should put a driver in a better position to reach necessary controls. However, use of the vehicle seat does require the ability to complete a transfer relatively easily. Generally, a seating system will provide the user with a better functional position than a vehicle seat will.[27] The most important limitation of using the vehicle seat concerns individuals at risk for pressure ulcers. Vehicle seats are not designed with tissue integrity in mind and over a long trip, a pressure ulcer could easily develop. Chapter 4 discusses principles of seating for tissue integrity. In this regard, it is important to consider information about risk indicators for the development of a pressure ulcer. The benefits and limitations of remaining in a wheelchair during transportation are the reverse of the above with some additional factors. The wheelchair seating system is designed to give better postural control and trunk stability than a vehicle seat, which are important safety considerations for either a driver or a passenger.[27,31] However, any vehicle tie-down system will not be as safe a restraint as the OEM's system. A less apparent consideration is the suspension system of the wheelchair. Vehicle seats do not have suspension systems, so the seat does not move independently of the vehicle. Such is not the case with a wheelchair with a suspension system. Travel in these chairs may have the uncomfortable side effect of motion sickness.[27]

Vehicle Access

Ingress and egress issues for an individual who transfers into a vehicle seat were considered previously. In this section we will discuss access issues for individuals who

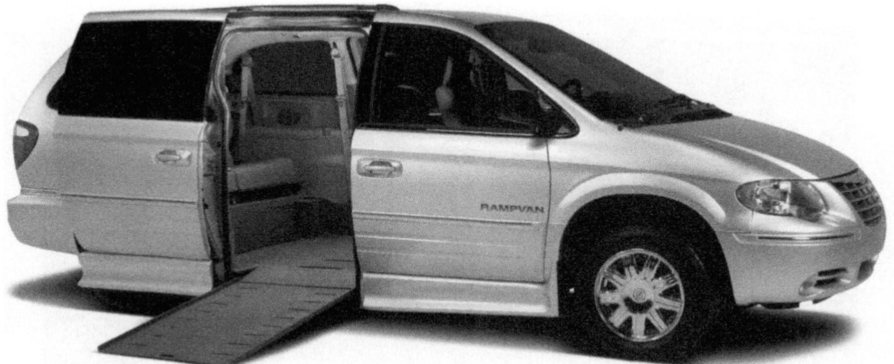

Figure 13-6 Side access ramp for transfer with wheelchair into and out of vehicle. (Courtesy of Braun Corporation: www.braunlift.com.)

remain in their wheelchairs for transportation. In these instances, the vehicle will be a modified van. We will also consider after-market devices that load and store the wheelchair once the user has transferred to a vehicle seat.

Van modifications typically involve provision of a ramp for access and a tie-down system to secure a wheelchair. The latter were discussed in an earlier section of this chapter. Ramps are either side- or rear-loading and either manual or power operated. They provide access through the sliding passenger door or the rear. Figure 13-6 shows a lowered floor that accesses the side sliding passenger door. Newer designs store the ramp in a recessed area on the van floor so they don't interfere with access inside the vehicle. Many car manufacturers provide reimbursement for after-market modifications required to make a vehicle accessible (e.g., Chrysler's Automobility* and GM's Mobility† programs). The Web addresses for the main van conversion companies are listed in Box 13-9.

Integration of the wheelchair with the van modifications is critical. A mismatch between these mobility devices is a very expensive mistake. The consumer needs to know the dimensions and configuration of his wheelchair before proceeding with van modifications. The following should be considered: (1) the width of the wheelchair for movement through the opening into the vehicle and maneuvering once inside the vehicle; (2) the height of the wheelchair for head clearance (remember that a tilt chair may increase the overall height); and (3) the length of the wheelchair and consequent turning radius (keep in mind that the front rigging and the need for a reclined position will increase the length of the wheelchair). If a person remains in their wheelchair to drive, there are further considerations. He must be able to fit into the space allocated for the driver and in between the driver and passenger seats. The seat height must not interfere with the travel of the steering wheel. He or she must be able to reach the necessary controls and be able to see out of the front and side windows and access the mirrors. In some situations, if the wheelchair seat height is too high, the driver will not be able to see out of the front window.[27] These are important considerations; a modified van that does not accommodate the user's wheelchair is of no benefit.

If it is not possible for the individual to load a wheelchair manually into the vehicle, there are powered wheelchair-loading devices that can assist with this function. These devices pick up and store a manual wheelchair in the back seat, in the trunk, or in a carrier attached to the roof or back of the car. Figure 13-7 shows an example of a loading device that folds and stores a conventional wheelchair inside a cover that is mounted on top of the car. The other advantage of this type of loading device is that the wheelchair does not take up room in the trunk or back seat. These devices can be operated either from outside or inside the vehicle.

* http://www.chryslergroupllc.com/enus/community/automobility/pages/automobility.aspx

† http://www.gm.com/vehicles/services/gm_mobility/

BOX 13-9 Van Conversion Companies

- Braun Corporation: www.braunlift.com
- Access Mobility Systems: www.accessams.com
- Ricon Corporation: www.riconcorp.com
- Access Unlimited: www.accessunlimited.com

MODIFICATIONS FOR DRIVING

The driver with a disability needs to be carefully evaluated for any modifications that are being considered. It is assumed here that the driver has been previously determined to be able to drive and has a valid driver's license. The assessment of an individual for driving modifications progresses in a logical manner, starting with an assessment of her ability to operate the primary controls, followed by an assessment of the use of the secondary controls. Once modifications are recommended, only a reputable dealer should install them. In most cases, an OTR/driver rehabilitation specialist will assess and make recommendations for driving modifications and provide training in their safe use, in collaboration with a driving instructor.

Primary Driving Controls

The **primary driving controls** are those that are used to stop (brakes), go (accelerator), and steer. Modifications are available to assist the driver to maintain a grip on the

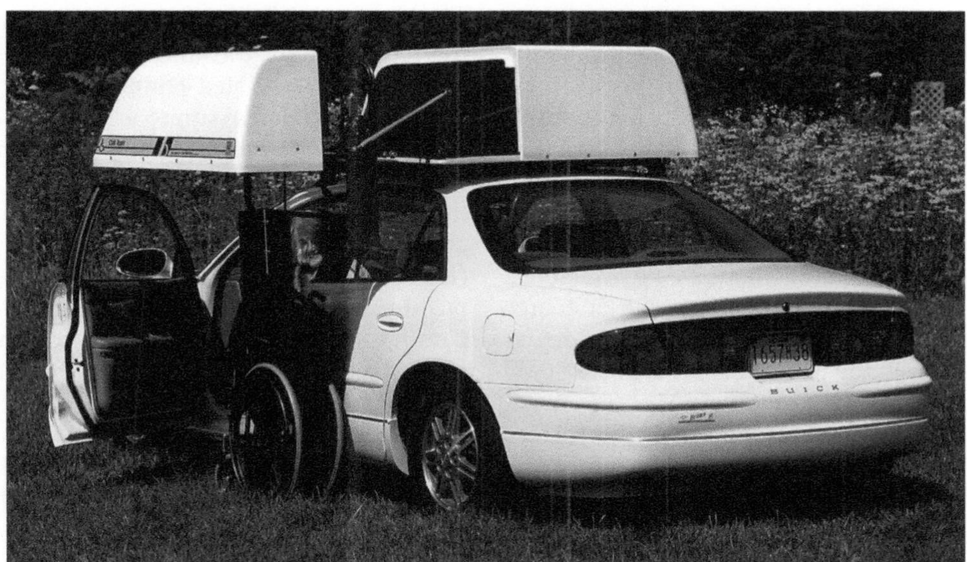

Figure 13-7 Wheelchair loading device for a sedan. (Courtesy of Braun Corporation: www.braunlift.com.)

steering wheel, to access the pedals, or to control the vehicle with the hands and arms only when the driver does not have use of his legs to control the vehicle. Each of these vehicle modifications will be considered in turn.

There are a number of options to consider for steering for drivers who use one arm, use a prosthetic arm, or have impaired arm and hand function. For a driver who uses one hand to steer, a steering device allows the driver to maintain control of the wheel at all times.[23] Evaluation of the client's hand function determines both the type and location of the device.[7] Steering devices attach directly to the steering wheel or to a bar that stretches across the inner diameter of the wheel and is attached to each side of the steering wheel. These devices are frequently removable so that another person can drive the vehicle.[7] Steering devices (shown clockwise in Figure 13-8) include palm grip, tri-pin, fork-grip or V-grip, spinner knob, and amputee ring (for use with prosthetic hooks). Additional modifications for steering may include a reduced-effort or zero-effort steering

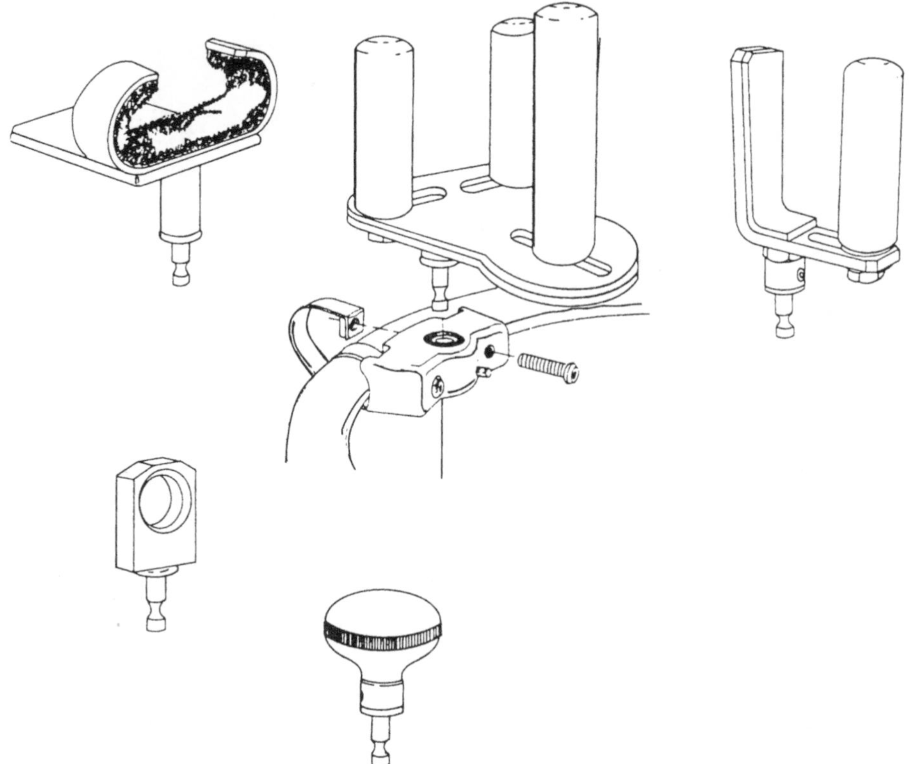

Figure 13-8 Different steering aids that accommodate a variety of consumer needs. (Courtesy of Mobility Products and Design.)

mechanism, a steering wheel of reduced diameter, height and angle adjustments to the steering column, and reduced gain (i.e., the number of turns of the steering wheel required to pivot the wheels from fully left to fully right). Reduced- or low-effort steering systems reduce the effort required for steering a vehicle by 40%, whereas zero-effort systems are able to reduce the effort required by 70%.[26]

Two primary types of pedal adaptations are available: a left foot accelerator and pedal extensions.[7] The latter are available from many OEMs and are used by individuals who are not able to reach the pedals. As the name would indicate, the left foot accelerator allows the driver to control both braking and acceleration with the left foot. This device is also removable for other drivers. It requires an automatic transmission vehicle.

Hand controls for accelerator and brake consist of a mechanical linkage connected to each pedal, a control handle, and associated connecting hardware. There are four common design approaches: push-pull, push-twist, push-right-angle-pull,[7,23,26] and push-tilt.[7] In each case the first designation (e.g., push) refers to activation of the brake and the second (e.g., pull or twist) is used for activation of the accelerator. When using a push control (Figure 13-9, *A*), the consumer activates the brakes by pushing on a lever in a direction directly away from him, parallel to the steering column. Acceleration is accomplished either by pulling back on the control, rotating it, or pulling downward at a right angle to the steering column. The weight of the user's hand is sufficient to maintain a constant velocity. When the accelerator control is released, it returns to the off position. These controls are

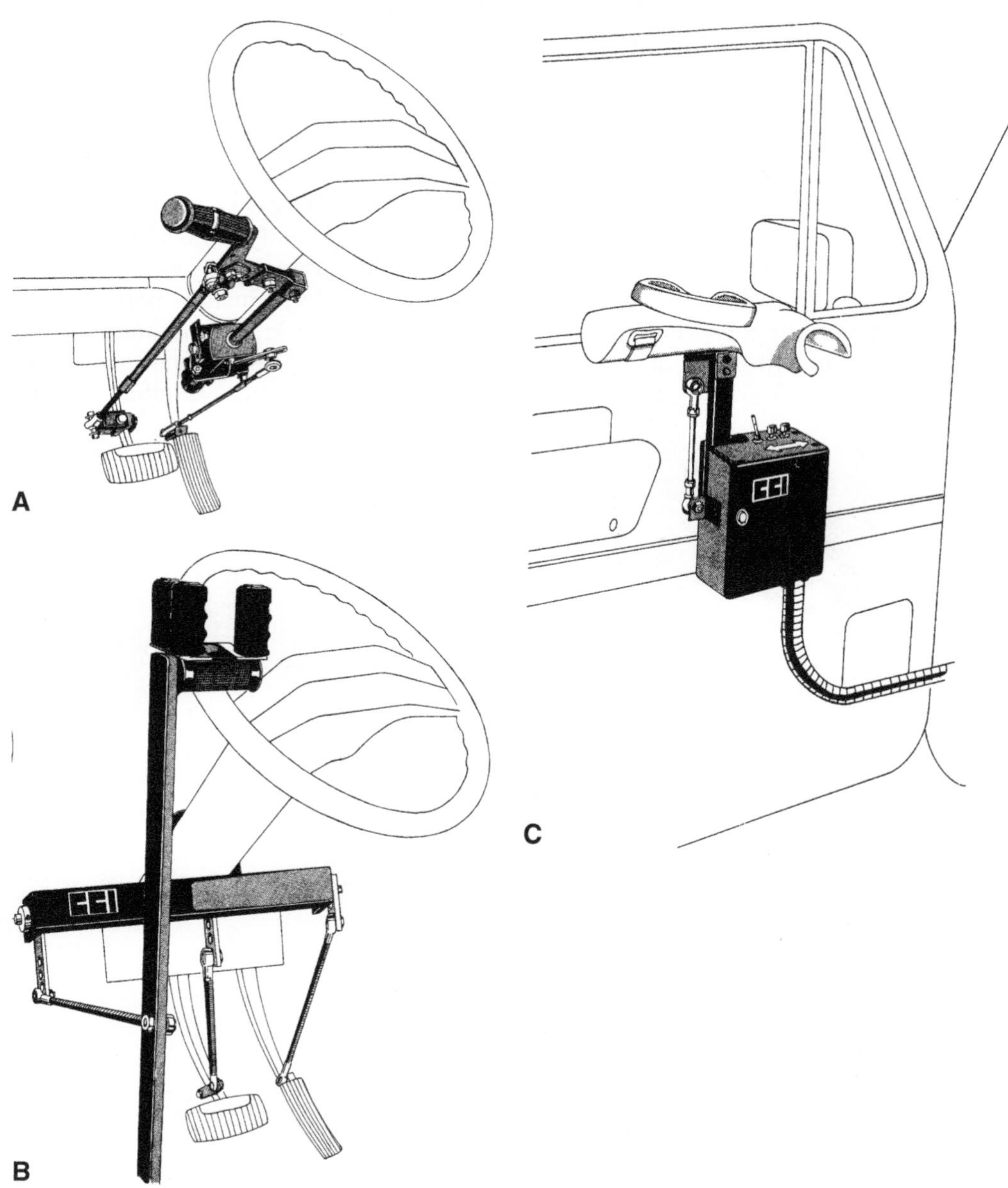

Figure 13-9 Hand controls for braking and acceleration. **A,** Push-twist hand control; **B,** Mechanically assisted manual system. **C,** Electrically assisted controller and interface. (Courtesy of Creative Controls, Inc.)

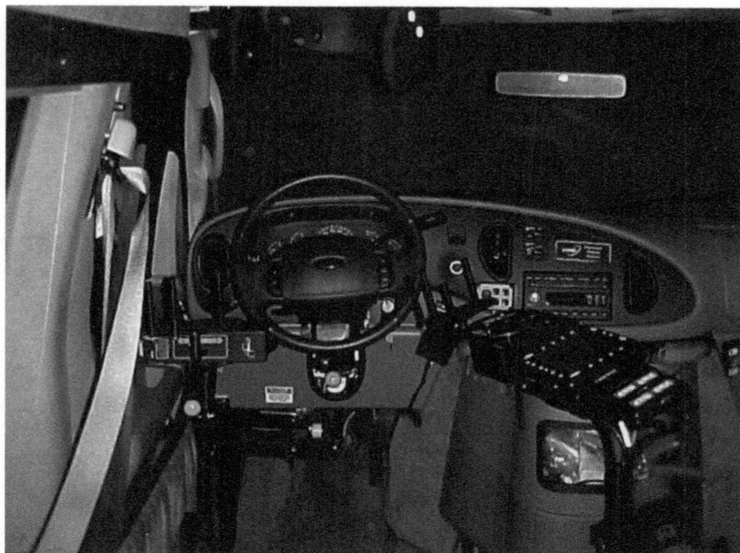

Figure 13-10 Control panel for primary and secondary driving control. (Courtesy of Access Mobility Systems: www.accessams.com.)

normally operated with the left hand, and the right hand is used for steering; however, right-hand mounting systems are also available from a variety of manufacturers.[7]

Additional assistance is required for persons with weak upper extremities (e.g., high-level spinal cord injury). There are two basic approaches: (1) mechanical assist and (2) power assist. Mechanical assist systems use one of the approaches described previously, but they provide a lever arm that affords a mechanical advantage (Figure 13-9, *B*). Instead of connecting the hand control directly to the accelerator and brake pedals, there is a mechanical linkage that magnifies the force applied by the user. Typically this linkage is a long arm, attached to the floor, which is pulled back for acceleration and pushed forward for braking. The arm is also linked to the pedals through connecting hardware. Power-assisted devices use either hydraulic or pneumatic assist (similar to power brakes or steering) or electronically powered systems. Electronically powered systems add servomotors that apply force to the brake and accelerator system. An electronically assisted brake and accelerator control is shown in Figure 13-9, *C*. One of the most recent developments is the use of a joystick that the driver pulls back for acceleration and pushes forward for braking.

Secondary Driving Controls

In addition to the controls necessary to maneuver the vehicle, **secondary driving controls** are needed for safe operation of a vehicle. These include devices that assist the driver to activate turn signals, parking brakes, lights, horn, the ignition, temperature control (heat and air conditioning), and windshield wipers. The mechanisms for operating secondary controls, as provided by the OEM, may not be within reach of the driver or may be of such a shape that the driver cannot operate them.[7] These mechanisms can be adapted by adding extensions or a differently shaped control or by relocating them so the driver can use them. A control panel that contains all these functions can also replace the standard controls. This panel is a special-purpose membrane keyboard that interfaces through a microcomputer to activate the secondary functions. It is mounted to either side of the steering wheel in a location that is within reach of the driver (see Figure 13-10). Drivers who only have the use of one hand have the option of a voice-activated control panel that activates the secondary functions through spoken commands.[7] Many recent advances in vehicle technology make use of these controls much more accessible; for example, the smart key and push-button system that switches on the ignition are available on many current vehicles.

SUMMARY

Access to a vehicle affords independence and the ability to participate in community activities. Technology relating to occupant protection and vehicle access needs to be considered in light of its ability to provide safety when traveling in the vehicle either as a driver or a passenger. In this chapter we considered assistive technology that aids safe transportation for individuals with disabilities. A primary concern is occupant protection, which includes selection and use of proper vehicle restraint systems for children who are not able to use the vehicle seat belt assembly and for individuals with mobility impairments who remain seated in wheelchairs while riding in adapted vehicles. The factors that need to be considered when determining whether an individual can transfer to a vehicle seat or needs to remain in a wheelchair were discussed. Further, the voluntary standards that guide the testing and labeling of wheelchairs for use during transportation and for vehicle tie-down and occupant restraint systems were also discussed. Vehicle modifications that assist driving were also described.

A case study, "Safe transportation while seated in a wheelchair" is included with this chapter. It illustrates a situation in which a rehabilitation assistant has a role. By answering the questions that accompany it, you will integrate some of the information that is found in this chapter.

CASE STUDY – SAFE TRANSPORTATION WHILE SEATED IN A WHEELCHAIR

You are a rehabilitation assistant in a school with a large number of children with special needs. Many of these children are transported to and from school in an adapted bus that has a four belt–type wheelchair tie-down system to secure the wheelchairs in the vehicle during transit. The bus driver and child's parent are responsible for properly securing the child in the morning, on the trip to school. You are responsible with the bus driver for properly securing the children for the trip home. Both power and manual wheelchairs are used by the children while riding the bus. Some children have peripheral equipment attached to their chair (e.g., laptray, AAC system). All of the children have some form of belting system associated with their seating system (e.g., lap belt or chest belt).

CASE STUDY QUESTIONS

1. What is a WC-19 chair? How would you determine if a child's chair is in this category?
2. Describe the proper use of a four-belt wheelchair tie-down system.
3. Which belting system (OEM seat belt or wheelchair seating system straps) provides protection for the child during a crash? What is the proper positioning of these belts?
4. Do you remove peripheral equipment or leave it in place while the child is riding in the vehicle? Justify your answer.

STUDY QUESTIONS

1. What are the three main categories of child restraint systems for vehicles? What are the indications for the use of each category in your jurisdiction?
2. Describe the common misuses of child vehicle restraint systems.
3. What modifications can be made to a child restraint system designed for a typically developing child that can accommodate the positioning needs of a child with a disability? What types of modifications cannot be made to these systems? Why?
4. Describe the advantages and disadvantages of transferring to the OEM vehicle seat for travel in a vehicle, rather than remaining in a wheelchair. Describe the advantages and disadvantages of remaining in a wheelchair when traveling in a vehicle.
5. Name the standards that set the criteria for crash testing and labeling of wheelchairs and seating systems. What are the requirements of these standards?
6. Define a wheelchair tie-down and occupant restraint system.
7. Describe the advantages and disadvantages of each of the two types of wheelchair securement systems for vehicles.
8. Describe the major considerations for selecting a vehicle for use by an individual with a disability, as either a driver or a passenger.
9. Describe the observations that you would make to determine that an individual's wheelchair is compatible with her modified vehicle.

REFERENCES

1. American Academy of Pediatrics, Committee on Injury and Poison Prevention: Selecting and using the most appropriate car safety seats for growing children: guidelines for counseling parents, *Pediatrics* 109(3):550–553, 2002.
2. American Academy of Pediatrics, Committee on Injury and Poison Prevention: Safe transportation of newborns at hospital discharge, *Pediatrics* 104(4):986–987, 1999a.
3. American Academy of Pediatrics, Committee on Injury and Poison Prevention: Transporting children with special health care needs, *Pediatrics* 104(4):988–992, 1999b.
4. ANSI/RESNA: *Wheelchairs/Volume 1: Requirements and test methods for wheelchairs (including scooters)*, Section 19: Wheelchairs used as seats in motor vehicles. Arlington, Va., 2000, American National Standards Institute (ANSI)/ Rehabilitation Society of North America (RESNA).
5. ANSI/RESNA: *Wheelchairs/Volume 4: Wheelchairs used in motor vehicle transportation*, Section 20: Seating devices for use in motor vehicles. Working draft June 2004.
6. Bertocci G, Karg P, Furhman S: Wheelchair seating systems for use in transportation. In Karg P, Schneider L, Hobson D, editors: *State of the science workshop on wheelchair transportation safety: final report 2005*, Pittsburgh, Pa., 2005, RERC on Wheelchair Transportation Safety, pp 35–56.
7. Bouman J, Pellerito JM: Preparing for the on-road evaluation. In Pellerito JM, editor: *Driver Rehabilitation and Community Mobility*, St. Louis Mo., 2005, Mosby, pp 239–253.
8. Decina LE, Lococo KH, Doyle CT: *Child restraint use survey: LATCH use and misuse*, Washington, D.C., 2006, NHTSA.
9. Durbin DR, Chen I, Smith R, et al: Effects of seating position and appropriate restraint use on the risk of injury to children in motor vehicle crashes, *Pediatrics* 115(3):e305–e309, 2005.
10. Ebel BE, Koepsell TD, Bennett EE, et al: Use of child booster seats in motor vehicles following a community campaign: a controlled trial, *JAMA* 289(7):879–884, 2003.
11. Eby DW, Molnar LJ, Kartje PS: *Maintaining safe mobility in an aging society*, Boca Raton, Fla., 2009, CRC Press.
12. Fox M, Sarno S, Potvin J: A biomechanical evaluation of child safety seat installation: forward facing. In *Proceedings of the Inaugural Ontario Biomechanics Conference*, Barrie ON, February 2004, p 53.
13. Hobson DA: Problem-solving the next generation of wheelchair securement for use in public transport vehicles. In Karg P, Schneider L, Hobson D, editors: *State of the science workshop on wheelchair transportation safety: final report 2005*, Pittsburgh, Pa., 2005, RERC on Wheelchair Transportation Safety, pp 57–78.

14. ISO: *ISO 7176-19: Wheelchairs: wheeled mobility devices for use in motor vehicles*, Geneva, Switzerland, October 2001a, International Standards Organization (ISO).
15. ISO: *ISO 10542-1: Technical systems and aids for disabled or handicapped persons—wheelchair tiedown and occupant-restraint systems—Part 1: Requirements and test methods for all systems*. Geneva, Switzerland, July 2001b, ISO.
16. ISO: *ISO 10542-2: Technical systems and aids for disabled or handicapped persons—Wheelchair tiedown and occupant-restraint systems—Part 2: Four-point strap-type tiedown systems*. Geneva, Switzerland, July 2001c, ISO.
17. ISO: *ISO 16840-4: Wheelchair seating—Part 4: Seating systems for use in motor vehicles*, Geneva Switzerland, February 2004, ISO.
18. ISO: *ISO 10542-3: Technical systems and aids for disabled or handicapped persons—Wheelchair tiedown and occupant-restraint systems—Part 3: docking-type tiedown systems*. Geneva, Switzerland, 2005, ISO.
19. Karg P, Schneider L, Hobson D: *State of the science workshop on wheelchair transportation safety: Final report 2005*. Pittsburgh, Pa., 2005, RERC on Wheelchair Transportation Safety. Available from: www.rercwts.pitt.edu.
20. Kohn M, Chausmer K, Flood MH: Anticipatory guidance about child safety seat misuse: lessons from safety seat "check-ups", *Arch Pediatr Adolesc Med* 154(6):606–609, 2000.
21. Korner-Bitensky N, Gélinas I, Man-Son-Hing M, et al: Recommendations of the Canadian Consensus Conference on driving evaluation in older drivers, *Phys Occup Ther Geriatr* 23(2/3):123–144, 2005.
22. Lane WG, Liu GC, Newlin E: The association between hands-on instruction and proper child safety seat installation, *Pediatrics* 106(4 Suppl):924–929, 2000.
23. Lillie SM: Driving with a physical dysfunction. In Pedretti LW, editor: Occupational therapy: practice skills for physical dysfunction, St. Louis, 1996, Mosby.
24. Marottoli RA: Mendes de Leon CF, Glass TA, et al: Consequences of driving cessation: decreased out-of-home activity levels, *J Gerontol B Psychol Sci Soc Sci* 55(6):S334–S340, 2000.
25. Murphy RF: *The body silent*, New York, 1990, W.W. Norton & Co.
26. Peterson WA: Transportation. In Galvin JC, Scherer JM, editors: Evaluating, selecting and using appropriate assistive technology, Gaithersburg, MD, 1996, Aspen Publishers.
27. Phillips K, Fisher K, Miller Polgar J: Transportation integration: thinking beyond the wheelchair. In *Proc 21 Int Seat Symp*, Orlando, Fla., January 2005, pp 97–98.
28. *SAE Recommended Practice J2249: Wheelchair tiedowns and occupant restraint systems for use in motor vehicles*, October 1996, Society of Automotive Engineers revised, January 1999.
29. Sarno S, Fox M, Potvin J: A biomechanical evaluation of child safety seat installation: rear facing. In *Proceedings of the Inaugural Ontario Biomechanics Conference*, Barrie ON, February, 2004, p 54.
30. Shaw, LS., Miller Polgar, J., Vrlkjan, B et al. (2010). Seniors' perceptions of vehicle safety risks and needs. *American Journal of Occupational Therapy*, 64(2):215–224.
31. Schneider LW, Manary MA: Wheeled mobility tiedown systems and occupant restraints for safety and crash protection. In Pellerito JM, editor: *Driver rehabilitation and community mobility: principles and practice*, St. Louis Mo., 2006, Mosby, pp 357–372.
32. Schneider L, Manary M, Bunning ME: Barriers to development, marketing, purchase and proper use of transit-safety technologies. In Karg P, Schneider L, Hobson D, State of Science Workshop on Wheelchair Transportation Safety, *Final Report*, p 4–30, 2005. Downloaded from: http://www.rercwts.org/RERC_WTS2_KT/RERC_WTS2_KT_SOS/WTS1_SOS_pdf/SOS_Final_05.pdf.
33. Stephens BW, McCarthy DP, Marsiske M, et al: International older driver consensus conference on assessment, remediation, and counseling for transportation alternatives: summary and recommendations, *Phys Occup Ther Geriatr* 23(2/3):103–121, 2005.
34. Thacker J, Shaw G: Safe and secure, Team Rehabil Rep 5: 26–30, 1994.
35. van Roosmalen L, Hobson D: Looking toward future wheelchair transportation–what should be our vision and how do we realize it? In Karg P, Schneider L, Hobson D, State of Science Workshop on Wheelchair Transportation Safety, *Final Report*, p 79–89, 2005. Downloaded from: http://www.rercwts.org/RERC_WTS2_KT/RERC_WTS2_KT_SOS/WTS1_SOS_pdf/SOS_Final_05.pdf.
36. Winston FK, Chen IG, Elliott MR, et al: Recent trends in child restrain practices in the United States, *Pediatrics* 113(5):e458–e464, 2004.
37. Winston FK, Durbin DR, Kallan MJ, et al: The danger of premature graduation to seat belts for young children, *Pediatrics* 105(6):1179–1183, 2000.
38. Yakupcin JP: Child passenger safety in the school-age population, *Pediatr Emerg Care* 21(4):286–290, 2005.

CHAPTER 14

Technologies That Aid Manipulation and Control of the Environment

CHAPTER OUTLINE

LEARNING OBJECTIVES

Upon completing this chapter, you will be able to do the following:

1. List functional manipulative tasks that can be aided by assistive technologies
2. Describe low-technology aids that are useful for self-care, school and work, and play and leisure activities
3. Describe the operation of electrically powered feeding aids
4. List the features and design properties of electronic page turners
5. List the functions carried out by electronic aids to daily living systems (EADL)
6. Describe an assessment process for determining the most appropriate EADL system
7. Describe the basic components of EADL systems and how they are implemented

KEY TERMS

Alternative
Augmentative
Continuous Control
Discrete Control
Electrically Powered Feeders
Electrically Powered Page Turners
Electronic Aid to Daily Living (EADL)
Fine Motor Functions
General-Purpose Manipulation Devices
Gross Motor Functions
Head Pointers
Infrared (IR) Transmission
Latched Switch
Momentary Switch
Mouthsticks
Programmable Controllers
Radio Frequency Transmission
Reachers
Remote Control
Specific-Purpose Manipulation Devices
Telephone Controllers
Trainable Controllers

One of the activity outputs described in Chapter 2 (see Figure 2-7) is manipulation. At the most basic level, *manipulation* refers to those activities that we normally accomplish using the upper extremities, particularly the fingers and hand. Many types of "manipulation" are required to use assistive devices, especially those that are electronically controlled. For example, keys must be pressed for computer entry, joysticks controlled for powered mobility, and switches activated for communication devices. We have discussed this type of manipulation in previous chapters, and we exclude it from the general discussion of manipulation in this chapter. In this chapter, we describe gross motor manipulation as reaching, grasping/releasing, lifting, carrying, and coordination of movements such as pushing, pulling, and turning. Fine motor manipulation includes pinch, point, and dexterity of finger movements. The end goal of the integration of these manipulation components is a person's actions in daily and life activities. For example, activities

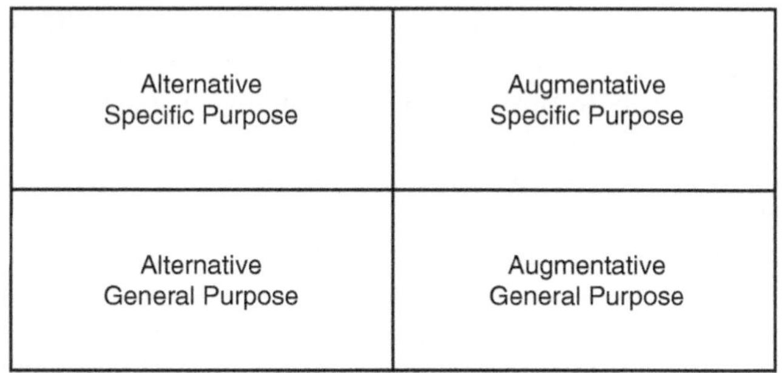

Figure 14-1 Assistive technologies for manipulation can be categorized in two dimensions: general purpose versus specific and alternative versus augmentative.

such as handwriting, food preparation, eating, reaching, using controls in the environment such as door handles and elevator buttons, and appliance control depend on manipulation of physical objects. These types of activities and the technology that supports them are our focus in this chapter.

Figure 14-1 is a characterization of assistive technology devices used for manipulation. As in many other areas of assistive technology application, we can provide manipulative aids that are either **alternative** (a different method of doing the same task) or **augmentative** (assistance in doing the task in the same manner as it is normally done). For manipulation, we can also distinguish devices as being either *specific purpose* or *general purpose.* **Specific-purpose manipulation devices** are designed for only one task, whereas **general-purpose manipulation devices** serve two or more manipulative activities (see Chapter 1). For example, an augmentative, specific-purpose approach to eating may include a modified fork with an enlarged handle. An alternative, special-purpose apparatus for eating is an electromechanical device that lifts food off the plate and up to mouth level when a switch is pressed. A hand splint that allows gripping of any utensil serves as a general-purpose augmentative aid, since it can be used to hold a fork for eating or a pen for writing. In this chapter we discuss all four categories of assistive technologies for manipulation shown in Figure 14-1.

The variety and choice of technology to assist with elements of manipulation have expanded greatly over the past several years. Often a commercially available tool or appliance will work very well for an individual with a disability to assist with manipulation. A commercially available gardening tool with an enlarged handle is an example of universal design, as described in Chapter 1, because it is useful by a wide range of individuals. Many implements for activities such as cooking and gardening are commercially available with enlarged or ergonomically designed handles. In a similar fashion, manufacturers are producing implements with telescoping or long handles. Follow the device selection guidelines described in Chapter 2 to identify devices that will assist a client with many manipulation tasks. Modification of implements they currently own or the purchase of commercially available implements is frequently a simple means to assist with manipulation.

MANIPULATION

The definition of manipulation that was given at the beginning of this chapter suggested that it involves what we do with our upper extremities. Generally, it involves **gross motor functions** (larger and more forceful movement and function) and **fine motor functions** (smaller and more delicate movements). Fine motor coordination is considered to be "the smooth and harmonious action of groups of muscles working together to produce a desired motion."[6] Let's look at the activity of dressing to illustrate gross and fine motor actions. Gross shoulder movements are needed to reach overhead, behind the back, across the midline of the body, and below the waist for lower extremity dressing. Elbow range of motion is needed to assist with reaching. Grasp and release are needed to grab and hold clothes while putting them on and taking them off. Strength is needed for grasp/release as well as to pull clothing up or down, on or off. Fine motor movements are necessary to use zippers, button and unbutton, tie shoelaces, and use fasteners behind the body (e.g., buttons or the hook and eye of a waistband). Gross motor functions important here include reaching; grasping/releasing an object; lifting and carrying an object; and actions such as pushing, pulling, and turning an object or control.

Manipulation can be affected by conditions that affect range of motion including those that limit strength, cause pain, or result in flexible or fixed deformities. Strength is also affected by conditions that result in pain or changes in muscle function. Dexterity and fine motor coordination can be affected by tremor and imbalances of muscle tone (e.g., hyper- or hypotonus). Examples of musculoskeletal conditions that affect manipulation include rheumatoid arthritis, osteoporosis, fracture, and amputation. Neuromuscular conditions that affect manipulation include cerebral palsy, spinal cord injury, stroke, traumatic brain injury, and progressive disorders such as amyotrophic lateral sclerosis, multiple sclerosis, and muscular dystrophy. Manipulation can also be affected by general conditions such as frailty and morbid obesity, primarily through loss of strength.

LOW-TECHNOLOGY AIDS FOR MANIPULATION

In Chapter 1 we define low-technology aids as inexpensive, simple to make, and easy to obtain. Many manipulative aids fall into the low-technology category. We group these aids into general- and specific-purpose devices. Within specific-purpose devices, we categorize devices according to the major performance areas of the Human Activity

Assistive Technology (HAAT) model: self-care, work or school, and play or leisure. The examples and other aids to daily living are available from many sources, including home health stores and online and mail-order catalogs.*

General-Purpose Aids

To be classified as general purpose, a manipulation aid must serve more than one need. Three general purpose aids are described here because they are commonly found in most environments: mouthsticks, head pointers, and reachers. The first two of these are often used as control enhancers in conjunction with control interfaces. **Head pointers** and **mouthsticks** are discussed in Chapter 5, including their use as control enhancers for activating control interfaces. Both mouthsticks and head pointers are used for direct manipulation. Turning pages is often accomplished with a mouthstick or a head pointer used in conjunction with a book or magazine mounted on a simple stand. A ballpoint pen tip or a pencil can also be attached to a mouthstick for writing. Additional attachments include a pincher that is opened or closed by tongue action and a suction cup end that can be used to grip objects (e.g., a page) by sucking on the end of the mouthstick. Many tasks require sliding objects (e.g., paper, pens) around on a desk or table. Both mouthsticks and head pointers can be used for this task. Mouthsticks or head pointers can also be used for such functions as dialing a telephone, typing, and turning lights on and off.

Many individuals need to extend their physical range. Often the need for extended range is a result of being seated in a wheelchair and wanting to reach an object on a counter or in a cabinet. In other cases it is a need to reach an object on the floor when bending is difficult or stability is poor. Reaching to the floor or in a forward direction is difficult following a hip replacement or a hip fracture when the individual has limitations in hip movements. In all these cases, reachers can be useful. A **reacher** consists of a handle grip that is used to control the jaws of the reacher in order to grasp an object. The grasp required to activate the grip may be of several types: squeeze with the whole hand, pistol grip with all the fingers, or trigger with the index finger. Overall length varies from 24 to 36 inches, and some models fold for ease of carrying. The gripper portion of the reacher may be circular for ease of gripping cans or pincher-like for picking up smaller objects. Rubber or other nonslip materials are often used for grippers on reachers. Reachers can be used to manipulate many objects, including food (e.g., cans, packages), cooking utensils (e.g., pans, pots, plates, dishes), office objects (e.g., paper, books, magazines), and recreational or leisure objects (e.g., books, tapes, CDs).

Reachers are used in many ways to manipulate different objects. They can act in similar ways to head pointers and sticks to push or pull objects into a space that is usable by the individual. Reaching devices can assist with activities such as dressing, hygiene, and other self-care activities and household activities (i.e., any activity that requires grasp and retention of an object that is outside of the individual's reach). Because a reaching device extends the length of the arm, it also extends the length of the lever arm, resulting in increased force required to lift the object. As an experiment, try lifting a book and holding it close to your body. Hold it in that position for about 30 seconds. Sense its weight. Now hold the book at arm's length. Hold it in this position for 30 seconds. Notice the difference in the sensation of weight. The book feels like it weighs much more when held away from the body; more force is required to hold it. Keep this consideration in mind when encouraging a client to use a reacher.

Specific-Purpose Aids

Because specific-purpose, low-tech aids are designed for one or two tasks only, they serve those tasks very well. However, because they are so specialized, it may be necessary to have several of these available to meet the demands of self-care, work, and leisure.

Most specific-purpose adaptations of products involve one of four things: (1) lengthening a handle or reducing the reach required, (2) modifying the handle of a utensil for easier grasping or manipulation, (3) converting two-handed tasks to one-handed ones (providing an alternative method of stabilizing the tools that are being used), and (4) amplifying the force that a consumer can generate with her hands. These include enlarged grips for easier grasping, cuffs that hold a utensil and circle the fingers, angled handles for ease of scooping (for people with limited wrist movement), swivel handles that allow the end to be oriented differently for different positions in space (e.g., on a table or near the mouth), and handles that require only limited grasp.

Self-Care

Self-care includes aids for assistance in several areas: food consumption, food preparation, dressing, and hygiene. Food consumption aids include a variety of modifications to utensils, such as enlargement and ergonomic shapes of handles, swivel handles so the bowl of the spoon retains a level orientation, lengthening of handles, and combinations of utensils called "sporks." Modifications to plates include suction cups for stability, enlarged rims that make it easier to scoop food onto a utensil (scoop dish), and removable rims that attach to any plate (plate guard). Drinking aids include cups with caps and "sipper" lids through which fluid can be sucked, nose cutouts that allow drinking to occur without tipping the head back, and double-handled cups for two-handed use. Figure 14-2 shows a number of low technology devices to assist with food consumption.

* Suppliers of the aids described in this section include: Maddak Ableware® (www.maddak.com) and Patterson Medical (www.pattersonmedical.com). Useful Web sites for further information on devices described in this section include: AbilityHub (www.abilityhub.com) and AbleData (www.abledatacom).

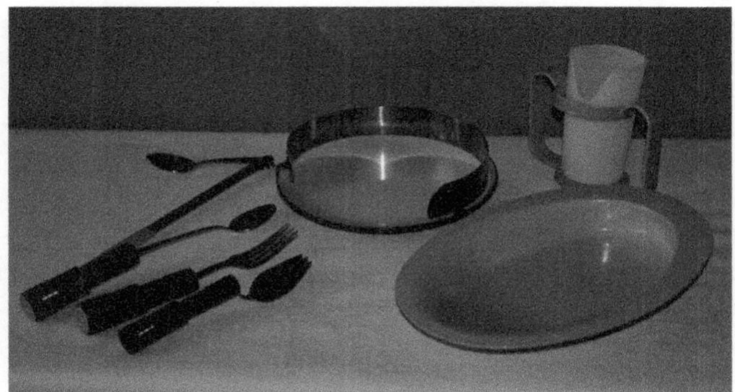

Figure 14-2 Low technology aids for food consumption. Left to right: long handled spoon with adjustable angle, utensils with built up handles, plate guard, scoop dish and cup holder.

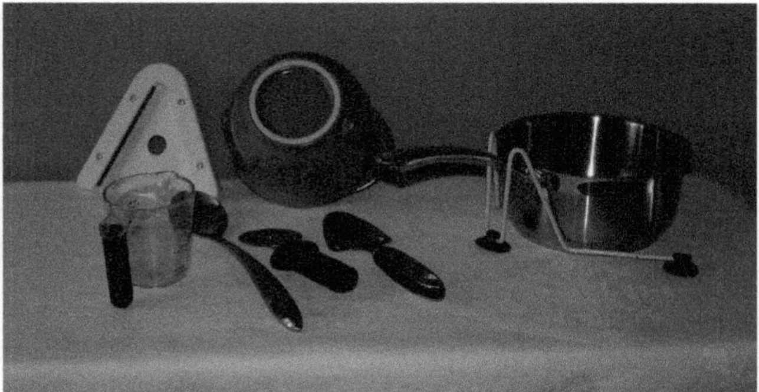

Figure 14-4 Low technology aids for food preparation. Rear left to right: one handed jar opener, and bowl with non-slip base. Front left to right: measuring cup with enlarged handle; commercially available kitchen implements with enlarged, ergonomic handles; and pot holder to stabilize pot for one-handed use.

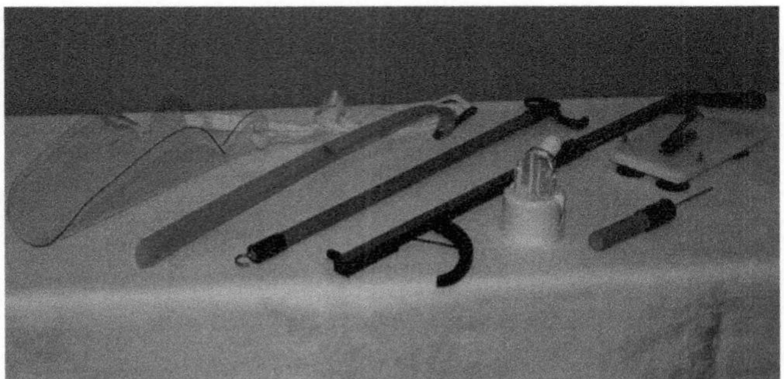

Figure 14-3 Low technology aids for dressing and hygiene. Left to right: sock aid, long-handled shoehorn, dressing stick, reacher, toothpaste holder, button hook, and nail clipper on stable base for one-handed use.

Dressing aids designed to compensate for poor fine motor control include adapted button hooks for single-handed buttoning and zipper pulls. These are available with enlarged, suction, and quad grip handles. For limited reach, there are aids for pulling on socks and pantyhose, long-handled shoe horns, and trouser pulls. A variety of dressing and hygiene aids are shown in Figure 14-3. A reacher is also shown in this figure.

Areas of hygiene that can be aided by special-purpose devices include: hair combing and brushing, teeth brushing, shaving, bathing, and toileting. Adaptive aids are available that enlarge, change the angle, or lengthen the handle of hairbrushes, combs, toothbrushes, bath sponges, and manual razors. Toothpaste and shaving cream containers can be adapted with a simple device that allows one-handed dispensing of the product. Devices are available that attach an implement such as nail clippers or an electric shaver to a base, thus stabilizing them for one-handed use.

Examples of food preparation adaptations include one-handed holders for opening cans and jars, brushes with suction cups for one-handed scrubbing of vegetables, bowls with suction cup bottoms for stability while stirring with one hand, bowl and pan holders (some of which tilt for pouring), and cutting boards that stabilize food during cutting. Modified handles are available for knives and serving spoons, as well as for other utensils. Many of these devices are shown in Figure 14-4, which includes both commercially available and rehabilitation products. Other self-care items intended for use in the home include cuffs that are used to grip brooms and mops, extended handles on household items such as dustpans and dusters, and key holders. Many of these products are commercially available.

Devices, such a universal cuff, are available for individuals unable to grasp (for example, following a spinal cord injury). These devices function in two ways: either as a cuff that is attached to the hand, or as a rigid, shaped bar that can be slid onto the hand, between the thumb and forefinger. When a universal cuff is used, implements such as a comb, toothbrush, or pen are inserted into a sleeve that crosses the palm to allow use of the implement without the need for grasp. Another common device that is used by individuals with weak or limited grasp is a tenodesis splint. This splint is constructed to employ the biomechanical action of finger flexion that occurs in conjunction with wrist extension.

Work and School

Throughout this book we have described assistive technologies that aid consumers in accomplishing work- and school-related tasks (e.g., computers, augmentative communication devices). In this section we discuss low-tech aids that specifically help work and school in the areas of writing and reading.

Handwriting is a major need in work and school environments. Special-purpose manipulative aids that assist handwriting focus on one of two problems: holding the pen or pencil and holding the paper. Some consumers lack the ability to grip a standard pen or pencil. Low-tech approaches to this problem include modified grippers that attach to the hand and clamp to the pen or pencil; wire, wooden, or plastic holders that support the pen or pencil off the paper and allow it to slide across the paper; weighted pens (with variable amounts of weight) that help reduce problems associated with tremor; and pens with enlarged bodies to make them easier to grasp. There are several different designs for holding paper in place for one-handed writing. Generally the paper is attached to the support surface using either clips or a magnet (in this case the surface is steel). Desks with small tops can also be modified using a rotating "lazy Susan" device that rotates to bring items within reach. File folders are often modified for easier grasping by putting hooks or loops on them. The loop or hook protrudes above the folder so that it can be grasped more easily. High-tech aids for writing are discussed in Chapter 11.

There are also low-tech reading aids. Book holders provide support for the reading material so the consumer does not have to hold it. Page turning is done either by hand or with a head pointer or mouthstick. In the next section we discuss electrically powered page turners and other electronic devices that aid reading. Figure 14-5 shows some low technology aids that can be used in work, school, or leisure settings.

Play and Leisure

As with other types of manipulative aids, lack of grasping ability in recreational or leisure aids is generally accommodated for by altering the type of handle. Recreation and leisure examples include cameras with modified shutter releases, modified grip scissors, modified handles on garden tools, and modified grasping cuffs for pool cues, racquets, or paddles. A person with limited manipulation strength can fly a kite by adding special wrist or hand cuffs for holding the string. Similarly, someone with limited grasp can use a cuff to hold a hockey stick or golf club in order to participate in these leisure activities. Computer access methods that were described in Chapter 7 enable an individual to play computer games in the same way they provide access to educational materials.

One example of a holder is a gooseneck arm attached at one end to a table clamp. At the other end is a bracket that holds an embroidery frame. Using this device, an individual can embroider, crochet, or mend using only one hand. Other examples of devices designed for one-handed assistance are playing card holders, knitting needle holders, and card shufflers. For individuals with limited two-hand function, there are handheld playing card holders. Devices that aid lack of reaching ability include a mobile bridge for holding the end of a pool cue off the table (a small bracket with wheels allows positioning of the pool cue), and ramps for use while bowling (the ball is placed at the top of the ramp and the user releases it after aiming the ramp toward the pins).

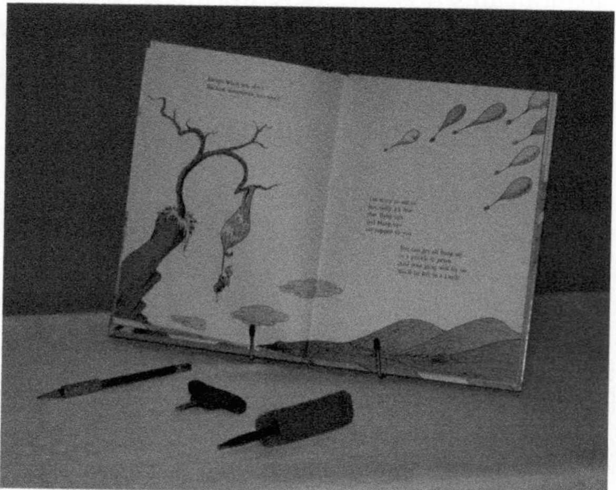

Figure 14-5 Low technology aids for play, school and work. Rear: book stand. Front left to right: pencil grip, key holder, and universal cuff holding a pen.

SPECIFIC-PURPOSE ELECTROMECHANICAL AIDS FOR MANIPULATION

There are two primary manipulative tasks for which electromechanical devices have been specifically designed and for which there are commercially available products: (1) feeding and (2) page turning. We discuss these specific-purpose alternative manipulation devices in this section.

Electrically Powered Feeders

One area of human activity in which independence is highly desirable is eating. Anyone who has been unable to feed himself (even for a brief period) knows the frustration of looking at one type of food on the plate and being fed another (e.g., expecting peas and getting potatoes). Being fed by another person can also create a feeling of dependency, and lack of independence in eating is often equated with childlike behavior. None of these stereotypes is accurate, and most persons who are fed by an attendant maintain control over the situation through direction of the attendant's actions. Nevertheless, many people would prefer to feed themselves if it were possible. Electromechanical feeders make this an option even for individuals who have very little motor control.

Use of an **electrically powered feeder** requires that the individual be able to control two separate functions. The first of these is location of the particular type of food that is to be eaten, and the second is picking up the food and moving it to mouth level. Currently available feeders require that the human operator be able to take food off a spoon, chew it, and swallow it safely. These requirements eliminate a large number of persons, but there are many who only lack the ability to pick up the food and get it to their mouths. It is this group for whom feeders are most beneficial.

The most commonly available feeder is the Winsford Feeder®,* which is marketed by several mail order equipment companies. This feeder is illustrated in Figure 14-6. This feeder has rechargeable batteries that are used to power it at many different settings. It has an adjustable height base that can accommodate varying spoon height requirements. A chin-activated dual switch is mounted on

* Both the Winsford Feeder® and the Meal Buddy are available from Patterson Medical (www.pattersonmedical.com).

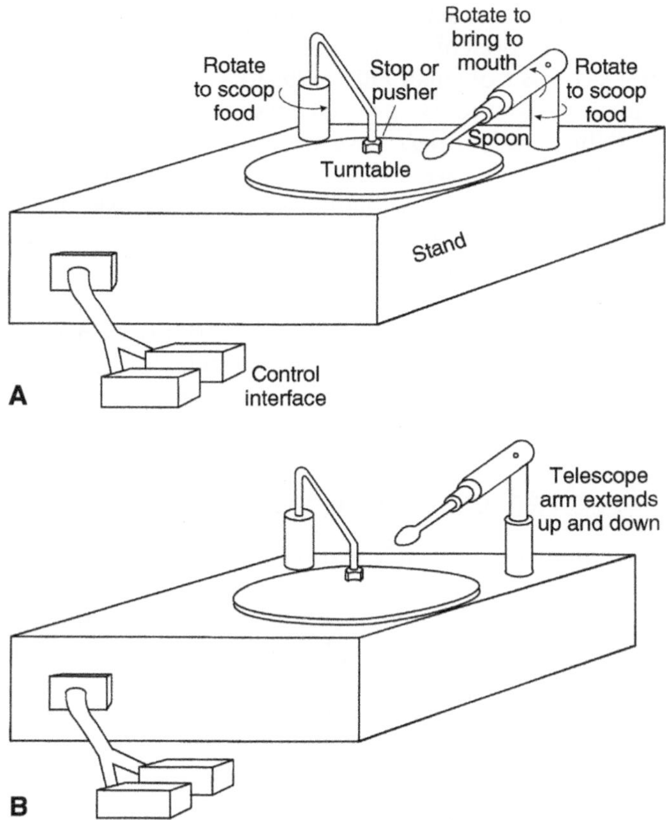

Figure 14-6 Winsford® Feeder

a long, solid wire. When it is pushed in one direction, plate rotation occurs; and when it is pushed in the opposite direction, food is pushed onto the spoon and elevated to mouth level. The device can also be controlled by a hand or foot adaptation. Other dual switches or two single switches may be adapted to work with this feeder. Although the device is portable, it does take considerable space on a table so its use in community settings such as restaurants may be limited.

Another dining device is the Meal Buddy, which incorporates a robotic arm to scoop food from the bowl and transport it to the consumer. The arm is activated with a single switch. A sip-n-puff option is available. The system includes three bowls for different food types or courses. It is also portable but, as with the Winsford Feeder®, it takes up considerable space on a table. The primary safety consideration of these devices is the avoidance of the spoon hitting the user in the face.

These feeders require assistance from another person for setup of the device and preparation of the food. Food must be prepared so that it is either mashed or pureed or cut into bite-size pieces. Liquids such as soup are difficult to consume using these systems. In addition to the space they take on a table, the devices are not always reliable, causing unwanted attention to the user if food falls off the spoon onto their clothing or the table. In addition, because the device is unusual and large, the novelty of this method of eating might bring unwanted attention. So, while the device affords independent eating, once setup has taken place, its use might only be acceptable to the user in his own home. In the community or another social setting, the individual may choose to receive assistance from another person. This influence of location is an example of the social context from the HAAT model as well as resource allocation, both discussed in Chapter 2.

Electrically Powered Page Turners

Access to books, magazines, and other reading material is important for the acquisition of information for school, work, or leisure. There are many individuals with disabilities who are able to read, but who cannot physically manipulate the pages of the reading material. There are several approaches that can be used to assist these individuals. A book holder and mouthstick (see the section on low-tech aids in this chapter) allow independence in page turning for some persons. The major limitation of this approach is the requirement that the book be set up by an aide and properly positioned for both visual and physical access. This method also requires a high degree of head control and the ability to hold a mouthstick. A mechanical head pointer eliminates the last requirement, but can result in neck fatigue if the user reads for a prolonged time.

Talking books, such as those made available for the blind, can also provide an alternative to physically manipulating pages. These are discussed in Chapter 8. Using a simple environmental control unit, a person with physical limitations can control the tape recorder and obtain access to the talking book at her own speed. Another approach is the use of books on computer disks. These can be loaded into a word processor, and the person needing access can use standard computer adaptations to turn the pages, scan through the material, find key words, and so on. This approach is also used by persons who have low vision or are blind, and we discuss it in Chapter 8. Both talking books and computer-based reading suffer from the limitation that not all reading material is available in these formats.

The recent advent of e-readers and tablet computers has significantly enhanced access to books and other reading materials. The user can download reading material directly to the device or through a computer. They can be positioned on a stand to relieve the need to hold the device. Most include a touch screen as a method of turning the pages, which is completed in a very intuitive manner. Others have buttons to advance the pages. A mouthstick or head pointer can be used to turn the pages, providing the device is well stabilized. Many of these products have options to change font size. As these products become more available, add-ons are being developed that make them more accessible. For example Airturn (www.airturn.com) has a wireless hands-free device that allows the user to change pages through the use of a foot switch. Some of the devices have text-to-speech applications, although with varying reliability. Apple products can use the VoiceOver feature that is part of the

Mac operating system. Others have proprietary software, which is inconsistently used by publishers of the material offered by the device manufacturer. A major limitation is that many of these devices do not have USB ports, which limits their modification through the connection to switches. However, third party applications are available that enable modifications to allow switch access.

A final alternative is an **electrically powered page turner**. From a manipulative point of view, page turning of print material requires two primary actions: (1) separating the page to be turned from the other pages and (2) physically moving the page from one side to the other (forward or backward). Additional useful but not essential features include scanning a number of pages, turning to a specific page, and locating a bookmark and turning to that page. Turning a single page is the most difficult for page turners, and its success for any page turner is a major indicator of the quality of the unit. Because reading materials differ widely in size, binding (e.g., uniform, spiral, loose leaf), and paper types (e.g., rough, slick, newsprint), it is important to evaluate any individual page turner with reading materials that vary in size, paper type, and binding style. Once the page to be turned is successfully isolated, the page turner must move it to the opposite side of the book or magazine.

The Gewa page turner* (Figure 14-7) uses a rotating roller to separate pages from each other and then moves the entire roller from one side of the book or magazine to the other after the page has been separated. The standard control for the Gewa is a four-direction joystick. Two joystick directions cause roller rotation either clockwise or counterclockwise, and the other two cause the roller to move forward or backward. Any other four-switch control interface can also be used. An additional accessory for the Gewa is a scanning selection method in which a single switch is used to select one of the four control functions as they are presented in sequence. The display of functions consists of small LED indicators, with each labeled function corresponding to one joystick direction.

* Distributed in North America by Zygo Industries, Portland, Ore. (http://www.zygo-usa.com/).

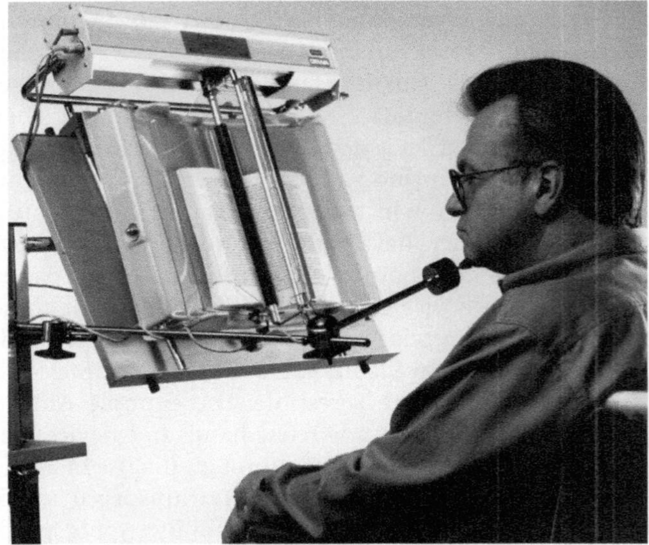

Figure 14-7 The Gewa page turner. (Courtesy Zygo Industries.)

Other page turners have different mechanisms. The Touch Turner* uses a rubber-coated wheel to separate the pages, and then a rotating semicircular disk pushes the separated page from one side to the other. As the disk rotates, the page is moved forward or backward, depending on the direction of rotation of the disk. The Touch Turner has both one-direction and two-direction models for standard books and a special model for paperback books and magazines. This device offers sip-n-puff and other switch access options.

ELECTRONIC AIDS TO DAILY LIVING

Daily activities routinely involve manipulation of appliances, controls, electronic devices, and environmental features such as doors and window coverings. Technology is readily available that replaces the need to physically manipulate the controls of many devices and features in our environment. For example, most of us have remote control devices that allow us to turn the TV or DVD player on and off, select the channel or disk, control the volume, program events such as recording a favorite show, and adjust other settings such as color contrast on the display. Similarly, many vehicles use a remote key entry system that eliminates the need to physically manipulate the key in the lock to open the car door. Some of these systems also remotely open the door. Simple security features are wired into new houses that automatically turn home lights on and off at preset times or when motion is detected. In the community, many buildings have at least one entrance where the door is controlled either through a mechanical switch or a sensor that detects when someone approaches. Voice control is an emerging means of controlling functions of phones and vehicle controls (e.g., temperature). All of these are examples of existing commercial means to control our environment.

Yet, many objects still need to be physically manipulated, including both electrically powered devices such as appliances (e.g., room lights, fans, and kitchen appliances such as blenders or food processors) and environmental features such as doors and windows, which can be modified by adding electrically powered control to them. The majority of these electrical appliances and controls are powered from standard house wiring (110-volt AC in North America, 220-volt AC in Europe and other countries). When an individual does not have sufficient motor skills to manipulate these devices directly, an **electronic aid to daily living (EADL)** can be used. We will describe the components of an EADL, including transmission and selection methods, assessment considerations, and integration of multiple-function EADLs with needs of the

* Touch Turner Company, Everett, Wash. (www.touchturner.com/).

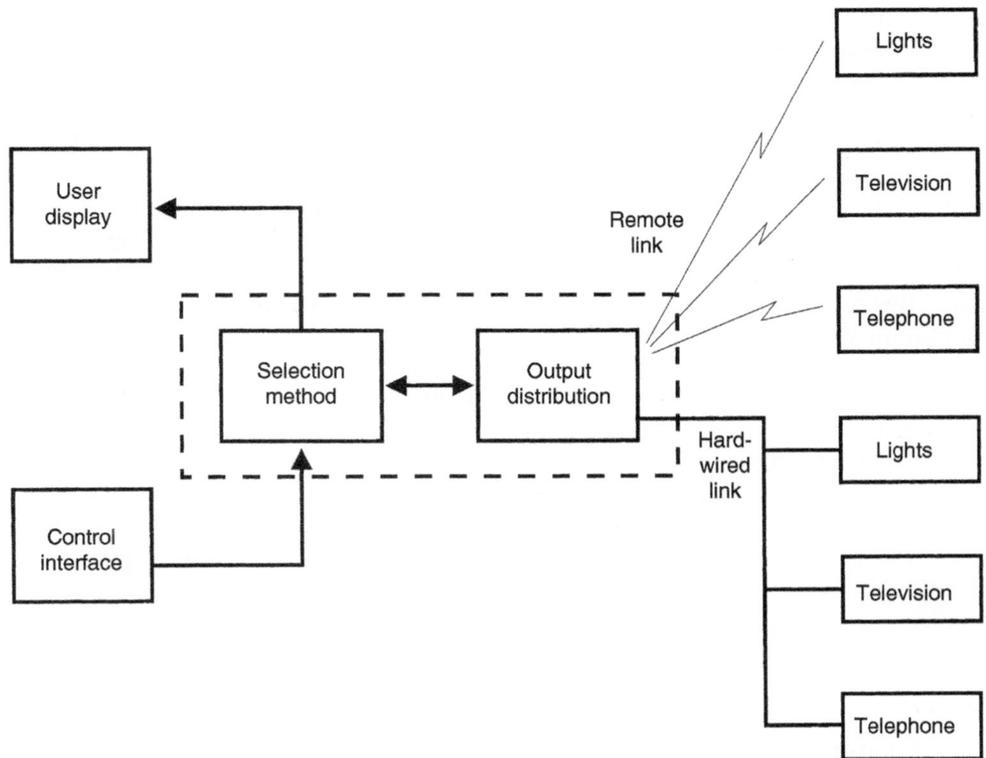

Figure 14-8 The major parts of an electronic aid to daily living. The *control interface* and *user display* constitute the human/technology interface. The components within the dotted box are the processor. The appliances listed on the right side of the figure are the activity output.

user. Figure 14-8 shows the different components of an EADL. It depicts a user who wants or needs to control a device, the device to be controlled, and the processor (the selection method and the output distribution unit). The means by which the user accesses the EADL is the *control interface* or *input device* (see Chapter 6), which can include a keyboard or keypad, joystick, or single and multiple switches. The *selection method* refers to how the user indicates his choice (e.g., direct selection or scanning). Feedback is provided to the user by some form of *user display*, which might be a monitor or screen, a light, or sound. The *output distribution* component translates the selection into some form of control of the device, which is connected to the output distribution component either directly (i.e., hard wired) or via a remote link. Together the selection method and the output distribution component make up the processor element of the HAAT model as described in Chapter 2, Figure 2-5. Examples of the appliances to be controlled via an EADL are shown on the right hand side of the diagram in Figure 14-8. The devices are hard wired to the home wiring and have some form of receiver (either integrated into the device as with a TV or connected to the device) that receives the signal from the output distribution unit.

The EADL may simply turn the appliance on/off or open/close a door or window covering. This simple function is referred to as **discrete control**. An on/off or open/close function is referred to as binary, since there are only two responses possible. Other examples of discrete control involve selection of a single event such as selection of a TV channel or a pre-stored telephone number. Each of these events is a discrete entry, and each selection produces a different result. The other type of control function employed in EADLs is continuous. **Continuous control** results in successively greater or smaller degrees of output. Examples of EADL continuous control are opening and closing draperies, controlling volume on a television or radio, and dimming or brightening lights.

There are two switch outputs available on most EADLs: (1) momentary and (2) latched. A **momentary switch** closure is active only as long as the switch is pressed. In the case of the EADL, this output remains active only as long as the control interface is activated (e.g., a switch is pressed). The momentary output mode is useful for continuous functions such as closing draperies. The output can be sustained as long as the person desires it to be (e.g., to open drapes half way). In the **latched** mode a switch closure is turned on by the first activation and off by the next activation, and it toggles between these two states with each activation. This feature can be useful when turning on an appliance such as a light or radio, or when sustained switch activation is difficult for the user.

Functions of Electronic Aids to Daily Living

Little (2010)[9] suggests four functions of EADLs: (1) environmental regulation, (2) information acquisition, (3) safety/security, and (4) communication. Environmental regulation allows the user to adjust the temperature, lighting, and some pressure relief devices. Individuals with spinal cord injuries, multiple sclerosis, and some other conditions are more sensitive to temperature changes than individuals without disabilities. Increases in temperature can have significant negative effects on their ability to function, so having a means to control the temperature independently is of great importance. Devices in this category may also open and close window coverings.

Devices that enable information acquisition are used to control audio-visual equipment, electric page turners, and other electronic devices. Perhaps the most commonly used devices in this category are those that are like the remote control that most of us use to control the TV, DVD, or MP3 player. EADLs for safety and security purposes notify the user that someone is at the entrance to their home or apartment and allows them to see that individual and to remotely unlock (and then relock) the door so it can be opened and closed. Other functions include systems that contact a service in the case of an emergency or monitor distant areas of a home. Communication functions enabled by EADLs include use of the telephone to both place and receive a call, intercom systems, and attendant calls.[9]

Transmission Methods

All EADL systems must transmit a signal to the appliance to be controlled. There are several methods used for this transmission. In the following sections we discuss three methods: direct connection, infrared transmission, and house wiring (X-10). We use the term **remote control** to mean the absence of a physical attachment among the various components shown in Figure 14-8. Typically, remote control occurs between the output unit and the appliances it controls. However, it is also possible to have remote links between the control interface and the processor.

Direct Connection

Direct wiring requires that the controlled devices be physically close together or necessitates the installation of special wiring just for the EADL. Devices wired to the EADL can include telephone lines, intercom systems, bed control, nurse call, and external speakers.[9] Benefits to this transmission method include increased reliability and control of devices not suitable for remote control methods. The primary disadvantage is that the device is tethered to what it controls.[9] Although it is theoretically possible to connect all the appliances to be controlled directly to the rest of the EADL via wires, this method is not practical.

House Wiring—X-10

The industry standard for communication among devices using home automation, also called the power line control method, uses the household wiring (power line) to carry short-wave radio frequency (RF) signals to devices that need to be controlled (i.e., the devices are plugged into the home wiring system).[9] Figure 14-9 shows how this approach works. Digital control signals are transmitted over the house wiring from the distribution control device to individual appliance modules, which are plugged into the standard electrical outlet. The distribution and control unit is also plugged into a wall outlet. This unit has a transmitter that sends out two codes over the house wiring. The first code identifies the device to be controlled, and the second selects the function to be performed (e.g., turn on or off, or dim or brighten a light). Each appliance to be controlled is plugged into a module, which is then plugged into the wall outlet. Each module contains a receiver that can interpret the codes sent out by the distribution and control unit. This type of appliance control was designed for use by the general population; consequently, it is common and inexpensive. Devices are available at many consumer electronic stores. This type of device can be a completely adequate EADL for individuals who are able to press the buttons on the control unit.

The major advantages of house wiring transmission are that no modification is needed to the home electrical system and the technology is relatively inexpensive.[9] Disadvantages include (1) the lack of privacy; (2) possible interference between systems on the same electrical power system (e.g., in an apartment building), resulting in unreliable performance; (3) the inability to transmit when multiple circuits are used for the wiring system; and (4) the lack of portability. Multiple circuits are often used in house and commercial wiring. Each circuit has a separate circuit breaker and they are physically separate from each other, which means that a module connected to one circuit does not receive the control signals from a transmitter connected to a different circuit.

Infrared Transmission

Another mode is based on the use of invisible **infrared (IR) light transmission** as the medium. This method is the most common in the control of home electronics (e.g., television set, cable television, DVD/CD player). Infrared remote controls are used for binary discrete and continuous types of control. Generally each remote device has a set of unique codes, and a remote unit manufactured by one company cannot be used with a system manufactured by someone else, which means that several remote controllers may be necessary to manage TV, cable, and other devices unless a "universal remote" is programmed to control all these appliances.

Infrared remote control is also used in EADLs. The remote link between the control interface and the distribution and control unit in Figure 14-10 is often implemented using IR in the same way that TV and other IR controls are used. Sometimes the link between the control and distribution unit and the remote appliances is also implemented using IR transmission.

The major advantages of the IR devices are no installation costs (as compared with hard wiring) and ease of portability.[9] A major disadvantage is that the signal, because it is a light wave, can be blocked by many materials; commonly a direct line of sight between the

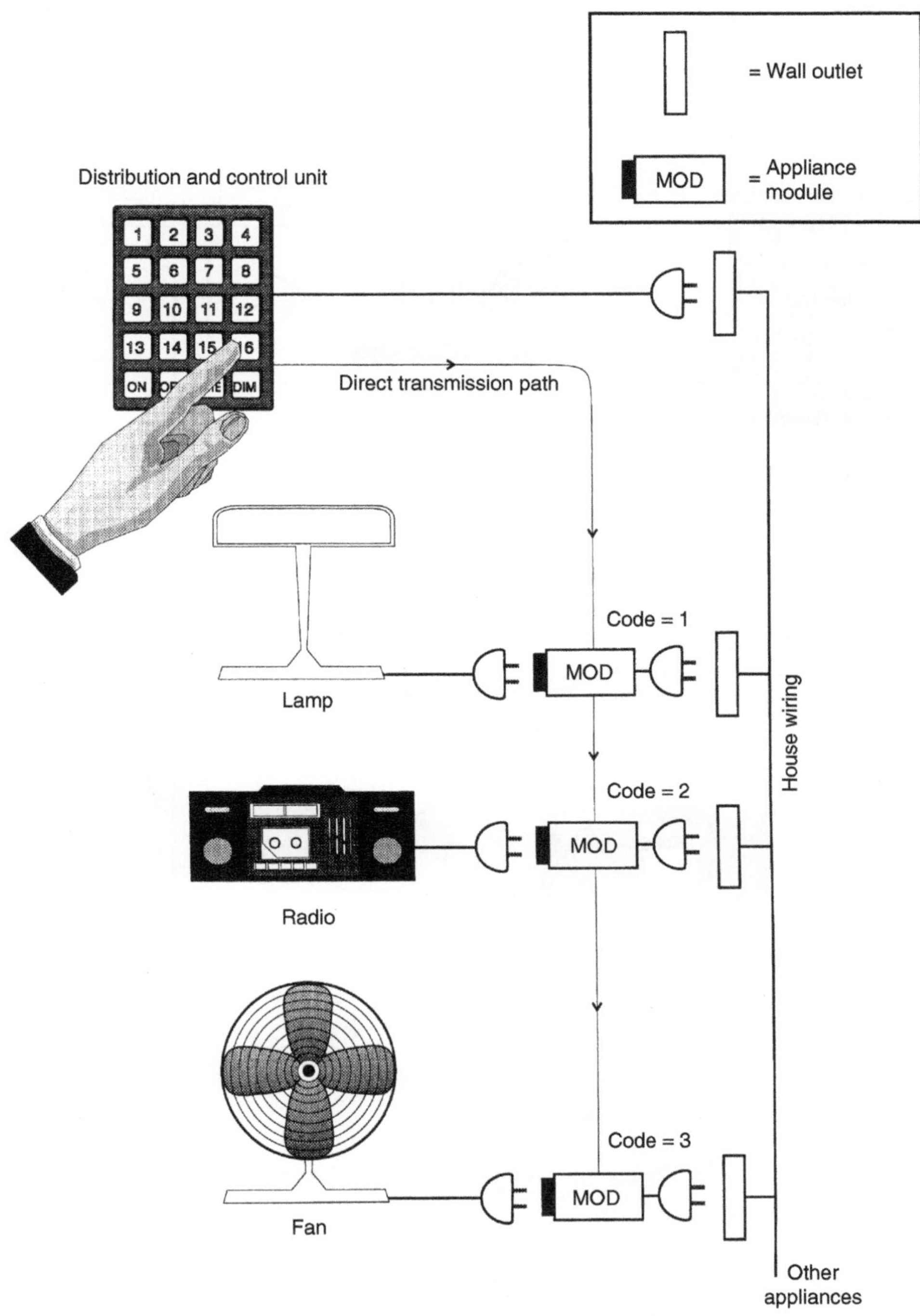

Figure 14-9 A direct-selection EADL. Each appliance has a numeric code, and the keypad is used to select the appropriate module. Control functions such as ON, OFF, and DIM are also activated by pressing the proper key on the keypad. This figure also illustrates the use of house wiring for distribution of the control signals to the appliance modules.

transmitter and receiver is required,[9] which means that the transmitter and receiver must be in the same room. Because the receiver must be connected to the controlled appliances (possibly through the house wiring), the line-of-sight requirement limits the range of application (e.g., outside, inside, different rooms). Because IR devices are light sensitive, they often do not work well in bright sunlight. Recall that the HAAT model includes a consideration of the physical context (see Chapter 2, Figure 2-4) in which a given activity is taking place. In this case the EADL is typically used in an interior location where light, heat, and sound can be controlled. However, interference from other appliances or interference caused by transmission from the EADL can affect the performance of these systems.

Radio Frequency Transmission

A final transmission approach is the use of radio frequency (RF) waves as the link between the distribution and control unit and the control interface, the controlled

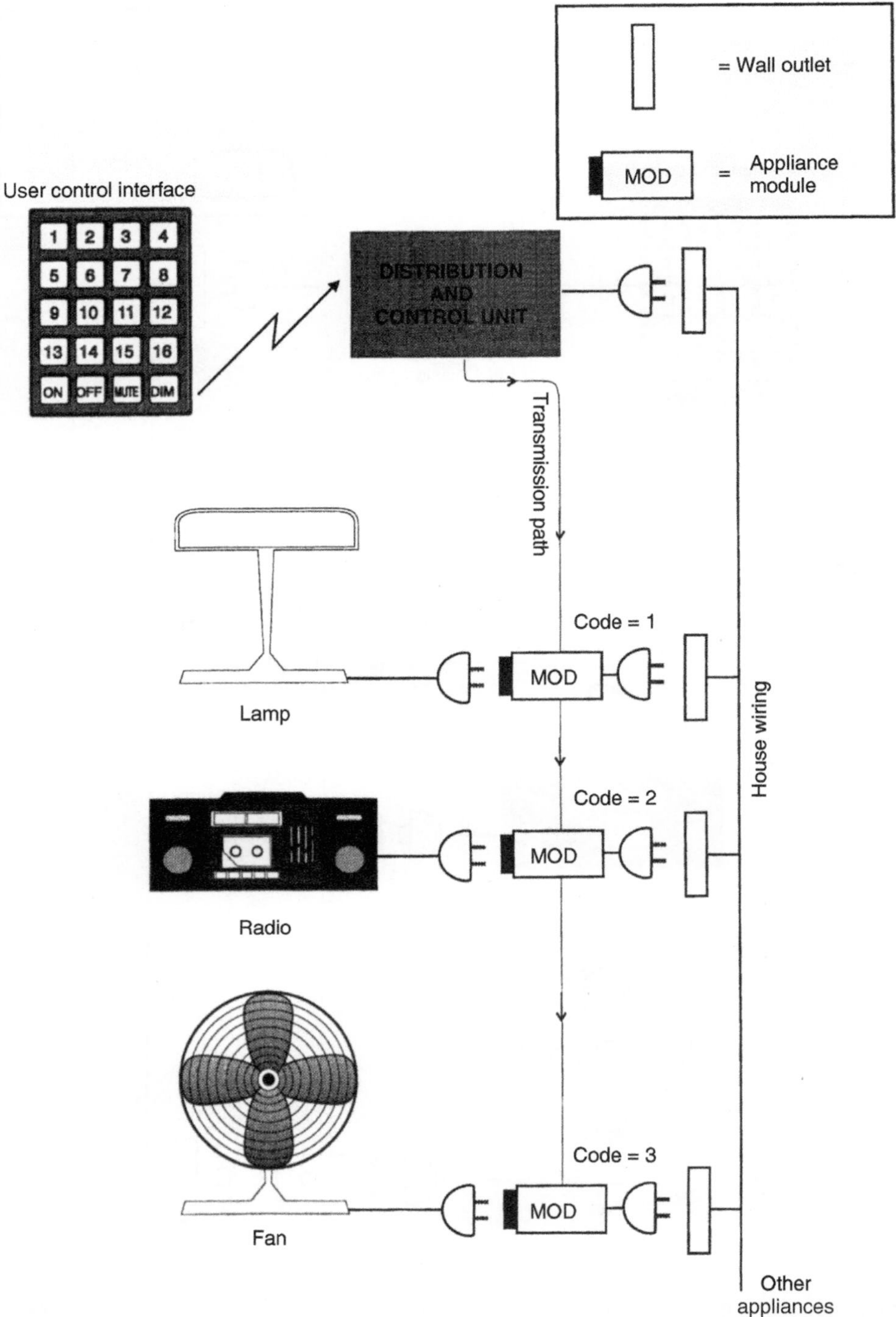

Figure 14-10 An EADL that employs infrared transmission from the control interface to the distribution and control unit. As in Figure 14-9, house wiring is used for transmission from the distribution and control unit to the appliance modules.

appliances, or both. The most common examples of this type of remote control are garage door openers and portable telephones. The term *RF transmission* is used because the signals are in the same range as broadcast FM radio. **Radio frequency transmission** is used as the link between the control interface and the processor.

The major advantage of RF transmission is that it is not blocked by common household materials (although it can be blocked by metal that is connected to the ground), and transmission can be over a relatively long distance throughout a house and yard. Because it is less restricted, it has the major disadvantages of interference and lack of privacy.[12] The interference problem is generally approached by reducing the distance between the transmitter and the receiver and by having several transmission channels available. The user can switch between channels (or the device will automatically scan) to find the strongest signal. Privacy is generally addressed by allowing the user to select a transmission code (often with a bank of small switches) and then matching the transmitter and receiver codes.

Selection Methods

Control of EADL is achieved through voice recognition, single or dual switch, touch screen, integration with controls used for other devices such as switches for AAC devices or joystick on a wheelchair or alternative computer access.[9] In Chapter 5 we define several selection methods used for control of assistive technology devices. These include direct selection, scanning, directed scanning, and coded access. Each of these can be used with EADLs. Direct selection occurs when the user of the system can choose any output directly. For example, an EADL for controlling a room light, a fan, and a radio on-off control may have one control interface (possibly a key on a small keyboard or speech recognition) for each of the three functions (Figure 14-9). If the same three-unit system is to be operated via scanning access, then the keyboard can be replaced by a scanning panel and each of the three items to be controlled has a corresponding light. When the light of the device to be activated comes on, the user activates a control interface to select that item. Finally, a code such as Morse code (see Chapter 5) can be used for one of the four output devices. The user enters a series of dots and dashes corresponding to the numerical code required to activate the desired appliance. Each of these selection systems is used in current EADLs, and some EADLs have multiple options available. We discuss specific selection methods in the remainder of this section. Choice of a control interface for use with an EADL is based on the considerations presented in Chapter 6.

Trainable or Programmable Devices

Remote devices that utilize either IR or RF typically are designed for operation with only one appliance (e.g., TV or VCR). If an individual owns several remotely controlled devices, this can lead to "controller clutter," with a separate control required for each device. To reduce this problem, several manufacturers produce remote control units that can be adapted to work with any appliance. Some of these are called **trainable controllers**. These devices operate by storing the control code for any specific appliance function (e.g., on/off). As shown in Figure 14-11, *A*, the storage is often accomplished by pointing the trainable controller at the controller for the specific appliance and sending the specific function code (TV ON in Figure 14-11). In the training mode the EADL device is aimed at the individual appliance controller, the function to be stored is pressed on the individual control, and the code is stored. This process is repeated for all functions and for all individual controllers. These trainable devices are relatively small, lightweight, and battery powered, and they can be hand carried or mounted to a wheelchair. When the stored code is sent to the appliance, it is received and used as if it had been sent by the appliance's own controller. This process is illustrated in Figure 14-11, *B*. In this manner, all the functions of the individual appliance controllers can be stored in one master controller and the user need only activate this one device. Most of these controllers have two modes: train and operate. Figure 14-12 shows a trainable EADL unit mounted to a wheelchair and used for controlling appliances such as the television.

Some controllers have codes for many appliances permanently stored in them. The user selects a code corresponding to his appliance (e.g., a television set made by a specific manufacturer). The user selects her appliance and looks up the controller code in a table. Once this code is entered into the controller, it is able to control the appliance. We refer to these as **programmable controllers**.

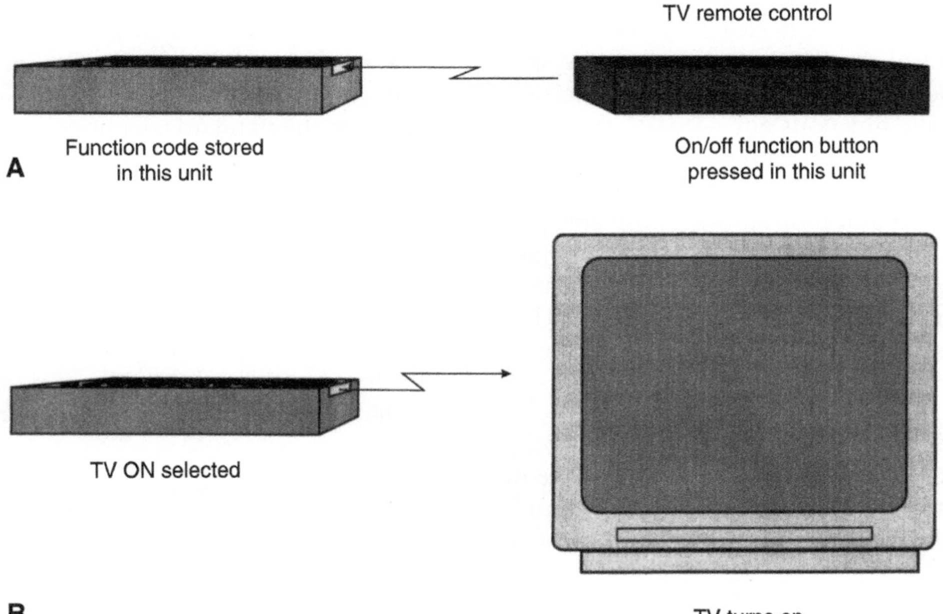

Figure 14-11 A trainable infrared controller. The trainable or programmable controller is shown on the left. **A,** Training is accomplished by aiming the device-specific control at the trainable controller and pressing the desired button (in this case, TV ON). **B,** The trained unit can then be used with the appliance to accomplish the desired function.

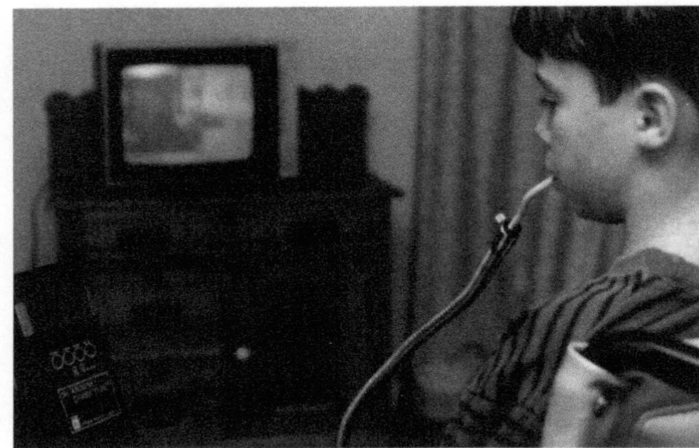

Figure 14-12 A trainable infrared EADL with scanning access. The EADL is shown mounted to a wheelchair. It is positioned so there is a line-of-sight link to the television for use of IR control. (Courtesy APT Technology, Inc., DU-IT CSG, Inc., Shreve, Ohio.)

Trainable or programmable controllers designed for the general home electronics market can be of benefit to persons with disabilities who are able to press the small keys associated with these devices. For those persons who cannot use standard controllers, there are specially adapted trainable or programmable units that provide both direct selection and scanning selection.* Control interfaces include expanded keyboards or a built-in keyboard or single switches for scanning access. In the latter case, one of two methods is typically used: (1) small lights that are located next to each button are sequentially illuminated or (2) alphanumeric labels or numeric codes for each function are sequentially displayed. For each of these approaches, the user presses the switch when the desired choice is presented.

Most of the trainable or programmable EADL devices can be interfaced to other electronic devices (e.g., AAC devices, computers, powered wheelchair controllers) via a USB port. To control the EADL, a code must be sent from the communication device or computer to the controller, and all specific functions and separate appliance codes must be stored in the communication device or computer. Several manufacturers include control software for EADL in their communication software programs (see Chapter 11). When the EADL is controlled by a computer or communication device, the software program generates the control signals and sends them through the USB port to the EADL.

Phone Control

Communication via telephone has changed drastically in the past few years, opening up options for the use of these devices by persons with significant physical disabilities. Individuals who did not have the physical capacity to manipulate a telephone need some form of assistive technology to allow them to lift the receiver, hold it during a conversation, retrieve and/or dial the desired number, and then replace the handset. Many options exist that provide alternative means of lifting, holding, and replacing the headset. These include simple holders that position a handset for hands-free operations, headsets that perform the same function, and mechanical switches that control the latch on a standard phone to answer a call and hang up once it is finished. A head pointer or mouthstick enables a user to dial a number, providing the phone is properly stabilized. Many of the new wireless phones are quite light and sit in a stand that makes it difficult to exert sufficient force to press a button without toppling the device.

Existing commercial technology can replace many of the manipulation requirements for telephone use. Speaker phones eliminate the need to lift, hold, and replace the headset. Stored numbers are readily available on most products along with a redial function. Cell phones or smart phones include many of these options as well as the option for voice commands. Voice over Internet protocols offer telephone use through the computer, opening up this mode of communication, using the variety of computer access methods described in Chapter 11. Despite all of these changes, some individuals still require an EADL to use the telephone.

Because modern telephones are actually sophisticated electronic devices, automation via electronic **telephone controllers** is relatively easy, and there are a variety of commercial products available to accomplish telephone access for persons with disabilities.* Many of the general-purpose EADLs have built-in telephone functions.† The functional components of a telephone controller are shown in Figure 14-13. Individual devices may group these components differently. Telephone controllers for a person with disabilities are built around standard telephone electronics. In some cases the controller is connected into the standard telephone, whereas in others the telephone is bypassed and the controller plugs directly into the telephone line. These devices enable several of the important functions common to consumer telephones, such as automatic dialing of stored numbers, redial, and the ability to answer the phone electronically.

Scanning as described in Chapter 5 is a common method to access and dial phone numbers, including both stored and novel numbers (i.e., a number that the user dials only once or on such an infrequent basis that

* For example, Gewa Link, Zygo Industries, Portland, Ore. (www.zygo-usa.com); Mini Relax and Relax II, TASH Inc., an AbleNet company (www.ablenetinc.com); U-Control III, Words Plus, Palmdale, Calif. (www.words-plus.com)

* For example, Relax II, Tash Inc., an AbleNet company, (www.ablenetinc.com); GewaTel 200 Speaker Telephone, an IR controlled telephone, Zygo Industries, Portland, Ore. (www.zygo-usa.com).

† For example, Ezra, KY Enterprises, Belgrade, Mont, (www.quadcontrol.com); EZ Control, Regenesis, North Vancouver, B.C., Canada; Simplicity Switch, Quartet Technology, Inc., Tyngsboro, Mass. (www.qtiusa.com); Imperium, SiCare Pilot, and Relax 3 from TASH, an AbleNet company (www.ablenetinc.com).

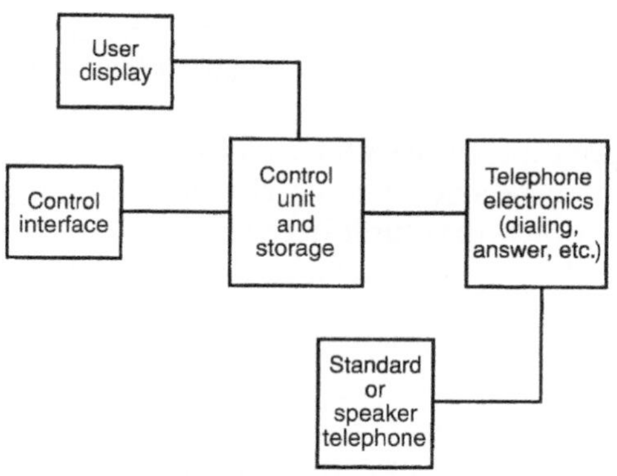

Figure 14-13 Functional components of an automatic telephone dialer. The *control interface* and *user display* constitute the human/technology interface, the *control unit and storage* and *telephone electronics* are the processor, and the *telephone* constitutes the activity output.

it is not stored). A control interface is required for users who require a single-switch access to the system (see Figure 14-13). The control interface is connected to a control unit that also interfaces with a display and with the telephone electronics. Although systems vary in their design, a typical approach is for the device to display digits sequentially. When the digit to be dialed is presented, the user presses his switch to select the number. Once a choice has been made, the scan begins again at zero. In this way, any phone number can be entered. Once the number is entered, it is sent to the telephone electronics for automatic dialing.

Many persons with disabilities respond slowly, and each switch press may take several seconds. For example, if we assume that it takes 2 seconds to respond, then we must display each number for at least 3 seconds, which may require scanning through 10 numbers (30 seconds) just to get to the desired number. If all the desired numbers were large (e.g., 7, 8, or 9), it could take almost 5 minutes (300 seconds) to dial one long-distance (11-digit) number. For this reason, all practical systems use stored numbers and automatic dialing. They also allow numbers to be entered and either stored or dialed using scanning. Redial also can speed things up, and this feature is normally included as well. Another unique feature in most telephone dialers designed for persons with disabilities is the inclusion of a HELP (e.g., a neighbor) or EMERGENCY (911) phone number that can be dialed quickly.

There are several modes of operation in automatic telephone dialers that require a selection by the user. First, the user must choose among dial, answer, or hang up. If dial is chosen, then the user must decide whether to access a stored number, redial, call for help, or dial an un-stored number. When single-switch devices are used as the selection method, this decision is generally made in one of two ways: (1) the system sequentially presents the choices to the user and the user waits until the desired choice is presented before pressing his switch, or (2) two switches are used: one to access the operational modes only (e.g., dial, answer, store) and the second switch to select numbers. In either method, if HELP is selected, it is automatically dialed with no further entry. Some units merely reserve the first place in the stored number directory for HELP, whereas others use a special selection scheme for it (e.g., a long switch press). The next place in the phone list is generally redial.

If redial is not chosen, then stored numbers are presented, usually by a code. Many new systems allow a picture of the person to be presented with their number, greatly simplifying the selection process. Most systems have a capacity for multiple stored numbers. The user merely waits until the code or picture for the number of the person he wants to call is presented and then presses the switch. At this point everything else is automatic. If the user wishes to dial or store a new number, he waits until that choice is presented and then activates the switch. Once in this mode, the method discussed previously is used to enter the number, and the user then tells the controller whether to enter it into memory or to dial it.

Because the telephone controller obtains access to the telephone lines in the course of its normal operation, it is relatively easy to include other telephone-based functions in the adapted controller's operation. For example, apartment buildings often use the telephone system for the intercom and front door latch, and the adapted telephone dialer can access these by including additional codes selected by the user.

When a computer is used as part of an EADL, the telephone dialing functions can be implemented using software programs coupled with an electronic telephone interface that connects to the telephone line. These software and electronics are common for use in modems for communication between computers (e.g., for Internet access), and they have been adapted for some EADL systems. Similarly, applications (apps) available for smart phones and tablet computers can augment the dialing functions.

Configuring Electronic Aids to Daily Living

Having looked at the components that normally make up EADLs, we now move to a discussion of how EADLs get selected and configured to meet the specific needs of a person with a disability. The first step in this process is to carry out an assessment of the person's needs and skills.

Assessment for EADL Use

As we discuss in Chapter 3, the initial assessment step is to determine the consumer's needs carefully, especially in the context of daily living demands (e.g., home, employment).[2] Bentham, Bereton and Sapacz (1992) discuss major considerations to be included in a careful needs assessment for EADL selection. This study emphasizes the need for a careful analysis of factors in addition to physical and cognitive ability, such as ease of use, displays, home modifications required, and equipment standardization. We discuss several of these later in this chapter.

Holme et al. (1997)[7] conducted a survey of occupational therapists (OTs) working in spinal cord injury and disease centers. Their study concluded that the top four reasons for recommending an EADL were: (1) empowerment of the client, (2) improvement in the client's quality of life, (3) increased access to call systems, and (4) decreased need for attendant care. They identified the major reasons for *not* recommending an EADL as: (1) lack of funding (64% of respondents), (2) high cost of EADLs (47%), (3) unavailability of EADLs for trial, and (4) lack of EADL knowledge by the OT responsible for the client's rehabilitation.

Activity

Application of the HAAT model indicates that the starting point in the determination of the most appropriate EADL is to consider the activities that the user wants or needs to do that can be supported by an EADL (see Chapter 2). For example, the user may need to use the telephone, respond to someone at the door to their home (and admit them as appropriate), use the TV/DVD player, and open/close window coverings. Consideration of the activities also includes an understanding of where these activities occur. For example, does she need to perform these activities in multiple locations (within the home, across the home and community, or at home and at work)? How frequently are these activities conducted? Activities that are repeated many times a day are more appropriate for control via an EADL than those that are infrequently performed and for which the user can receive assistance from another person. Time of day may also influence the EADL recommendation since an EADL may be required when the user is alone.

Human

Dickey and Shealey (1987)[4] describe an evaluation process that follows this first step. The first step in their process is to determine the person's physical abilities (see Chapter 3) and her ability to use a control interface (see Chapter 6). If she is also using an augmentative communication device (see Chapter 11) or a powered wheelchair (see Chapter 12), then EADL functions may be included in one of these other devices and a separate control interface may not be necessary.

The next step in Dickey and Shealey's[4] evaluation process is to determine the consumer's cognitive status, which includes such things as short-term and long-term memory, attention, and problem-solving skills. Motor planning skills also require evaluation. These abilities are all important in understanding and effectively using an EADL. In determining the feasibility of using an EADL, Dickey and Shealey[4] suggest that the consumer's ability to learn new tasks and her most reliable method of integrating new skills with old activities should be determined. These two areas can have a significant impact on the effectiveness of an EADL.

The HAAT model also indicates that psychosocial factors need to be considered during the evaluation. Affects such as motivation and feelings of competence and self-worth are examples of psychosocial elements that affect the use of EADLs. Another component to consider is the user's prior experience with technology. A novice user has a limited perspective on how technology can support her function, which may limit her willingness to try various devices and techniques that have the potential to enhance her activities.

Context

The setting and supports available in the setting influence the choice of an EADL. Three different settings are of primary importance: the acute care hospital, the rehabilitation center, and the client's home in the community. These settings differ in terms of the activities in which the client engages the support available, the environmental accessibility, and the user's level of recovery and rehabilitation. The purpose and types of EADLs are different across these settings.

In the acute care setting, the client has experienced a sudden change in her ability to engage in daily activities (e.g., loss of motor skills and sensation following a spinal cord injury), changes in motor control and cognitive function following a traumatic brain injury, or change in the underlying condition of a progressive disease such as amyotrophic lateral sclerosis. The client has limited physical abilities and, in the case of a spinal cord injury, no longer knows what her body can do or how she can control her environment. Her world is limited to her bed and hospital room for extended lengths of time. Necessarily activities in this context include use of the call bell for nursing assistance and perhaps controlling a TV. At this point, provision of a simple EADL that offers control of these two devices can demonstrate to the client that she can still engage in some activities and control her environment with a degree of independence. The acute care setting may be able to provide professionals with expertise in EADLs to support the client's use of the technology.

At the point when a client moves to a rehabilitation context, she typically is learning how to engage in many more activities and may have regained some motor function. This setting is more likely to employ professionals with EADL expertise who will be involved in assessment, recommendation, setup, and training of the technology. The client will have greater mobility and will be learning to use a powered wheelchair, enabling her independence to move about the facility and its grounds. During the rehabilitation period, the client also has the opportunity to go out into the community. The rehabilitation period affords the client the opportunity to learn how to use EADLs that support more complex functions, such as using a telephone or controlling different appliances.

Once the client returns to the community, either to her own home or to some form of supported living, she needs to engage in many more activities. The focus of EADL use in the home is to enable engagement in daily activities.

For example, if she returns to her own home, she needs to identify someone at the door, unlock/open the door to admit the person as appropriate, and then close the door. This activity is an example of something that was not required in either of the other two settings. Similarly, she needs to control different aspects of the environment—such as temperature and lighting, using a phone in an emergency, or controlling window coverings—that were not required in the previous two settings. The support and training of a caregiver or support personnel in the home is less than what is available in the rehabilitation setting, particularly in the initial period following return home. The home environment does provide the opportunity to determine the requirements for EADLs in a stable environment and how this technology needs to be integrated into the user's daily life.

The institutional aspect of the context is also considered during an assessment. Funding is an important consideration in the acquisition of an EADL. Often these devices are not considered eligible under many government-funded programs. They may be available through health care insurance or insurance benefits if the client needs to use an EADL as the result of a motor vehicle or industrial accident (i.e., an accident for which an insurance or legal claim can be made). In addition to funding, it is important to determine whether the device belongs to the client, so it moves with him across different settings, and who bears the responsibility for maintaining and insuring the device.

Technology

The listing of other electronic devices should include both consumer electronic devices, such as a TV, CD/DVD player, computer, and speaker telephone (all with brand names and model numbers), and assistive technologies, such as communication devices and powered wheelchairs. Information should be documented on the appliances that the consumer wishes to control in his environment.

Little (2010)[9] describes several issues that affect the introduction of EADLs. In the acute phase, post-trauma, the responses to the EADL may vary and the devices may be rejected because the client needs time to adjust to his altered function and to recognize how technology can enhance his function. Arguments for introduction of the EADL during the acute hospital phase of rehabilitation include developing a sense of control and possible independence in the patient and providing the system while there is significant support available for setup and training.[1] Early introduction of a device to someone with a progressive disease gives him the opportunity to become proficient with the use of the device so he isn't both learning how to use it and adapting to loss of function at the same time. Little (2010)[9] suggests the introduction of a device early in rehabilitation but to wait before actually obtaining it until the person has returned to the community so there is a better sense of what he can and needs to do as well as the environmental support for these devices. The exact specifications and configuration of an EADL requires an assessment of the home environment and the recommendation should wait until the person has returned home (Ability Research Centre, 1999[1]).

Studies of EADL Users

Several studies have been conducted to determine the preferred features and factors influencing successful application of EADLs. Most of the studies were conducted before some of the current features (e.g., trainable or programmable IR controllers) became available, but they still reflect basic preferences of users. The results of these studies are summarized in Box 14-1, reflecting themes of factors that influence use or abandonment, outcomes of use of the device, and issues of device recommendation.

Implementation of EADLs for Manipulation

The discussion up to this point has described different aspects of the technology and aspects that need to be considered during an assessment. In order to understand implementation of an EADL for manipulation, let's consider the case of Eileen, a 62-year-old woman who had a brainstem stroke (Case Study 14-1). The case study describes the role of the rehabilitation assistant in providing training in the use of a new EADL device, the Relax II, which Eileen has just received. This device allows Eileen to use scan through a series of selections in order to make a choice. She can also control her lamp and the attendant call button using this device to remotely control X-10 modules. Let's make two assumptions with this case: that Eileen is currently familiar with scanning from her use of a communication device and that the Relax II has been programmed for control of the TV and DVD player.

CASE STUDY 14-1 – EADLS FOLLOWING A STROKE

Eileen, a 62-year-old woman, had a brainstem stroke which left her with minimal reliable physical function. She requires maximum assistance for activities of daily living and lives in a supportive living facility, where she has her own room. Eileen's cognitive abilities are intact. She seems withdrawn at times, preferring to remain in her room rather than joining in group activities. Her head control is good so she uses her head to control devices. She lost her ability to speak following the stroke, although her receptive language is intact. She has no functional movement below the level of her shoulders due to muscle weakness as a result of the stroke.

Her main activities include watching TV, listening to music on a DVD, and talking to friends on the telephone. She also needs to control the attendant call button in her room and turn the bedside lamp on/off.

She currently uses a power wheelchair with head controls. In addition to controlling the movement of the chair,

CASE STUDY 14-1 – EADLS FOLLOWING A STROKE—cont'd

she can also control power tilt and recline features on the chair. She uses a Medentec Tracker® light pointer, mounted to a head band, to control a communication device.

Eileen has just received a scanning, trainable infrared remote (Relax II) with a single switch that is mounted near her head. She will be able to control the TV directly with this EADL. An IR sensitive switch is used to control both the lamp and attendant call system via two X-10 modules, one attached to the lamp and one that is located at the attendant's station on her floor. She can activate the switch by using head movement without having to take the light pointer off. You are a rehabilitation assistant employed by the facility. You have been asked to work together with Eileen to help her learn to use the new device.

Madentec Tracker® from Madentec: www.madentec.com

Relax II from Tash Inc., an AbleNet company: www.ablenetinc.com

The case study indicates that Eileen plans to use the EADL when watching TV or listening to music. Discussion with Eileen can uncover when she wants to do these activities: are there certain times of day when she engages in these activities? Are there certain shows that she wants to watch? Does she want to be able to record her favorite shows to watch at another time? The rehabilitation assistant should also explore the setup with Eileen to ensure that she can access the device when needed and that she is in a good position to view the TV. Because she uses tilt and recline functions on her power chair, the TV needs to be positioned so she can see it. The rehabilitation assistant should also interact with Eileen at different times during the day to determine if there is any change in her head control over the course of the day. For example, does she get fatigued after being up in her chair for a certain length of time, resulting in difficulty maintaining head control that allows her to access her devices?

The rehabilitation assistant should determine what other activities might affect Eileen's use of the EADL. For example, the switch is mounted near her head, on the

BOX 14-1 What the Research Says: Consumers' Use of Electronic Aids to Daily Living (EADLs)

Factors that influence use of EADLs:

- Training and ongoing support are available for the user, caregivers, and staff.[1,10,11,16,18]
- The device is reliable, consistently doing what it is intended to do with few errors or malfunctions.[1]
- The user has the opportunity to try the device for a period of time (e.g., 2 weeks) before purchase.[3]
- The device affords the user an enhanced sense of security and comfort, allowing them to spend longer periods of time alone.[11]
- The user identifies applications of the device for communication, safety/security, household, employment, and educational tasks.[11]

Factors that influence the discontinuation or lack of use of EADLs:

- When the situations described above are not present, the device is more likely to be abandoned in the short or long term.
- The user may prefer to have another person (caregiver, personal attendant) provide assistance for the tasks that could be completed with the use of an EADL.[7]

Outcomes of EADL use:

- Functional Outcomes:
  - Users and caregivers reported greater independence with the use of EADLs.[5,17,18]
  - Greater privacy is achieved because the user does not need to ask for assistance with many tasks.[16]
  - More use of devices such as TV and DVD when independent control is enabled.[10]
  - Higher scores on standardized measures of functional independence.[13]
- Psychosocial Outcomes:
  - Greater feeling of control in the environment.[16]
  - Greater feelings of self-worth and self-esteem.[13,16]
  - Heightened sense of competence.[13]
  - Improved perception of quality of life.[8]
  - Psychosocial changes rise just prior to acquiring an EADL, decrease shortly after acquisition, and then return to the same level as prior to acquisition. Challenges and temporary loss of function that result from learning to use the device are considered to explain the decrease in the early stages.[15]
  - Satisfaction with performance of daily activities when using EADLs remains stable over long periods of time (e.g., 2 years).[14]

Primary reasons for recommendation of EADLs[7]

- Empowerment of the client.
- Improvement of the client's quality of life.
- Reduce the need for attendant care.
- Provide access to attendant call systems and other devices in the environment.

Primary reasons why EADLs are not recommended[7]

- Lack of external funding, paired with the high cost of the devices.
- Limited availability of different types of devices due to the infrequency with which many providers make recommendations for these devices.
- When service providers do not regularly recommend these devices, their knowledge may be limited to only a narrow range of devices.
- The expense of the equipment and the complexity of setup restricts opportunities users have to trial the devices.

BOX 14-2 Tips for Setting Up and Using EADLs

- Make sure that the EADL and the device to be controlled are linked.
  - IR controlled devices: make sure there is line of sight between the EADL and the controlled device—sometimes the signal can be bounced off a bright wall if line of sight is difficult to obtain.
  - For X-10 devices: be sure that the device code set on the EADL matches the number on the coded receiver.
- For each appliance, test the selection of each function (e.g., channel change, volume, on/off) and the individual controls within each function (e.g., turning volume up and down).
- Train the user to control each function in a step-by-step fashion:
  - Choosing the devices to be controlled.
  - Controlling the individual functions.
- Provide instructions and a training demonstration of the EADL for use with an existing IR controller (TV, DVD, etc.).
- If the user is controlling the EADL with an augmentative communication device, make sure that it is understood how to change between communications and EADL and make sure that all of the required EADL functions are programmed into the AAC device (including any training of the IR output for a particular device to be controlled).
- Provide written, step-by-step instructions for daily setup of the EADL for care staff. Attach these instructions to the case of the EADL. Include setting up the control interfaces (switch, keypad, AAC device) for controlling the EADL.

head array of her power wheelchair. This position is suitable when she uses her chair. However, if she takes a nap or requires some time out of her chair for pressure relief purposes, Eileen then needs access to controls while in bed. Consideration of access to controls while in bed will have occurred during the assessment; however, the rehabilitation assistant needs to determine that the setup is adequate at this stage.

Training activities should be graded to enable Eileen to gain competence in simpler control aspects before proceeding to more complex ones. They should also meet Eileen's priorities for control of specific devices. Since Eileen already uses scanning with her communication device, she will not need to relearn this control method. She will need to learn the scanning pattern on the Relax II and remember which selection controls specific functions. The rehabilitation assistant needs to ensure that the scanning rate and time allotted to make a selection meet Eileen's physical needs. A training sequence might involve learning to use the EADL to control the on/off, channel selection, and volume control TV functions. Recording functions might follow.

Eileen is an experienced user of assistive technology via head controls. Consequently, training likely needs to focus on familiarization with the functions of the devices. She also needs troubleshooting options (e.g., access to someone with the technical expertise to assist her if the device does not work as expected). Eileen's family and friends should also be engaged in the training program so they are familiar with its use and can provide assistance as needed.

In this case study, the rehabilitation assistant provides the primary training support in the use of a new EADL device. He needs sufficient training in order to teach Eileen how to use the device. Box 14-2 provides some tips for ensuring that the EADL device use is successful. He also needs background information about her functional skills. This case study highlights some of the considerations the rehabilitation assistant needs to be aware of when engaging with the client for the purpose of training in the use of an EADL device. It also gives some direction for the actual training. Now look at Case Study 14-2 and think about the questions related to EADL use by a client who has a progressive disorder.

CASE STUDY – EADL AND A PROGRESSIVE CONDITION

Dorothy, a 45-year-old woman who has amyotrophic lateral sclerosis (ALS), lives with her son, daughter, and husband. She receives attendant care daily. Dorothy uses a computer for written communication and an EADL for telephone, door, electrical bed, and appliance control. For writing, she uses a trackball with a virtual keyboard software program for text entry (see Chapter 7). She uses a power wheelchair, with a joystick control on her right side. The power chair includes power tilt and recline functions to assist with pressure management and comfort.

Appliance and telephone control were implemented with a stand-alone EADL accessed with a single-touch switch. This approach was taken, instead of combining the communication and environmental control functions, because Dorothy generally does not need access to the EADL functions while she is writing. Automatic telephone dialing is accomplished by the scanning approach described previously. Dorothy's needs for controlling augmentative communication appliances are met by using X-10 modules plugged into the house wiring. The EADL also plugs into the house wiring to communicate with the modules. These can control lights, appliances, or a call signal. The electric door opener is controlled by a switch output on the EADL.

CASE STUDY – EADL AND A PROGRESSIVE CONDITION—cont'd

QUESTIONS:

1. What are the important features of ALS that affect the use of EADLs?
2. What are the implications of a progressive condition on the use of EADLs in the future?
   a. Describe indicators that suggest the current EADL system needs to be modified.
3. What social supports does Dorothy have in her home environment?
4. What additional information is important for the rehabilitation assistant to gather?
   a. What are her daily activities? Are there important activities she does on a less frequent basis?
   b. What is the location of these activities?
   c. Are there times when Dorothy is alone?
   d. What is Dorothy's perception of her use of these devices and her role in the family?
5. What factors affect the setup and position of the EADL devices?
6. Describe training strategies used by a rehabilitation assistant for learning to use the devices when they are first received.

SUMMARY

Assistive technologies designed to aid manipulation help consumers in accomplishing tasks for which they normally use their upper extremities. Some manipulative aids are general purpose, meaning they serve multiple functions; some are specific purpose, designed for one task. In some cases the manipulative aid assists with normal hand function (e.g., handwriting aids); we refer to these as *augmentative.* In other cases an *alternative* method is used (e.g., remote control of an X-10 module to turn a lamp on/off). In addition, special-purpose and general-purpose devices may be either high or low tech.

Low-tech general-purpose manipulation aids include mouthsticks, head pointers, and reachers. Specific-purpose devices are available to meet needs in the general performance areas of self-care, work or school, and recreation or leisure.

Commercially available specific-purpose electrically powered devices serve two primary functions: self-feeding and page turning. These may be controlled by many different control interfaces and selection methods. Electronic aids to daily living (EADLs) are general purpose electrically powered devices that include appliance control; telephone access; TV, DVD, and CD control; and remote access to doors, drapes, and windows. EADLs are controlled by computers and may be accessed by a variety of control interfaces and selection methods. Both mainstream technologies and technologies directed to persons with disabilities were discussed in this chapter.

The role of the rehabilitation assistant is highlighted in the assessment and data-gathering process leading to the recommendation of an assistive technology to support manipulation functions. The rehabilitation assistant needs to be familiar with the operation of these devices and the indications for their use. She needs to be observant for the indications that a low-tech device would be useful (e.g., observing that a client has difficulty bending to reach an object that has fallen on the floor, indicating the need for a reacher). Understanding how more complex devices operate, such as electrically powered feeding systems and EADLs will enable her to select and employ effective training strategies. Appropriate support by a rehabilitation assistant for the use of technology that aids manipulation is an important element in the integration of these devices into the daily lives of the client.

STUDY QUESTIONS

1. Define gross motor and fine motor function. List examples of each type of function and apply these to the activity of eating a sandwich.
2. Describe four specific purpose adaptations for manipulation devices.
3. List three examples of self-care adaptations provided by low-tech manipulation aids.
4. List three examples of work or school adaptations provided by low-tech manipulation aids.
5. List three examples of play and leisure adaptations provided by low-tech manipulation aids.
6. Describe the control of an electrically powered feeder.
7. What are the major approaches used to support turning pages when reading?
8. Describe the four functions of electronic aid to daily living devices.
9. What are the three major transmission modes used in EADL systems? Describe the advantages and disadvantages of each.
10. What is the difference between a trainable and a programmable IR controller?
11. Discuss the effect of setting on EADL selection and use.
12. Describe the assessment process for determining the most appropriate EADL.
13. List the top four reasons for recommending an EADL.
14. What issues are considered important for the introduction of EADL devices?

REFERENCES

1. Ability Research Centre: Environmental control systems for people with spinal cord injuries, 1999, retrieved from http://www.abilitycorp.com.
2. Bentham JS, Bereton DS, Sapacz RA: The selection of environmental control systems. In *Proc RESNA 13th Ann Conf,* June 1992, pp 108–109.
3. Croser R, Garrett R, Seeger B, et al: Effectiveness of electronic aids to daily living: increased independence and decreased frustration, *Aust Occup Ther J* 48(1):35–44, 2001.

4. Dickey R, Shealey SH: Using technology to control the environment, *Am J Occup Ther* 41(11):717–721, 1987.
5. Efthimiou J, et al: Electronic assistive devices: their impact on the quality of life of high level quadriplegic persons, *Arch Phys Med Rehabil* 62(3):131–134, 1981.
6. Giuffrida G, Rice MS: Motor skills and occupational performance: assessments and interventions. In Blesedell Crepeau E, Cohn ES, Boyt Schell BA, editors: *Willard and Spackman's Occupational Therapy*, ed 11, Philadelphia, 2009, Lippincott, Williams & Wilkins, pp 681–714.
7. Holme SA, et al: The use of environmental control units by occupational therapists in spinal cord injury and disease, *Am J Occup Ther* 51(1):42–48, 1997.
8. Jutai J, et al: Psychosocial impact of electronic aids to daily living, *Assist Technol* 12(2):123–131, 2000.
9. Little R: EADL, *Phys Med Rehabil Clin N Am* 21(1):33–42, 2010. Doi: 10:1016/j.pmr.2009.07.008.
10. Mann WC: Use of environmental control devices by elderly nursing home patients, *Assist Technol* 4(2):60–65, 1992.
11. McDonald DW, Boyle MA, Schumann TL: Environmental control unit utilization by high-level spinal cord injured patients, *Arch Phys Med Rehabil* 70(8):621–623, 1989.
12. Mills R: Impact of standards on future environmental control systems. In *Proc 10th RESNA Conf*, June 1987, pp 679–682.
13. Rigby P, Ryan S, Joos S, et al: Impact of electronic aids to daily living on the lives of persons with cervical spinal cord injuries, *Assist Technol* 17(2):89–97, 2005.
14. Ripat J: Function and impact of electronic aids to daily living for experienced users, *Tech Disabil* 18(2):79–87, 2006.
15. Ripat J, Strock A: Users' perceptions of the impact of electronic aids to daily living throughout the acquisition process, *Assist Technol* 16(1):63–72, 2004.
16. Symington DC, et al: Environmental control systems in chronic care hospitals and nursing homes, *Arch Phys Med Rehabil* 67(5):322–325, 1986.
17. Von Maltzahn WW, Daphtary M, Roa RL: Usage patterns of environmental control units by severely disabled individuals in their homes, *IEEE Trans Rehabil Eng* 3(2): 222–227, 1995.
18. Woods BM, Jones RD: Environmental control systems in a spinal injuries unit: a review of 10 years' experience, *Int Disabil Stud* 12(4):137–140, 1990.

Index

Note: Page numbers followed by *b* indicate boxes, *f* indicate figures, and *t* indicate tables.